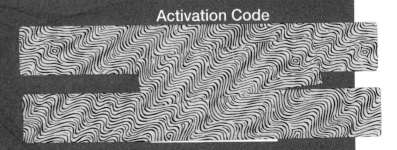

MILLER'S ANESTHESIA REVIEW

THIRD EDITION

MILLER'S ANESTHESIA REVIEW

THIRD EDITION

Lorraine M. Sdrales, MD

Assistant Professor of Anesthesiology, Cedars-Sinai Medical Center, Los Angeles, California

Ronald D. Miller, MD

Professor Emeritus of Anesthesia, Department of Anesthesia and Perioperative Care, University of California, San Francisco, School of Medicine, San Francisco, California

ELSEVIER

ELSEVIER

1600 John F. Kennedy Blvd.
Ste 1800
Philadelphia, PA 19103-2899

MILLER'S ANESTHESIA REVIEW, THIRD EDITION

ISBN: 978-0-323-40054-1

Previous editions copyrighted in 2013, 2001.
Library of Congress Cataloging-in-Publication Data

Names: Sdrales, Lorraine M., editor. | Miller, Ronald D., 1939-editor. |
    Preceded by (work): Sdrales, Lorraine M. Miller's anesthesia review.
Title: Miller's anesthesia review / [edited by] Lorraine M. Sdrales, Ronald
    D. Miller.
Other titles: Anesthesia review
Description: Third edition. | Philadelphia, PA : Elsevier, [2018] | Preceded
    by Miller's anesthesia review / Lorraine M. Sdrales, Ronald D. Miller.
2nd
    ed. 2013. | Includes bibliographical references and index.
Identifiers: LCCN 2017004618 | ISBN 9780323400541 (pbk. : alk. paper)
Subjects: | MESH: Anesthesia | Examination Questions
Classification: LCC RD82.3 | NLM WO 218.2 | DDC 617.9/6076--dc23 LC record available at
https://lccn.loc.gov/2017004618

Executive Content Strategist: Dolores Meloni
Senior Content Development Specialist: Ann R. Anderson
Publishing Services Manager: Patricia Tannian
Senior Project Manager: Sharon Corell
Book Designer: Ryan Cook

CONTRIBUTORS

Amr E. Abouleish, MD, MBA
Professor
Department of Anesthesiology
The University of Texas Medical Branch
Galveston, Texas

Meredith C.B. Adams, MD, MS
Assistant Professor
Department of Anesthesiology
Director
Pain Medicine Fellowship
Medical College of Wisconsin
Milwaukee, Wisconsin

Clayton Anderson, MD
Anesthesiologist
Salt Lake City, Utah

Dean B. Andropoulos, MD, MHCM
Professor
Department of Anesthesiology and Pediatrics
Vice Chair
Department of Anesthesiology
Baylor College of Medicine
Houston, Texas

Jeffrey L. Apfelbaum, MD
Professor and Chair
Department of Anesthesia and Critical Care
University of Chicago Medicine
Chicago, Illinois

Sheila R. Barnett, MD
Associate Professor of Anaesthesia
Harvard Medical School
Vice Chair
Perioperative Medicine
Department of Anesthesiology, Critical Care, and Pain Medicine
Beth Israel Deaconess Medical Center
Boston, Massachusetts

Charles B. Berde, MD, PhD
Professor of Anaesthesia (Pediatrics)
Harvard Medical School
Chief
Division of Pain Medicine
Department of Anesthesiology, Perioperative and Pain Medicine
Boston Children's Hospital
Boston, Massachusetts

Michael P. Bokoch, MD, PhD
Clinical Insructor and Liver Transplant Anesthesia Fellow
Department of Anesthesia and Perioperative Care
University of California, San Francisco, School of Medicine
San Francisco, California

Kristine E.W. Breyer, MD
Assistant Professor
Department of Anesthesia and Perioperative Care
University of California, San Francisco, School of Medicine
San Francisco, California

Richard Brull, MD, FRCPC
Professor
Department of Anesthesia
University of Toronto
Toronto, Ontario, Canada

Vincent W.S. Chan, MD, FRCPC, FRCA
Professor
Department of Anesthesia
University of Toronto
Toronto, Ontario, Canada

Emily L. Chanan, BA, MD
Critical Care Fellow
Department of Anesthesia and Perioperative Care
University of California, San Francisco, Department of Medicine
San Francisco, California

Tony Chang, MD
Staff Anesthesiologist
Swedish Medical Center
Seattle, Washington

Frances Chung, MBBS, FRCPC
Professor
Department of Anesthesiology
University Health Network
Toronto Western Hospital
Toronto, Ontario, Canada

Neal H. Cohen, MD, MPH, MS
Vice Dean
School of Medicine
Professor
Department of Anesthesia and Perioperative Care
University of California, San Francisco
San Francisco, California

Daniel J. Cole, MD
Professor of Clinical Anesthesiology
Department of Anesthesiology
Ronald Reagan UCLA Medical Center
Los Angeles, California

Wilson Cui, MD, PhD
Assistant Professor
Department of Anesthesia and Perioperative Care
University of California, San Francisco, School of Medicine
San Francisco, California

Andrew J. Deacon, B Biomed Sci (Hons), MBBS, FANZCA
Staff Specialist
Department of Anaesthesia and Pain Medicine
The Canberra Hospital
Garran, ACT, Australia

Jennifer DeCou, MD
Associate Professor
Anesthesiology
University of Utah
Salt Lake City, Utah

David M. Dickerson, MD
Assistant Professor
Department of Anesthesia and Critical Care
University of Chicago Medicine
Chicago, Illinois

Kenneth Drasner, MD
Professor Emeritus
Department of Anesthesia and Perioperative Care
University of California, San Francisco, School of Medicine
San Francisco, California

Helge Eilers, MD
Professor
Department of Anesthesia and Perioperative Care
University of California, San Francisco, School of Medicine
San Francisco, California

John Feiner, MD
Professor
Department of Anesthesia and Perioperative Care
University of California, San Francisco, School of Medicine
San Francisco, California

Alana Flexman, MD
Clinical Assistant Professor
Department of Anesthesia, Pharmacology, and Therapeutics
University of British Columbia
Vancouver, British Columbia, Canada

Elizabeth A.M. Frost, MD
Professor
Department of Anesthesiology, Perioperative and Pain Medicine
Icahn School of Medicine at Mount Sinai
New York, New York

William R. Furman, MD, MMHC
Professor and Acting Chair
Department of Anesthesiology
Dartmouth College
Geisel School of Medicine
Vice President
Regional Perioperative Service Line
Dartmouth Hitchcock Medical Center
Lebanon, New Hampshire

Steven Gayer, MD, MBA
Professor of Anesthesiology and Ophthalmology
Department of Anesthesiology
University of Miami Miller School of Medicine
Miami, Florida

Sarah Gebauer, MD, BA
Assistant Professor
Department of Anesthesiology and Critical Care Medicine and Department of Internal Medicine
Division of Palliative Care
University of New Mexico
Albuquerque, New Mexico

Rebecca M. Gerlach, MD, FRCPC
Assistant Professor
Department of Anesthesia and Critical Care
Interim Director for Anesthesia Perioperative Medicine
Clinic
University of Chicago Medicine
Chicago, Illinois

David B. Glick, MD, MBA
Professor
Department of Anesthesia and Critical Care
Medical Director
Post-Anesthesia Care Unit
University of Chicago Medicine
Chicago, Illinois

Erin A. Gottlieb, MD
Assistant Professor
Department of Anesthesiology
Baylor College of Medicine
Director of Clinical Operations
Division of Pediatric Cardiovascular Anesthesiology
Texas Children's Hospital
Houston, Texas

Tula Gourdin, MBA
Analyst
Department of Anesthesia and Perioperative Care
University of California, San Francisco, School of
Medicine
San Francisco, California

Andrew T. Gray, MD, PhD
Professor
Department of Anesthesia and Perioperative Care
University of California, San Francisco, School of
Medicine
San Francisco, California

Jin J. Huang, MD
Assistant Professor
Department of Anesthesia and Perioperative Care
University of California, San Francisco, School of
Medicine
San Francisco, California

Lindsey L. Huddleston, MD
Assistant Professor
Department of Anesthesia and Perioperative Care
University of California, San Francisco, School of
Medicine
San Francisco, California

Robert W. Hurley, MD, PhD
Professor and Vice Chairman
Department of Anesthesiology
Director
F&MCW Comprehensive Pain Program
Medical College of Wisconsin
Milwaukee, Wisconsin

Andrew Infosino, MD
Professor
Department of Anesthesia and Perioperative Care
University of California, San Francisco, School of
Medicine
San Francisco, California

Ken B. Johnson, MD
Professor
Department of Anesthesiology
University of Utah School of Medicine
Salt Lake City, Utah

Rami A. Kamel, MBBCh
Department of Anesthesiology
Toronto Western Hospital
University Health Network
Toronto, Ontario, Canada

Kerry Klinger, MD
Assistant Professor
Department of Anesthesia and Perioperative Care
University of California, San Francisco, School of
Medicine
San Francisco, California

Anjali Koka, MD
Instructor in Anaesthesia
Harvard Medical School
Department of Anesthesiology, Perioperative and Pain
Medicine
Boston Children's Hospital
Boston, Massachusetts

Catherine Kuza, MD
Assistant Professor
Department of Anesthesiology and Critical Care
Medicine
Keck School of Medicine of the University of Southern
California
Los Angeles, California

Benn Lancman, MBBS, MHumFac, FANZCA
Visiting Clinical Instructor
Department of Anesthesia and Perioperative
Care
University of California, San Francisco, School of
Medicine
San Francisco, California
Associate Clinical Instructor
School of Medicine
University of Sydney
Sydney, NSW, Australia

Chanhung Z. Lee, MD, PhD
Professor
Department of Anesthesia and Perioperative
Care
University of California, San Francisco, School of
Medicine
San Francisco, California

Theresa Lo, MD
Fellow
Department of Anesthesia and Critical Care
University California, San Francisco, School of
Medicine
San Francisco, California

Jennifer M. Lucero, MD
Assistant Professor
Department of Anesthesia and Perioperative Care
University of California, San Francisco, School of
Medicine
San Francisco, California

Alan J.R. Macfarlane, BSc (Hons), MBChB (Hons),
MRCP, FRCA
Consultant Anaesthetist
Department of Anaesthesia
Glasgow Royal Infirmary and Stobhill Ambulatory
Hospital
Honorary Senior Clinical Lecturer
Department of Anaesthesia, Critical Care, and Pain
Medicine
University of Glasgow, Great Britain

Dermot P. Maher, MD, MS
Assistant Professor
Department of Anesthesia and Critical Care
Medicine
Chronic Pain Medicine Division
The Johns Hopkins Hospital
Baltimore, Maryland

Vinod Malhotra, MD
Professor and Vice-Chair for Clinical Affairs
Department of Anesthesiology
Professor of Anesthesiology in Clinical Urology
Weill Cornell Medical College
Clinical Director of the Operating Rooms
New York-Presbyterian Hospital
Weill Cornell Medical Center
New York, New York

Mitchell H. Marshall, MD
Clinical Professor and Chief of Anesthesiology Service
New York University Langone Hospital for Joint Diseases
Department of Anesthesiology, Perioperative Care, and
Pain Medicine
New York University School of Medicine
New York, New York

Mary Ellen McCann, MD, MPH
Senior Associate in Perioperative Anesthesia
Associate Professor of Anaesthesia
Harvard Medical School
Department of Anesthesiology, Perioperative Care,
and Pain Medicine
Boston Children's Hospital
Boston, Massachusetts

Joseph H. McIsaac, III, MD, MS
Associate Clinical Professor
Department of Anesthesiology
University of Connecticut School of Medicine
Farmington, Connecticut
Chief of Trauma Anesthesia
Department of Anesthesiology
Hartford Hospital
Hartford, Connecticut

Rachel Eshima McKay, MD
Professor
Department of Anesthesia and Perioperative Care
University of California, San Francisco, School of Medicine
San Francisco, California

Lingzhong Meng, MD
Professor of Anesthesiology and Neurosurgery
Chief
Division of Neuro Anesthesia
Department of Anesthesiology
Yale University School of Medicine
New Haven, Connecticut

Ronald D. Miller, MD, MS
Professor Emeritus of Anesthesia
Department of Anesthesia and Perioperative Care
University of California, San Francisco, School of Medicine
San Francisco, California

Cynthia Newberry, MD
Assistant Professor
Department of Anesthesiology
University of Utah School of Medicine
Salt Lake City, Utah

Dorre Nicholau, MD, PhD
Professor
Department of Anesthesia and Perioperative Care
University of California, San Francisco, School of
Medicine
San Francisco, California

Howard D. Palte, MBChB, FCA(SA)
Assistant Professor
Department of Anesthesiology
University of Miami
Miami, Florida

Anup Pamnani, MD
Assistant Professor of Anesthesiology
Department of Anesthesiology
Weill Cornell Medical College
New York, New York

Krishna Parekh, MD
Assistant Professor
Department of Anesthesia and Perioperative Care
University of California, San Francisco, School of
Medicine
San Francisco, California

Amy C. Robertson, MD, MMHC
Assistant Professor
Department of Anesthesiology
Vanderbilt University Medical Center
Nashville, Tennessee

David L. Robinowitz, MD, MHS, MS
Associate Professor
Department of Anesthesia and Perioperative Care
University of California, San Francisco, School of
Medicine
San Francisco, California

Mark D. Rollins, MD, PhD
Professor
Department of Anesthesia and Perioperative Care
Director
Obstetric and Fetal Anesthesia
University of California, San Francisco, School of
Medicine
San Francisco, California

Andrew D. Rosenberg, MD
Professor and Chair and Dorothy Reaves Spatz, MD,
Chair
Department of Anesthesiology, Perioperative Care, and
Pain Medicine
New York University School of Medicine
New York, New York

Patricia Roth, MD
Professor
Department of Anesthesia and Perioperative Care
University of California, San Francisco, School of
Medicine
San Francisco, California

Scott R. Schulman, MD, MHS
Professor of Anesthesia, Surgery, and Pediatrics
Department of Anesthesia and Perioperative Care
University of California, San Francisco, School of
Medicine
San Francisco, California

Lorraine M. Sdrales, MD
Assistant Professor of Anesthesiology
Cedars-Sinai Medical Center
Los Angeles, California

David Shimabukuro, MDCM
Professor
Anesthesia and Perioperative Care
University of California, San Francisco, School of
Medicine
San Francisco, California

Mandeep Singh, MBBS, MD, MSc, FRCPC
Assistant Professor
Department of Anesthesiology
Toronto Western Hospital
University Health Network
Toronto, Ontario, Canada

Peter D. Slinger, MD, FRCPC
Professor
Staff Anesthesiologist
Department of Anesthesia
University of Toronto
Toronto General Hospital
Toronto, Ontario, Canada

Wendy Smith, MD
Fellow
Department of Anesthesia and Perioperative Care
University of California, San Francisco, School of
Medicine
San Francisco, California

Scott Richard Springman, MD
Professor
Department of Anesthesiology
Medical Director
Outpatient Surgical Services
University of Wisconsin School of Medicine and Public Health
Madison, Wisconsin

Randolph H. Steadman, MD, MS
Professor and Vice Chair of Education
Director
Liver Transplant Anesthesiology
Department of Anesthesiology and Perioperative Medicine
University of California, Los Angeles
David Geffen School of Medicine
Los Angeles, California

Erica J. Stein, MD
Associate Professor
Department of Anesthesiology
Wexner Medical Center at The Ohio State University
Columbus, Ohio

Marc Steurer, MD, DESA
Associate Professor
Department of Anesthesia and Perioperative Care
University of California, San Francisco, School of Medicine
Vice Chief
Department of Anesthesia and Perioperative Care
Zuckerberg San Francisco General Hospital and Trauma Care
San Francisco, California

Bobbie Jean Sweitzer, MD, FACP
Professor of Anesthesiology
Director
Perioperative Medicine
Northwestern University Feinberg School of Medicine
Chicago, Illinois

James Szocik, MD
Clinical Associate Professor
Department of Anesthesiology
University of Michigan
Ann Arbor, Michigan

Magnus Teig, MB, ChB, MRCP, FRCA
Clinical Associate Professor
Department of Anesthesiology
University of Michigan
Ann Arbor, Michigan

Kevin K. Tremper, PhD, MD
Professor and Chair
Department of Anesthesiology
University of Michigan
Ann Arbor, Michigan

Avery Tung, MD, FCCM
Professor and Quality Chief for Anesthesia
Department of Anesthesia and Critical Care
University of Chicago
Chicago, Illinois

John H. Turnbull, MD
Assistant Professor
Department of Anesthesia and Perioperative Care
University of California, San Francisco, School of Medicine
San Francisco, California

Arthur W. Wallace, MD, PhD
Professor
Department of Anesthesia and Perioperative Care
Chief
Anesthesiology Service
San Francisco Veterans Affairs Medical Center
University of California, San Francisco
San Francisco, California

Stephen D. Weston, MD
Assistant Professor
Department of Anesthesia and Perioperative Care
University of California, San Francisco, School of Medicine
San Francisco, California

Elizabeth L. Whitlock, MD, MSc
Clinical Instructor and Postdoctoral Research Fellow
Department of Anesthesia and Perioperative Care
University of California, San Francisco, School of Medicine
San Francisco, California

Victor W. Xia, MD
Clinical Professor
Department of Anesthesiology and Perioperative Medicine
University of California, Los Angeles
David Geffen School of Medicine
Los Angeles, California

Edward N. Yap, MD
Assistant Professor
Department of Anesthesia and Perioperative Care
University of California, San Francisco, School of Medicine
San Francisco, California

PREFACE

The first edition of Miller's *Anesthesia Review* was published in 2001 to fulfill the need for a question-and-answer style review of basic anesthesia principles. There were many textbooks that provided the student of anesthesiology with the information needed to practice anesthesia. What had been lacking was a book with which students at every level could actively participate in their own learning.

Miller's Anesthesia Review is a study guide that allows readers to evaluate their own knowledge and formulate answers alone or in groups, and it provides an alternate means of study of the information. This book is a companion book to Miller's *Basics of Anesthesia*. The two books have matching chapters and are organized in a logical progression from basic anesthesia principles and concepts to more complex issues. These include the delivery of anesthesia in various settings and the administration of anesthesia to patients with organ system dysfunction and disease states. In all but a few chapters, the author is the same for the corresponding chapters in *Basics of Anesthesia* and *Anesthesia Review*.

As with *Basics of Anesthesia*, this edition of *Anesthesia Review* has added four new chapters that reflect the expanding practice of anesthesia: "Anesthetic Neurotoxicity," "Palliative Care," "Sleep Medicine and Anesthesia," and "New Models of Anesthesia Care: Perioperative Medicine, the Perioperative Surgical Home, and Population Health." The remaining chapters have been extensively edited to challenge the reader to provide up-to-date information on evolving concepts in anesthesia. All the answers are current and self-explanatory. The page number references provided at the end of each question refer the reader to the seventh edition of *Basics*

of *Anesthesia*, where further information on the given topic can be found.

There are several ways this study guide can be used. The first-year anesthesia resident may use it for self-study to solidify information read. Anesthesia residents at every level may use it to prepare for specific clinical situations that they may face on a subspecialty rotation or with given cases on a particular day. Anesthesia residents can also use this study guide for group study in which they will be required to answer questions on given topics. Similarly, faculty may use the study guide to quiz residents orally in a coherent, progressive manner in formal or informal settings. Finally, anesthesiologists in practice may find the study guide useful to refresh their knowledge base and to review information that they may not have been taught during their residencies. The multiple uses of this study guide make it an appropriate choice for students, teachers, and clinicians of anesthesiology at every level. Our intention is that *Anesthesia Review* will facilitate learning and retention of current fundamental anesthesia concepts necessary for a solid knowledge base and clinical competence.

We are thankful to the authors of the current and previous edition of *Anesthesia Review*. We also acknowledge Elsevier, our publisher, and their staff. Special thanks to executive content strategists William R. Schmitt and Dolores Meloni, senior content development specialist Ann Ruzycka Anderson, and senior project manager Sharon Corell.

Lorraine M. Sdrales
Ronald D. Miller

CONTENTS

1 SCOPE OF ANESTHESIA PRACTICE

Ronald D. Miller

1. When did the specialty of anesthesiology become recognized?
2. How was anesthesia primarily used initially, and how has it evolved?
3. Name the two medical organizations whose approval allowed anesthesiology to be recognized as a medical specialty.

DEFINITION OF ANESTHESIOLOGY AS A SPECIALTY

4. Besides monitoring and maintenance of normal physiology during the perioperative period, what are some areas of the practice of anesthesiology as defined by the American Board of Anesthesiology (ABA)?
5. Name some of the organizations within the American system of anesthesiology.

EVOLUTION OF ANESTHESIA AS A MULTIDISCIPLINARY MEDICAL SPECIALTY

6. Name the five subspecialties of anesthesiology that require an additional certification process from the ABA.
7. In pain management, anesthesia providers are usually part of a multidisciplinary team. Name some of the other specialties that provide services that support pain management.
8. Describe an "open" versus a "closed" critical care unit.
9. Which other anesthesiology subspecialties are evolving toward a separate certification process?
10. What are some certifications offered by the National Board of Echocardiography?
11. Why has obstetric anesthesia been an essential component of anesthesia training programs?

PERIOPERATIVE PATIENT CARE

12. What are the components of perioperative care?
13. What was the impetus behind the creation of preoperative clinics, and who generally manages these clinics?
14. Describe the standard perioperative pathway.
15. What is throughput?

TRAINING AND CERTIFICATION IN ANESTHESIOLOGY

16. Which clinical anesthesia subspecialties are studied during the anesthesiology postgraduate training years (residency)?
17. Describe the fundamental steps that lead to being a "board-certified anesthesiologist."
18. What is the emphasis of the Maintenance of Certification in Anesthesiology (MOCA)?
19. What are some other specialties in anesthesiology that the ABA certifies?
20. Name the three new professional performance concepts developed by the Accreditation Council for Graduate Medical Education (ACGME) and the American Board of Medical Specialties (ABMS).

OTHER ANESTHETIC PROVIDERS

21. What are the training differences between a certified registered nurse anesthetist and an anesthesiologist assistant?

QUALITY OF CARE AND SAFETY IN ANESTHESIA

22. The Joint Commission (TJM) provides quality improvement guidelines in anesthesia for health care organizations. What three areas do these guidelines address?
23. Continuous quality improvement (CQI) programs may focus on both critical incidents and sentinel events. Describe critical incidents versus sentinel events.
24. What are some of the key factors in preventing patient injuries related to anesthesia?
25. Provide two examples of Patient Safety Practices and the Suggested Penalties for Failure to Adhere to the Practice as published in the *New England Journal of Medicine.*

ORGANIZATIONS WITH EMPHASIS ON ANESTHESIA QUALITY AND SAFETY

26. Anesthesiology has the distinction of being the only specialty in medicine with a foundation dedicated to issues of safety in patient care. Name the foundation.
27. What is the role of the Anesthesia Quality Institute?
28. What is the role of the American Society of Anesthesiologists Closed Claims Project and its registries?
29. What is the role of the Foundation for Anesthesia Education and Research (FAER)?

PROFESSIONAL LIABILITY

30. Is negligence on the part of the anesthesiologist implied when complications occur during the course of an anesthetic procedure?
31. What is the anesthesiologist's best protection against medicolegal action?
32. What actions should the anesthesiologist take in the event of an accident or complication related to the administration of anesthesia?

RISKS OF ANESTHESIA

33. What is the estimated mortality rate from anesthesia?
34. What are some of the factors that have contributed to the increased safety of anesthesia?
35. What are some of the anesthesiologist's greatest anesthesia patient safety issues?
36. What effects do sleep loss and fatigue have on the anesthesiologist's ability to perform the task of vigilance?

HAZARDS OF WORKING IN THE OPERATING ROOM

37. Name some of the most prevalent hazards encountered in the operating room.

ANSWERS*

1. The concept of providing analgesia, and eventually anesthesia, became increasingly possible in the early 19th century. Anesthesiology eventually evolved into a recognized medical specialty, and the first diplomates of anesthesiology were certified in 1939. (3)
2. The major emphasis of anesthesia practice was initially in surgical anesthesia. It then evolved into airway management including endotracheal intubation, which led to the development of critical care medicine, regional anesthesia, and pain medicine. The practice of anesthesiology continues to evolve. (3)
3. The two organizations whose approval allowed anesthesiology to be recognized as a medical specialty are the American Medical Association (AMA) and the American Board of Medical Specialties (ABMS). (3)

---

*Numbers in parentheses refer to pages, figures, boxes, or tables in Pardo MC, Miller RD, eds. *Basics of Anesthesia.* 7th ed. Philadelphia: Elsevier; 2018.)

DEFINITION OF ANESTHESIOLOGY AS A SPECIALTY

4. The American Board of Anesthesiology (ABA) defines anesthesiology as a discipline within the practice of medicine that deals with the following: assessment of, consultation for, and preparation of patients for anesthesia; relief and prevention of pain during and following surgical, obstetric, therapeutic, and diagnostic procedures; monitoring and maintenance of normal physiology during the perioperative period; management of critically ill patients including those receiving their care in an intensive care unit (ICU); diagnosis and treatment of acute, chronic, and cancer-related pain; management of hospice and palliative care; clinical management and teaching of cardiac, pulmonary, and neurologic resuscitation; evaluation of respiratory function and application of respiratory therapy; conduct of clinical, translational, and basic science research; supervision, instruction, and evaluation of performance of both medical and allied health personnel involved in perioperative or periprocedural care, hospice and palliative care, critical care, and pain management; and administrative involvement in health care facilities and organizations and medical schools as appropriate to the ABA's mission. (3-4)

5. As with other medical specialties, anesthesiology is represented by professional societies (American Society of Anesthesiologists, International Anesthesia Research Society), scientific journals (*Anesthesiology, Anesthesia & Analgesia*), a residency review committee with delegated authority from the Accreditation Council for Graduate Medical Education (ACGME) to establish and ensure compliance of anesthesia residency training programs with published standards, and the ABA, which establishes criteria for becoming a certified specialist in anesthesiology. Other countries have comparable systems of training and certifying mechanisms, and some work in a collective manner to educate and certify specialists in anesthesiology (e.g., European Society of Anesthesia). (4)

EVOLUTION OF ANESTHESIA AS A MULTIDISCIPLINARY MEDICAL SPECIALTY

6. In addition to board certification in anesthesiology, the ABA has an additional certification process for critical care medicine, pain medicine, pediatric anesthesiology, hospice and palliative medicine, and sleep medicine. (4)

7. Many other supportive services are involved in the pain management specialty of anesthesiology, including neurology, internal medicine, psychiatry, and physical therapy. (4)

8. Regarding critical care units, usually a "closed" system means that full-time critical care physicians take care of the patients. An "open" system means that the patient's attending physician continues to provide the care in the ICU. (4)

9. The American Board of Pediatrics and the ABA have commenced a combined integrated training program in both pediatrics and anesthesiology that would take 5 years instead of the traditional 6 years. In addition, cardiac anesthesiologists who now serve both pediatric and adult cardiac patients may move toward a separate certification process. (5)

10. Certifications offered by the National Board of Echocardiography include transthoracic echocardiography, transesophageal echocardiography, transthoracic plus stress echocardiography, and basic and advanced perioperative transesophageal echocardiography. The ACGME began to accredit adult cardiothoracic anesthesia fellowships, which led to increasing structure and standardization of the fellowships, including the requirement for echocardiography training. (5)

11. Because of the unique physiology and patient care issues, and the painful nature of childbirth, obstetric anesthesia experience has always been an essential component of anesthesia training programs. (5)

PERIOPERATIVE PATIENT CARE

12. Perioperative care includes preoperative evaluation, preparation in the immediate preoperative period, intraoperative care, management in the postanesthesia care unit (PACU), acute postoperative pain management, and possibly ICU care. (5)

13. Initially preoperative clinics were formed when patients were no longer admitted to the hospital the day before surgery. The increased complexity of patient medical risks and surgical procedures prompted the creation of preoperative clinics that allowed patients to be evaluated before the day of surgery. These clinics are often multidisciplinary (e.g., nursing, hospitalists, internists) and led by anesthesiologists. (5)

14. The standard perioperative pathway includes preoperative evaluation, the accuracy of predicting length and complexity of surgical care, and patient flow in and out of PACUs. (5)

15. Throughput is the term used to describe the efficiency of each patient's perioperative experience. This can be influenced by such things as operating room availability, length of surgery scheduling times, availability of beds in the PACU, and many other issues. At some institutions, perioperative or operating room directors are appointed to manage this perioperative process. (5)

TRAINING AND CERTIFICATION IN ANESTHESIOLOGY

16. All aspects of clinical anesthesia are covered in postgraduate training for anesthesiology, including obstetric, pediatric, and cardiothoracic anesthesia; neuroanesthesia; anesthesia for outpatient surgery and recovery room care; regional anesthesia; and pain management as well as at least 4 months of training in critical care medicine. (6)

17. To become a certified diplomate of the ABA, one must complete an accredited postgraduate training program, pass a written and oral examination, and meet licensure and credentialing requirements. (6)

18. Maintenance of Certification in Anesthesiology (MOCA) emphasizes continuous self-improvement and evaluation of clinical skills and practice performance to ensure quality and public accountability. In 2000, board certification became a 10-year, time-limited certificate that emphasizes participation in MOCA. In 2016 MOCA was redesigned as MOCA 2.0. Diplomates who are not time-limited (certificate issued before January 1, 2000) can voluntarily participate in MOCA certification. (6)

19. The ABA issues certificates in Pain Medicine, Critical Care Medicine, Hospice and Palliative Medicine, Sleep Medicine, and Pediatric Anesthesiology to diplomates who have completed 1 year of additional postgraduate training in the respective subspecialty, meet licensure and credentialing requirements, and pass a written examination. (7)

20. Evaluation of a clinician's professional performance as established by the ACGME and the ABMS now includes data regarding General Competences, Focused Professional Practice Evaluation, and Ongoing Professional Practice Evaluation. (7)

OTHER ANESTHETIC PROVIDERS

21. A certified registered nurse anesthetist (CRNA) must first be a registered nurse, spend 1 year as a critical care nurse, and then complete 2 to 3 years of didactic and clinical training in the techniques of the administration of anesthetics in an approved nurse anesthesia training program. The American Association of Nurse Anesthetists is responsible for the curriculum and criteria for certification of CRNAs. An anesthesiologist assistant completes a graduate-level 27-month program leading to a master of medical science degree in anesthesia from an accredited training program. (7)

QUALITY OF CARE AND SAFETY IN ANESTHESIA

22. The Joint Commission (TJM) guidelines evaluate quality improvement programs and evaluate care based on the measurement and improvement of the following three areas: structure (personnel and facilities used to provide care), process (sequence and coordination of patient care activities such as performance and documentation of a preanesthetic evaluation, and continuous attendance to and monitoring of the patient during anesthesia), and outcome. (7)

23. Critical incidents (e.g., ventilator disconnection) are events that cause or have the potential to cause injury if not noticed and corrected in a timely manner. Measurement of the occurrence rate of important critical incidents may serve as a substitute for rare outcomes in anesthesia and lead to improvement in patient safety. Sentinel events are isolated events that may indicate a systematic problem (e.g., syringe swap because of poor labeling, drug administration error related to keeping unnecessary medications on the anesthetic cart). (8)

24. Some key factors for the prevention of patient injuries related to anesthesia are vigilance, up-to-date knowledge, adequate monitoring, and adherence to the standards endorsed by the American Society of Anesthesiologists. (8)

25. The following are examples of patient safety practices and suggested penalties for not following them as published by the *New England Journal of Medicine*: (a) Hand hygiene. Initial penalty: Education and loss of patient care privileges for 1 week. (b) Following an institution's guidelines regarding provider-to-provider sign-out at the end of a shift. Initial penalty: Education and loss of patient care privileges for 1 week. (c) Performing a time-out before surgery. Initial penalty: Education and loss of operating room privileges for 2 weeks. (d) Marking the surgical site to prevent wrong-site surgery. Initial penalty: Education and loss of operating room privileges for 2 weeks. (e) Using the checklist when inserting central venous catheters. Initial penalty: Counseling, review of evidence, and loss of catheter insertion privileges for 2 weeks. (8)

ORGANIZATIONS WITH EMPHASIS ON ANESTHESIA AND SAFETY

26. The Anesthesia Patient Safety Foundation (APSF) is dedicated to patient safety issues in anesthesia and has a quarterly newsletter that provides discussion on this topic. (8)

27. The Anesthesia Quality Institute (AQI) provides a retrospective database of patient and safety data that can be used to assess and improve patient care. It is the primary source of information for quality improvement in the practice of anesthesiology. AQI provides the National Anesthesia Clinical Outcomes Registry (NACOR) on its website. (8)

28. The American Society of Anesthesiologists Closed Claims Project and its Registries provide a retrospective analysis of legal cases with adverse outcomes. Its investigations have helped identify patient and practice areas of risk that tend to have difficulties and require added attention regarding quality and safety. (8)

29. The Foundation for Anesthesia Education and Research (FAER) encourages and supports research, education, and scientific innovation in anesthesiology, perioperative medicine, and pain management. FAER has funded numerous research grants and supported the development of academic anesthesiologists. (8)

PROFESSIONAL LIABILITY

30. If a complication occurs during the course of an anesthetic, negligence is not immediately implied if ordinary and reasonable care was implemented by the anesthesiologist. Anesthesiologists are not expected to guarantee a favorable outcome to the patient. They are expected to make medical judgments consistent with national standards and with the skills expected of other anesthesiologists. (8-9)

31. The anesthesiologist's best protection against medicolegal action is by practicing within current standards of anesthesia, along with interest in the patient's outcome through preoperative and postoperative visits. Detailed records of the course of anesthesia should also be maintained. (9)

32. In the event of an accident or complication related to the administration of anesthesia, the anesthesiologist should promptly document the facts and patient treatment on the patient's medical record, as well as obtain consultations with other physicians when appropriate. The anesthesiologist should immediately notify the appropriate agencies, beginning at the department level and continuing with one's own medical center quality improvement administration and risk

management office. In addition, the anesthesiologist should provide the hospital and the company that writes the physician's professional liability insurance with a complete account of the incident. (9)

RISKS OF ANESTHESIA

33. Currently, it is estimated that the mortality rate from anesthesia is approximately 1 in 250,000 patients. This is based on a series of 244,000 surviving patients who underwent anesthesia and surgery. (9)
34. The increased safety of anesthesia is presumed to reflect the introduction of improved anesthesia drugs and monitoring, as well as the training of increased numbers of anesthesiologists. In addition, persuading patients to stop smoking, lose weight, avoid excess intake of alcohol, and achieve optimal medical control of essential hypertension, diabetes mellitus, and asthma before undergoing elective surgery can lead to improved safety in anesthesia practice. (10)
35. Difficult airway management is perceived to be the greatest anesthesia patient safety issue. Other examples of possible adverse outcomes besides death include peripheral nerve damage, brain damage, airway trauma, intraoperative awareness, eye injury, fetal/newborn injury, and aspiration of gastric contents. (10)
36. Sleep loss and fatigue can affect an anesthesiologist's vigilance by known detrimental effects on work efficiency and cognitive tasks, such as monitoring and clinical decision making. (10)

HAZARDS OF WORKING IN THE OPERATING ROOM

37. Hazards anesthesiologists are exposed to in the operating room include vapors from chemicals, ionizing radiation, and infectious agents. There is psychological stress from demands of the constant vigilance required for patients under anesthesia. In addition, interactions with members of the operating team may introduce varying levels of interpersonal stress. Other hazards include latex sensitivity from exposure to latex gloves, substance abuse, mental illness, and suicide. Blood-borne infection transmission is a risk of accidental needlestick injuries that can be reduced using universal precautions in the care of every patient. (10)

2 LEARNING ANESTHESIA

Lorraine M. Sdrales

Lorraine M. Sdrales

COMPETENCIES AND MILESTONES

1. What are some competencies and milestones described by the Accreditation Council for Graduate Medical Education (ACGME) that must be met during the 4 years of anesthesia residency?
2. What are some goals of the preoperative evaluation the anesthesia resident should achieve during the preoperative phase of anesthesia care?
3. What are some aspects of the anesthetic plan the anesthesia resident should be prepared to discuss with the supervising anesthesia provider?
4. What are some operating room preparation responsibilities of the anesthesia resident?
5. What are some aspects of the administered anesthetic that the anesthesia resident should address with the patient in the follow-up visit?

LEARNING STRATEGIES

6. What are the various methods that can be used for teaching in the anesthesia training program?
7. What is the learning goal in the "learning orientation" approach to a learning challenge? How does this compare to the "performance orientation" approach?

TEACHING ANESTHESIA

8. Is there a role for anesthesia residents to teach medical students?

ANSWERS*

COMPETENCIES AND MILESTONES

1. The Outcome Project developed by the Accreditation Council for Graduate Medical Education (ACGME) describes six core competencies: patient care, medical knowledge, professionalism, interpersonal and communication skills, systems-based practice, and practice-based learning and improvement. Milestones involve five progressive levels of patient care competency at five selected intervals during the 4 years of the anesthesia residency training program. Milestones measured are for creating an anesthetic plan as well as for resident conduct. These ultimately lead to the final level of ability to independently formulate and execute anesthetic plans for complex patients. (12)
2. Goals of the preoperative evaluation the anesthesia resident should achieve during the preoperative phase of anesthesia care include the assessment of the patient's

---

*Numbers in parentheses refer to pages, figures, boxes, or tables in Pardo MC, Miller RD, eds. *Basics of Anesthesia*. 7th ed. Philadelphia: Elsevier; 2018.

coexisting diseases, assessing the patient's perioperative risk, addressing the patient's questions, and discussing the options for anesthesia. (13)

3. Aspects of the anesthetic plan the anesthesia resident should be prepared to discuss with the supervising anesthesia provider include anesthetic technique and alternatives and drug choices and specific doses. Drug choices should include premedication as well as induction, intraoperative, and postoperative phases. Finally, the anesthesia resident should be prepared to discuss any potential adverse events that may occur and the plan for management. (13-14)

4. Standard operating room preparation responsibilities of the anesthesia resident include checking the anesthesia machine and circuit, suction, oxygen, intravenous supplies, monitors, and preparing drugs. The drugs should be drawn, labeled, dated, timed, and initialed. In addition, the resident should prepare any special anesthetic supplies or equipment based on the anesthetic plan or contingent plans. (14)

5. In the follow-up visit with the patient, the anesthesia resident should address general patient overall satisfaction with the anesthetic as well as any potential anesthetic complications. Anesthetic complications that may be addressed include dental injury, nausea, nerve injury, and intraoperative recall. (15)

LEARNING STRATEGIES

6. The mainstay of the approach to teaching anesthesia is through direct patient contact and case-based learning. Various additional methods that can be used for teaching in the anesthesia training program include lectures, group discussions, simulations, independent reading, journal clubs, quality assurance conferences, and problem-based discussions. In some cases, videos presenting information or scenarios can be viewed online prior to meeting for discussion. (15-17)

7. The learning goal in the "learning orientation" approach to a learning challenge is achieved through mastery of a situation. In this approach residents are given feedback on their mastery and are more likely to thrive in a challenging and demanding learning environment. This is in contrast to the "performance orientation" approach, which focuses more on the resident's abilities rather than proficiency. (17)

TEACHING ANESTHESIA

8. Both anesthesia residents and medical students benefit from anesthesia residents having a role in teaching medical students. (17)

3 ANESTHESIA AND HEALTH INFORMATION TECHNOLOGY

David L. Robinowitz and Scott Richard Springman

1. What is medical informatics? How has the growth in electronic clinical data systems transformed anesthesia education?
2. What is "health IT"?

HISTORY OF ANESTHESIA DOCUMENTATION AND AIMS

3. Who pioneered anesthesia records and when did it occur? What was the purpose of these records?
4. What key documentation elements form the basis of anesthesia records?
5. When introduced in the 1980s, what were considered to be the advantages of the anesthesia automated record keeper?

THE DEMAND FOR DATA

6. Which anesthesia organization in 2001 endorsed the adoption of the Anesthesia Information Management System (AIMS) as a patient safety system?
7. Which U.S. government act of 2009 catalyzed the rapid implementation of health IT in the United States?
8. What subsequent U.S. federal program of 2011 provided economic incentives for the adoption of health IT?
9. List some benefits of data collection and reporting for health care organizations.
10. What is a *data warehouse*?
11. What is a data registry, and what are some examples?
12. What are some barriers to full, effective use of data registries?
13. What is "Big Data" and what might be its use in health IT?

PROFESSIONAL PERFORMANCE DATA REPORTING WITH HEALTH IT

FEATURES OF THE ELECTRONIC HEALTH RECORD IN ANESTHESIA AND PERIOPERATIVE CARE

14. What are two professional electronic quality and value-based reporting systems administered by the Centers for Medicare & Medicaid Services (CMS)?
15. Name two organizations that are members of the CMS-approved qualified clinical data registry. What is the benefit of being members of this group?

16. What is a definition of an EHR (electronic health record)?
17. What data should be included in an AIMS?
18. What are fundamental EHR requirements for the clinician user?

HEALTH CARE INFORMATION PRIVACY AND SECURITY

19. Name some important U.S. legislation that regulates the privacy and security of EHRs.
20. What critical features of EHRs support protected health information privacy and security rules?
21. List some protected health information privacy and security recommended practices for health care providers.

SELECTED KEY TOPICS FOR HEALTH IT

INTEROPERABILITY

22. What two general approaches can be used to meet both core organizational and subspecialty health IT needs?
23. What is interoperability? What are some benefits of interoperability in health IT?
24. What are some methods by which health IT applications share data?

SYSTEM DESIGN, USER INTERFACE, AND USABILITY

25. What is *usability*, and why is it important to clinicians?
26. What is the user interface, and why is it important?
27. What are the "hierarchy of controls" safety practices and principles from other industries that have been applied to health IT design to reduce clinical hazards?
28. The American Medical Informatics Association has recommended clinician usability principles in building EHRs. List some core recommended principles.
29. How can clinician usability of a health IT system be assessed?

CLINICAL DECISION SUPPORT

30. Computerized clinical decision support (CDS) is an important feature of effective modern health IT and one of the most touted reasons for organizations to purchase health IT. Describe what CDS does and what tools are often used.
31. What are some reasons CDS may not function as intended?
32. What is "automation-induced complacency"?
33. What is one negative repercussion of too many alerts or warnings, especially if they are overly sensitive?

TRANSITIONING TO HEALTH IT: FROM PAPER RECORDS TO AN AIMS, AND BEYOND

34. What are some possible undesired effects of using health IT?
35. What kind of leadership is needed for a health IT rollout project?
36. Who should take the lead in reducing the risk of organizational tension and backlash with the implementation of a new health IT project?

LEGAL ISSUES AND RESPONSIBILITIES OF THE AIMS USER

37. How have AIMS data artifacts, unnoticed data dropouts, and inaccurate autodocumentation affected medicolegal risk to anesthesia providers?
38. During a case, the automated recording of hemodynamic variables is accidentally interrupted for 2 hours. What is the proper response by the anesthesia clinician in cases of AIMS failure such as this one?

ANSWERS*

1. Medical informatics is the branch of information science that relates to health care and biomedicine. Medical informatics encompasses health informatics, medical computer science, and computers in medicine. In 2014 it was estimated that 84% of U.S. academic medical centers would have an Anesthesia Information Management System (AIMS) installed by the end of that year. Soon few anesthesia trainees will graduate from residency having used a paper anesthetic record! AIMS is also used to track educational milestones such as numbers of subspecialty case and quality of care measures. (19)
2. *Health IT* (health information technology) is a global term that incorporates electronic health records and the growing number of adjunct electronic and computer devices and software. (19)

---

*Numbers in parentheses refer to pages, figures, boxes, or tables in Pardo MC, Miller RD, eds. *Basics of Anesthesia*. 7th ed. Philadelphia: Elsevier; 2018.

HISTORY OF ANESTHESIA DOCUMENTATION AND AIMS

3. Famous neurosurgeon and physiologist, Harvey Cushing, and his then medical school classmate, E. A. Codman, introduced anesthesia records in 1895, 50 years after the inception of anesthesia care. They believed that by documenting anesthesia management they could look for associations and patterns that correlated with good and bad outcomes, and so improve their anesthetic care. (20)

4. Documentation of significant events during the case coupled with automated real-time recordings of hemodynamic vital signs forms the foundation of anesthesia records and the modern AIMS. (20)

5. The anesthesia automated record keeper introduced in the 1980s automated recording of hemodynamic data and was the precursor to the modern AIMS. The touted advantages of the automated record keepers included correction of some of the disadvantages of paper records—namely, recall bias, illegible records, missing data or whole records (with regulatory and billing implications), and lack of an "audit" trail for medical/legal purposes. Clinical studies of anesthesia automated record keepers also revealed that they produced a more accurate record of hemodynamic variables than handwritten charts. (20)

THE DEMAND FOR DATA

6. In a very significant event, in 2001 the Anesthesia Patient Safety Foundation (APSF) endorsed the concept of AIMS to support the retrieval and analysis of automated anesthesia data to improve patient safety. This added even more credibility to the move toward the adoption of computerized records in anesthesiology. (20)

7. The Health Information Technology for Economic and Clinical Health (HITECH) Act of 2009 encouraged the adoption and appropriate use of health IT. The act included provisions for monetary rewards and penalties. (20)

8. In 2011, the U.S. Department of Health & Human Services Centers for Medicare & Medicaid Services (CMS) initiated the Medicare and Medicaid EHR Incentive Programs. Their "Meaningful Use" criteria encourage health care providers and organizations to adopt health IT through a staged process, via variable payments or penalties. (20)

9. Health care organization data collection and reporting support analysis of workflows; guide improvement in utilization, scheduling, and resource management; permit the measurement of costs, quality, and clinical outcomes; satisfy compliance regulations; serve research studies; and may be required by external public and private agencies. (21)

10. A data warehouse is a central repository of data, pooled from one or more sources or systems. (21)

11. A data registry is a national or international aggregation of data from many centers. Examples include the Anesthesia Quality Institute (AQI), National Anesthesia Clinical Outcomes Registry (NACOR), Multicenter Perioperative Outcomes Group (MPOG), Society for Ambulatory Anesthesia (SCOR) database, Pediatric Regional Anesthesia Network, and Society for Cardiovascular Anesthesiologists Adult Cardiac Anesthesia Module. (21)

12. Barriers to effective use of data registries include the need for concept mapping, the lack of a universally accepted taxonomy (or data dictionary), missing or inaccurate data in clinical documentation, use of clinicians as data-entry sources, and large amounts of data in unstructured, and noncategorized, text. (21)

13. "Big Data" are large-scale datasets such as those collected from national registries. Big data may be analyzed using methods developed by big business in other fields. These methods can then be applied to health care and anesthesia to find novel relationships among patient types, diseases, and therapies to predict outcomes and guide medical care to the most effective path. (21)

PROFESSIONAL PERFORMANCE DATA REPORTING WITH HEALTH IT

14. CMS administers the Physician Quality Reporting System (PQRS) and Meaningful Use (MU) quality and value-based assessment systems. The PQRS receives quality

information from individual eligible professionals and group practices, whereas MU pertains to how providers and organizations use health IT to further quality of care. CMS intends to combine these two systems in the future and create new payment systems. (21)

15. The ASA's Anesthesia Quality Institute (AQI) and the Multicenter Perioperative Outcomes Group (MPOG) are both members of a CMS-approved qualified clinical data registry. Qualified clinical data registries have a high level of medicolegal discovery protection to encourage accurate reporting. (21)

FEATURES OF THE ELECTRONIC HEALTH RECORD IN ANESTHESIA AND PERIOPERATIVE CARE

16. The EHR has been described as a longitudinal electronic record of patient health information generated by one or more encounters in any care delivery setting. The fundamental purpose of the EHR is to support required clinical and administrative activities. (21)

17. Data that should be included in an AIMS are the recording of device data (creating a permanent record of data from hemodynamic monitors, anesthesia machines, and other clinical devices) metadata such as case events, documentation of the preoperative evaluation, management of perioperative orders, and integration with the patient's EHR. Aspects of the patient's EHR that should be integrated in the AIMS include the medication record (integrated with pharmacy systems), laboratory and radiology tests, vital signs, provider and consultant notes, nursing documentation, billing functions, patient tracking, perioperative management systems, and admissions/discharge transfer functions. (21)

18. An EHR should be intuitive and guide users through their workflows, as well as provide access to the right information at the right time. An EHR should be reliable and fault-tolerant (i.e., network, hardware, or simple software "bugs" should not prevent system function). (22)

HEALTH CARE INFORMATION PRIVACY AND SECURITY

19. The Health Insurance Portability and Accountability Act (HIPAA) Privacy, Security, and Breach Notification Rules regulate the privacy and security of EHRs in the United States. The Privacy Rule sets standards for how protected health information may be used and disclosed in electronic, written, or verbal form. The Security Rule requires certain precautions so that access to health IT systems is limited to those with legitimate purposes and proper authorization. The Breach Notification Rule requires health care providers and organizations to report any violation of privacy and security. (22)

20. EHR features that support HIPAA rules include login requirements, security settings for individuals and groups, and extensive audit trails and integrity checks to detect intrusions, access, and unauthorized alterations of data. (23)

21. Some recommended health care provider practices to improve protected health information security include not sharing passwords under any circumstances, using a "strong" password (minimum of six characters, mix in uppercase, numbers, and symbols), and password use on all computing devices including smartphones. Health care providers should log out of computer systems when not in use. Papers containing protected health information should not be left unattended in an insecure location and should be destroyed in a shredder or locked disposal bin. Better yet, perhaps protected health information should not be printed at all. Protected health information should not be sent over an unsecure email system, in social media, or left on voicemail. (23-24)

SELECTED KEY TOPICS FOR HEALTH IT

INTEROPERABILITY

22. To meet health IT needs, some organizations take a "modular" approach, in which they employ many separate applications from multiple vendors that

need to be "stitched together" (e.g., a laboratory system, orders system). Other organizations predominantly use a single vendor, in hopes of creating an "out of the box" integrated "enterprise system." (24)

23. Interoperability is the capability to communicate among health IT modules. This can apply to modules within a health IT application, outside health IT applications, and with various data sources—both within and external to an organization. Benefits of interoperability are its replacement of inefficient paper workflows, reduction of duplicated testing, and reduced medication errors. Interoperability also facilitates better preventive care and chronic disease management and improves health care provider communication. (24)

24. Health IT applications may share data with built-in functionality (e.g., sharing the same database), using application-application interfaces with standardized data formats, or through use of application programming interfaces. Health IT applications may interface remotely via health information exchanges (HIEs)—large data stores that aggregate data from various health care organizations. In addition, the newest trend—the "Internet of Things"—allows a wide array of electronic devices (from home appliances, to vehicles, to personal health devices) to be interconnected via the Internet. (24)

SYSTEM DESIGN, USER INTERFACE, AND USABILITY

25. *Usability* is the extent to which a technology helps users achieve their goals in a satisfying, effective, and efficient manner within the constraints and complexities of their work environment. Usability is vital to the clinician users of the EHR because of the nature of clinical information and human factors. A large variety of information is necessary to assemble a clinical picture of the patient's health status. This information may be found in several virtual "locations" within the EHR. Cognitive and memory burdens on the clinician can negatively impact human performance. These "human factors" should inform health IT designers, resulting in a good design that fosters a high degree of clinical "situational awareness" (a term originally derived from aviation human factors research). (25)

26. The user interface includes all aspects of an information device with which a user may interact, including when and how the system invites interaction and responds to it. A good health IT user interface allows clinicians to quickly comprehend and process large amounts of information safely and efficiently. (25)

27. A "hierarchy of controls" has been applied to health IT design to reduce clinical hazards. These controls can include those that eliminate risk, such as a hard stop that does not allow ordering a lethal dose of medication. Another control is a substitution, such as replacing free text with specific check boxes or buttons. Lower levels of intervention rely on administrative or organizational policies (e.g., policies or checklists). The lowest level of control is the least effective, as it relies on individual user education. By defining the levels of interventions of a health care design process, health IT engineers can more effectively work with clinical and institutional leadership to eliminate, replace, or "engineer" hazards away. (25)

28. The American Medical Informatics Association recommended clinician health IT usability principles of *minimalism, reversibility, memory, flexibility,* and *standardization. Minimalism* is the ability to access core function quickly. *Reversibility* is the functionality to undo simple user errors. *Memory* refers to memory load reduction, to reduce the cognitive burden of operating the system, preserving memory capacity for critical tasks. *Flexibility* refers to system customization to suit the individual user needs, balanced with the benefits of *standardization* according to local and national norms. (25)

29. There is no single accepted metric for measuring clinician usability of health IT systems, but several techniques have been employed. They include user questionnaires, simulation, screen and video recording (of system and user behavior), charting accuracy metrics, situational awareness assessment (a measure of effectiveness), and number of "clicks" or time to complete a task (a measure of efficiency). Usability testing should be done prior to health IT implementation, and

periodically afterward, especially around the time of system updates or upgrades. Close attention should be given to how users "work around" system constraints and their general level of satisfaction with the user interface. (25)

CLINICAL DECISION SUPPORT

30. Computerized clinical decision support (CDS) provides patient specific information and recommendations for clinical care, ideally intelligently filtered and presented at appropriate times. CDS tools include (but are not limited to) computerized alerts and reminders to health care providers and patients; easy access to clinical guidelines; condition-specific order sets; focused patient data reports and summaries; documentation templates; diagnostic support; and contextually relevant reference information. CDS may be *passive*, providing information at the right time to assist with decision making. CDS can also be *active*—for example, monitoring for a specific set of conditions and then generating a warning, alert, or automated action in response to the conditions. (26)

31. CDS cannot be informed by information that is not integrated within the CDS application. For example, CDS cannot respond to information that resides in a nonintegrated system, even if that information may in some way be "visible" to the user, nor can it use information that is not yet in the medical record. For instance, if an anesthesia provider administers a medication prior to ordering and documenting it, the resultant pop-up warning that there is a critical history of a medication contraindication would be of limited utility. (26)

32. "Automation-induced complacency" is a cognitive error in which a clinician becomes dependent on automated processes, such as CDS alerts, and does not perform the same recommended clinical action in situations if automation is not active or has failed (e.g., CDS did not warn of medication interaction because the patient's medical history was not stored in an integrated system). (26)

33. "Alert fatigue" is the phenomenon of clinician conditioning by excessive system alerts to ignore important alerts or warnings. This results in ignoring, or "clicking through," alerts. Alert fatigue is more common when alerts are calibrated to be overly sensitive, generating a high frequency of false positive alerts—that is, alerts or warnings in response to a situation that is not critical or not true. The clinicians are then effectively trained to ignore alerts altogether. It has thus been described as "the boy who cried wolf" fable applied to clinical monitoring. (26)

TRANSITIONING TO HEALTH IT: FROM PAPER RECORDS TO AN AIMS, AND BEYOND

34. There are many possible undesirable effects of health IT. Health IT may paradoxically reduce direct communication among providers. It can produce new and excessive documentation work for clinicians, cognitive errors due to information overload, and errors due to changed and fragmented traditional workflows. With health IT, erroneous documentation or ordering interventions for the wrong patient may occur more frequently. "E-work" may cause provider distraction away from clinical work or from patient interaction, and copy-paste overuse may result in out-of-date information and "note bloat." Patient data may be lost or corrupted, and information transfer may be lost. Health IT can be associated with excessive costs, including the initial cost of the system, ongoing costs for hardware and software licenses, network costs support, licenses and updates, facility IT support, and further development. Any "hold harmless" clause in health IT vendor contracts may leave organizations liable for health IT-related clinical problems. There may be a persistence of paper work-arounds leading to dual systems and resultant confusion and complexity. There can be unwanted, unanticipated changes in status of orders, patient electronic location, or task lists. In addition to alert fatigue, there can be poor clinical correlation for medication or other alerts. A poor health IT user interface and usability can lead to errors and low user satisfaction and morale, as well as negative attitudes. (27)

35. A health IT project needs strongly committed leadership, including a project champion or leadership group with strong political and social skills as well as the political authority to make appropriate changes in policy to support the rollout (e.g., mandate training, change patient check-in sequence). Early and

frequent inclusion of clinician users in the project, coordination with other stakeholders, and transparency from the initial design process to final evaluation should result in a system with higher usability. (27)

36. It is the role of health IT governance and clinical leaders to prioritize system design and modification requests according to institutional priorities, as well as to advocate for overall clinician usability. The use of the technology should not degrade patient care. (28)

LEGAL ISSUES AND RESPONSIBILITIES OF THE AIMS USER

37. Proper use of the AIMS, including data artifacts, unnoticed data dropouts, and inaccurate autodocumentation, has not resulted in significant medicolegal negative consequences to anesthesia providers. (28)

38. It is the responsibility of the anesthesia provider/AIMS user to follow institutional, local, and national standards to create a complete and accurate anesthetic record. Users should be aware of reasonable gaps in the record, and if necessary, enter in missing data manually during times of system failure or downtime. An appropriate note or comment should be entered into the record describing the charting defect and what actions, exactly, were taken to remedy it. These steps, as well as reporting the system issue to the responsible entity (e.g., clinical engineering), should be taken as soon as possible. (28-29)

4 BASIC PHARMACOLOGIC PRINCIPLES

Jennifer DeCou, Clayton Anderson, and
Ken B. Johnson

PHARMACOKINETIC PRINCIPLES

1. Define pharmacokinetics.
2. What are three fundamental processes that govern pharmacokinetics?
3. Define volume of distribution.
4. What is a basic mathematical expression to describe volume of distribution?
5. Does the transfer of a drug to peripheral tissues increase or decrease the drug's total volume of distribution?
6. What are two properties of a drug that influence its distribution to peripheral tissues?
7. Is the volume of distribution constant over time?
8. Define drug clearance.
9. What is a basic mathematical expression to describe clearance?
10. What is the difference between systemic clearance and intercompartmental clearance?
11. What is drug elimination? How does drug elimination compare to drug clearance?
12. Define extraction ratio.
13. What is a basic mathematical expression to describe extraction ratio?
14. When is the extraction of a drug "flow limited"?
15. When is the extraction of a drug "capacity limited"?
16. Define front-end kinetics.
17. What is a compartmental pharmacokinetic model?
18. How are compartmental pharmacokinetic models created?
19. What are the three distinct phases of rate of drug concentration decline over time that are illustrated in the three-compartment model?
20. How are compartmental pharmacokinetic models used?
21. Define back-end kinetics.
22. Define decrement time and context-sensitive half-time.
23. How does the duration of a continuous infusion of drug influence the drug's decrement time?
24. Define biophase.

PHARMACODYNAMIC PRINCIPLES

25. Define pharmacodynamics.
26. What is a pharmacodynamic model?
27. How is a pharmacodynamic model created?
28. How is a pharmacodynamic model used?
29. What is drug potency?
30. What is drug efficacy?
31. What is an anesthetic drug interaction?
32. Distinguish among additive, antagonistic, and synergistic drug interactions.

<table>
<tr><td>

SPECIAL POPULATIONS

</td><td>

33. What are some examples of weight scalars, and how are they used clinically?
34. Do volatile anesthetics accumulate more in obese patients than in lean patients, thus prolonging emergence in obese patients?
35. How does age influence anesthetic dosing in the elderly?

</td></tr>
</table>

ANSWERS*

PHARMACOKINETIC PRINCIPLES

1. Pharmacokinetics describes the relationship between drug dose and drug concentration in plasma or, at the site of drug effect, over time. It can be thought of as "what the body does to the drug." (33)
2. Three fundamental processes that govern pharmacokinetics are absorption, distribution, and elimination (metabolism and excretion). (33)
3. Volume of distribution refers to the distribution of an administered drug into various tissues throughout the body. (34)
4. This basic mathematical expression can be used to describe volume of distribution:

$$\dot{V}/\dot{Q} \quad (34)$$

5. The transfer of a drug to peripheral tissues increases the drug's total volume of distribution. The peripheral tissues can be thought of as peripheral volume. (34)
6. Two properties of a drug that influence its distribution to peripheral tissues are its solubility and drug binding. The more soluble a drug is, and the more it binds to peripheral tissues, the greater the total volume of distribution. (34)
7. The volume of distribution is not constant over time, due to transfer of drug to the peripheral tissues (increases the total volume of distribution) and elimination (decreases the total volume of distribution). (35)
8. Clearance is the rate of drug removal from the plasma. It is defined in units of flow, that is, the volume completely cleared of drug per unit of time (e.g., liters/minute). (35)
9. This basic mathematical expression is used to describe clearance:

$$\bar{v} \quad (37)$$

10. Clearance can be either systemic or intercompartmental. Systemic clearance is permanent drug removal from the body, whereas intercompartmental clearance is drug movement between plasma and peripheral tissues. (36)
11. The drug elimination rate (mg/min) is the removal of drug in proportion to drug concentration. Clearance is drug elimination normalized to concentration. Drug elimination is high in the presence of high drug concentrations and low in the presence of low concentrations. Clearance is the same regardless of drug concentration. (36)
12. The extraction ratio is the fraction of inflowing drug extracted by an organ. (36-37)
13. A basic mathematical expression to describe extraction ratio (using C_{in} and C_{out} to represent the drug concentration moving into and out of an organ, respectively) is $(C_{in} - C_{out})/C_{in}$. (37)
14. The extraction of a drug by an organ is "flow limited" when the organ has a tremendous capacity to metabolize the drug and metabolism is limited only by the amount of blood flow to the organ. In this case, clearance depends on delivery of the drug to the tissue. An example of this is the hepatic clearance of propofol, whose extraction ratio is nearly 1. (37)

---

*Numbers in parentheses refer to pages, figures, boxes, or tables in Pardo MC, Miller RD, eds. *Basics of Anesthesia.* 7th ed. Philadelphia: Elsevier; 2018.

15. The extraction of a drug by an organ is "capacity limited" when the organ is limited in its capacity to take up and metabolize the drug. In this case, clearance of the drug can be influenced by liver disease or enzymatic induction and is independent of blood flow to the organ. An example of this is the hepatic clearance of alfentanil, whose extraction ratio is very low. (37)

16. Front-end kinetics describes intravenous drug behavior immediately following its administration. Front-end kinetics account for how drug concentration changes over time as drug distributes throughout the circulatory system and into peripheral tissues following injection. (37)

17. A compartmental pharmacokinetic model is a schematic rendering or illustration of a complex exponential equation used to describe drug concentrations over time. There are several types; for example, there are pharmacokinetic models with one, two, or three compartments. The number of compartments reflects the complexity of the exponential equations (e.g., the number of times the slope changes over time). (38)

18. To create a compartmental pharmacokinetic model, a drug is administered and plasma drug concentrations are measured and charted immediately and at various points of time. Data from several individuals are collected. Using sophisticated modeling software, compartmental pharmacokinetic models are built that consist of parameters for a complex exponential equation. In order for these compartmental model parameters to be better understood by the clinician, they are converted into terms such as distribution volume, clearance, and intercompartmental clearance. These terms, although more descriptive, are fictitious and do not represent any real body compartment or organ tissue. (38)

19. For many drugs there are three distinct phases of rate of drug concentration decline. For example, just after a bolus dose, the drug concentration may have a rapid decline. A few minutes later, it may have a moderate decline. Several minutes later, it may have a slow decline. This drug behavior would be best described by a three-compartment model. In this model the three compartments would correspond to the central compartment (plasma, where drug is injected), the rapidly equilibrating peripheral compartment, and the slowly equilibrating peripheral compartment. The rates of decline of drug concentration correspond to three phases. The first is the "rapid-distribution" phase (beginning immediately after intravenous bolus) when there is rapid movement of drug from the plasma to the rapidly equilibrating tissues. The second is the "slow-distribution" phase, when drug moves to the more slowly equilibrating tissues. And finally in the "elimination" phase, or terminal phase, drug returns from the tissues to the plasma and is permanently removed from the plasma by metabolism or excretion. (38)

20. Compartmental pharmacokinetic models are used to explore drug concentrations over time for various drug doses. Some models have been used to program infusion pumps. Using special infusion pumps, practitioners enter in a desired drug concentration and the model predicts how much drug is required to reach and maintain a target concentration. This technology is known as target-controlled infusions. (40-41)

21. Back-end kinetics describes how plasma drug behaves during a continuous infusion and how concentrations decrease once the continuous infusion is terminated. (41)

22. Decrement time is the time required to reach a specified plasma concentration once an infusion is terminated. The context-sensitive half-time is the 50% decrement time. (41)

23. During a continuous infusion drug accumulates in peripheral tissues, prolonging the decrement time; the longer the continuous infusion, the longer the decrement time. This makes decrement times useful as a tool to compare drug behavior within a drug class, such as comparing the decrement times of various opioids or sedatives. (41)

24. Biophase refers to the time delay between changes in plasma concentration and drug effect. Biophase accounts for the time required for drug to diffuse from the plasma to the site of action plus the time required, once drug is at the site of action, to elicit a drug effect. An increase in drug effect lags behind an increase in plasma drug concentrations. The opposite holds true for decreasing plasma concentrations. Pharmacokinetic models are modified to account for this lag time with an "effect site" compartment added to the central compartment. The "effect site" compartment represents the fictional compartment where drugs exert effects. There is no "volume" estimate to the effect site compartment. (41)

PHARMACODYNAMIC PRINCIPLES

25. Pharmacodynamics is the relationship between drug concentration and pharmacologic effect. It can be thought of as "what the drug does to the body." (42)

26. A pharmacodynamic model describes the relationship between drug concentration (most frequently the effect site concentration) and drug effect.
The relationship is typically described by a sigmoid curve. At low concentrations, there is no effect with increasing concentrations. This segment of the curve is flat. At high concentrations, there is no increase in maximal effect with increasing drug concentrations. This segment of the curve is also flat. In between, the curve has an increasing slope that tracks the rise in drug effect with the rise in drug concentration. (42)

27. To create a pharmacodynamic model a specific drug effect (such as analgesia or loss of responsiveness) is measured at various drug concentrations. Data are combined from several individuals, and measured concentrations are plotted versus the observed effect along all three portions of the sigmoid curve. Using sophisticated modeling software, models are built that consist of estimates for a complex exponential equation. Some of the common estimates include the C_{50} and γ (gamma). C_{50} is defined as the estimate for effect site concentration at which there is a 50% probability of effect (e.g., the C_{50} for fentanyl is 1 ng/mL, which represents the concentration at which 50% of people will experience analgesia). Gamma is defined as the rise in the slope that tracks the rise in drug effect with the rise in drug concentration. (43)

28. A pharmacodynamic model is used to predict drug effects from measured or estimated concentrations. Pharmacodynamic models are often used in conjunction with pharmacokinetic models to estimate drug effect from a given concentration. With combined pharmacokinetic and pharmacodynamic models, the onset and duration of effect can be estimated. (43)

29. Drug potency describes the amount of drug required to elicit an effect, with C_{50} as a commonly utilized metric for the comparison of potency between drugs. (43)

30. Drug efficacy describes the effectiveness of a drug to elicit an action when attached to a receptor. Drugs that achieve maximal effect are known as full agonists, and those with an effect less than maximal are known as partial agonists. (44)

31. Drugs from one class of anesthetics (e.g., opioids) interact with drugs from another class of anesthetics (e.g., sedatives) to enhance the effects of one another. A variety of effects have been characterized for interactions between inhaled agents and opioids, as well as sedatives and opioids. Some of these include responses to verbal, tactile, or painful stimuli; loss of response to laryngoscopy and tracheal intubation; and hemodynamic or respiratory effects. (45)

32. Drug interactions can be additive, synergistic, or antagonistic. For additive drug interactions, when the drugs are coadministered their overall effect is the sum of the two individual drug effects. For synergistic drug interactions, administering both drugs leads to an effect greater than the sum of their individual effects. With antagonistic drug interactions, the overall drug effect is less than if the drug combination was additive. (45)

SPECIAL POPULATIONS

33. Examples of weight scalars include lean body mass, ideal body weight, and fat-free mass. Weight scalars are used to dose drugs administered to obese patients to avoid excessive or underdosing these patients. In general, the purpose of using weight scalars is to match dosing regimens for obese patients with what is required for patients of normal size. Several weight scalars have been used for anesthetic agents, each with advantages and limitations. The scientific foundation for weight scalars is relatively immature. Clinical trials are warranted to validate their use to improve dosing obese patients. (47)

34. Contrary to perception, volatile anesthetics do not accumulate more in obese patients than in lean patients, and emergence in obese patients has not been confirmed to be prolonged. Blood flow to adipose tissue decreases with increasing obesity. In addition, the time required to fill adipose tissue with enough volatile anesthetic to significantly prolong emergence is much longer than the duration of most anesthetics. (47-49)

35. Both pharmacokinetics and pharmacodynamics are altered with age. In the elderly a decrease in cardiac output slows drug circulation time and decreases perfusion of metabolic organs. This results in higher peak plasma drug concentrations and decreased clearance for a given dose. Smaller doses of most anesthetic drugs are needed in elderly patients to produce the same therapeutic effect noted in younger counterparts based on pharmacokinetic and pharmacodynamic models. For example, to achieve an equipotent dose of remifentanil in an 80-year-old, the dose should be reduced by 55% of what would be administered to a 20-year-old. An analysis for propofol had similar results. The dose of propofol for an 80-year-old should be reduced by 65% of what would be administered to a 20-year-old for an equipotent effect. Dosing adjustments in elderly patients should account for their overall physical status (physiologic age) as well as their actual age. (50)

5 CLINICAL CARDIAC AND PULMONARY PHYSIOLOGY

John Feiner

HEMODYNAMICS

1. What is mean arterial pressure (MAP)?
2. What is the relationship of MAP to cardiac output and systemic vascular resistance (SVR)?
3. What is the "pulse pressure"?
4. What factors affect pulse pressure?
5. What pathologic factors may decrease SVR?
6. How is SVR calculated?
7. How is resistance related to the radius of the blood vessel?
8. Where is most of the resistance in the vascular system?
9. Which monitors allow calculation of cardiac output?
10. How is stroke volume (SV) calculated?
11. What is the cardiac index?
12. How might changes in heart rate or rhythm affect stroke volume?
13. Define ejection fraction (EF).
14. What is a normal value for EF?
15. Describe factors that may affect EF.
16. Define preload.
17. How can preload be measured clinically?
18. When will central venous pressure (CVP) poorly reflect filling pressures in the left side of the heart?
19. How does pulmonary capillary wedge pressure (PCWP) reflect left-sided heart filling pressures?
20. What is the Frank-Starling mechanism?
21. What are common causes of low preload?
22. What are systolic pressure variation (SPV) and pulse pressure variation (PPV), and how might they be useful in analyzing hypotension?
23. What is contractility?
24. What are some important clinical causes of low contractility?
25. Which monitors might best identify low contractility?
26. Define afterload.
27. What does low SVR or afterload do to EF?
28. What does low SVR or afterload do to cardiac filling pressures?
29. What does low SVR or afterload do to end-systolic volume, and how might this best be detected by monitoring?

CARDIAC REFLEXES

30. What are the physiologic effects of the parasympathetic and sympathetic nerves on the cardiovascular system?
31. What is the normal heart rate response to hypotension or hypertension?

32. Where are the baroreceptors located, and what is their response to increased blood pressure?
33. What is the effect of chemoreceptors in the carotid sinus?
34. What are the Bainbridge, oculocardiac, and Cushing reflexes?
35. What effects do anesthetic agents have on cardiac reflexes?

CORONARY BLOOD FLOW

36. What is the usual myocardial oxygen extraction, and how does this compare to whole-body oxygen extraction?
37. What is the physiologic coronary response to increased oxygen demand?
38. What are some endogenous regulators of coronary blood flow?
39. When is the myocardial subendocardium perfused?
40. What is the perfusion pressure of the left ventricle?

PULMONARY CIRCULATION

41. What is the function of the bronchial circulation?
42. How does the pulmonary artery (PA) pressure compare to systemic blood pressure?
43. How is pulmonary vascular resistance (PVR) calculated?
44. How does PVR respond to increased cardiac output?
45. How does lung volume affect PVR?
46. What drugs modify PVR?
47. What is the effect of hypoxia on PVR?
48. What are some pathologic causes of elevated PVR?
49. How does gravity affect pulmonary blood flow in West's zones 1, 2, and 3 of the lung?
50. What are the two main types of pulmonary edema?

PULMONARY GAS EXCHANGE

51. How does arterial hypoxemia differ from hypoxia?
52. How is blood oxygen measured?
53. How is arterial oxygen content calculated?
54. Why is $Pa_{O_2}/F_{I_{O_2}}$ (P/F ratio) useful for measuring oxygenation?
55. What is the P_{50}? What is a normal value?
56. What are common clinical factors that shift the oxyhemoglobin dissociation curve left and right?
57. What are the benefits of a rightward shift in the oxyhemoglobin dissociation curve?
58. What is the equation describing the effect of ventilation on oxygenation?
59. How does increased $F_{I_{O_2}}$ improve oxygenation during hypercapnia?
60. Is it possible to deliver hypoxic gas mixtures with a modern anesthesia machine?
61. How is the A-a gradient useful clinically with respect to a problem in oxygenation?
62. What is intrapulmonary shunt?
63. What does the shunt equation describe?
64. What does $\dot{V}/\dot{Q}$ (ventilation-perfusion) mismatch describe?
65. Is diffusion impairment a significant clinical cause of hypoxemia?
66. Which causes of hypoxemia are very responsive to supplemental oxygen and therefore easily treated with higher $F_{I_{O_2}}$?
67. How does low mixed venous oxygen saturation affect arterial oxygenation?
68. What are the three forms in which carbon dioxide is carried in the blood?
69. Why is hypercapnia a problem clinically?
70. What are some physiologic effects of hypercapnia on the lungs, kidneys, central nervous system, and heart?
71. What are the four physiologic causes of hypercapnia?
72. What are significant causes of increased CO_2 production under anesthesia?
73. Define dead space. What are the types of dead space?
74. What pathologic conditions may increase dead space?
75. What is a normal value for physiologic dead space?
76. What does the Bohr equation describe?
77. How can dead space be estimated under general anesthesia?
78. What is the effect on Pa_{CO_2} if alveolar ventilation decreases by one half?
79. How quickly can apnea increase Pa_{CO_2}?

PULMONARY MECHANICS	80. What are pulmonary mechanics?
	81. What factors contribute to the static pressure in the lung?
	82. How is surface tension reduced in the lungs?
	83. Define static compliance.
	84. What is functional residual capacity (FRC) with respect to the static mechanical properties of the lung and chest wall?
	85. What determines airway resistance?
	86. How can one distinguish clinically between elevated airway pressure produced from resistance and that caused by static compliance?
	87. List important clinical causes of elevated airway resistance.
CONTROL OF BREATHING	88. Where are the central chemoreceptors located?
	89. What is the main stimulus for the central chemoreceptors?
	90. How would the central chemoreceptors respond to lactic acidosis?
	91. What are the primary peripheral chemoreceptors?
	92. What factors stimulate the peripheral chemoreceptors?
	93. Why do peripheral chemoreceptors effectively sense arterial, not venous, blood values?
	94. What is the hypercapnic ventilatory response?
	95. What receptors drive the hypercapnic ventilatory response?
	96. What is an apneic threshold?
	97. How quickly does a CO_2 ventilatory response develop?
	98. What is the hypoxic ventilatory response?
	99. What receptors are responsible for hypoxic stimulation of ventilation?
	100. How does hypoxia depress ventilation?
	101. How quickly does the hypoxic ventilatory response develop?
	102. What is the effect of P_{CO_2} on hypoxic drive?
	103. Do opioids, sedative-hypnotics, and volatile anesthetics depress hypercapnic ventilatory drive, hypoxic ventilatory drive, or both?
	104. What ventilatory problems are neonates of low postconceptual age at risk for?
	105. What is Ondine's curse?
	106. When is periodic breathing most likely to occur?
INTEGRATION OF THE HEART AND LUNGS	107. Write the Fick equation.
	108. Define oxygen delivery.
	109. Why is examining oxygen extraction clinically useful?
	110. What is normal mixed venous oxygen saturation?
	111. How does the normal mixed venous oxygen saturation value change with hemoglobin level?
	112. How would the arterial to venous oxygen content difference change with higher F_{IO_2}?
	113. Why is the oxygen extraction ratio useful?
	114. How can the body respond physiologically to anemia or increased metabolic demand (oxygen consumption)?

ANSWERS*

HEMODYNAMICS	1. Mean arterial pressure (MAP) is the time-weighted average blood pressure. On modern monitors, MAP is calculated from electronically integrating the arterial

*Numbers in parentheses refer to pages, figures, boxes, or tables in Pardo MC, Miller RD, eds. *Basics of Anesthesia.* 7th ed. Philadelphia: Elsevier; 2018.

waveform over time. Automated blood pressure cuffs estimate the MAP by the point of maximum amplitude of the pressure oscillations. MAP can also be estimated by adding one third of the pulse pressure to the diastolic blood pressure. (53)

2. MAP is the product of cardiac output (CO) and systemic vascular resistance (SVR), or MAP = CO × SVR. This relationship is similar to Ohm's law in electricity, where voltage = current × resistance. If we were to be exactly correct, we would use the pressure drop across the systemic vascular system, or MAP – CVP (central venous pressure). (54)

3. Pulse pressure is the difference between systolic and diastolic blood pressures. (54)

4. Pulse pressure is produced from the stroke volume being pushed into the aorta on top of the diastolic blood pressure. The compliance features of the aorta therefore have a very significant effect on pulse pressure so that a stiff aorta results in a higher pulse pressure, a common feature of aging. A lower diastolic pressure can reduce pulse pressure by shifting to a more compliant part of the aortic compliance curve. A higher stroke volume generally increases pulse pressure. Lower SVR can decrease pulse pressure because part of the stroke volume "runs off" rapidly during ejection. Aortic insufficiency can increase pulse pressure as the diastolic pressure drops significantly during backward flow into the left ventricle. (54)

5. Classic pathologic causes of low SVR include sepsis, anaphylactic and anaphylactoid reactions, liver failure, and reperfusion of ischemic organs. Many antihypertensive medications, anesthetic drugs, and neuraxial anesthetics also lower SVR. (54)

6. SVR = 80 × (MAP – CVP)/CO, where MAP is mean arterial pressure, SVR is systemic vascular resistance, CVP is central venous pressure, and CO is cardiac output. The factor 80 converts the SVR to the proper units. (54)

7. Resistance is inversely proportional to the fourth power of the radius of the vessel. (54)

8. Most of the resistance in the vascular system is in the arterioles. Despite capillaries having smaller diameters than arterioles, there are large numbers of capillaries in parallel, resulting in overall lower resistance at this level of the vascular tree. (54)

9. Cardiac output is the amount of blood (L/min) pumped by the heart. Cardiac output can be determined by thermodilution with a pulmonary artery (PA) catheter and is the dominant technique. In addition, transesophageal echocardiography (TEE) may be used to estimate cardiac output. A variety of other noninvasive monitors are available and are being developed that estimate cardiac output, including Doppler of the ascending aorta and arterial pressure waveform analysis. The Fick equation can also be used to calculate cardiac output from the oxygen consumption and arterial and mixed venous oxygen content. (54)

10. Stroke volume (SV) is the cardiac output (CO) divided by heart rate (HR): SV = CO/HR. It is important to calculate stroke volume, because a high heart rate may make cardiac output appear normal despite inadequate stroke volume. (54)

11. Because the appropriate cardiac output changes with body size, the cardiac index is used to normalize for body size by dividing cardiac output by body surface area. (54)

12. Both tachycardia and bradycardia can affect stroke volume. An excessively rapid heart rate might not leave sufficient time to fill the ventricle. Loss of sinus rhythm, as reflected by the lack of a p wave on the ECG, will also lead to inadequate ventricular filling from loss of atrial contraction. This is particularly true in patients with a poorly compliant ventricle. A slow heart rate may allow for enhanced ventricular filling and stroke volume, but an excessively low heart rate results in an inadequate cardiac output. (54)

13. Ejection fraction (EF) is the percentage of ventricular blood volume that is pumped during a single contraction, or stroke volume/end-diastolic volume (SV/EDV). (54)

14. A normal EF is 60% to 70%. Unlike stroke volume, EF does not change with body size. Poor cardiac function is indicated by a low EF, although with dilated cardiomyopathy, the stroke volume can improve despite the lower EF. (54)

15. Hyperdynamic states with low SVR, such as sepsis and liver failure, are reflected by an elevated EF. Increased SVR can decrease EF, particularly in patients with poor cardiac function. (54)

16. Preload refers to the amount the heart muscle is "stretched" before contraction. Preload is best defined clinically as the EDV of the heart. (54)

17. The EDV of the heart, or preload, can be measured directly by transesophageal echocardiography (TEE). Ventricular filling pressures can be measured on the right side of the heart with central venous pressure and on the left side of the heart by pulmonary capillary wedge pressure. A complete picture of preload would still require both pressure and volume information to more fully understand the compliance of the heart. Systolic pressure variation (SPV) may also be an important indicator of preload. (54)

18. Central venous pressure will poorly reflect filling of the left ventricle in a number of pathologic conditions. With pulmonary disease and elevated peripheral vascular resistance (PVR), right-sided heart failure may increase CVP despite poor filling of the left ventricle. With left ventricular failure, CVP may be normal despite elevated left-sided heart filling pressures as long as right ventricular function is preserved. Therefore, CVP correlates with filling pressures on the left side of the heart in the absence of pulmonary disease and when cardiac function is normal. (54)

19. Pulmonary capillary wedge pressure (PCWP) reflects the filling pressure of the left side of the heart, becoming nearly equivalent to left atrial pressures. By using a balloon to stop flow in a pulmonary artery, pressure equilibrates within the system. (55)

20. The Frank-Starling mechanism describes how the heart responds to increased filling by increasing contraction and stroke volume. A larger preload results in an increased contraction necessary to eject the added ventricular volume, resulting in a larger SV and similar EF. Small increases in preload may have dramatic effects on SV and CO, although at higher filling pressures little benefit may be derived. This is described by cardiac function curves. (55)

21. Hypovolemia or low circulating blood volume is a key cause of low preload. Blood loss and fluid loss from other sources are commonly faced during surgery. Low preload can also occur with venodilation from anesthetic agents and neuraxial anesthesia. Pathologic problems such as pericardial tamponade and tension pneumothorax may result in low preload (inadequate filling of the heart) despite normal blood volume and high CVP. Pulmonary embolus and pulmonary hypertension are examples of pathologic problems that may prevent the right side of the heart from pumping sufficient volume to fill the left side of the heart, also resulting in low preload. (55)

22. Systolic pressure variation (SPV) describes the regular changes in systolic pressure that occur with ventilation. During mechanical ventilation, significant SPV reflects low preload. In cases of hypotension, high SPV may indicate low preload. Extreme SPV may indicate other important causes of hypotension, such as pericardial tamponade or tension pneumothorax. Pulse pressure variation (PPV), which is closely related to SPV, requires computer calculation. Many monitoring systems will compute both. Both SPV and PPV are the most sensitive and specific indicators of which patients will respond appropriately to fluid administration. Although cardiac filling pressures (CVP and PCWP) reflect preload, a single number may not adequately determine whether an individual patient requires more or less fluid. (55)

23. Contractility, or inotropic state, describes the force of myocardial contraction independent of preload and afterload. It is reflected in the rate of rise of pressure over time. Graphically, it is reflected in the systolic pressure-volume relationships. (55)

24. Important causes of poor myocardial contractility that may be associated with hypotension include myocardial ischemia, previous myocardial infarction, cardiomyopathy, and myocardial depression from a number of different drugs. In addition, when considering a differential diagnosis of hypotension, valvular heart disease can be reflected as low contractility. (55)

25. Low myocardial contractility is most easily observed with TEE, where it may be quite obvious even to the untrained observer. The rate of rise of the arterial pressure on arterial waveform, although theoretically reflective of low contractility, is not usually adequate. (55)

26. Afterload is the resistance to ejection of blood from the left ventricle with each contraction. Clinically, afterload is largely determined by the SVR. (55)

27. Low SVR or afterload increases EF, which can approach 75% or even 80% in low SVR states. This is a classic feature of low SVR conditions such as liver failure. (56)

28. Low SVR or afterload lowers cardiac filling pressure (CVP or PCWP) via the Frank-Starling mechanism. Vasodilation can therefore cause relative hypovolemia and a volume-responsive condition. Likewise, high SVR or afterload increases cardiac filling pressure. (56)

29. Low SVR or afterload leads to low end-systolic left ventricular volume (which can also occur with very low preload!). This is a pathognomonic sign of low SVR on TEE. (56)

CARDIAC REFLEXES

30. The parasympathetic nervous system primarily affects the cardiovascular system by decreasing heart rate through vagal innervation of the sinoatrial node via muscarinic acetylcholine receptors. It also decreases conduction through the atrioventricular node. Mild negative effects on contractility are probably less important. The sympathetic nervous system can increase heart rate (via activation of β_1-adrenergic receptors), increase conduction through the atrioventricular node, and increase contractility. The sympathetic nervous system also causes peripheral vasoconstriction. (56)

31. Although anesthetic agents and other medications may blunt autonomic reflex responses, significant hypotension will usually increase heart rate, and hypertension will decrease it. (57)

32. Baroreceptors are present in the carotid sinus and aortic arch. Increased blood pressure will stimulate stretch receptors, leading to parasympathetic stimulation via the vagus and glossopharyngeal nerves and a decrease in heart rate. Sympathetic nervous system activity is also decreased, resulting in a decrease in myocardial contractility and reflex vasodilation. (57)

33. Chemoreceptors in the carotid sinus respond to arterial hypoxemia with respiratory and cardiovascular effects. Sympathetic nervous system is stimulated by arterial hypoxemia, although more profound and prolonged arterial hypoxemia can result in bradycardia, possibly through central mechanisms. (57)

34. The Bainbridge reflex describes the increase in heart rate from atrial stretch. This helps increase cardiac output in response to increased venous return. The oculocardiac reflex describes bradycardia in response to ocular pressure. The Cushing reflex describes bradycardia in response to increased intracranial pressure. (57)

35. Anesthetic agents blunt cardiac reflexes in a dose-dependent manner. This increases the likelihood of hypotension under anesthesia. (57)

CORONARY BLOOD FLOW

36. The myocardium extracts a higher percentage of oxygen than other tissues in the body, up to 60% to 70%. Normal whole-body oxygen extraction is approximately 25%. (57)

37. The physiologic coronary response to increased oxygen demand is by coronary vasodilation and increased coronary blood flow, because increased oxygen extraction is not possible. (57)

38. Endogenous regulators of coronary blood flow include adenosine, nitric oxide, and adrenergic stimulation. (57)

39. Intramural pressure of the myocardium during systole stops blood flow to the subendocardium. Therefore, blood flow to the subendocardium occurs predominantly during diastole. (57)

40. The perfusion pressure of the left ventricle is DBP – LVEDP, where DBP is diastolic blood pressure and LVEDP is left ventricular end-diastolic pressure. LVEDP may exceed CVP and is therefore used as the downstream pressure. (57)

PULMONARY CIRCULATION

41. The bronchial circulation supplies nutrients to lung tissue and empties into the pulmonary veins and left atrium. (57)

42. The pulmonary circulation has much lower pressures than the systemic circulation. This is due to lower pulmonary vascular resistance compared to the systemic vascular resistance, because both systems accept the entire cardiac output. Because these pressures are reported for right-sided heart catheterization, and can be measured clinically with a PA catheter, the anesthesiologist should be familiar with normal and pathologic values. (57)

43. Similar to SVR, PVR is calculated as 80 × (mean PA pressure – PCWP)/CO. (57)

44. PA pressure stays remarkably constant over a wide range of cardiac output. PVR accommodates to increased cardiac output by *distention* and *recruitment* of capillaries, so that resistance decreases as cardiac output increases. (57)

45. Both high and low lung volumes increase PVR. At high lung volumes, intra-alveolar vessels are compressed. At low lung volumes, extra-alveolar vessels are compressed. Increased PVR at low lung volumes may be physiologically helpful in diverting blood flow from a collapsed lung, thereby improving gas exchange. (58)

46. Elevated PVR can be very difficult to treat. Inhaled nitric oxide, prostaglandins, and phosphodiesterase inhibitors may lower PVR, but cannot always completely reverse elevated PA pressure. (58)

47. Hypoxia increases PVR through hypoxic pulmonary vasoconstriction (HPV). This process may significantly improve gas exchange by lowering blood flow to areas of poor ventilation. However, global hypoxia, such as occurs at high altitude, can result in increased PA pressure through HPV. (58)

48. Pathologic elevation in PVR may occur with pulmonary emboli (blood clots, air, amniotic fluid, carbon dioxide, fat). In addition, arteriolar hyperplasia may occur with certain congenital cardiac diseases (Eisenmenger syndrome), idiopathically (primary pulmonary hypertension), and associated with cirrhosis (portopulmonary hypertension). Intrinsic lung disease from a variety of causes can also increase PVR. (58)

49. Because the PA pressure is low, hydrostatic changes due to gravity can have significant effects on pulmonary blood flow. For every 20-cm change of height there is a 15-mm Hg pressure difference. This has minimal effect for systemic pressure but can be significant in the lung. Notable effects are in West's zone 1 of the lung, where airway pressure is higher than PA pressure, leading to no perfusion and therefore dead space. This zone normally does not exist, but with positive-pressure ventilation or low PA pressures zone 1 develops. In zone 2, airway pressure is more than pulmonary venous pressure but not more than PA pressure. Therefore, blood flow is proportional to the difference between PA pressure and airway pressure. In zone 3, PA pressure and venous pressure exceed airway pressure, and blood flow is proportional to their difference. This can be useful clinically, by positioning the patient such that areas of poor gas exchange are in an elevated position where there is also lower perfusion, improving gas exchange. In lung surgery, the lower PA pressure in the nondependent collapsed lung helps gas exchange. (58)

50. Pulmonary edema can be due to hydrostatic leak or capillary leak. Hydrostatic leak can occur in the lung when pulmonary capillary pressure is elevated. Pulmonary edema results when lymphatic system removal of fluid is overwhelmed by the degree of hydrostatic leak. The risk of pulmonary edema increases as PCWP exceeds 20 mm Hg. Pulmonary edema due to capillary leak can also occur with pulmonary injury from a variety of causes, such as aspiration, sepsis, or blood transfusion (transfusion-related acute lung injury). The acute respiratory distress syndrome (ARDS) represents very significant lung injury with a high risk of mortality. (59)

PULMONARY GAS EXCHANGE

51. Arterial hypoxemia, which reflects pulmonary gas exchange, is defined as a low partial pressure of oxygen in the blood. Mild and even moderate arterial hypoxemia (e.g., high altitude) can be tolerated and may not result in substantial injury or adverse outcomes. Hypoxia is a more general term including tissue hypoxia, which also reflects circulatory factors. Anoxia is a nearly complete lack of oxygen. (59)

52. Three measurements of blood oxygen are used clinically: the partial pressure (Pa_{O_2} in mm Hg), oxyhemoglobin saturation (Sa_{O_2} in %), and arterial oxygen content (Ca_{O_2} in mL O_2/dL). (59)

53. Arterial oxygen content (Ca_{O_2}) is really a concentration and is the sum of the amount of oxygen bound to hemoglobin (1.39 mL O_2/dL/g hemoglobin fully saturated) and dissolved in the plasma (0.003 mL O_2/mm Hg/dL). The contribution of dissolved oxygen to the Ca_{O_2} can be clinically important at high F_{IO_2} levels and with hyperbaric oxygen therapy. (59)

54. Pa_{O_2}/F_{IO_2} ratio (P/F ratio) is a common clinical index of arterial oxygenation that is less affected by variations in the F_{IO_2} than is Pa_{O_2} or A-a gradient. (59)

55. The oxyhemoglobin dissociation curve relates Pa_{O_2} and Sa_{O_2}, or oxygen partial pressure and oxyhemoglobin saturation. The P_{50} is the partial pressure of oxygen (P_{O_2}) at which hemoglobin is 50% saturated, normally 26.8 mm Hg. Sigmoidal curves are defined by such midpoints. (59)

56. The most important factors shifting the oxyhemoglobin dissociation curve to the right are metabolic acidosis and hypercapnia. Metabolic alkalosis and hypocapnia shift the curve to the left. Lower 2,3-DPG in stored blood and the presence of fetal hemoglobin lead to a significant left shift. (59)

57. Rightward shifts of the oxyhemoglobin dissociation curve improve unloading of oxygen in the tissues. For the same tissue P_{O_2} more oxygen will be unloaded because of a rightward shift, improving tissue oxygenation. Because of the sigmoidal shape of the curve, little change in loading of oxygen in the lungs will occur because of the rightward shift. (59)

58. The *alveolar gas equation* is used most commonly to determine the effect of ventilation on oxygenation. The equation describes the transfer of oxygen from the environment to the alveoli and therefore contains all the determinants of alveolar oxygen: barometric pressure (P_B), F_{IO_2}, and ventilation in respiratory quotient (RQ). The respiratory quotient is the ratio of carbon dioxide production to oxygen consumption and is assumed to be 0.8 on a normal diet. The alveolar gas equation is $PA_{O_2} = F_{IO_2} \times (P_B - P_{H_2O}) - Pa_{CO_2}/RQ$. (60)

59. F_{IO_2} is a determinant of alveolar oxygen, and it can overcome the effect of higher CO_2 on alveolar oxygen as can occur during hypoventilation. The alveolar gas equation can be used to describe this effect of supplemental oxygen improving arterial oxygenation. (60)

60. Modern anesthesia machines can effectively prevent delivery of hypoxic gas mixtures. Multiple features are necessary, including pin indexing of tanks and gas hoses, shut-off valves for nitrous oxide, and use of oxygen to drive the bellows. These safety mechanisms might be overcome if a gas other than oxygen were delivered through the oxygen piping, which has occurred because of construction mishaps. A monitor measuring F_{IO_2} is therefore still critical. Hypoxemia still occurs because of unintentional delivery of room air in patients

requiring supplemental oxygen, such as might occur with an exhausted oxygen transport cylinder. (60)

61. Calculation of an A-a gradient ($P_{AO_2} - Pa_{O_2}$) divides the potential causes of hypoxemia into two groups of causes. The first group of causes includes all the factors that determine alveolar oxygen: FI_{O_2}, barometric pressure (altitude), and ventilation. Hypoxemia in the presence of a normal A-a gradient (5 to 10 mm Hg) would indicate that this first group is the problem. An abnormal A-a gradient indicates a gas exchange issue, usually $\dot{V}/\dot{Q}$ (ventilation-perfusion) mismatch or shunt. A-a gradients are simple to calculate but are clinically most useful at room air. The P/F ratio is more consistent and clinically useful at higher FI_{O_2}. (61)

62. Intrapulmonary shunt describes the passage of mixed venous blood through the lung, unexposed to alveolar gas. This commonly occurs because alveoli are collapsed (atelectasis) or filled with fluid such as in pneumonia or pulmonary edema. Mixed venous blood combines with blood passing through normal lung, lowering the Pa_{O_2}, which is the end result of the mixture. An intracardiac shunt can occur in various congenital types of heart diseases and sometimes in adults with blood flow through a patent foramen ovale. (62)

63. The shunt equation quantitatively describes the physiologic effect of shunt on oxygenation. The equation calculates the shunt fraction, or shunt flow relative to total flow. Because $\dot{V}/\dot{Q}$ mismatch may also be present, the shunt equation really describes a simple two-compartment model analyzing oxygenation as if it were all pure shunt. (62)

64. Ventilation-perfusion mismatch describes the disparity between the ventilation and perfusion in various alveoli. Well-ventilated alveoli are described as having a high $\dot{V}/\dot{Q}$, whereas a low $\dot{V}/\dot{Q}$ describes alveoli that are poorly ventilated and, if this reflects a significant portion of the lungs, may result in a low Pa_{O_2} and arterial hypoxemia. (62)

65. Diffusion impairment is not a major clinical cause of hypoxemia. However, diffusion impairment is often misunderstood and is not equivalent to a low diffusing capacity. Diffusion impairment occurs when a partial pressure gradient still exists between the alveolus and the capillary blood after the blood has passed through. Diffusion impairment is rare because there is usually sufficient time for diffusion, with equilibration occurring early in the process. If an alveolus is filled with fluid, such that no diffusion of oxygen occurs, this is *shunt*, not diffusion impairment. Even alveolar thickening, which may slow diffusion, does not usually result in diffusion impairment because equilibration of P_{O_2} between the alveolus and capillary blood does occur. Diffusion impairment may be a clinically significant physiologic problem at extreme altitude during exercise because of both a smaller driving oxygen partial pressure and the limited time for equilibrium due to the rapid transit of blood through the pulmonary capillaries. (62)

66. Hypoventilation, diffusion impairment, and $\dot{V}/\dot{Q}$ mismatch are all very responsive to supplemental oxygen. High FI_{O_2} can effectively eliminate hypoxemia from these causes. Shunt is much more resistant to supplemental oxygen. At shunt fractions over 30%, hypoxemia may remain despite administration of 100% oxygen. Higher FI_{O_2} does improve oxygenation with intrapulmonary shunt by adding more dissolved oxygen in the normally perfused alveoli. Arterial hypoxemia remaining despite administration of 100% oxygen is always caused by the presence of an intrapulmonary shunt. (62)

67. Low mixed venous oxygen levels may affect Pa_{O_2} but only in the presence of shunt. For the same shunt, lower mixed venous oxygen results in a lower Pa_{O_2}. (62)

68. In the blood, carbon dioxide is carried as dissolved gas, as bicarbonate, and bound to hemoglobin as carbaminohemoglobin. The greatest total quantity of CO_2 is as bicarbonate, which is in fairly rapid equilibrium with CO_2. Equilibrium occurs because of the enzyme carbonic anhydrase, through carbonic acid.

Despite being the smallest total, the CO_2 from carbaminohemoglobin represents about one third of the venous to arterial CO_2 movement. (63)

69. Hypercapnia can be well tolerated, although at higher levels, probably approaching 80 mm Hg or greater, hypercapnia can cause CO_2 narcosis. The most significant problem is what hypercapnia represents. A major cause of hypercapnia is oversedation or narcotization. This could progress to apnea and anoxia. Hypercapnia may also represent impending respiratory failure from a variety of causes. (63)

70. Hypercapnia affects the lungs (pulmonary vasoconstriction, right shift of the hemoglobin-oxygen dissociation curve), kidneys (renal bicarbonate resorption), central nervous system (somnolence, cerebral vasodilation), and heart (coronary artery vasodilation, decreased cardiac contractility). (63)

71. Hypercapnia is caused by increased production or decreased removal. Physiologically, hypercapnia can be caused by (1) rebreathing (elevated inspired CO_2), (2) hypoventilation, (3) elevated CO_2 production, and (4) elevated dead space. (63)

72. The most concerning cause of significant CO_2 production under general anesthesia is malignant hyperthermia (MH). Although fever alone will increase CO_2 production, the increase is not dramatic. MH may increase CO_2 production severalfold. Thyroid storm may increase CO_2 production. Absorption of CO_2 introduced during laparoscopy may be quite significant for certain procedures, particularly if subcutaneous CO_2 emphysema develops. The CO_2 removed through the lungs appears as if it is CO_2 production. Other causes of increased CO_2 under anesthesia include malfunctioning expiratory valves on the anesthesia machine, exhausted CO_2 absorbents, and, although temporary effects, the administration of sodium bicarbonate and the release of an extremity tourniquet. (64)

73. Dead space is "wasted ventilation," or areas receiving ventilation that do not participate in gas exchange. Dead space is described as anatomic, alveolar, or physiologic (total). Anatomic dead space consists of the conducting airways, which are not involved in gas exchange, plus the larynx and pharynx. Alveolar dead space consists of alveoli that are not involved in gas exchange, usually from lack of blood flow. Physiologic or total dead space consists of all dead space and is the easiest to measure. "Equipment" dead space may be produced by the addition of tubing beyond the Y-connector of the anesthesia circuit. (64)

74. Many forms of end-stage lung disease, such as emphysema and cystic fibrosis, are characterized by elevated dead space. Pulmonary emboli of any source increase dead space. Hypovolemic shock increases dead space, because very low PA pressures result in more zone 1 of the lung, where alveoli are not perfused and therefore represent dead space. Increased airway pressure and positive end-expiratory pressure (PEEP) can also increase dead space. (64)

75. Normal dead space is 25% to 30% and consists almost entirely of anatomic dead space. (64)

76. The Bohr equation is used to calculate the amount of dead space, expressed as a ratio of the volume of dead space relative to tidal ventilation, V_D/V_T. It requires measuring Pa_{CO_2} and mixed-expired CO_2 by collecting exhaled gas. Because collection of exhaled gas may be difficult, devices have been developed to measure dead space from exhaled CO_2 and expiratory flow and also CO_2 production. (64)

77. Clinically, the gradient from Pa_{CO_2} to end-tidal Pa_{CO_2} is a reflection of alveolar dead space and is a simple way of evaluating dead space under general anesthesia. However, even when dead space is constant the gradient will change with hyperventilation or hypoventilation. (64)

78. The Pa_{CO_2} should double when alveolar ventilation decreases by one half. This change occurs over several minutes as a new steady state develops. (64)

79. CO_2 jumps up fairly rapidly during the first 30 seconds to 1 minute of apnea. This jump is due to rapid transition to mixed venous CO_2 levels, which usually

means an increase of about 6 mm Hg. This occurs because the lungs do not continue to store CO_2, so once equilibration of CO_2 occurs across the alveoli, Pa_{CO_2} will jump to mixed venous levels. Thereafter, CO_2 increases as a result of metabolism at a slower rate of about 2 to 3 mm Hg/min. (65)

PULMONARY MECHANICS

80. Pulmonary mechanics describes the pressure, volume, and flow relationships of gas within the lungs and the tracheobronchial tree. (65)
81. The static pressure in the lung is determined by the interplay between the elastic properties of the lung, the pressure effect of the chest wall and abdominal cavity, and alveolar surface tension, which exists at any air-fluid interface. (65)
82. Surfactant reduces surface tension in the lungs and makes the alveoli more compliant. Without surfactant the lungs would be much stiffer, and alveoli would be less stable and would tend to collapse. (65)
83. Static compliance is the change in volume divided by the change in pressure. By static, this means that the pressure and volume measurements are made at a point of no gas flow, which would contribute a resistive pressure component. Low or poor compliance would indicate that more pressure is needed to inflate the lungs. True static compliance would require measurement of intrapleural pressures to isolate just the lung, whereas measurement of airway pressure reflects additional factors outside the lung. (65)
84. The functional residual capacity (FRC) is simply the balance point between the lungs collapsing and the chest wall expanding. Stiffer lungs will produce a lower FRC, because this balance point will occur at a lower lung volume. On the other hand, a disease such as emphysema, with loss of elastic recoil, results in a higher FRC. (65)
85. Similar to the vascular system, resistance is largely determined by airway diameter. However, turbulent gas flow can add a significant resistance component, which can happen at airway narrowing points. (65)
86. Pressure from resistance only occurs during gas flow. By ceasing gas flow with an inspiratory pause (a feature of most ventilators), the pressure on the airways contributed by resistance and flow disappears, and one can determine the static or "plateau" pressure. (65)
87. High airway resistance can be caused by a number of common clinical conditions. A useful differential might trace the potential resistance anatomically, starting with airway equipment, including the endotracheal tube. Causes of resistance in the upper airways can include compression, foreign bodies, and secretions. In the lower airway, bronchoconstriction becomes the dominant cause. (66)

CONTROL OF BREATHING

88. The central chemoreceptors are located on the ventral surface of the brainstem (medulla). (66)
89. Carbon dioxide is the main stimulus for the central chemoreceptors. Carbon dioxide crosses the blood-brain barrier and rapidly equilibrates with carbonic acid. Although the signal for the chemoreceptors is transduced by protons produced through local changes in the pH, for clinical purposes the chemoreceptors are considered responsive to CO_2. (66)
90. The central chemoreceptors are protected from metabolic acid by the blood-brain barrier. Cerebrospinal fluid pH will change in response to peripheral blood pH changes, but this may take days. An acute lactic acidosis will therefore have no effect on central chemoreceptors, except due to decreases in Pa_{CO_2} that may occur from the ventilatory response to the peripheral acidosis. (66)
91. The carotid bodies are the primary peripheral chemoreceptors in humans. Aortic bodies do not appear to have a significant clinical effect (which was studied in humans who had carotid body denervation). (66)
92. The peripheral chemoreceptors are stimulated by low pH, high Pa_{CO_2}, and low Pa_{O_2}. Unlike the central chemoreceptors, the peripheral chemoreceptors are not

protected from an acute metabolic acidosis, which will cause stimulation and hyperventilation (the lower Pa_{CO_2} from this hyperventilation will affect the central chemoreceptors). (66)

93. High blood flow relative to metabolic rate creates a tissue with hardly any arterial to venous P_{O_2} difference. This allows the carotid bodies to effectively "sense" arterial values. (66-67)

94. The hypercapnic ventilatory response describes increases in ventilation in response to increases in Pa_{CO_2}. Although a variety of techniques are used to obtain ventilatory data, the slope of CO_2 versus minute ventilation is the primary measure of hypercapnic ventilatory responsiveness. The slope is the change in minute ventilation divided by the change in CO_2 and is moderately linear except at the extremes. Minute ventilation does not tend to go to "zero" because of an "awake" drive to breathe, whereas at high P_{CO_2} levels minute ventilation is eventually limited by maximal minute ventilation. Usually end-tidal P_{CO_2} is used clinically because a noninvasive measurement can be preferable. (67)

95. The central chemoreceptors are the major receptor system responsible for hypercapnic drive. However, in room air, approximately one third of the CO_2 response is from peripheral chemoreceptor drive. Usually hypercapnic drive is measured at higher $F_{I_{O_2}}$ where the majority of the response will then be from central chemoreceptors. (67)

96. Below a certain value of Pa_{CO_2}, ventilation usually ceases. In an awake person, this can be difficult to measure due to an awake drive to breath. Under general anesthesia, this phenomenon is easy to observe. With mechanical ventilation, if a patient is hyperventilated, spontaneous ventilatory efforts cease at a P_{CO_2} about approximately 5 mm Hg lower than the setpoint. As CO_2 is allowed to build up again, ventilation begins slowly and will stabilize again at the setpoint. (67)

97. CO_2 ventilatory drive is a slow response, with a time constant (one time constant is 63% toward equilibrium) of approximately 2 minutes. It takes 5 minutes to reach 90% of steady-state ventilation. This is rarely appreciated, although it is easy to observe that ventilation takes noticeable time to stabilize as CO_2 rises to a patient's setpoint. (67)

98. The hypoxic ventilatory response describes increases in ventilation in response to decreases in Pa_{O_2} and Sa_{O_2}. The hypoxic ventilatory drive can be measured from a plot of P_{O_2} versus minute ventilation or Sa_{O_2} versus minute ventilation. Because the relationship of P_{O_2} to minute ventilation is nonlinear, more complex parameters would be needed to describe the relationship, which then are not very clinically useful. A plot of Sa_{O_2} (Sp_{O_2} is conveniently and noninvasively measured by pulse oximetry) versus minute ventilation is linear. Hypoxic responsiveness can then be measured by a simple slope (which will be negative), the change in minute ventilation divided by the change in Sp_{O_2}. (67)

99. Hypoxic ventilatory stimulation is from the peripheral chemoreceptors in the carotid bodies. (67)

100. Central nervous effects of hypoxia lead to a slower development of ventilatory depression known as hypoxic ventilatory decline. The carotid bodies initially lead to increased minute ventilation, but if hypoxia is prolonged, ventilation drops to a level lower than peak ventilation to an intermediate plateau in about 15 to 20 minutes but still above baseline. This drop in ventilation is due to hypoxic ventilatory decline. This central response is a regulated response probably involving several inhibitory neurotransmitters. (67)

101. Hypoxic drive from the peripheral chemoreceptors develops extremely rapidly. The time constant is 10 to 20 seconds. Peak ventilation will therefore usually occur within 1 minute. The response is rapid enough that carotid body output will actually vary in response to the small oscillations of P_{O_2} and P_{CO_2} that occur with tidal breathing. (67)

102. The hypoxic drive is significantly higher with a higher Pa_{CO_2}. This synergistic response between P_{O_2} and P_{CO_2} is a prominent feature of apnea. The hypoxic drive is dramatically decreased by low Pa_{CO_2} levels. (67)

103. Opioids, sedative-hypnotics, and volatile anesthetics work on neurons in the integratory area of the brainstem. They do not affect detection of hypoxia or hypercapnia per se. The clinically observed respiratory depression therefore affects both hypercapnic and hypoxic ventilatory drive equally in a dose-dependent fashion. (67)

104. Neonates less than 60 weeks of postconceptual age can be at risk of apnea following general anesthesia. (68)

105. Originally described following surgery near the high cervical spinal cord, Ondine's curse describes patients with a nearly absent drive to breath. While awake, they may breathe fairly normally. But asleep, or under general anesthesia, breathing can be significantly depressed. This is due to abnormalities in the central integratory system that seem to blunt the hypoxic and hypercapnic ventilatory responses. Idiopathic forms of Ondine's curse, which present in childhood, are usually referred to as primary central alveolar hypoventilation syndrome. (68)

106. Periodic breathing occurs frequently when some degree of hypoxia is present, such as can occur during drug-induced sedation. This is most likely caused by the peripheral chemoreceptors responding to mild arterial hypoxemia leading to overcorrection and undercorrection of the Pa_{O_2}. Oscillations of the Pa_{CO_2} and Sa_{O_2} result. This is a major cause of sleep disturbance at high altitudes. Some patients with central sleep apnea have problems primarily with periodic breathing. Periodic breathing will not usually be observed in patients who are awake. (68)

INTEGRATION OF THE HEART AND LUNGS

107. The Fick equation describes the relationship between cardiac output, oxygen consumption (V_{O_2}), and arterial to venous oxygen content difference: $V_{O_2} = CO \times (Ca_{O_2} - Cv_{O_2})$. This value reflects oxygen needs at the tissue level. (68)

108. Oxygen delivery (D_{O_2}) is the total amount of oxygen supplied to the tissues. It is defined as the product of cardiac output (CO) and arterial oxygen content (Ca_{O_2}), $D_{O_2} = CO \times Ca_{O_2}$. Decreased cardiac output or arterial oxygen content (anemia, hypoxemia) can result in decreased oxygen delivery. (68)

109. Examining oxygen extraction provides a better global indication of whether cardiac output is matched to the body's oxygen needs. Oxygen extraction may provide clinically and diagnostically useful clues as to disease state. In cardiogenic shock, oxygen extraction is high because cardiac output is insufficient for oxygen consumption. In sepsis and liver failure, oxygen extraction may be very low. (68)

110. Normal whole-body mixed venous oxygen saturation is about 75%. Individual organs and tissues can differ significantly. (68)

111. Cardiac output increases in response to anemia so that oxygen delivery is maintained. Therefore, the mixed venous oxygen saturation remains relatively constant. But this means that arterial to venous oxygen content difference necessarily decreases with anemia. At some level of hemoglobin, cardiac output does not completely compensate and increased oxygen extraction occurs. Under anesthesia, with a blunted heart rate response, increased extraction may occur earlier. (68)

112. Arterial to venous oxygen content difference ($Ca_{O_2} - Cv_{O_2}$) is independent of $F_{I_{O_2}}$, whereas the mixed venous oxygen saturation ($S\bar{v}_{O_2}$) can increase significantly with higher Pa_{O_2}. Arterial to venous oxygen content difference decreases with anemia, because not as much oxygen can be extracted without excessively desaturating mixed venous blood. (68)

113. The oxygen extraction ratio is probably the most reliable index of oxygen extraction. It is the oxygen extraction value most independent of $F_{I_{O_2}}$ and hemoglobin level. (68)

114. The two major compensatory mechanisms for increased demand or less availability of oxygen are (1) increased cardiac output and (2) increased extraction. This is readily apparent by examining the Fick equation. In anemia without general anesthesia, the primary compensation is increased cardiac output. Increased extraction occurs with more severe anemia. Under anesthesia, the cardiac output compensation may be blunted, and oxygen extraction is more important. In exercise, for the increased metabolic demand and oxygen consumption both increased cardiac output and increased extraction are utilized. (68)

6 AUTONOMIC NERVOUS SYSTEM

Erica J. Stein and David B. Glick

1. What are the two principal branches of the autonomic nervous system (ANS)?
2. What is the primary function of the sympathetic nervous system (SNS)?
3. What is the primary function of the parasympathetic nervous system (PNS)?
4. The heart, the vasculature, the bronchial tree, the uterus, the gastrointestinal tract, and the pancreas all have dual innervation from the SNS and PNS. Which response, sympathetic or parasympathetic, predominates in each of these organs?

ANATOMY OF THE AUTONOMIC NERVOUS SYSTEM

5. Where do the preganglionic fibers of the SNS originate?
6. Where are the ganglia of the SNS located?
7. How are sympathetic signals amplified to create a broad and diffuse response?
8. What neurotransmitter and receptor are involved in the autonomic ganglia?
9. What is the most common neurotransmitter released by the postganglionic sympathetic neurons when they synapse with their target organs?
10. What are the other classic neurotransmitters of the SNS?
11. What are some of the common cotransmitters released at the terminal of the postganglionic sympathetic fibers, and what do they do?
12. What receptor types do the various classic sympathetic neurotransmitters bind to at the target organ?
13. Where are α_2-receptors located, and what happens when they are stimulated?
14. What postsynaptic receptors does dopamine bind to?
15. What are the chemical intermediates in the synthesis of norepinephrine from tyrosine substrate, and where does this process occur?
16. What is the rate-limiting step in the synthesis of norepinephrine, and what enzyme catalyzes this step?
17. Where is epinephrine synthesized?
18. What percent of the norepinephrine reserve stored in vesicles at the sympathetic nerve terminal is released with each depolarization of the postganglionic nerve?
19. How is the action of norepinephrine at the synapse terminated?
20. Where do the preganglionic fibers of the PNS originate?
21. Where are the ganglia of the PNS located?
22. What is the primary neurotransmitter of the PNS?
23. How are the postganglionic neurons of the PNS different from the postganglionic neurons of the SNS?
24. What happens to acetylcholine (ACh) after it is released into the synaptic cleft?

ADRENERGIC PHARMACOLOGY

25. Which adrenergic effect of norepinephrine predominates, the α or the β? What are the usual clinical responses seen with the administration of norepinephrine?
26. What risks are associated with the administration of norepinephrine?

27. What receptors does epinephrine stimulate?
28. What life-threatening events are treated with epinephrine?
29. Name two ways that the local vasoconstrictive effects of epinephrine are used clinically.
30. What are the therapeutic effects of intravenous epinephrine?
31. What are the primary endocrine and metabolic effects of epinephrine administration?
32. What are the usual infusion rates for the catecholamines dopamine, norepinephrine, epinephrine, and dobutamine?
33. In what circumstances is an intravenous dose of 1.0 mg of epinephrine appropriate?
34. What are epinephrine's primary effects at low, medium, and high infusion rates?
35. What are the mechanisms of action of epinephrine for the treatment of bronchospasm? How is the epinephrine administered? What is the dosing?
36. What is the concern when giving epinephrine to a patient during a halothane-based anesthetic?
37. What receptors bind dopamine?
38. In what two ways does dopamine exert its sympathomimetic effects?
39. How is dopamine metabolized?
40. How does the dose of dopamine administered affect the receptors it binds and its clinical effect?
41. Does dopamine provide a clinical benefit to patients in shock?
42. What receptors are stimulated by isoproterenol?
43. What are two clinical uses for isoproterenol?
44. Which adrenergic receptors are stimulated by dobutamine?
45. What patients are most likely to benefit from treatment with dobutamine?
46. What is the problem with prolonged administration of dobutamine?
47. Which receptors are stimulated by fenoldopam?
48. What are the pharmacologic effects of fenoldopam?
49. What are the clinical uses for fenoldopam?
50. Through what two mechanisms do most noncatecholamine sympathomimetic amines exert their effects?
51. Name three noncatecholamine sympathomimetic amines.
52. What are the advantages and disadvantages of using ephedrine to treat hypotension in pregnancy?
53. What is the cause of tachyphylaxis after repeat doses of ephedrine?
54. Should ephedrine be used to treat life-threatening events?

α-ADRENERGIC RECEPTOR AGONISTS

55. What is the primary effect of phenylephrine, and when is its use common?
56. What is the usual dosing for intravenous phenylephrine?
57. Besides its effects on the cardiovascular system, what other pharmacologic actions does phenylephrine have?
58. What is the mechanism of action of the α_2-adrenergic agonists?
59. What are the clinical effects of administering α_2-agonists?
60. What is "clonidine withdrawal"?
61. What drug is commonly used to treat clonidine withdrawal?
62. How does the administration of an α_2-agonist affect a patient's anesthetic requirements?
63. What effect do the α_2-agonists have on perioperative mortality risk?
64. What is the indication for epidural clonidine?
65. How is clonidine used in the treatment of chronic pain?
66. What is the distribution half-life of dexmedetomidine?
67. What is the dosing for a dexmedetomidine infusion?
68. What makes dexmedetomidine an attractive agent for use in awake fiberoptic endotracheal intubations?

β₂-ADRENERGIC RECEPTOR AGONISTS

69. What makes dexmedetomidine an attractive agent for use in patients with obstructive sleep apnea?

70. What are two common uses for β_2-adrenergic agonist drugs?

α-ADRENERGIC RECEPTOR ANTAGONISTS

71. What side effects are commonly associated with the use of α_1-antagonists as antihypertensive therapies?
72. What must happen before there is complete recovery from α_1-blockade with phenoxybenzamine?
73. What are the primary clinical effects of treatment with phenoxybenzamine?
74. Phenoxybenzamine is most often used to treat what disease?
75. What is the treatment for phenoxybenzamine overdose?
76. What effect does prazosin have on serum lipid levels?
77. Why are episodes of intraoperative hypertension more common in patients receiving prazosin as compared to phenoxybenzamine during pheochromocytoma resection?

β-ADRENERGIC RECEPTOR ANTAGONISTS

78. What are some of the clinical indications for β-blocker therapy?
79. What are the current recommendations for initiating β-blockade perioperatively according to the American College of Cardiology/American Heart Association?
80. What is the effect of β-blocker therapy in patients who have heart failure with reduced ejection fraction?
81. What are the significant characteristics that differentiate the intravenous β-blockers commonly used in anesthetic practice?
82. What are the primary effects of the cardioselective (β_1-selective) β-blockers?
83. What are the cardiac side effects of β-blockade?
84. What are the risks of treating diabetics with β-blockers?
85. What is the role of β-blockers in patients who have pheochromocytomas?
86. How should a β-blocker overdose be treated?
87. Which drug-drug interactions are particularly concerning when a patient is on β-blockers?
88. How is propranolol metabolized?
89. What effect does propranolol have on the oxyhemoglobin dissociation curve?
90. What is the intravenous dosing for the cardioselective β-blocker metoprolol?
91. What adrenergic receptors are antagonized by labetalol?
92. What is the dosing for labetalol?
93. Why is labetalol used to treat hypertension during pregnancy?
94. What accounts for the short half-life of esmolol?
95. When is cardioselective esmolol an especially good choice for β-blockade?

CHOLINERGIC PHARMACOLOGY

96. What are the pharmacologic effects of the muscarinic antagonists?
97. How does the tertiary structure of atropine affect its clinical actions?
98. In what kinds of cases are muscarinic antagonists still commonly given as premedications?
99. Why is glycopyrrolate given when neuromuscular blockade is reversed with the anticholinesterase drugs?
100. What are the common uses and side effects of a scopolamine patch?
101. What is the central anticholinergic syndrome, and how is it treated?
102. What is the mechanism of action of the cholinesterase inhibitors (anticholinesterases)?
103. What is the clinical use for the cholinesterase inhibitors in the perioperative period?
104. What is the anesthetic risk for patients who use echothiophate eye drops?

ANSWERS*

ANATOMY OF THE AUTONOMIC NERVOUS SYSTEM

1. The two principal branches of the autonomic nervous system (ANS) are the sympathetic and parasympathetic nervous systems. (70)
2. The sympathetic nervous system (SNS) is responsible for increasing cardiac output and shunting blood to the skeletal muscles to enable the "fight or flight" response necessary when an organism is threatened. (70)
3. The parasympathetic nervous system (PNS) is responsible for the body's maintenance functions such as digestion and genitourinary function. (70)
4. Most organs receive dual innervation from the SNS and PNS. When an organ receives these dual inputs one or the other normally predominates. In the heart, the rate and force of the contraction are mainly determined by the cholinergic (PNS) response. Vascular tone is determined solely by adrenergic (SNS) inputs. The tone of the smooth muscle of the bronchial tree is predominantly controlled by PNS inputs. Uterine tone is primarily controlled by SNS inputs. The gastrointestinal tract's primary inputs are from the PNS. The pancreas's insulin release is controlled exclusively by the SNS. (70)
5. The preganglionic fibers of the SNS originate from the thoracolumbar (T1-L2/L3) neurons of the spinal cord. (70)
6. Most of the ganglia of the SNS are distributed in paired ganglia, creating the sympathetic chains that are immediately lateral to the left and right borders of the vertebral column. Other sympathetic fibers extend to ganglia along the midline in the celiac or mesenteric plexuses. (70)
7. The initial sympathetic signal is amplified as the preganglionic fibers not only synapse at the ganglion of the level of their origin but also course up and down the sympathetic chain, activating ganglia of the adjacent spinal levels as well, thereby widening the body's response to the sympathetic signal. (70)
8. The neurotransmitter released at both sympathetic and parasympathetic ganglia is acetylcholine (ACh), and the postganglionic receptors that bind the ACh in both the SNS and the PNS are nicotinic receptors. (72)
9. The neurotransmitter released at the terminal end of the postganglionic sympathetic fibers at the synapse with its target organ is usually norepinephrine. (72)
10. Besides norepinephrine, the other classic neurotransmitters of the SNS are epinephrine and dopamine. (72)
11. Identified sympathetic cotransmitters include adenosine triphosphate (ATP) and neuropeptide Y. These molecules are released into the sympathetic synapse at the target organ and modulate the sympathetic activity. (72)
12. Norepinephrine and epinephrine bind to postsynaptic adrenergic receptors located on the target organ. These receptors include α_1-, β_1-, β_2-, and β_3-receptors. (72)
13. α_2-Receptors are located presynaptically on the terminal end of the postganglionic nerve fiber. When norepinephrine binds to the α_2-receptor, subsequent norepinephrine release is decreased, creating a negative feedback loop. (72)
14. Dopamine binds postsynaptically to dopamine-1 (D_1) receptors, α-receptors, and β-receptors. (72)
15. Tyrosine is converted to dihydroxyphenylalanine (DOPA), DOPA is converted to dopamine, and dopamine is converted to norepinephrine. These transformations occur in the postganglionic sympathetic nerve ending. (72)

---

*Numbers in parentheses refer to pages, figures, boxes, or tables in Pardo MC, Miller RD, eds. *Basics of Anesthesia*. 7th ed. Philadelphia: Elsevier, 2018.

16. The rate-limiting step in the synthesis of norepinephrine is the conversion of tyrosine to DOPA. The enzyme that catalyzes this reaction is tyrosine hydroxylase. (72)

17. Norepinephrine is converted to epinephrine in the adrenal medulla. The enzyme that catalyzes the methylation of norepinephrine to epinephrine is phenylethanolamine N-methyltransferase. (72)

18. Approximately 1% of the stored norepinephrine is released with each depolarization, so there is a tremendous functional reserve of norepinephrine at the sympathetic nerve terminal. (72)

19. After being released from the adrenergic receptor(s), most of the norepinephrine in the synaptic cleft is actively taken up at the presynaptic nerve terminal and transported to vesicles for reuse. Norepinephrine that escapes reuptake and makes its way into the bloodstream is metabolized by either the monoamine oxidase (MAO) or catechol-O-methyltransferase (COMT) enzyme in the blood, liver, or kidney. (72)

20. The preganglionic fibers of the PNS arise from cranial nerves III, VII, IX, and X and from sacral nerve roots (S1-S4). (72)

21. Unlike the ganglia of the SNS that are located in ganglionic chains on either side of the vertebral column, the ganglia of the PNS are located close to or within their target organs. (72)

22. ACh is released from both the presynaptic and postsynaptic receptors, making it the primary neurotransmitter of the PNS. (73)

23. The postganglionic neurons of the PNS are short (because the PNS ganglia are close to or within the target organs), and they release ACh from their terminal end when the postganglionic neuron depolarizes. (73)

24. ACh released from the parasympathetic neuron binds to postsynaptic muscarinic receptors on the target cell. Upon release from these receptors, ACh is rapidly metabolized within the synapse by the cholinesterase enzyme. (73)

ADRENERGIC PHARMACOLOGY

25. Norepinephrine's stimulatory effects on α_1-adrenergic receptors predominate. This leads to an increase in systemic vascular resistance and a resultant increase in diastolic, systolic, and mean arterial pressure. The increase in systemic vascular resistance can also lead to a reflex bradycardia. (73)

26. Besides the acute risks associated with severe hypertension that can occur with the administration of norepinephrine, the vasoconstriction caused by norepinephrine can decrease the blood flow to the pulmonary, renal, and mesenteric circulations so infusions must be carefully monitored to decrease the risk of injury to these vital organs. Additionally, prolonged norepinephrine infusions can cause ischemia of the fingers because of the marked peripheral vasoconstriction. (73)

27. Epinephrine binds to and stimulates α- and β-adrenergic receptors. (73)

28. Exogenous epinephrine is given intravenously to treat cardiac arrest, circulatory collapse, and anaphylaxis. (73)

29. Epinephrine is commonly added to local anesthetics to decrease the spread of the local anesthetic. It can also be injected locally to decrease surgical blood loss from the soft tissue (as in tumescent anesthesia for liposuction). (73)

30. Among the therapeutic effects of intravenous epinephrine are positive inotropy, chronotropy, and enhanced conduction through the heart (β_1-mediated); smooth muscle relaxation in the vasculature and bronchial tree (β_2-mediated); and vasoconstriction (α_1-mediated). The predominant effect depends on the dose of epinephrine administered. (73)

31. Epinephrine's primary endocrine and metabolic effects are increased blood glucose (via decreased insulin release), increased lactate, and increased free fatty acids. (73)

32. All the exogenous catecholamines have short half-lives, so they are administered as continuous infusions. The usual dose for dopamine is 2 to

20 µg/kg/min. The usual dose of norepinephrine is 0.01 to 0.1 µg/kg/min. The usual dose of epinephrine is 0.03 to 0.15 µg/kg/min. The usual dose of dobutamine is 2 to 20 µg/kg/min. (73)

33. An intravenous dose of 1.0 mg epinephrine is given for cardiovascular collapse, asystole, ventricular fibrillation, electromechanical dissociation, or anaphylactic shock. This dose of epinephrine is chosen because it constricts the peripheral vasculature while maintaining myocardial and cerebral perfusion. (73)

34. At low infusion rates (1 to 2 µg/min), epinephrine's primary action is a β_2-mediated decrease in airway resistance and vascular tone. At medium doses (2 to 10 µg/min) of epinephrine one usually sees an increase in heart rate, an increase in myocardial contractility, and increased conduction through the AV node. At high doses (>10 µg/min), the α_1-effects predominate and there is a generalized vasoconstriction with a reflex bradycardic response. (73)

35. Epinephrine is effective therapy for bronchospasm both because of its direct effect as a bronchodilator (via relaxation of the bronchial smooth muscle) and because it decreases antigen-induced release of bronchospastic substances (as may occur during anaphylaxis) by stabilizing the mast cells that release these substances. When using epinephrine to treat bronchospasm, it can be given subcutaneously. The usual subcutaneous dose is 300 µg every 20 minutes, with a maximum of three doses. (74)

36. Epinephrine decreases the myocardial refractory period, so giving epinephrine during a halothane-based anesthetic increases the risk of cardiac arrhythmias associated with the administration of halothane. This risk seems to be lower in pediatric cases (the population in which halothane is still used), and the arrhythmic risk increases with hypocapnia. (74)

37. Dopamine is bound by α-, β-, and dopaminergic receptors. (75)

38. Dopamine binds to the adrenergic receptors on target cells to cause a *direct* adrenergic effect. Dopamine also causes the release of endogenous norepinephrine from storage vesicles. This is referred to as dopamine's *indirect* sympathomimetic effect. (75)

39. Dopamine, like the other endogenous catecholamines, is rapidly metabolized by MAO and COMT. The rapid metabolism by these enzymes results in dopamine's half-life of 1 minute. (75)

40. At doses between 0.5 and 2 µg/kg/min the dopamine-1 receptors are stimulated, resulting in renal and mesenteric vascular dilation. At doses between 2 and 10 µg/kg/min, the β_1-adrenergic effects predominate with increases in cardiac contractility and cardiac output. At doses greater than 10 µg/kg/min, the α_1-adrenergic effects predominate, and there is generalized vasoconstriction negating any benefit to renal perfusion. (75)

41. Whereas previous literature suggested that low-dose dopamine infusions protected the kidneys and aided in diuresis, more recent studies have shown that dopamine does not provide a beneficial effect on renal function. Its use for patients in shock has been called into question as it may increase mortality risk and can be associated with arrhythmic events. (75)

42. Isoproterenol is bound by the β_1- and β_2-adrenergic receptors, with its β_1-adrenergic effects predominating. Because it is not taken up into the adrenergic nerve ending like the endogenous catecholamines, its half-life is longer than that of the endogenous catecholamines. (75)

43. Isoproterenol can be used as a chronotropic agent after heart transplantation as well as to initiate atrial fibrillation during cardiac electrophysiology ablation procedures. (75)

44. Dobutamine stimulates β_1-adrenergic receptors without significant effects on β_2-, α-, or dopaminergic receptors. (75)

45. Dobutamine is particularly useful in patients with congestive heart failure (CHF) or myocardial infarction complicated by low cardiac output. Doses lower than 20 µg/kg/min usually do not cause tachycardia. Because dobutamine has no

indirect adrenergic action, it is effective even in catecholamine-depleted states such as chronic CHF. (76)

46. Prolonged treatment with dobutamine causes downregulation of β-receptors, and tolerance to its hemodynamic effects is significant after 3 days. To avoid this problem of tachyphylaxis, intermittent infusions of dobutamine have been used in the long-term treatment of heart failure. (76)

47. Fenoldopam is a selective dopamine-1 agonist. (77)

48. Fenoldopam is a potent vasodilator that increases renal blood flow and diuresis. It is usually administered as a continuous infusion at 0.1 to 0.8 μg/kg/min. (77)

49. Because of unconvincing data from clinical trials, fenoldopam is no longer used to treat CHF or chronic hypertension. It is still used as an alternative to sodium nitroprusside to treat severe acute hypertension because it has fewer side effects and improved renal function. Its peak effects occur in 15 minutes. (77)

50. Noncatecholamine sympathomimetic amines exert their effects on the α- and β-receptors via both *direct* and *indirect* actions. The direct effects result from the binding of these compounds to the adrenergic receptors like other sympathomimetic agents. The indirect effects result from the release of endogenous norepinephrine stores that these compounds induce. (77)

51. Mephentermine, metaraminol, and ephedrine are all noncatecholamine sympathomimetic amines. The only one widely used today is ephedrine. (77)

52. Animal models suggest that ephedrine does not decrease uterine blood flow significantly, and as a result, it has been the drug of choice for treating hypotension in the parturient for many years. Recent studies, however, suggest that phenylephrine causes less fetal acidosis than ephedrine, and so the use of phenylephrine to treat hypotension in pregnant patients is on the rise. (77)

53. The response to the indirect sympathomimetic effects of ephedrine wanes as the body's stores of norepinephrine available for release become depleted. (77)

54. Although ephedrine is widely used as a first-line drug to treat intraoperative hypotension, data from the closed claims database suggest that relying on ephedrine in situations in which there is life-threatening hypotension rather than switching earlier to epinephrine may contribute to an increase in morbidity from these events. (77)

α-ADRENERGIC RECEPTOR AGONISTS

55. The primary effect of the α_1-agonists such as phenylephrine is to cause vasoconstriction. The rise in blood pressure that results leads to a reflex slowing of the heart rate. These agents are used when blood pressure is low and cardiac output is adequate (e.g., to treat the hypotension that can accompany the delivery of a spinal anesthetic). Phenylephrine is also used when a decrease in afterload compromises coronary perfusion in the context of aortic stenosis. (77)

56. Phenylephrine has a rapid onset of action and a short duration of action (5 to 10 minutes). It can be given as a bolus of 40 to 100 μg or as an infusion starting at 10 to 20 μg/min. (77)

57. Phenylephrine is also a mydriatic and nasal decongestant. It can be applied topically to the nostril to prepare the nose for nasotracheal intubation. (77)

58. The α_2-agonists bind the presynaptic α_2-receptor on the postganglionic sympathetic neuron and decrease the release of norepinephrine. This results in a decrease in the overall sympathetic tone of the patient. (77)

59. Besides the decrease in blood pressure, the α_2-agonists have sedative, anxiolytic, and analgesic effects. (77)

60. Acute stoppage of chronic clonidine therapy can lead to a rebound hypertensive crisis, so clonidine should be continued throughout the perioperative period. If a patient is unable to take clonidine orally, administration can be topical via a transdermal patch. (78)

61. Labetalol is commonly used to treat clonidine withdrawal syndrome. (78)

62. α_2-Agonists reduce the requirements for other intravenous or inhaled anesthetics as part of a general or regional anesthetic technique. (78)

63. The α_2-agonists have been shown to decrease the incidence of myocardial infarction and reduce the perioperative mortality risk in patients undergoing vascular surgeries. (78)

64. Epidural clonidine is indicated for the treatment of intractable pain. (78)

65. Clonidine is used to treat chronic pain in patients with reflex sympathetic dystrophy and other neuropathic pain syndromes. (78)

66. The distribution half-life of dexmedetomidine is less than 5 minutes, making its clinical effect quite short. (78)

67. Because of its short clinical effect, dexmedetomidine is run as a continuous infusion of 0.3 to 0.7 µg/kg/h either with or without a 1-µg/kg loading dose given over 10 minutes. (78)

68. Dexmedetomidine increases sedation, analgesia, and amnesia when used in conjunction with agents that produce those effects. The relatively minor impact of α_2-induced sedation on respiratory function combined with its short duration of action has made dexmedetomidine a popular sedative agent for awake fiberoptic endotracheal intubations. (78)

69. Infusions of dexmedetomidine in the perioperative period in obese patients with obstructive sleep apnea minimize the need for narcotics while providing adequate analgesia. (78)

β_2-ADRENERGIC RECEPTOR AGONISTS

70. β_2-Adrenergic agonists (metaproterenol and albuterol) are used to treat reactive airway disease. Ritodrine (another β_2-agonist) is used to interrupt premature labor. All these agents lose their β_2-selectivity when given at higher doses, which leads to β_1-associated adverse effects. (78)

α-ADRENERGIC RECEPTOR ANTAGONISTS

71. The common side effects of α_1-blockers used for antihypertensive therapy are orthostatic hypotension, fluid retention, and nasal stuffiness. (78)

72. Because phenoxybenzamine irreversibly binds α_1-receptors, new receptors must be synthesized before complete recovery can occur. (78)

73. The primary clinical effects of treatment with phenoxybenzamine are decreased blood pressure and increased cardiac output (both are the result of decreased peripheral vascular resistance). Its primary adverse effect is orthostatic hypotension that can lead to syncope. (78)

74. Phenoxybenzamine is most often used to create a "chemical sympathectomy" ahead of resection of a pheochromocytoma (a catecholamine-secreting tumor). Effective α-adrenergic blockade in these patients makes arterial blood pressure less labile intraoperatively and has decreased the surgical mortality rate dramatically. (78)

75. When exogenous sympathomimetic drugs are given following α-blockade, their effects are inhibited. Nevertheless, a phenoxybenzamine overdose is treated with an infusion of norepinephrine. Presumably, this is effective because some of the α-receptors remain free of the phenoxybenzamine. Vasopressin can also be used to overcome the effects of phenoxybenzamine. (78)

76. Prazosin lowers low-density lipid levels and raises high-density lipid levels. (78-79)

77. Prazosin provides competitive antagonism to α-receptors, as compared to the irreversible binding that occurs with phenoxybenzamine. Therefore, intraoperative hypertension can be seen in patients who received prazosin when an increase in circulating catecholamines occurs, such as during direct surgical manipulation of the pheochromocytoma. (79)

β-ADRENERGIC RECEPTOR ANTAGONISTS

78. β-Blocker therapy is used in ischemic heart disease, postinfarction management, arrhythmias, hypertrophic cardiomyopathy, hypertension, heart failure, migraine prophylaxis, thyrotoxicosis, and glaucoma. (79)

79. According to the American College of Cardiology/American Heart Association (ACC/AHA), the continuation of perioperative β-blockade started 1 day or less

before noncardiac surgery in high-risk patients prevents nonfatal myocardial infarction, but it increases the rate of death, hypotension, bradycardia, and stroke. Additionally, there are insufficient data regarding the continuation of β-blockers started 2 days or more before noncardiac surgery. The current ACC/AHA guideline for perioperative noncardiac surgery management is that chronic β-blocker therapy continue in the perioperative period, but β-blocker therapy should not be started on the day of surgery. (79)

80. In patients with heart failure and reduced ejection fraction, β-blocker therapy has been shown to reverse ventricular remodeling and reduce mortality risk. (79)

81. The β-blockers commonly used during anesthesia are propranolol, metoprolol, labetalol, and esmolol. These intravenous agents are differentiated based on their duration of action and cardioselectivity. (79)

82. With β_1-selective blockade, velocity of atrioventricular conduction, heart rate, and cardiac contractility all decrease. Renin release and lipolysis also decrease with β_1-blockade. At higher doses, the cardioselectivity of the β_1-blockers is lost and β_2-receptors are also blocked, which can lead to bronchoconstriction, vasoconstriction, and decreased glycogenolysis. (79)

83. Life-threatening bradycardia or asystole may occur with β-blockade. In addition, β-blockade can precipitate heart failure in patients with compromised cardiac contractility. (79)

84. Diabetes mellitus is a relative contraindication to the long-term use of β-blockers because warning signs of hypoglycemia (tachycardia and tremor) can be masked and because compensatory glycogenolysis is inhibited. (79)

85. To avoid worsening the hypertension in patients with pheochromocytomas, β-blockers should only be given after the patient is fully α-blocked. (79)

86. A β-blocker overdose may be treated with atropine. Isoproterenol, dobutamine, glucagon, or cardiac pacing may also be necessary depending on the patient's symptoms and response to initial therapy. (79)

87. The combination of a β-blocker with either verapamil or digoxin can lead to life-threatening effects on heart rate (verapamil or digoxin) and contractility (verapamil) or conduction (digoxin). (79)

88. Propranolol is highly lipid soluble and extensively metabolized in the liver, so changes in liver function or hepatic blood flow can profoundly affect propranolol's clinical response and duration of action. (80)

89. Propranolol shifts the oxyhemoglobin dissociation curve to the right. (80)

90. Intravenous dosing for metoprolol is 2.5 to 5 mg every 2 to 5 minutes up to a total dose of 15 mg. The doses are titrated to the patient's heart rate and blood pressure. (80)

91. Labetalol is a competitive antagonist of the α_1- and β-adrenergic receptors. (80)

92. Five to 10 mg of labetalol can be given intravenously every 5 minutes. Because, like propranolol, it is metabolized in the liver, changes in hepatic blood flow affect its clearance. (80)

93. Labetalol is used acutely and chronically to treat hypertension during pregnancy because uterine blood flow is not affected by labetalol therapy, even with significant reductions in blood pressure. (80)

94. Esmolol is hydrolyzed by plasma esterases, resulting in a half-life for the drug of only 9 to 10 minutes. (80)

95. Because of its short half-life, esmolol is particularly useful when the duration of β-blockade desired is short or in critically ill patients in whom the adverse effects of bradycardia, heart failure, or hypotension may require rapid discontinuation of the drug. (80)

CHOLINERGIC PHARMACOLOGY

96. The muscarinic antagonists cause an increase in heart rate, sedation, and dry mouth. (80)

97. The tertiary structure of atropine and scopolamine (as opposed to the quaternary structure of glycopyrrolate) makes it possible for them to cross the

blood-brain barrier. As a result, atropine and scopolamine have more central nervous system (CNS) effects than glycopyrrolate. (80)

98. Preoperative use of muscarinic antagonists continues in some pediatric and otorhinolaryngologic cases or when planning fiberoptic endotracheal intubation to dry the oral secretions. (80)

99. Glycopyrrolate is given along with the reversal agent to block the adverse effects (bradycardia) of the anticholinesterase. Glycopyrrolate is used because it has a longer duration of action than atropine and because, unlike atropine or scopolamine, it does not cross the blood-brain barrier, so there are fewer CNS side effects (sedation or delirium). (80)

100. A scopolamine patch is used prophylactically to protect against postoperative nausea and vomiting. It can be associated with adverse eye, bladder, skin, and psychological effects. (81)

101. The distortion of mentation (delusions and/or delirium) that can result from atropine or scopolamine's effects on the CNS has been labeled the "central anticholinergic syndrome." It is treated with physostigmine, a cholinesterase inhibitor that has a tertiary structure that allows it to cross the blood-brain barrier. (81)

102. The cholinesterase inhibitors inhibit the cholinesterase enzyme that normally catalyzes the inactivation of ACh at the nicotinic and muscarinic receptors. As a result, these drugs sustain cholinergic agonism at the cholinergic receptors. (81)

103. The cholinesterase inhibitors are used clinically in the perioperative period to reverse muscle relaxation produced by nondepolarizing neuromuscular blocking drugs. The accumulation of ACh that results from the administration of the anticholinesterases allows ACh to more effectively compete with nondepolarizing neuromuscular blocking drugs for sites on the nicotinic receptor, thereby overcoming the effects of the paralytic agents. They are also used for the treatment of myasthenia gravis. (81)

104. Echothiophate iodine irreversibly binds the cholinesterase enzyme and can interfere with the metabolism of succinylcholine (as the anticholinesterases impair the function of the pseudocholinesterase enzyme as well), leading to a marked prolongation of succinylcholine's paralytic effects. (81)

Chapter

7 INHALED ANESTHETICS

Rachel Eshima McKay

THE FIRST INHALED ANESTHETICS

1. According to written documentation, what were the first three drugs used to provide general anesthesia to patients undergoing painful surgical procedures?
2. Was the first public demonstration of anesthesia considered successful? What property of the anesthetic administered to the patient may have been responsible? How did this compare to the second public demonstration in the same institution with a different anesthetic?
3. Describe the advantages and disadvantages of each of the three first anesthetics.

INHALED ANESTHETICS BETWEEN 1920 AND 1940

4. What were the principal disadvantages of anesthetics developed during the early 20th century?

FLUORINE CHEMISTRY AND MODERN INHALED ANESTHETICS

5. Name the six modern potent inhaled anesthetics.
6. What innovation in synthetic chemistry permitted development of modern inhaled anesthetics? How does the characteristic molecular structure of anesthetics synthesized in this manner confer clinical advantage?
7. What are some advantages and disadvantages of halothane?
8. What are some disadvantages of methoxyflurane?
9. What are some advantages and disadvantages of enflurane?
10. What are some advantages and disadvantages of isoflurane?
11. What are some advantages and disadvantages of sevoflurane and desflurane?

MECHANISM OF ACTION

12. What characterizes the anesthetic state?
13. Which characteristics of the anesthetic state are achieved by the administration of inhaled volatile anesthetics?
14. Which characteristics of the anesthetic state are achieved by the administration of nitrous oxide?
15. What is the mechanism of action of inhaled anesthetics in the central nervous system?

PHYSICAL PROPERTIES

16. Why are vaporizers required for the inhaled administration of volatile anesthetics?
17. Describe how a vaporizer for volatile anesthetics works.
18. What is the potential effect of tilting or overfilling a vaporizer?
19. What are the characteristics of desflurane that preclude its delivery in the conventional variable-bypass vaporizer?
20. What considerations must be taken into account when administering inhaled anesthetics at high altitude?
21. How should the dialed concentration of desflurane be adjusted by the clinician when administering desflurane at high altitude?

22. What are the advantages of using low fresh gas flow rates when administering inhaled anesthetics?
23. What are nonrebreathing fresh gas flow rates? What are advantages and disadvantages of administering inhaled anesthetics at this rate?
24. How do inhaled anesthetics affect the environment?
25. What characteristics of any given inhaled anesthetic determine its potential environmental impact?
26. Which inhaled anesthetic has the most atmospheric longevity?
27. Which volatile anesthetic has the greatest carbon dioxide equivalent impact on the environment? Which volatile anesthetic has the lowest?
28. What are two potentially toxic compounds that can be produced as a result of the degradation or metabolism of volatile anesthetics?
29. What is a potentially toxic compound that can be produced as a result of the interaction between sevoflurane and the carbon dioxide absorbent? What factors may increase this risk?
30. What is the potential risk of human exposure to compound A? How can this risk be minimized?
31. What is a potentially toxic compound that can be produced as a result of the interaction between desflurane and the carbon dioxide absorbent? What factors may increase this risk?
32. What is the potential risk of carbon monoxide production from the carbon dioxide absorbent?
33. What is the potential risk resulting from the temperature increase in the carbon dioxide absorbent canister? How can this risk be minimized?

RELATIVE POTENCY OF INHALED ANESTHETICS

34. How are relative inhaled anesthetic potencies compared?
35. What are minimum alveolar concentration (MAC) values for isoflurane, sevoflurane, desflurane, and nitrous oxide in a person whose age is between 30 to 55 years?
36. What concentration of anesthetic is sufficient to provide amnesia in volunteers? How does this value relate to surgical patients?
37. What factors increase MAC?
38. What factors decrease MAC?

PHARMACOKINETICS OF INHALED ANESTHETICS

39. Describe the process by which induction of anesthesia is achieved by an inhaled anesthetic.
40. What six factors determine the alveolar partial pressure of anesthetic?
41. Describe a strategy that allows maintenance of stable anesthetic partial pressure in the brain after the induction of anesthesia.
42. What is the concentration effect?
43. What is the "second gas effect"?
44. How might hyperventilation lead to inhaled anesthetic overdose?
45. What are some characteristics of the anesthetic breathing system that influence the rate of increase of the alveolar partial pressure of anesthetic?
46. How is anesthetic solubility expressed?
47. How does anesthetic solubility in blood influence speed of induction?
48. What is the clinical relevance of the tissue-blood partition coefficient?
49. What is the clinical relevance of anesthetic transfer by intertissue diffusion?
50. How does nitrous oxide affect the enzyme methionine synthase? How might this relationship affect patients receiving nitrous oxide?
51. How does nitrous oxide affect closed air-filled spaces in the body? What is the clinical relevance of this?
52. How does cardiac output affect the rate of induction of an inhaled anesthetic?
53. How does a shunt affect the rate of induction of an inhaled anesthetic?
54. How does wasted ventilation affect the rate of induction of an inhaled anesthetic?
55. What does the alveolar-to-venous anesthetic partial pressure difference reflect?
56. What are some differences between the induction of inhaled anesthesia and recovery from anesthesia?

57. How are volatile anesthetics metabolized?
58. What factors influence the context-sensitive half-time of inhaled anesthetics?
59. What is the clinical impact of vessel-poor tissue reservoirs of inhaled anesthetic on recovery?
60. What is diffusion hypoxia?

EFFECTS ON ORGAN SYSTEMS

61. Why might an individual patient's responses vary in the circulatory effects of equipotent doses of a given inhaled volatile anesthetic?
62. How do inhaled volatile anesthetics affect arterial blood pressure? What is the mechanism by which this effect occurs?
63. How does the substitution of nitrous oxide for an equipotent portion of volatile anesthetic affect arterial blood pressure at a given anesthetic dose?
64. How do inhaled volatile anesthetics affect heart rate? What is the mechanism by which this occurs?
65. How do inhaled volatile anesthetics affect the cardiac index?
66. How does the rapid concentration increase of volatile anesthetics affect hemodynamics?
67. How do inhaled volatile anesthetics affect myocardial rhythm?
68. How do inhaled volatile anesthetics affect myocardial conduction?
69. How do inhaled volatile anesthetics affect coronary artery blood flow? What is coronary artery steal syndrome? What is its clinical relevance?
70. What is ischemic preconditioning? How does this apply to volatile anesthetics and myocardial protection?
71. How is the rate of breathing affected by inhaled volatile anesthetics?
72. How is the tidal volume affected by inhaled volatile anesthetics?
73. How is the minute ventilation affected by inhaled volatile anesthetics? How is the overall pattern of ventilation affected by inhaled volatile anesthetics?
74. How is the ventilatory drive affected by inhaled volatile anesthetics?
75. How does the addition of nitrous oxide to a volatile anesthetic affect the ventilatory drive and the resultant Pa_{CO_2}?
76. How do inhaled volatile anesthetics affect hypoxic pulmonary vasoconstriction?
77. How do inhaled volatile anesthetics affect bronchial tone?
78. How do inhaled anesthetics differ in their capacity to cause airway irritation? How do these differences affect their use in various clinical situations?
79. How does nitrous oxide affect cerebral blood flow and intracranial pressure?
80. How do inhaled volatile anesthetics affect cerebral blood flow and intracranial pressure?
81. How do inhaled volatile anesthetics affect cerebral metabolic oxygen requirements?
82. How do inhaled volatile anesthetics affect intracranial pressure?
83. How do inhaled volatile anesthetics affect cerebral autoregulation?
84. How do inhaled volatile anesthetics affect evoked potentials?
85. What electroencephalographic (EEG) changes occur with increasing concentration of inhaled volatile anesthetics?
86. How do inhaled volatile anesthetics affect neuromuscular function?
87. Which inhaled anesthetics have the potential to trigger malignant hyperthermia?
88. How do inhaled volatile anesthetics affect the liver?
89. How do inhaled volatiles anesthetics affect the kidneys?

ANSWERS*

THE FIRST INHALED ANESTHETICS

1. The first three drugs in recorded history used to facilitate an anesthetic state for surgical procedures were nitrous oxide, diethyl ether, and chloroform. (83)

*Numbers in parentheses refer to pages, figures, boxes, or tables in Pardo MC, Miller RD, eds. *Basics of Anesthesia.* 7th ed. Philadelphia: Elsevier; 2018.

2. The first public demonstration of anesthesia involved administration of nitrous oxide to a patient undergoing dental extraction at the Massachusetts General Hospital. Many attendees at the demonstration were skeptical because the patient vocalized and moved during the procedure. Because nitrous oxide is not potent, its delivered concentration is limited. The second demonstration of anesthesia, performed with diethyl ether, was considered successful because the patient was quiet and still (note that ether is roughly 100 times more potent than nitrous oxide). (84)

3. Advantages of nitrous oxide were its lack of odor, nonflammability, and apparent absence of toxicity. Its principal disadvantage was its low potency. Advantages of diethyl ether were its potency, providing excellent conditions for surgery. Its disadvantages were flammability, unpleasant odor, and association with nausea and vomiting. Chloroform had the advantage of a more rapid induction, lack of flammability, and less risk of postoperative nausea. Its disadvantage was related to adverse outcome in many patients, including hepatotoxicity and death after surgery. (83-85)

INHALED ANESTHETICS BETWEEN 1920 AND 1940

4. Anesthetics developed and promoted during the first half of the 20th century had properties of pleasant odor and faster induction and emergence but had disadvantages of flammability (divinyl ether, ethylene, cyclopropane) and toxicity (chloroform, ethyl chloride, and trichloroethylene, all fully chlorinated). (85)

FLUORINE CHEMISTRY AND MODERN INHALED ANESTHETICS

5. The six modern potent inhaled anesthetics, all introduced after 1950, are halothane, methoxyflurane, enflurane, isoflurane, sevoflurane, and desflurane. (85)

6. Early inhaled anesthetics were halogenated strictly with chlorine. Modern inhaled anesthetics are partly or wholly halogenated with fluorine. Fluorination conferred the more favorable characteristics to the modern inhaled anesthetics of greater stability and lesser toxicity. (85)

7. At the time it was introduced into clinical practice in 1956, halothane was advantageous because of its nonflammability, pleasant odor, and faster induction and emergence than previous anesthetics. Halothane's disadvantages are its sensitization of the myocardium to the dysrhythmogenic effects of catecholamines and its potential to cause postoperative liver injury. (85)

8. A major disadvantage of methoxyflurane is its dose-related nephrotoxicity due to an inorganic fluoride resulting from its metabolism. (86)

9. Enflurane, introduced into clinical practice in 1972, was advantageous over halothane in that it did not sensitize the myocardium to catecholamines, nor was it associated with hepatotoxicity. Its major disadvantage was that its metabolism could lead to EEG-confirmed seizure activity, especially when administered in high concentrations and in the presence of hypocapnia. (86)

10. At the time of its introduction into clinical practice in 1980, isoflurane's advantages included its lack of association with cardiac dysrhythmias, lack of organ toxicity, and rapid induction and emergence properties. There were no clear disadvantages of isoflurane at that time. (86)

11. Sevoflurane and desflurane are both wholly halogenated with fluorine, which accounts for its low blood solubility and its rapid induction and emergence. Although expensive and hard to synthesize, the increase in outpatient anesthesia cases led to demand for its use. (86)

MECHANISM OF ACTION

12. No single, accepted definition is used to constitute the anesthetic state. Characteristics of the anesthetic state include immobility, amnesia, analgesia, and skeletal muscle relaxation. (86)

13. Characteristics of the anesthetic state that are achieved by inhaled volatile anesthetics include immobility, amnesia, and skeletal muscle relaxation.

Analgesia is difficult to define in an amnestic, immobile patient, but surrogate measures of perception of painful stimuli (i.e., increases in heart rate or blood pressure at the time of incision or intubation) suggest that inhaled anesthetics do not possess analgesic characteristics at concentrations typically used in clinical practice. (87)

14. Immobility is a characteristic of the anesthetic state that is achieved by nitrous oxide, but nitrous oxide is not reliable in doing so when administered alone. It has amnestic effects at higher concentrations (although these are difficult to assure) and, in contrast to potent inhaled anesthetics, does not contribute to skeletal muscle relaxation. (87)

15. Inhaled anesthetics are thought to produce central nervous system depression by enhancing inhibitory ion channels and blocking excitatory ion channels. Anesthetics may also affect the release of neurotransmitters. (87)

PHYSICAL PROPERTIES

16. Volatile anesthetics exist as liquids at room temperature and at atmospheric pressure. The inhaled delivery of these anesthetics requires that the anesthetics be vaporized. Vaporizers allow not only the vaporization of liquid anesthetics, but they also reliably and accurately deliver the specified concentration of anesthetic to the common gas outlet and ultimately to the patient. Nitrous oxide exists as a gas at room temperature and therefore does not require a vaporizer for inhaled delivery to a patient. (87)

17. Conventional volatile anesthetic vaporizers are classified as agent-specific, variable-bypass, flow-over, temperature-compensated, and out-of-circuit. Vaporizers are agent-specific, designed and calibrated for a specific gas. The vapor pressure of the anesthetic gas, a physical property that is unique to each anesthetic, determines the quantity of anesthetic in the gas phase. The concentration of anesthetic vaporizer output is controlled by the clinician adjusting the dial on the vaporizer.

    Fresh gases pass through the flowmeters, mix in the common manifold, and then enter the vaporizers. Once in the vaporizer there are two different streams of flow that the gases can take. The gases may be diverted to the bypass chamber, or they may enter the vaporizing (sump) chamber where it comes into contact with a reservoir of liquid anesthetic. The bypass valve adjusts the amount of gas that enters each of the two chambers, and the concentration of anesthetic is determined by the splitting ratio of the flow stream as controlled by the clinician.

    The vaporizer compensates for temperature, such that when the temperature of the vapor is warm, more gas is directed to the vaporizer outlet via the bypass chamber than when the temperature is relatively cooler. The opposite occurs when the temperature of the vapor is relatively cooler. That is, more of the gas is directed toward the vaporizing chamber. This allows the vaporizer to compensate for changes in temperature, so the desired concentration of volatile anesthetic is maintained.

    Typically, about 20% of the gas flows through the vaporizing chamber. A higher dialed concentration will result in more gas going to the vaporizing chamber than otherwise. In the vaporizing chamber, there are a series of wicks that have been saturated with the liquid anesthetic. As the gas passes over the series of wicks, the gas becomes saturated with the anesthetic vapor. The gas, now saturated with anesthetic vapor, enters the mixing chamber. In the mixing chamber, the saturated gas mixes with the unsaturated gas that has been diverted there. Together the gases pass through the vaporizer outlet toward the common gas outlet at the desired concentration of volatile anesthetic. (87)

18. The potential effect of tilting or overfilling a vaporizer is the delivery of an overdose of anesthetic. (87)

19. The volatility of desflurane precludes its delivery in a conventional variable-bypass vaporizer. At 20° C, the vapor pressure of desflurane is 700 mm Hg (near boiling state at room temperature), whereas those of isoflurane and sevoflurane

are 238 mm Hg and 157 mm Hg, respectively. Because of its volatility, unpredictable and possibly dangerously high concentrations of desflurane would be delivered if a conventional variable-bypass vaporizer were to be used. The Tec 6 heated vaporizer is specifically designed for desflurane. It heats the desflurane gas to 2 atm pressure to accurately measure and deliver the desire concentration of desflurane to the patient. (88)

20. No adjustment needs to be made for variable-bypass vaporizers when administering sevoflurane or isoflurane at high altitude, but an adjustment is needed when administering desflurane. Although vaporizer output is conventionally expressed in volumes percent, the pharmacologically relevant measure is anesthetic partial pressure. Administration of anesthesia at high altitude will result in higher volumes percent vaporizer output when a variable-bypass vaporizer is used. However, the increase in anesthetic partial pressure will be minimized by the overall decrease in ambient pressure, and the clinical effect will be very small. On the other hand, the Tec 6 vaporizer maintains constant volumes percent output. Therefore, at high altitude, although the volumes percent output will be unaffected, the anesthetic partial pressure will be substantially smaller and an adjustment must be made to avoid unintentional delivery of partial pressures below those clinically needed. (88)

21. When administering desflurane at high altitude, the clinician must adjust the vaporizer setting using the following equation:

$$\text{required vaporizer setting} = (\text{desired vaporizer setting at sea level} \times 760\ \text{mm Hg}) / \text{local barometric pressure (in mm Hg)}$$

(88)

22. Use of low fresh gas flow rates (0.5 to 1 L/min) minimizes waste of anesthetic into the environment, decreases cost, and helps conserve body temperature. (88)

23. Nonrebreathing fresh gas flow rates meet or exceed the patient's minute ventilation. The administration of inhaled anesthetic at nonrebreathing gas flow rates allows rapid titration of anesthetic but promotes loss of anesthetic to the environment. (88)

24. Inhaled anesthetics are greenhouse gases and are concerning for their contribution to trapping heat within the atmosphere and to climate change. Inhaled anesthetics are largely vented out to the environment to avoid accumulation within the indoor workspace. Clinical practice that minimizes environmental impact includes use of as low as possible fresh gas flows during maintenance of anesthesia. (88)

25. The potential environmental impact for any given inhaled anesthetic is determined by both its atmospheric lifetime gas, as well as its unique infrared absorption spectrum. (88)

26. Nitrous oxide gas has the most atmospheric longevity, with 114 estimated years. The other inhaled gases are much less, at 10, 3.6, and 1.2 estimated years for desflurane, sevoflurane, and isoflurane, respectively. (88)

27. Of the volatile anesthetics, desflurane has the greatest carbon dioxide equivalent impact on the environment, and sevoflurane has the lowest. (88)

28. Two potentially toxic compounds that can be produced as a result of the degradation or metabolism of volatile anesthetics include compound A and carbon monoxide. (88)

29. A potentially toxic compound that can be produced as a result of the interaction (alkaline degradation) between sevoflurane and the carbon dioxide absorbent is compound A. This can occur with either soda lime or Baralyme, but the risk appears to be higher with Baralyme. Other factors that may increase the risk of compound A production include the low inflow of fresh gases, high concentrations of sevoflurane, and higher absorbent temperatures. (88)

30. The concern with exposure to compound A is for nephrotoxicity. Compound A has been shown to be nephrotoxic in animals. Indeed, in humans prolonged exposure to sevoflurane at low fresh gas flows (1 L/min) has been shown to result in transient proteinuria, enzymuria, and glycosuria. There has been no evidence for increased serum creatinine levels or prolonged deleterious effects, however. This is evidenced by the millions of anesthetics that have been administered with sevoflurane without harm. Regardless, according to manufacturer recommendation, administration of sevoflurane at fresh gas flow rates < 2L/m should be restricted to no more than 2 minimum alveolar concentration (MAC) hours. This is calculated by MAC × duration of anesthesia. (88)

31. A potentially toxic compound that can be produced as a result of the interaction between all volatile anesthetics, but especially desflurane, and carbon dioxide absorbent is carbon monoxide. Carboxyhemoglobin concentrations can reach as high as 30% with either soda lime or Baralyme, but the production of carbon monoxide appears to be greater with Baralyme. Other factors that appear to increase the production of carbon monoxide include higher anesthetic concentrations, an increased temperature, and greater desiccation of the absorbent. The majority of cases of carbon monoxide toxicity occurred after 2 days of disuse of the absorbent, particularly with continued airflow through the circle system. (88)

32. The production of carbon monoxide from the interaction between volatile anesthetics and carbon dioxide absorbent can result in the inhaled delivery of carbon monoxide to the patient. The potential risk is for undiagnosed carbon monoxide poisoning. The diagnosis of carbon monoxide poisoning under these conditions can be difficult because the toxicity may be masked by the anesthesia itself, and the pulse oximetry readings are likely to be unchanged. (88)

33. The exothermic reaction between desiccated carbon dioxide absorbent and volatile anesthetic increases the temperature in the absorbent canister. The temperature increase can be very high and can lead to explosion and fire in the canister or anesthetic circuit. Although the risk is remote, it can be avoided by avoiding desiccation of the carbon dioxide absorbent, i.e., changing the absorbent regularly, turning down or off fresh gas flow when the anesthesia machine is not in use, limiting the rate of fresh gas flow during anesthesia, and changing the absorbent if there is any concern. (88)

RELATIVE POTENCY OF INHALED ANESTHETICS

34. Relative potency among inhaled anesthetics is most commonly described by the dose required to suppress movement in 50% of patients in response to surgical incision, known as MAC. Because this dose has a standard deviation of approximately 10%, 95% of patients should not move in response to incision at 1.2 MAC, and 99% should not move at 1.3 MAC. (89)

35. In persons aged 30 to 55 years, MAC of isoflurane is 1.15%, sevoflurane 1.85%, desflurane 6%, and nitrous oxide 104%. MAC values are additive. For example, 0.5 MAC of nitrous oxide administered with 0.5 MAC isoflurane has the same effect as 1 MAC of any inhaled anesthetic in preventing movement in response to incision. (89)

36. The expired concentration of isoflurane that prevented recall of a verbal stimulus in 50% of volunteers was 0.20 MAC, and the concentration preventing recall in 95% of volunteers was 0.40 MAC. Assuming a standard normal distribution in dose response and a standard deviation of 0.10 MAC, the calculated highest anesthetic concentration required by 1 in 100,000 subjects with the highest requirement would be 4.27 standard deviations above the mean, or 0.627 MAC or more. Extrapolation of this value to the context of surgery must be made with caution, however, because (1) the dose required to prevent recall of painful stimulation as opposed to verbal stimulation may be considerably larger, and (2) the ratio of concentration necessary to prevent recall versus MAC differs

substantially between volatile inhaled anesthetics and nitrous oxide (recall occurs with as much as 0.6 MAC of nitrous oxide). (89)

37. Age has a large influence on MAC, being highest at 6 months of age. After 6 months of age, MAC declines, increases again during adolescence, and thereafter declines until the end of life. Other factors that increase MAC include acute amphetamine use, cocaine, ephedrine, and chronic alcohol use. Hyperthermia, hypernatremia, and red hair color also increase MAC. (89)

38. Older age decreases MAC. Hyponatremia, anemia, hypothermia, hypoxia, and pregnancy all decrease MAC, as does acute alcohol ingestion and chronic amphetamine use. The concomitant administration of certain drugs such as propofol, etomidate, barbiturates, ketamine, opioids, local anesthetics, benzodiazepines, α_2-agonists, lithium, and verapamil all decrease MAC. (89)

PHARMACOKINETICS OF INHALED ANESTHETICS

39. The induction of anesthesia relies on delivery of inhaled anesthetic from the alveoli to the brain via the arterial blood. By controlling the inspired partial pressure, a gradient is created among the machine, the alveoli, the arterial blood, and the brain. Higher inspired anesthetic partial pressure is needed during inhaled induction to offset the impact of anesthetic uptake into the blood and tissues. The delivery of higher fresh gas flow allows the avoidance of rebreathing anesthetic-depleted gases. Anesthetic present in the alveoli is taken up by the blood and carried to the tissues, including the brain; initially the uptake of anesthetic in the blood limits the rate at which the partial pressure in the brain can rise. As the gradient diminishes, alveolar partial pressure approaches equilibrium with blood and vessel-rich tissue, and the partial pressure in the alveoli begins to reflect partial pressure in the brain. The primary objective of inhalation anesthesia is to establish equilibrium between the alveoli and the brain, such that there is a constant, optimal partial pressure of anesthetic in the brain. This can be reflected in the partial pressure of anesthetic in the alveoli or the end-tidal anesthetic value. (89)

40. The alveolar partial pressure is determined by input of anesthetic into the alveoli minus the uptake of anesthetic into the pulmonary arterial blood. The input of anesthetic into the alveoli is determined by the inspired partial pressure of anesthetic, alveolar ventilation, and the characteristics of the breathing circuit. The uptake of anesthetic from the alveoli is determined by the anesthetic solubility in blood and tissues, cardiac output, and the alveolar-to-venous partial pressure difference. For a high partial pressure in the alveoli, and thus a rapid induction of anesthesia, the following should occur: a high inspired partial pressure of anesthetic, a high minute ventilation, a low-volume breathing circuit, high fresh gas flows, a low solubility of anesthetic in the tissues, a low cardiac output, and a small alveolar-venous partial pressure difference. (90)

41. A higher inspired anesthetic partial pressure is needed during an inhaled induction to offset the impact of anesthetic uptake into the blood, and higher fresh gas flow allows for the avoidance of rebreathing. Uptake diminishes as the anesthetic partial pressure in the blood approaches that in the alveoli. This results in narrowing of the alveolar-venous difference, reduced uptake, and if inspired anesthetic concentration is maintained, a rapid increase in brain concentration. To achieve maintenance of a stable anesthetic partial pressure in the brain, once uptake in the blood is reduced and approaching equilibration, the dialed concentration of inhaled anesthetic must be decreased. The decrease in delivered anesthetic may be achieved by decreasing vaporizer concentration, fresh gas flows, or both. (90)

42. The effect of a higher inspired partial pressure offsetting the impact of uptake of anesthetic into the blood, and therefore accelerating the induction of anesthesia, is known as the concentration effect. (90)

43. The second gas effect describes the influence of one gas, administered at high volume, on the uptake of a companion gas. The process occurs when a large volume of "first" gas (e.g., nitrous oxide) is taken up during induction, and this

uptake effectively concentrates the "second" gas (oxygen or potent inhaled anesthetic) into a smaller alveolar volume. Pharmacokinetic models have proved the second gas effect, but its clinical importance is doubtful. (90)

44. Hyperventilation can lead to inhaled anesthetic overdose during controlled ventilation through its effects of increased anesthetic input (increased alveolar ventilation) and decreased anesthetic uptake (decreased venous return resulting in decreased cardiac output). This may be mitigated by the decrease in cerebral blood flow, and therefore anesthetic delivery to the brain, that occurs with hyperventilation. Anesthetic overdose from hyperventilation may cause myocardial depression. Hyperventilation itself may limit venous return to the heart and impair coronary blood flow. (90)

45. Characteristics of the anesthetic breathing system that influence the rate of increase of the alveolar partial pressure of anesthetic include the volume of the system, solubility of the inhaled anesthetic in the rubber or plastic components of the system, and gas inflow into the anesthesia machine. The solubility of the components of the anesthetic breathing system act as a buffer; high gas flows from the anesthesia machine negate this buffer effect. (91)

46. Anesthetic solubility in blood and tissues is denoted by partition coefficients. A partition coefficient can be viewed as the affinity of anesthetic for one particular tissue versus another, indicating the quantitative ratio of anesthetic distributed between two phases when partial pressures are equal. For example, a blood-gas partition coefficient of 0.65 means that the concentration of sevoflurane in the alveolus is 1 and 0.65 in blood at equilibrium. Partition coefficients are dependent upon temperature and, unless otherwise stated, are given for 37° C. (91)

47. When an anesthetic has a high solubility in blood, it means that a large amount of inhaled anesthetic must be dissolved in the blood before equilibration with the gas phase is reached. The blood can be considered a pharmacologically inactive reservoir, and the size of this reservoir is directly related to the solubility of the anesthetic in blood. Therefore, greater inhaled anesthetic solubility in blood slows induction. This can be offset somewhat by increasing the inhaled partial pressure of anesthetic. (91)

48. The tissue-blood partition coefficient determines the time to equilibration of inhaled anesthetic between the tissue (e.g., brain) and blood. The speed at which this equilibration takes place is expressed as a time constant. The time constant related to a tissue group is correlated to the amount of anesthetic that can be dissolved in that tissue divided by the blood flow received by the tissues. One time constant reflects about 67% equilibration between blood and tissue, and complete equilibration is achieved in three time constants. The vessel-rich tissue group (i.e., brain, heart, kidneys, and liver) accounts for less than 10% of the body mass, but it receives 75% of cardiac output. The brain time constant for isoflurane is 3 to 4 minutes, whereas those of sevoflurane and desflurane are about 2 minutes. Therefore, complete equilibration between alveoli and the brain may be achieved as quickly as 6 to 10 minutes. (91)

49. Anesthetic uptake can occur from direct transfer of anesthetic from a tissue with lower affinity (lean tissue) to a tissue with higher affinity (adipose tissue) and not just through blood flow. Clinically, larger people with more areas of lean tissue/adipose tissue interface may have a greater uptake of anesthetic in adipose tissue. (92)

50. Nitrous oxide inactivates methionine synthase, the enzyme that regulates vitamin B_{12} and folate metabolism. Although this inactivation may not usually produce clinically evident change, patients with an underlying critical illness, exposure to chemotherapy, or preexisting vitamin B_{12} deficiency may suffer neurologic or hematologic sequelae. Another consequence of methionine synthase inactivation is increased serum homocysteine concentration because the enzyme is needed to convert cysteine to methionine. Elevated homocysteine levels and increased frequency of ischemic episodes have been concurrently demonstrated in patients undergoing carotid endarterectomy while receiving nitrous oxide. (92)

51. Nitrous oxide is 34 times more soluble than nitrogen in blood, as reflected by their respective blood-gas partition coefficients of 0.46 versus 0.014. As a result, nitrous oxide can more readily diffuse out of the circulation and occupy an air-filled compartment than the nitrogen in the compartment can diffuse from the compartment into the circulation. The result of this imbalance is an increase in the gas contents of a closed air-filled space. The space and volume of gas will expand if the walls of the space are compliant (e.g., intestinal gas, pneumothorax, air embolism), or the pressure in the space will increase if the walls of the space are noncompliant (e.g., middle ear, eye, cerebral ventricles, supratentorial subdural space). The magnitude of volume or pressure increase in the air-filled space will be influenced by the alveolar partial pressure of nitrous oxide, blood flow to the compartment, and the duration of nitrous oxide administration. Presence of a closed pneumothorax is a contraindication to nitrous oxide administration. Difficulty with ventilation encountered in the setting of chest trauma may reflect nitrous oxide expansion of a previously unrecognized pneumothorax. Indeed, inhalation of 75% nitrous oxide has been shown to double the volume of a pneumothorax in 10 minutes. Air bubbles associated with venous air embolism expand rapidly when exposed to nitrous oxide. (92)

52. Cardiac output influences uptake in the pulmonary artery blood and thus the amount of anesthetic carried away from the alveoli. A high cardiac output results in more anesthetic uptake into the blood, and a lower alveolar partial pressure, resulting in a slower induction of anesthesia. The converse is also true, that is, a low cardiac output results in a faster induction of anesthesia. (92)

53. A right-to-left shunt slows the rate of the induction of an inhalation anesthetic through the dilutional effect of shunted blood (without anesthetic) mixing with blood that has passed by ventilated alveoli (with anesthetic) before delivery to the tissues. The clinical impact of this is probably negligible, however. (92)

54. Wasted ventilation, or ventilation of nonperfused alveoli, does not affect the rate of induction of an inhaled anesthetic because the partial pressure of anesthetic in the blood is not diluted. (93)

55. The alveolar-to-venous anesthetic partial pressure difference reflects tissue uptake of inhaled anesthetics. The highly perfused tissues (i.e., brain, heart, kidneys, and liver) equilibrate rapidly with the partial pressure in the blood. After 6 to 12 minutes, 75% of returning venous blood has the same anesthetic partial pressure as the alveolus, resulting in narrowing of the alveolar-venous difference. Tissues with less blood flow (skeletal muscle, fat) act as inactive reservoirs and continue to uptake anesthetic for several hours. (93)

56. The recovery from anesthesia differs from the induction of anesthesia in several ways. First, there cannot be a concentration effect to accelerate recovery. For example, the inhaled pressure of anesthetic cannot be less than zero to augment the anesthetic partial pressure of gradient from the brain to the alveoli. Second, there are variable concentrations of anesthetic in multiple tissue reservoirs at the end of surgery, when anesthetic administration is discontinued. These concentrations are affected by duration of anesthetic plus affinity of anesthetic for each specific reservoir (tissue compartment). Finally, metabolism of anesthetic has modest impact on recovery from halothane but minimal impact on newer anesthetics that undergo negligible metabolism. (93-94)

57. All volatile anesthetics are biotransformed to a variable extent in the liver. Halothane, isoflurane, and desflurane all undergo oxidative metabolism (15% to 40%, 0.2%, and 0.02%, respectively) by cytochrome P-450 enzymes to produce trifluoroacetate. Sevoflurane is metabolized (5% to 8%) to hexafluoroisopropanol. (94)

58. The context-sensitive half-time of inhaled anesthetics is the time required to decrease the anesthetic concentration in the central nervous system to a fraction of what it is at the start for any given time. Computer simulations are used to determine context-sensitive decrement times for inhaled anesthetics and are

based upon the presence of each potential tissue reservoir compartment within the body (i.e., blood, vessel-rich group, muscle, fat), the relative size of each compartment, the proportional blood flow received by each compartment, and the solubility of each specific anesthetic in the tissue composing the compartment. (94)

59. Vessel-poor tissue reservoirs (i.e., skeletal muscle, fat) of inhaled anesthetic have a longer context-sensitive half-time on recovery and therefore require more time to deplete anesthetic stores. The residual anesthetic in these reservoirs may manifest clinically as prolonged time to regain coordinated protective functions, such as the ability to swallow, and for an intact chemical ventilatory drive. (94)

60. Diffusion hypoxia is a term used to describe the dilution of oxygen in the alveoli due to the presence of another gas. This can occur at the conclusion of a nitrous oxide anesthetic when there is an initial high-volume output of nitrous oxide diffusing from the blood to the alveoli and filling the alveoli. If the patient is breathing room air at the time, the partial pressure of oxygen in the alveoli can be diluted to the extent that hypoxia results. Diffusion hypoxia at the conclusion of a nitrous oxide anesthetic can be avoided through the inhaled delivery of 100% oxygen. (95)

EFFECTS ON ORGAN SYSTEMS

61. The circulatory effect of an inhaled anesthetic for a given patient is influenced by multiple factors. These can include the effects of age, surgical stimulation, coexisting diseases such as myocardial dysfunction and stenotic valve lesions, intravascular fluid volume status, and concurrent drug administration. (95)

62. The volatile anesthetics all produce a dose-dependent decrease in mean arterial blood pressure, although the mechanism by which they exert their effects varies. Halothane primarily acts to decrease blood pressure by decreasing myocardial contractility and cardiac output. Isoflurane, desflurane, and sevoflurane primarily decrease blood pressure through their effects of peripheral vasodilation and an associated decrease in systemic vascular resistance. Nitrous oxide, when administered alone, causes minimal if any alteration in blood pressure. (95)

63. Nitrous oxide, when administered alone, causes little if any alteration of blood pressure. The substitution of nitrous oxide for an equipotent dose of a volatile anesthetic therefore results in a smaller decrease in arterial blood pressure than would have otherwise occurred if the volatile anesthetic were administered alone. This is in part the basis for the administration of nitrous oxide in combination with a volatile anesthetic. The combination of nitrous oxide with a volatile anesthetic allows for an increase in the MAC of anesthesia delivered with less circulatory depression than would occur if an equivalent dose of anesthetic composed of a volatile agent alone were to be used. (95)

64. Halothane has minimal effect on heart rate. Isoflurane, sevoflurane, and desflurane all tend to increase heart rate, but each behaves in a somewhat different manner. At concentrations as low as 0.25 MAC, isoflurane induces a linear, dose-dependent heart rate increase. Heart rate shows minimal increase with desflurane below 1 MAC, but above 1 MAC a steep dose-dependent increase in heart rate and blood pressure may be observed. In contrast to desflurane and isoflurane, heart rate in the presence of sevoflurane does not increase until the concentration exceeds 1.5 MAC. The tendency for desflurane to stimulate the circulation (i.e., increase mean arterial pressure and heart rate) is attenuated with the administration of β-adrenergic blocker (esmolol), opioid (fentanyl), and the passage of time (10 to 15 minutes). The increase in heart rate seen with isoflurane and sevoflurane is a baroreceptor reflex response to decreased mean arterial pressure. An exception to this is during an inhaled induction of anesthesia with 8% sevoflurane when tachycardia is noted in both children and adults. In this case, the tachycardia may be associated with sympathetic nervous system stimulation associated with epileptiform brain activity. The transient increase in heart rate that occurs above 1 MAC of desflurane results from sympathetic nervous system stimulation. (96)

65. Halothane produces a dose-dependent decrease in the cardiac index that parallels the decrease in blood pressure that is seen with its administration. In contrast, cardiac index is minimally influenced by the administration of isoflurane, sevoflurane, and desflurane over a wide range of concentrations in young healthy adults. (96-97)

66. The rapid concentration increase of desflurane above 1 MAC causes increases in heart rate and blood pressure, as does isoflurane, though to a lesser extent. This hemodynamic stimulation is associated with increases in plasma epinephrine and norepinephrine concentrations and sympathetic nervous system activity. The hemodynamic response is only seen when anesthetic delivery is in the absence of concomitant opioids, adrenergic blockers, or other analgesic medicines, as these medicines can profoundly attenuate the response. An initial increase in desflurane concentration from 4% to 8% within 1 minute can result in a doubling of the heart rate and blood pressure above baseline. A second rapid increase in concentration of desflurane from 4% to 8% 30 minutes later does not have the same hemodynamic effect, suggesting adaptation to the response. Rapid increases in concentration of sevoflurane, halothane, and enflurane do not result in circulatory stimulation. (97)

67. The only inhaled volatile anesthetic that has any effect on myocardial rhythm is halothane. The administration of halothane may be accompanied by a junctional rhythm, and halothane sensitizes the myocardium to premature ventricular extrasystoles, especially in the presence of catecholamines. Sensitization of the myocardium to ventricular extrasystoles is exaggerated in the presence of hypercarbia. In contrast, isoflurane, sevoflurane, and desflurane do not affect myocardial rhythm. (97)

68. Inhaled volatile anesthetics all prolong the QT interval on the electrocardiogram, particularly halothane and sevoflurane. Although malignant arrhythmias have been reported in patients receiving halothane who were subsequently found to have congenital long QT syndrome, the clinical significance of sevoflurane's QT interval prolongation is unclear. Regardless, sevoflurane should be avoided in patients with known congenital long QT syndrome. (98)

69. Isoflurane has been shown to selectively dilate small coronary arterioles in animal models. If coronary arterioles undergo vasodilation and blood flow is diverted from narrowed arterioles that are already maximally dilated to healthy arterioles with less resistance, this theoretically could result in ischemia in the areas supplied by the narrowed arterioles, and this process is known as *coronary steal*. However, these concerns turned out not to be valid. Isoflurane, sevoflurane, and desflurane all appear to exert a protective effect on the heart, limiting the area of myocardial injury and preserving function after exposure to ischemic insult. (98)

70. Ischemic preconditioning refers to the protective mechanism in all tissues and species in which exposure to brief episodes of ischemia can confer myocardial protection against reversible or irreversible injury with a subsequent prolonged ischemic event. The time period of myocardial protection appears to be 1 to 2 hours and again 24 hours up to 72 hours following the brief ischemic episode. This response is mediated by K_{ATP} channels. Volatile anesthetics appear to also protect the myocardium through this same mechanism, which is referred to as *anesthetic preconditioning*. In the setting of compromised myocardial perfusion, volatile anesthetics (unlike propofol) appear to provide similar myocardial protective benefits. (99)

71. Inhaled volatile anesthetics produced a dose-dependent increase in the rate of breathing. Although the exact mechanism for this is unclear, it is believed to result from central nervous system stimulation by the anesthetic. (99)

72. Inhaled volatile anesthetics decrease the tidal volume of patients breathing the anesthetic, leading to an increase in dead space ventilation in a dose-dependent manner. (99)

73. Inhaled anesthetics increase breathing frequency and decrease tidal volume in a dose-dependent manner. The pattern of breathing is regular, rapid, and shallow.

The decrease in tidal volume is not sufficiently compensated by the increase in respiratory rate, however. This results in a decrease in the minute ventilation of individuals breathing an inhaled anesthetic. The resting $Paco_2$ of these patients is increased as a result. The resting $Paco_2$ is therefore used as an index to evaluate the degree of respiratory depression that is produced by inhaled anesthetics. (99)

74. Inhaled anesthetics produce a dose-dependent depression of the ventilatory drive. The mechanism by which this occurs is thought to be due to direct depression of the medullary ventilatory centers, along with a lesser contribution from depressant effects on chest wall mechanics. Normally, minute ventilation should increase by 1 to 3 L/min for every 1 mm Hg increase in carbon dioxide, but in anesthetized patients there is a blunting of carbon dioxide responsiveness. This effect of inhaled anesthetics results in a progressive increase in carbon dioxide as anesthetic concentration rises. Indeed, at 1 MAC, carbon dioxide responsiveness is two to four times less than baseline values. At 1.7 MAC of desflurane in 100% oxygen, volunteer subjects become apneic. Volatile anesthetics all blunt or abolish the ventilatory stimulation evoked by arterial hypoxemia, even at a partial pressure below that when patients are awake. This is of great clinical importance during early recovery, when the concomitant effects of opioid and unresolved neuromuscular weakness may interact to compound ventilatory depression. (99)

75. The administration of nitrous oxide to patients does not change their $Paco_2$ levels from awake levels. Although there is an increase in the anesthetic depth when nitrous oxide is added to a volatile anesthetic, the patient's $Paco_2$ does not change with the addition of nitrous oxide to the volatile anesthetic. Similarly, the substitution of nitrous oxide for an equivalent dose of volatile anesthetic results in less of an increase in the $Paco_2$ than that which would have otherwise occurred with the volatile anesthetic alone. (99-100)

76. Hypoxic pulmonary vasoconstriction is a reflex response of pulmonary arterioles to vasoconstrict in areas of low alveolar Pao_2 in an attempt to decrease perfusion to underventilated alveoli, as in atelectasis. Although inhaled volatile anesthetics alter pulmonary blood flow, inhibition of hypoxic pulmonary vasoconstriction is minimal. (100)

77. All potent inhaled anesthetics promote some degree of bronchodilatation and attenuate bronchospasm. Bronchodilatation may be achieved by attenuation of CNS vagal activity, in addition to direct relaxation of bronchial smooth muscle. (100)

78. Sevoflurane, halothane, and nitrous oxide are all nonpungent, causing minimal or no irritation over a broad range of concentrations. For this reason, sevoflurane and halothane are selected most frequently for inhaled induction of anesthesia, because very high concentrations can be introduced to overcome the initial uptake of anesthesia into the blood. Both desflurane and isoflurane are pungent and can irritate the airway at concentrations above 1 MAC when given without opioids or propofol. However, isoflurane and desflurane may be administered via laryngeal mask airway (LMA) after propofol induction without greater incidence of coughing, breath holding, laryngospasm, or desaturation compared with sevoflurane or propofol. This is probably because anesthetic maintenance usually does not require concentrations in excess of 1 MAC, and small doses of opiate (1 µg/kg of fentanyl) attenuate or abolish the irritating effects. Because of their pungency, isoflurane and desflurane are not practical for inhaled induction of anesthesia. (100)

79. Nitrous oxide increases cerebral blood flow through cerebral vasodilation. The effect of nitrous oxide appears to be blunted in the presence of intravenous anesthetics. Nitrous oxide has less of an effect on cerebral blood flow than volatile anesthetics. Limitation of the inspired concentration of nitrous oxide to less than 0.7 MAC minimizes its effect of cerebral vasodilation. (100)

80. Potent inhaled anesthetics, at concentrations above 0.6 MAC, increase cerebral blood flow in a dose-dependent manner through vasodilatation. Cerebral blood

flow increase is greater with equipotent doses of halothane compared with isoflurane, sevoflurane, or desflurane. Intracranial pressure increases with all inhaled anesthetics above 1 MAC. Inhaled anesthetics do not abolish the cerebral vascular responsiveness to changes in Pa_{CO_2}. (100)

81. Inhaled volatile anesthetics decrease the cerebral metabolic oxygen requirement. Volatile anesthetics also increase cerebral blood flow. Normally, cerebral blood flow parallels the cerebral metabolic oxygen requirement, such that as the cerebral metabolic oxygen requirement increases, so does cerebral blood flow. This remains true at volatile concentrations less than 0.5 MAC. At concentrations greater than 1 MAC, the vasodilating effects of volatile anesthetics predominate and cerebral blood flow is increased despite the decrease in cerebral metabolic oxygen requirements. Given that volatile anesthetics increase cerebral blood flow and decrease the cerebral metabolic oxygen requirement, it has been said the volatile anesthetics uncouple these two physiologic characteristics. (100)

82. Intracranial pressure increases with all volatile anesthetics at concentrations of more than 1 MAC. (100)

83. Cerebral autoregulation is impaired by all inhaled volatile anesthetics at concentrations of less than 1 MAC. Cerebral autoregulation is the brain's adaptive ability to normalize cerebral blood flow over a wide range of systemic arterial blood pressures. (100-101)

84. All volatile anesthetics and nitrous oxide depress the amplitude and increase the latency of somatosensory evoked potentials in a dose-dependent manner, and the somatosensory evoked potentials may be abolished at 1 MAC. Motor evoked potentials become unreliable at concentrations as low as 0.2 to 0.3 MAC. (101)

85. Increasing depth of anesthesia with inhaled volatile anesthetics is characterized by increased amplitude and synchrony of EEG waveforms. Periods of electrical silence begin to occupy a greater proportion of time as depth increases (i.e., burst suppression), predominantly at 1.5 to 2.0 MAC. Sevoflurane and enflurane have been associated with the appearance of epileptiform EEG activity at high concentrations, although the clinical implications of these observations are not clear. (101)

86. All the inhaled volatile anesthetics produce mild dose-related skeletal muscle relaxation, and their administration may be helpful in achieving optimum surgical conditions. Use of an inhaled volatile anesthetic will likewise potentiate the effect of neuromuscular blocking drugs. The clinician may minimize or avoid the use of neuromuscular blocking drugs by virtue of the inhaled anesthetic's effects on skeletal muscle tone. At the conclusion of surgery, the presence of inhaled volatile anesthetic will delay the recovery of neuromuscular function when the effects of muscle relaxants are no longer desired. Nitrous oxide does not provide skeletal muscle relaxation. (101)

87. All of the inhaled volatile anesthetics have the potential to trigger malignant hyperthermia in susceptible patients. Studies in animals suggest that this risk may be greater with the use of halothane than with the use of isoflurane, sevoflurane, or desflurane. Nitrous oxide is not a trigger for malignant hyperthermia. (101)

88. All inhaled volatile anesthetics have the potential to cause severe hepatic injury, leading to death or the need for liver transplantation. The mechanism for this injury appears to be immunologic, usually requiring previous exposure to a volatile anesthetic. Trifluoroacetate, produced by metabolism of halothane, isoflurane, and desflurane, binds covalently to hepatocyte proteins and acts as a hapten. Subsequent volatile anesthetic exposure that results in the production of trifluoroacetate can provoke the immune response and lead to hepatic necrosis. Hexafluoroisopropanol, produced by sevoflurane metabolism, does not appear to have the same antigenic behavior as trifluoroacetate. A clinically milder form of liver injury, characterized by elevation of transaminases, can occur after exposure to halothane. This effect on the liver may be mediated by reductive

metabolism and related to conditions in which hepatic blood flow is compromised. (101)

89. Historical observations lead to the belief that increases in serum inorganic fluoride, from anesthetic metabolism, resulted in renal insufficiency. Methoxyflurane, the first nonflammable potent inhaled anesthetic, was developed after the Second World War. It undergoes extensive metabolism via two separate pathways (O-demethylation and dechlorination). Its clinical use was associated with renal injury, and the degree of injury was positively correlated with magnitude of plasma fluoride concentration. Subsequent investigations have shown the renal toxicity of methoxyflurane to be specifically associated with the O-demethylation pathway rather than increased plasma fluoride concentration per se. There is no clinical evidence that fluoride accumulation, in the ranges at or higher than those observed in conjunction with anesthesia after sevoflurane, results in renal injury in humans. (102)

8 INTRAVENOUS ANESTHETICS

Michael P. Bokoch and Helge Eilers

1. Name some examples of intravenous anesthetics. What are the potential clinical uses of intravenous anesthetics?
2. Explain the concept of "balanced anesthesia." In addition to intravenous anesthetics, what classes of drugs may be used to provide balanced anesthesia?
3. What is similar about the mechanism of action of propofol, barbiturates, benzodiazepines, and etomidate?

PROPOFOL

4. Describe the chemical structure and physical properties of propofol.
5. Why is it necessary for the manufacturer to include a preservative in propofol emulsions, and why is strict aseptic technique a must during handling?
6. Which patients may be at risk for a life-threatening allergic reaction to propofol?
7. If the elimination half-life of propofol is slow (4 to 24 hours), why do patients awaken rapidly, within 8 to 10 minutes, after a single bolus injection?
8. How is propofol cleared from the plasma?
9. What degree of metabolism does propofol undergo? How should the dose of propofol be altered when administered to patients with liver dysfunction?
10. Define the context-sensitive half-time for a drug. How does the context-sensitive half-time of propofol compare to other intravenous anesthetics?
11. What is the mechanism of action of propofol?
12. How does the emergence from a propofol anesthetic or propofol induction differ from the emergence seen with the other induction agents?
13. How does propofol affect the central nervous system?
14. How does propofol affect the seizure threshold?
15. How does propofol affect the cardiovascular system?
16. How does propofol affect ventilation?
17. How does propofol affect the upper airway and airway reflexes?
18. What is the propofol infusion syndrome, and what clinical findings should prompt investigation for it?
19. How can the pain associated with the intravenous injection of propofol be attenuated?
20. What is a typical induction dose of propofol? Describe at least two patient populations in which this dose should be adjusted.
21. How is propofol administered for maintenance anesthesia?
22. What is total intravenous anesthesia (TIVA)?
23. How is propofol administered for sedation?
24. What is the relationship between propofol and nausea and vomiting?

FOSPROPOFOL

25. How are the structure and physicochemical properties of fospropofol different from propofol?

26. What are the advantages and disadvantages of fospropofol compared with propofol?
27. What are the clinical uses of fospropofol?

BARBITURATES

28. Name some of the barbiturates. From what chemical compound are they derived?
29. What other drug formulations and fluids are incompatible to inject with barbiturates?
30. How are barbiturates cleared from the plasma?
31. Describe the metabolism of barbiturates and their interactions with the microsomal P450 system.
32. What is the effect-site equilibration time of barbiturates relative to other intravenous anesthetics?
33. What is the context-sensitive half-time of barbiturates relative to other intravenous anesthetics?
34. How do methohexital and thiopental compare with regard to induction doses, duration of action, and clinical utility?
35. What is the mechanism of action of barbiturates?
36. How do barbiturates affect the central nervous system? How do barbiturates affect an electroencephalogram?
37. How do barbiturates affect the arterial blood pressure?
38. How do barbiturates affect the heart rate?
39. How do barbiturates affect ventilation?
40. How do barbiturates affect laryngeal and cough reflexes?
41. What are some potential adverse complications of the injection of thiopental?
42. What is the risk of a life-threatening allergic reaction to barbiturates?
43. What are the various routes and methods for the administration of barbiturates in clinical anesthesia practice?
44. How should thiopental be administered and dosed for cerebral protection in patients with persistently elevated intracranial pressures?
45. What is barbiturate coma? What are some potential complications?

BENZODIAZEPINES

46. Name some of the commonly used benzodiazepines. What are some of the clinical effects and properties of benzodiazepines that make them useful in anesthesia practice?
47. How does water-soluble midazolam cross the blood-brain barrier to gain access to the central nervous system?
48. How are benzodiazepines metabolized? How does the metabolism of lorazepam differ from that of other benzodiazepines?
49. How do the metabolites of diazepam and midazolam differ?
50. What is the effect-site equilibration time of benzodiazepines relative to other intravenous anesthetics?
51. How do the context-sensitive half-times of the benzodiazepines compare to each other and to other classes of intravenous anesthetics?
52. What is remimazolam? Name two other commonly used drugs that are metabolized by a similar mechanism.
53. What is the mechanism of action of benzodiazepines?
54. Where are benzodiazepine receptors located?
55. Describe the overall macromolecular structure of the γ-aminobutyric acid type A (GABA$_A$) receptor. Is the structure typically constant or subject to variation?
56. How do midazolam, diazepam, and lorazepam compare with regard to affinity for the benzodiazepine receptor?
57. How do benzodiazepines affect the central nervous system?
58. How do benzodiazepines affect the cardiovascular system?
59. How do benzodiazepines affect ventilation and the upper airway?
60. Which organic solvent is used to dissolve diazepam into solution? What are some of the effects of this solvent?

61. How common are allergic reactions to benzodiazepines?
62. What are some clinical uses of benzodiazepines in anesthesia practice?
63. How do midazolam, diazepam, and lorazepam compare with regard to time of onset and degree of amnesia when administered for sedation?
64. What are some considerations the anesthesiologist should be aware of when deciding whether or not to use midazolam as premedication before elective or outpatient procedures?
65. Describe some features of the amnesia induced by midazolam and its importance to anesthesiologists and surgeons when counseling patients and families.
66. Describe dosage and strategies for induction of general anesthesia with midazolam. Why is midazolam preferred over other benzodiazepines for this purpose? What are some advantages and disadvantages of benzodiazepines for use as induction agents?
67. How can the effects of benzodiazepines be reversed?
68. What is the optimal choice, dose, and route of benzodiazepine for treatment of status epilepticus in hospitalized patients? How does it differ in prehospital treatment of status epilepticus?

KETAMINE

69. What chemical compound is ketamine a derivative of?
70. How does the anesthetic state induced by ketamine differ from other intravenous anesthetics?
71. How do patients appear clinically after an induction dose of ketamine?
72. What is the mechanism by which the effects of ketamine are terminated?
73. What is the mechanism of action of ketamine?
74. How does ketamine affect the central nervous system?
75. How does ketamine affect the cardiovascular system?
76. How does ketamine affect ventilation?
77. How does ketamine affect skeletal muscle tone? How does this affect the upper airway?
78. What are the induction doses for ketamine given by the intravenous and intramuscular routes? What is the time of onset for each route?
79. What does the emergence delirium associated with ketamine refer to? What is the incidence? How can it be prevented?
80. What are some common clinical uses of ketamine?
81. What can the repeated administration of ketamine lead to? How does it manifest clinically?
82. How common are allergic reactions to ketamine?
83. Name a common psychiatric condition that ketamine may be used to treat.

ETOMIDATE

84. What type of structure is etomidate? Name another intravenous anesthetic that shares this structure.
85. How is etomidate cleared from the plasma?
86. What degree of metabolism does etomidate undergo?
87. What is the context-sensitive half-time of etomidate relative to other intravenous anesthetics? What is the effect-site equilibration time of etomidate relative to other intravenous anesthetics?
88. What is its mechanism of action of etomidate?
89. How does etomidate affect the central nervous system?
90. How does etomidate affect the seizure threshold?
91. How does etomidate affect the cardiovascular system?
92. How does etomidate affect ventilation?
93. What are the endocrine effects of etomidate?
94. Name specific patient populations that may benefit from choice of etomidate as an induction agent.
95. What are some potential negative effects associated with the administration of etomidate?

DEXMEDETOMIDINE

96. What type of structure is dexmedetomidine? How is it cleared from the plasma?
97. What is the mechanism of action for dexmedetomidine?
98. How does the sedation produced by dexmedetomidine differ from that of other intravenous anesthetics?
99. What are the effects of dexmedetomidine on cerebral blood flow?
100. How does dexmedetomidine affect the electroencephalogram?
101. How does dexmedetomidine infusion affect the cardiovascular system?
102. Compare the hemodynamic effects of a bolus injection or rapid loading dose of dexmedetomidine with the hemodynamic effects of an infusion.
103. How does dexmedetomidine affect the respiratory system?
104. What are the typical doses for dexmedetomidine when used as infusion in the operating room?
105. What are some common clinical uses for dexmedetomidine?

ANSWERS*

1. Examples of intravenous (IV) anesthetics include the barbiturates, benzodiazepines, opioids, etomidate, propofol, ketamine, and dexmedetomidine. These drugs can be used as induction agents or, in combination with other anesthetics, for the maintenance of anesthesia. Some, particularly propofol and dexmedetomidine, are appropriate for sedation of mechanically ventilated patients in the intensive care unit (ICU). (104)

2. "Balanced anesthesia" is the idea of combining various classes of drugs to achieve hypnosis, amnesia, analgesia, and immobility. This allows smaller doses of each agent to be used and limits side effects. Inhaled anesthetics, neuromuscular blocking agents, and opioids are often combined with IV anesthetics to achieve balanced anesthesia. (104)

3. Propofol, barbiturates, benzodiazepines, and etomidate all work predominantly by activating or potentiating inhibitory currents through the γ-aminobutyric acid type A (GABA$_A$) chloride channel, leading to a decrease in synaptic transmission in the central nervous system (CNS). However, the exact electrophysiologic effects and GABA$_A$ receptor binding sites differ among the drugs. (105)

PROPOFOL

4. Propofol is a phenol ring derivatized at both *ortho*- positions (2 and 6) by isopropyl groups (an alkylphenol). It is highly lipid soluble and is formulated as an emulsion with soybean oil, glycerol, and purified egg yolk phosphatide. (105)

5. Propofol emulsions are a rich media that readily support bacterial growth. The manufacturer adds ethylenediaminetetraacetic acid (EDTA) or metabisulfite as a preservative. Vials or syringes of propofol should be discarded within 12 hours after opening, and strict aseptic technique should be followed when drawing up the drug. Failure to follow these recommendations may lead to fever or sepsis in the patient. (105)

6. Patients at risk for a life-threatening allergic reaction to propofol are those with a history of atopy or allergy to other drugs that also contain a phenyl nucleus or isopropyl group. Patients with confirmed IgE-mediated allergy to egg, soy, or peanut are not at increased risk, and propofol may be used normally. If a patient is known to have sulfite allergy or very reactive airways, it may be better to choose a propofol formulation with EDTA as the preservative.

*Numbers in parentheses refer to pages, figures, boxes, or tables in Pardo MC, Miller RD, eds. *Basics of Anesthesia.* 7th ed. Philadelphia: Elsevier; 2018.

Anaphylactoid reactions to the propofol compound itself and separate from the lipid emulsion are rare but have been reported. (105)

7. Awakening after a single bolus of propofol is determined by the kinetics of redistribution (movement between tissue compartments) and not elimination (removal from the body). After an IV bolus, propofol rapidly distributes to the brain due to high blood flow. It crosses the blood-brain barrier rapidly due to its high lipophilicity, leading to loss of consciousness within 30 seconds. Over the next few minutes, propofol rapidly redistributes from the brain to less well-perfused tissues such as skeletal muscle. The rapid decay of plasma propofol concentration leads to awakening within minutes. This process applies to most IV anesthetics given as a single bolus. (105)

8. Propofol is rapidly cleared from the plasma by redistribution to inactive tissue sites and rapid metabolism by the liver. Propofol clearance exceeds hepatic blood flow, suggesting that organs other than liver contribute to metabolism. Indeed, the lungs probably play a major role in the extrahepatic metabolism of propofol and likely account for the elimination of up to 30% of a bolus of propofol. (105)

9. Propofol is rapidly metabolized by the liver to inactive, water-soluble metabolites, which are then excreted in the urine. Less than 1% of propofol administered is excreted unchanged in the urine. Patients with liver dysfunction appear to rapidly metabolize propofol as well, lending some proof that extrahepatic sites of metabolism exist. In patients with advanced liver dysfunction, such as cirrhosis, the volume of distribution is increased, but protein binding is reduced (due to hypoalbuminemia). Taken as a whole, propofol bolus dosing does not need to be routinely altered in patients with liver disease. (105)

10. The context-sensitive half-time refers to the time needed for the plasma concentration of a particular drug to drop by 50% after discontinuation of an IV infusion. This time is "context-sensitive" because it depends on the duration for which the infusion was given. As an infusion is administered for a longer time, more tissue compartments accumulate the drug and the context-sensitive half-time will rise. The context-sensitive half-time depends mostly on the drug's lipid solubility and clearance mechanisms. Compared with most barbiturates and benzodiazepines, propofol has a shorter context-sensitive half-time for a given infusion duration. This explains the rapid recovery to consciousness of ICU patients, even after several days of sedation. (106)

11. The mechanism by which propofol exerts its effects is not fully understood, but it appears to be mostly through the $GABA_A$-activated chloride ion channel. Evidence suggests that propofol may interact with the $GABA_A$ receptor and maintain it in an activated state for a prolonged period, thereby resulting in greater inhibitory effects on synaptic transmission. (106)

12. After the administration of propofol, patients experience a rapid return to consciousness with minimal residual CNS effects. Patients who are to undergo brief procedures or outpatient surgical patients may especially benefit from the rapid wake-up associated with propofol anesthesia. Propofol also tends to result in the patient awakening with a general state of well-being and mild euphoria. Patient excitement has also been observed. (106)

13. Propofol decreases the cerebral metabolic rate for oxygen ($CMRO_2$), along with cerebral blood flow (CBF) and intracranial pressure (ICP), in a dose-dependent manner. However, given the relationship between mean arterial pressure (MAP) and cerebral perfusion pressure (CPP), patients with an elevated ICP may experience critical reductions in CBF due to arterial hypotension after an IV bolus of propofol. In large doses propofol produces burst suppression on the electroencephalogram (EEG), making it useful for neuroprotection during selected neurosurgical procedures. (106)

14. Propofol is an anticonvulsant and can be used to treat seizures. Excitatory effects that cause muscle twitching are not uncommon but do not indicate seizure activity. (106)

15. An induction dose of propofol results in a profound decrease in systolic blood pressure greater than any other induction agent. This effect appears to be primarily due to venous and arterial vasodilation, resulting in decreased preload and systemic vascular resistance (SVR). There is no clear evidence of direct myocardial depression. Hypotension is dose-dependent and worse with rapid injection, with hypovolemia, and in elderly patients. In contrast to barbiturates, compensatory increases in heart rate usually do not occur. Propofol inhibits the normal baroreceptor reflex, and profound bradycardia may result. (107)

16. The administration of an induction dose of propofol (1.5 to 2.5 mg/kg) almost always results in apnea through a dose-dependent depression of ventilation. The apnea that results appears to last for 30 seconds or greater and is followed by a return of ventilation that is characterized by rapid, shallow breathing such that the minute ventilation is significantly decreased for up to 4 minutes. During maintenance infusions propofol decreases minute ventilation through decreases in both the respiratory rate and, to an even greater extent, the tidal volume. Propofol also reduces the ventilatory response to hypoxia and hypercapnia. (107)

17. Propofol causes a greater reduction in airway reflexes than any other induction agent, making it a better choice as the sole agent for instrumentation of the airway. It also increases the collapsibility of upper airway musculature, predisposing patients to airway obstruction during emergence from propofol anesthesia or while undergoing sedation. (107)

18. Propofol infusion syndrome is a heterogeneous disorder that occurs rarely during administration of high-dose infusions (>4 mg/kg/h). Although it was first described in pediatric patients, it also occurs in adults. The most typical features are metabolic acidosis, rhabdomyolysis, and hyperkalemia. Fever, arrhythmia, electrocardiogram (ECG) changes, hypertriglyceridemia, hepatomegaly, renal failure, or heart failure may also occur. Otherwise unexplained metabolic acidosis, hyperkalemia, elevated creatine kinase, new-onset arrhythmias, or ECG changes in a patient receiving propofol infusion should prompt a full evaluation and consideration of switching the infusion to another sedative-hypnotic. (107)

19. Injection of propofol intravenously can cause pain and dissatisfaction in awake patients. The most effective method to attenuate injection pain is by using large antecubital veins for its administration. Prior administration of lidocaine, premedication with an opioid, or mixing lidocaine with propofol are also helpful techniques. (107)

20. Propofol is typically administered in the range of 1 to 2.5 mg/kg intravenously for induction of general anesthesia. There is high variability in dosing depending on the clinical situation and other concomitantly administered anesthetic agents. The propofol dose should probably be adjusted routinely in certain populations. This includes the elderly (decreased dose due to decreased anesthetic requirements and a smaller volume of distribution), morbidly obese patients (the dose should be based on lean body weight to prevent overdose), and children (increased dose due to higher anesthetic requirements, larger volume of distribution, and more rapid propofol clearance). (107)

21. Propofol may be administered for maintenance of anesthesia through a continuous IV infusion at a rate of 100 to 200 µg/kg/min. The clinician may use signs of light anesthesia such as hypertension, tachycardia, diaphoresis, or skeletal muscle movement as indicators for the need to increase the infusion rate of propofol. (107)

22. Total intravenous anesthesia (TIVA) is a technique by which an IV anesthetic, most typically propofol at a dose of 100 to 200 µg/kg/min, is combined with other IV sedative-hypnotics, opioids, or analgesics to provide general

anesthesia. Volatile anesthetics are not used as part of the technique. Propofol-based TIVA generally results in stable hemodynamics, good conditions for electrophysiologic monitoring such as evoked potentials during spine surgery, and decreased postoperative nausea and vomiting (PONV). Vigilance is required to ensure IV catheters delivering TIVA do not infiltrate, and adequate doses of hypnotic are delivered to prevent recall, particularly if neuromuscular blockade is used. (107)

23. Propofol may be administered for sedation through a continuous IV infusion at a rate of 25 to 75 µg/kg/min. At these doses, propofol will provide sedation, and likely amnesia, without complete hypnosis. Because of the pronounced respiratory depressant effect, propofol, even for sedation, should only be administered by individuals trained in airway management. (107)

24. Propofol appears to have a significant antiemetic effect, given the lower incidence of nausea and vomiting in patients who have received a propofol TIVA. In addition, propofol administered in subhypnotic doses has successfully treated nausea both postoperatively and in patients receiving chemotherapy. (107-108)

FOSPROPOFOL

25. Fospropofol is a water-soluble phosphate ester prodrug of propofol. It is metabolized by alkaline phosphatase in a reaction that produces propofol, phosphate, and formaldehyde. Formaldehyde is then further metabolized. (108)

26. There are several advantages of fospropofol when compared to propofol. First, it can be injected without the need for a lipid emulsion, thereby reducing the risk of bacterial contamination. There is also less pain upon IV injection. Theoretically, a bolus of fospropofol should result in a lower peak plasma concentration of the active metabolite (propofol), with reduced hypotension and respiratory depression. These advantages have not yet been clearly proved in human studies. A disadvantage of fospropofol is that it frequently causes a perineal burning sensation or pruritus after injection, likely related to the phosphate component. Also, the onset of sedation is slower and recovery is prolonged compared with propofol. (108)

27. In the United States, fospropofol is currently approved for sedation during monitored anesthesia care. It is best studied for procedural sedation during endoscopy, bronchoscopy, and minor surgical procedures. (108)

BARBITURATES

28. Thiopental and methohexital are the most commonly used barbiturates in the practice of anesthesia. Other barbiturates include pentobarbital, phenobarbital, and thiamylal. The barbiturate compounds are derivatives of barbituric acid. Barbiturates can be further classified as oxybarbiturates (e.g., methohexital) or thiobarbiturates (e.g., thiopental) depending on the substitution at the 2 position (oxygen or sulfur). (108)

29. Barbiturates are acidic molecules. They are formulated as sodium salts mixed with carbonate buffer, which forms an alkaline solution (pH higher than 10) when reconstituted in water or normal saline. If barbiturates are mixed with acidic drug preparations, rapid precipitation may occur. This particular problem may arise during rapid sequence induction and clog IV lines. Examples of drugs that should not be coadministered with barbiturates for this reason include neuromuscular blockers, ketamine, midazolam, some opioids (alfentanil, sufentanil), and some catecholamines (dopamine, dobutamine). Lactated Ringer solution will also precipitate barbiturates. (109)

30. Barbiturates are cleared from the plasma primarily through rapid redistribution to inactive tissue sites after bolus administration. (109)

31. Barbiturates are highly metabolized in the liver. They undergo oxidation, N-dealkylation, desulfuration, and ring breakdown. The resulting polar compounds are readily excreted in the urine or conjugated to glucuronic acid and excreted in the bile. Less than 1% of the drug is excreted unchanged by the kidneys. Drugs that induce microsomal oxidases increase the metabolism of

barbiturates, and barbiturates themselves are P450 inducers when chronically administered. Induction of hepatic enzymes by barbiturates can drive synthesis of aminolevulinic acid, the first step in porphyrin synthesis, and precipitate attacks of acute intermittent porphyria. (109)

32. Barbiturates are often used for the IV induction of general anesthesia. Maximal brain uptake and onset of effect take place within 30 seconds after rapid IV injection. Thus, the effect-site equilibration time for these agents is short and comparable to propofol. Methohexital has a slightly faster effect-site equilibration time than thiopental because it exists in a higher un-ionized fraction at pH 7.4 and crosses the blood-brain barrier more quickly. Acidosis and hypoalbuminemia contribute to an increased free un-ionized fraction of barbiturate and more rapid induction. Rapid awakening follows the administration of an induction dose of a barbiturate due to rapid redistribution to lean tissue (mostly skeletal muscle). The duration of action of a barbiturate after a single bolus dose is dictated by this redistribution from plasma to inactive sites. (110-111)

33. Repeated doses or infusions of lipid-soluble barbiturates can result in saturation of inactive sites (muscle and adipose tissue), accumulation of the drug, and prolonged effects upon discontinuing an infusion. The context-sensitive half-time of barbiturates is larger than that of propofol for an infusion of comparable duration. (110-111)

34. The induction dose of methohexital is 1 to 1.5 mg/kg intravenously, whereas the induction dose of thiopental is 3 to 5 mg/kg intravenously. Methohexital undergoes greater hepatic metabolism than thiopental, resulting in a shorter duration of action and more rapid awakening. Based on the shorter duration of action of methohexital, it is sometimes chosen over thiopental for the induction of anesthesia for patients undergoing outpatient procedures when rapid awakening is desired. An example of a procedure in which methohexital is frequently chosen for induction is electroconvulsive shock therapy. This is due to not only the short duration of action of methohexital but also its epileptogenic property. (110-111)

35. Barbiturates act at the $GABA_A$ receptor, which is a pentameric ion channel. GABA is the main inhibitory neurotransmitter in the CNS. Opening of the $GABA_A$ channel causes influx of chloride ions. Barbiturates potentiate the action of endogenous GABA, increase the duration of channel opening, and prolong the influx of chloride. The chloride current hyperpolarizes the cell and inhibits synaptic transmission. Barbiturates may also work through a separate mechanism to inhibit excitatory transmission. (110-111)

36. Barbiturates are potent cerebral vasoconstrictors. This results in a decrease in CBF, a decrease in cerebral blood volume, a decrease in ICP, and a decrease in $CMRO_2$. Barbiturates are also thought to depress the reticular activating system, which is believed to be important in maintaining wakefulness. Thiopental produces a dose-dependent depression of the EEG. A flat EEG may be maintained with a continuous infusion of thiopental. Methohexital is the only barbiturate that does not decrease electrical activity on an EEG. In fact, methohexital activates epileptic foci and is often used intraoperatively to identify epileptic foci during surgical ablation. The effects of barbiturates on the CNS suggest utility for patients in whom elevated ICP is a concern. Examples of patients who may benefit from the administration of a barbiturate as an induction agent or as maintenance anesthesia include patients with intracranial space-occupying lesions. No data support using barbiturates to lower ICP after head trauma, as reduction of MAP, CPP, and CBF may impair cerebral oxygen delivery and counteract potential benefits. (110-111)

37. The administration of barbiturates typically results in a modest decrease in arterial blood pressure. This decrease in blood pressure primarily results from peripheral vasodilation (decreased SVR and decreased preload). Vasodilation arises from a combination of depression of the vasomotor

center in the medulla and a decrease in sympathetic nervous system outflow from the CNS. Exaggerated blood pressure decreases may be seen in patients with chronic hypertension, whether or not they are being treated by antihypertensives. The administration of barbiturates should also be undertaken with caution in patients who are dependent on the preload to the heart to maintain cardiac output, as in patients with ischemic heart disease, pericardial tamponade, congestive heart failure, heart block, or hypovolemia. (110-111)

38. The administration of barbiturates results in an increase in heart rate. This increase in heart rate is thought to be due to a baroreceptor-mediated reflex response to a drop in blood pressure and helps to limit hypotension. Tachycardia may increase myocardial oxygen demand during a time when significant decreases in blood pressure may compromise coronary artery blood flow as well. Given this, barbiturates must be used with extreme caution in patients with ischemic heart disease. Although the administration of barbiturates typically results in an increase in heart rate, the cardiac output may be decreased. This is in part due to direct depression of myocardial contractility. The decreased cardiac output seen with barbiturates is rarely of clinical significance except in patients with cardiac disease or hypovolemia. (110-111)

39. Barbiturates depress ventilation centrally by depressing the medullary ventilatory centers. This is manifest clinically as a decreased responsiveness to the ventilatory stimulatory effects of hypercapnia and hypoxia. Depending on the dose administered, the patient will have a slow breathing rate and small tidal volumes to the extent that apnea follows. Transient apnea typically occurs after an induction dose of barbiturate and mandates controlled ventilation of the lungs. When spontaneous ventilation is resumed, it is again characterized by a slow breathing rate and small tidal volumes. (110-111)

40. Induction doses of thiopental alone do not reliably depress laryngeal and cough reflexes. Stimulation of the upper airway, as with the placement of an oral airway or an endotracheal tube, can result in laryngospasm or bronchospasm. It is therefore recommended that adequate suppression of these reflexes be obtained before instrumenting the airway. This can be accomplished with increased doses of a barbiturate, by the administration of a neuromuscular blocking drug, or by the addition of another preoperative medicine, such as opioids, to augment the anesthetic effects of thiopental during stimulation of the upper airway. (110-111)

41. Potential adverse complications of the injection of thiopental may result from accidental intra-arterial, subcutaneous, and even appropriate venous administration of thiopental. The accidental intra-arterial injection of barbiturates results in excruciating pain and intense vasoconstriction that can last for hours. It is believed that barbiturate crystal formation in the blood causes the occlusion of distant small-diameter arteries and arterioles. There are several treatment modalities for this potential problem, including the intra-arterial injection of papaverine or lidocaine, sympathetic nervous system blockade by stellate ganglion block of the involved upper extremity, and the administration of heparin to prevent thrombosis. Despite aggressive therapy, gangrene of the extremity often results. The accidental subcutaneous injection of barbiturates results in local tissue irritation. The irritation may proceed to pain, edema, erythema, or even tissue necrosis, depending on the volume and concentration injected. It has been recommended that 5 to 10 mL of 0.5% lidocaine be injected locally when the subcutaneous injection of thiopental occurs in an attempt to dilute the barbiturate. Venous thrombosis has been seen after the IV administration of thiopental. It is presumed that the thrombosis results from the deposition of barbiturate crystals in the vein. The crystallization of barbiturates is more likely to occur when the pH of the blood is too low to keep the barbiturate in solution. (110-111)

42. Life-threatening allergic reactions to barbiturates are rare. The risk has been estimated to be 1 in 30,000. (111)

43. There are various routes and methods for the administration of barbiturates in clinical anesthesia practice. For instance, the rapid IV administration of a bolus of barbiturate is indicated for a rapid sequence induction of anesthesia. The bolus of barbiturate should be immediately followed by the administration of succinylcholine or a nondepolarizing neuromuscular blocking drug to produce skeletal muscle paralysis and facilitate tracheal intubation under these conditions (although the neuromuscular blocking drug should not be mixed or injected simultaneously with the barbiturate as precipitation may occur). Alternatively, small doses of IV thiopental, in the range of 0.5 to 1 mg/kg, may be administered to adult patients who have difficulty accepting the application of an anesthesia mask or the inhalation of a volatile anesthetic. The rectal administration of the barbiturate methohexital can be used to facilitate the induction of anesthesia in young or uncooperative patients. (111)

44. In patients with persistently elevated ICP, barbiturates may be administered intravenously in high doses to decrease the ICP. Persistently elevated ICP is usually defined as greater than 20 cm H_2O despite mannitol, hyperosmolar therapies, hyperventilation, and CSF drainage. Care must be taken to avoid decreases in MAP that would compromise the CPP under these conditions. To ascertain the optimal dose of barbiturate administered for these patients, an EEG can be obtained. The dose of barbiturate can be uptitrated until burst suppression is seen, followed by an isoelectric or "flat-line" EEG. When the EEG is isoelectric, there is no benefit to increasing doses of barbiturate as cerebral metabolism and $CMRO_2$ cannot be further reduced. This allows the clinician to administer the dose of barbiturate that provides the maximal benefit with minimal adverse effects. Barbiturates may offer some protection for patients with regional cerebral ischemia such as from stroke or a space-occupying lesion. Patients with global cerebral ischemia, such as from cardiac arrest, are not thought to derive any protection from the administration of barbiturates. (111)

45. "Barbiturate coma" refers to the administration of a barbiturate (usually thiopental) to maximally suppress the EEG (isoelectric or "flat-line"). This is performed in a patient with brain injury, persistently elevated ICP, or focal ischemia in an attempt to provide neuroprotection. The benefits are thought to include a reduction in $CMRO_2$, cerebral oxygen consumption, and ICP, as well as antiepileptic effects. Potential side effects include hemodynamic instability, hypothermia, hypo- or hyperkalemia, liver dysfunction, arrhythmias, and immunosuppression. Invasive hemodynamic monitoring and frequent laboratory checks are indicated. Infusion of vasopressors to maintain MAP and CPP is often required. (111)

BENZODIAZEPINES

46. Benzodiazepines that are commonly used in the perioperative period include midazolam, diazepam, and lorazepam. The most common effects of benzodiazepines are their anxiolytic, sedative, and anterograde amnestic effects. When administered at higher doses, benzodiazepines may also produce unconsciousness. Other properties of benzodiazepines include a lack of retrograde amnesia, minimal cardiopulmonary depression, anticonvulsant activity, antiemetic effects, and relative safety when taken in overdose (as compared with barbiturates). Clinical uses of benzodiazepines include their use for preoperative medication, for IV sedation, for the IV induction of anesthesia, and for the suppression of seizure activity. In addition to the IV route of administration, benzodiazepines can be administered via intramuscular, intranasal, and sublingual routes. (112)

47. Midazolam is a hydrophilic drug stored at low pH in an open-ring form. When midazolam is exposed to the pH of the blood, it undergoes ring closure and

becomes highly lipid soluble. This change in structure allows it to rapidly cross the blood-brain barrier and gain access to the CNS. (112)

48. Benzodiazepines are highly lipophilic drugs. Most undergo oxidative metabolism (*N*-dealkylation and hydroxylation) by microsomal P450 enzymes, followed by glucuronidation and excretion. As such, benzodiazepine metabolism is highly susceptible to conditions that alter the activity of the microsomal P450 system, such as liver disease and drug-drug interactions with P450 inducers or inhibitors. Lorazepam, along with less common temazepam and oxazepam, do not undergo oxidation and are excreted after a single-step conjugation to glucuronic acid. This property makes lorazepam less susceptible to P450 interactions. (112)

49. Diazepam is oxidatively metabolized to long-acting active compounds, desmethyldiazepam and oxazepam, leading to prolonged sedation. The elimination half-life of desmethyldiazepam is at least 100 hours. Midazolam has a single active metabolite, 1-hydroxymidazolam, which is rapidly cleared from plasma in healthy patients (half-life for elimination about 1 hour). 1-Hydroxymidazolam may accumulate and contribute to prolonged sedation in patients with hepatic dysfunction, with renal dysfunction, or after prolonged infusion. (112)

50. Benzodiazepines are highly lipid-soluble drugs. This allows them to gain rapid entrance into the CNS by crossing the blood-brain barrier, where they are able to exert their effects. Thus the effect-site equilibration time of benzodiazepines is short, although it is slower than propofol or thiopental. As for propofol and barbiturates, the duration of action of benzodiazepines after a single IV bolus is dependent on the redistribution of the drug from the brain to inactive tissue sites. (112)

51. Continuous infusion or repeated boluses can result in saturation of inactive tissue sites (muscle and adipose) and a prolongation of drug effect, particularly for the benzodiazepines that have active metabolites. For instance, diazepam undergoes hepatic metabolism to long-lasting active metabolites, whereas midazolam has a single active metabolite that is rapidly cleared. The context-sensitive half-times for diazepam and lorazepam are prolonged when compared with that of midazolam. The context-sensitive half-time of midazolam is shorter than that of thiopental but longer than propofol for an infusion of similar duration. (112)

52. Remimazolam (CNS 7056) is a new ultra-short-acting benzodiazepine that is entering clinical trials. It contains a carboxylic ester moiety that is rapidly hydrolyzed by blood and tissue esterases to an inactive metabolite. It is predicted to have an extremely short context-sensitive half-time that does not increase significantly with prolonged infusion. Remifentanil (an opioid) and esmolol (a β-blocker) are both short-acting drugs broken down by ester hydrolysis. (112)

53. Benzodiazepines exert their effects through their actions on the $GABA_A$ receptor. When $GABA_A$ receptors are stimulated by the inhibitory neurotransmitter GABA, the channel opens, allowing chloride ions to flow into the cell. This results in hyperpolarization of the neuron and a resistance of the neuron to subsequent depolarization. Benzodiazepines enhance the effect of GABA by binding to subunits of the $GABA_A$ receptor and maintaining the chloride channel open for a longer period of time. Unlike barbiturates, benzodiazepines do not directly activate the $GABA_A$ receptor, even at high doses. This property may contribute to their relative safety as compared with barbiturates. (112-113)

54. Benzodiazepine receptors, the $GABA_A$ ion channel, are located primarily on postsynaptic nerve endings in the CNS. The greatest density of benzodiazepine receptors is in the cerebral cortex. The distribution of benzodiazepine receptors is consistent with the minimal cardiopulmonary effects of these drugs. (113)

55. GABA$_A$ receptors are ligand-gated ion channels formed with five subunits. They are found embedded in the cell membrane of neurons. A pore through which chloride ions pass is found at the center of the five-membered assembly (also known as a pentamer). The most common channel arrangement is two α-subunits, two β-subunits, and one γ-subunit. Benzodiazepines are thought to bind at the interface between α- and γ-subunits. However, there are at least 19 different subunits expressed in the mammalian brain, and the exact arrangement is highly variable. GABA, benzodiazepines, and other IV anesthetics likely bind to different sites on the receptors. Subunit diversity likely contributes to GABA$_A$ receptor function in the CNS. (113)

56. Midazolam has about twice the affinity for benzodiazepine receptors (i.e., GABA$_A$ receptors) as diazepam. Lorazepam has even higher affinity than midazolam. Therefore, the order of affinity (and potency) is lorazepam > midazolam > diazepam. (113)

57. Benzodiazepines decrease CBF and CMRO$_2$ in a dose-dependent manner, but there is a ceiling to this effect. This makes benzodiazepines safe for use in patients with intracranial space-occupying lesions. However, administration of benzodiazepines to patients with CNS disease may make subsequent neurologic evaluation difficult secondary to prolonged sedation. Benzodiazepines also have anticonvulsant effects that are thought to occur through the enhancement of the inhibitory effects of the neurotransmitter GABA in the CNS. Benzodiazepines have been shown to increase the seizure threshold and are first-line treatment for seizures due to local anesthetic toxicity, alcohol withdrawal, and epilepsy. It is not possible to achieve an isoelectric EEG by administration of benzodiazepines. (113)

58. Induction doses of midazolam may lead to decreases in systemic blood pressure that are greater than those seen with the induction dose of diazepam. This effect of midazolam may be particularly pronounced in patients who are hypovolemic. The decrease in systemic blood pressure is believed to be due to decreases in SVR. (113)

59. In general, benzodiazepines alone produce dose-dependent ventilatory depressant effects. Transient apnea may occur with the rapid administration of induction doses of midazolam, particularly if an opioid has been used for premedication. Benzodiazepines may impair pharyngeal coordination and increase the risk of pulmonary aspiration. (113)

60. Propylene glycol is an organic solvent used to dissolve lipid-soluble diazepam into solution. Propylene glycol is likely responsible for the unpredictable absorption of diazepam when administered intramuscularly. It is also responsible for the pain and possible subsequent thrombophlebitis experienced by patients on the IV injection of diazepam. (113)

61. Allergic reactions to benzodiazepines are extremely rare. (113)

62. Clinical uses of benzodiazepines in anesthesia practice include preoperative medication, IV sedation, the IV induction of anesthesia, and the suppression of seizure activity. (114)

63. When administered for sedation, midazolam has a more rapid onset and produces a greater degree of amnesia than diazepam. When given orally, peak plasma concentrations occur within about 30 minutes for midazolam, 60 minutes for diazepam, and 2 hours for lorazepam. The slow onset and greater duration of action of lorazepam limit its usefulness as a preoperative medication. All benzodiazepines may have prolonged and more pronounced sedative effects in the elderly. (114)

64. Midazolam is useful for providing anxiolysis, amnesia, and sedation. When given in combination with propofol, it may improve sedation and operating conditions during minor procedures such as colonoscopy. Midazolam has an antiemetic effect and may lower the incidence of PONV. Anterograde amnesia may be desirable, but caution is advised when providing important

information to patients. Finally, routine premedication with benzodiazepines has not been shown to improve patient satisfaction after elective surgery. (114-115)

65. Midazolam and other benzodiazepines produce anterograde but not retrograde amnesia. This means that formation of new memories should only be impaired after administration of the drug. Memories formed prior to drug administration should be unaffected. However, it has been found that many patients receiving midazolam in the preoperative holding area do not have recall of that time period. Anesthesiologists, surgeons, and other providers should be aware of this effect when counseling patients. Important information related to diagnosis, treatment, or follow-up care should be provided in a manner that ensures this information is not lost or misinterpreted. For example, written instructions may be provided when the patient is in recovery. Alternatively, information may be provided to a family member as long as the patient agrees and privacy rules such as those set forth by the Health Insurance Portability and Accountability Act (HIPAA) are followed. Benzodiazepines are probably superior to other IV anesthetics for the prevention of awareness under anesthesia in high-risk populations (e.g., trauma, cardiac surgery). (115)

66. The IV induction dose of midazolam is 0.1 to 0.3 mg/kg. The time of onset is anywhere between 30 and 80 seconds, depending on the dose and premedication. Midazolam has a shorter time of onset than diazepam. The speed of onset of both agents can be enhanced by prior administration of opioids. Benzodiazepines are advantageous over barbiturates potentially due to less circulatory effects and greater reliability for the production of amnesia. A disadvantage of benzodiazepines is their lack of analgesic properties. Additional medicines would need to be administered to blunt the cardiovascular and laryngeal responses to direct laryngoscopy. The major disadvantage of benzodiazepines for the induction of anesthesia is delayed awakening, which limits their usefulness for this purpose. Midazolam is the shortest acting of the benzodiazepines in current use and therefore the most appropriate choice for induction. Even so, awakening after a single induction dose of midazolam in healthy volunteers takes more than 15 minutes. Diazepam and lorazepam require even greater periods of time before awakening, precluding their use as anesthesia induction agents. (115)

67. The effects of benzodiazepines can be reversed by a specific antagonist drug, flumazenil. Flumazenil is a competitive antagonist that binds to the benzodiazepine receptor but has little intrinsic activity. Flumazenil should be titrated to effect by administering 0.2 mg intravenously every 60 seconds up to a total dose of 1 to 3 mg. Flumazenil binds tightly to the benzodiazepine receptor but is cleared rapidly from the plasma. This results in a duration of action of only about 20 minutes. The short duration of action mandates that the patient be closely monitored for resedation after a dose of flumazenil, and repeat dosing may be necessary. Alternatively, an infusion of flumazenil may be started and titrated to the desired effect to maintain a constant plasma level of this reversal agent. (115)

68. Benzodiazepines are potent anticonvulsant drugs that can terminate continuous seizure activity (status epilepticus). For status epilepticus occurring in hospitalized patients, lorazepam 0.1 mg/kg intravenously is the drug of choice. Diazepam 0.2 mg/kg intravenously is also effective and should be administered if it is more readily available than lorazepam. In the prehospital setting, emergency medical technicians and paramedics are often the first responders, and seizing patients usually do not have IV access. In this situation, intramuscular midazolam should be given in a dose of 5 to 10 mg. The intramuscular route decreases time to therapy and may decrease the need for hospitalization. In either situation, providers must be ready to manage the airway because respiratory compromise may occur. (115)

KETAMINE

69. Ketamine is a derivative of phencyclidine, also known as PCP. (115)

70. The administration of ketamine produces unconsciousness and hypnosis, but the quality of this state is quite different from that of other IV anesthetics. Ketamine hypnosis is characterized by unresponsiveness, amnesia, and profound analgesia. The anesthesia derived from ketamine administration has thus been termed a *dissociative anesthesia*. The dose-dependent analgesia produced by ketamine is unique among IV anesthetics. No drugs have yet been isolated that are able to antagonize the effects of ketamine. (115)

71. After an induction dose of ketamine the patient appears to be in a cataleptic state. The appearance of the patient may be characterized as eyes remaining open with a slow nystagmic gaze; the maintenance of cough, swallow, and corneal reflexes; moderate dilation of the pupils; lacrimation; salivation; and an increase in skeletal muscle tone, with apparently coordinated but purposeless movements of the extremities. Induction doses of ketamine provide an intense analgesia and amnesia in patients despite the patient's appearing as if he or she may be awake. (115)

72. The redistribution of highly lipid-soluble ketamine to inactive tissue sites allows for rapid awakening after the administration of a bolus of ketamine. Ketamine undergoes extensive hepatic metabolism to norketamine for its elimination. Norketamine has between 20% and 30% of the potency of ketamine and may contribute to some of the delayed effects of ketamine when administered as a continuous infusion. (115)

73. The exact mechanism by which ketamine exerts its effects remains unknown and likely involves several receptor and neurotransmitter systems. The most significant pathway is inhibition of the *N*-methyl-D-aspartate (NMDA) receptor complex, which is believed to mediate the general anesthetic actions of ketamine. The NMDA receptor is an ion channel that is gated by the excitatory neurotransmitter glutamate. Ketamine also occupies some μ-opioid receptors in the brain and spinal cord, which may partially explain its analgesic effects. Other receptors that ketamine interacts with include monoaminergic receptors, muscarinic receptors, and calcium channels. Functionally, ketamine is believed to cause selective depression of the projections from the thalamus to the limbic system and cortex. (115-116)

74. Ketamine has excitatory effects on the CNS that are opposite those of most other IV anesthetics. Ketamine is a cerebral vasodilator and increases cerebral metabolism, CBF, ICP, and $CMRO_2$. The excitatory effects of ketamine are reflected by the development of beta and gamma (higher frequency) wave activity on the EEG when ketamine is administered. Because of the CNS excitatory effects of ketamine, it is not recommended as an induction agent in patients with space-occupying intracranial lesions or after head trauma when increases in ICP can be detrimental. However, if ventilation is controlled and normocapnia maintained, any elevation in ICP caused by ketamine can usually be attenuated. (116)

75. Ketamine increases systemic blood pressure, pulmonary artery pressure, heart rate, and cardiac output. The systemic blood pressure may increase by 20 to 40 mm Hg over the first 5 minutes after induction doses of ketamine are administered. The rise in blood pressure is often sustained for over 10 minutes. The hemodynamic changes are not clearly dose-dependent and can be blunted by the prior administration of barbiturates, benzodiazepines, or opioids. These cardiovascular effects of ketamine are most likely mediated centrally through the activation of sympathetic nervous system outflow. Endogenous norepinephrine release has been found to accompany the administration of ketamine. This property of ketamine may make it useful as an induction agent in hypovolemic patients in whom hemodynamic support is beneficial. Conversely, patients with a history of myocardial ischemia may be adversely affected by the increases in myocardial oxygen demand, making ketamine a poor choice for induction in this patient population. Of note, the cardiovascular stimulatory effects of ketamine may not be as pronounced and may even be

absent in patients who are catecholamine depleted. In catecholamine-depleted states such as trauma or septic shock, the myocardial depressant effect of ketamine may be unmasked and lead to large drops in systemic blood pressure after an induction dose. (116)

76. The administration of ketamine can result in a transient depression of ventilation or even apnea with large doses. However, the resting Pa_{CO_2} is typically unaltered when ketamine is used as a single agent. Ketamine relaxes bronchial smooth muscle, resulting in bronchodilation. This effect of ketamine is most likely mediated by its sympathomimetic effects and may make it useful as an induction agent in patients with bronchial asthma. Ketamine also induces an increase in airway secretions. When ketamine is used as an induction agent, preoperative administration of an antisialagogue such as glycopyrrolate may be useful to decrease secretions. (116)

77. Ketamine preserves and may even increase skeletal muscle tone. Patients have varying degrees of purposeful skeletal muscle movement and hypertonus after an induction dose of ketamine. The preservation of skeletal muscle tone results in maintenance of a patent upper airway and the preservation of cough and swallow reflexes. Despite this, airway protection by these reflexes against regurgitation or vomiting cannot be assumed, and there is a risk of laryngospasm. (116)

78. For the induction of anesthesia, the IV dose of ketamine is 1 to 2 mg/kg, whereas the intramuscular dose is 5 to 10 mg/kg. The induction of anesthesia after IV administration is achieved within 60 seconds. The induction of anesthesia after intramuscular administration is achieved within 2 to 4 minutes. Return of consciousness after an IV induction dose of ketamine usually requires 10 to 20 minutes, whereas full orientation may take 60 to 90 minutes. Ketamine may also be administered orally or rectally. (116)

79. Recovery from ketamine administraton has been associated with a delirium, often referred to as an "emergence delirium." This state is characterized by vivid dreaming, visual and auditory illusions, and a sense of floating outside the body. These sensations may be associated with confusion, excitement, or fear. They may be unpleasant to the patient or result in euphoria. Emergence delirium typically occurs in the first hour of recovery and persists for 1 to 3 hours. The incidence has been estimated as high as 30%, and the severity may vary. Emergence delirium is more likely to occur when ketamine is used as the sole anesthetic agent. The risk may be reduced with preoperative or postinduction administration of benzodiazepines. (116)

80. Some common clinical uses of ketamine include induction of anesthesia in hypovolemic patients, intramuscular injection for induction of anesthesia in children or developmentally disabled patients who are difficult to manage, and for dressing changes and débridement procedures in burn patients. Small boluses of ketamine may be titrated for analgesia, or a low-dose infusion (3 to 5 µg/kg/min) may be given as an adjunct to general anesthesia or to reduce opioid-induced hyperalgesia. (116)

81. The repeated administration of ketamine may result in development of tolerance to the analgesic effects. Clinically, this would manifest as an increase in the dose of ketamine required with each subsequent anesthetic to provide sufficient analgesic effects. An example in which this situation may arise is in burn patients who are being administered ketamine while undergoing recurrent dressing changes. (116)

82. Allergic reactions to ketamine are uncommon. (116)

83. Ketamine has recently shown promise as a therapy for treatment-resistant major depression. (117)

ETOMIDATE

84. Etomidate is an imidazole derivative. Imidazole is a five-membered aromatic ring containing two nitrogens. Dexmedetomidine also contains an imidazole group, as does midazolam. (117)

85. The induction dose of etomidate is 0.2 to 0.3 mg/kg. Unconsciousness results in less than 30 seconds. The duration of action of etomidate after an induction dose is very short, owing to its rapid clearance from the plasma through redistribution to inactive tissue sites. (117)

86. Etomidate rapidly undergoes nearly complete ester hydrolysis to pharmacologically inactive metabolites by the liver, with less than 3% of the drug being excreted in the urine unchanged. (117)

87. Like thiopental and propofol, etomidate is highly lipid soluble, which allows it to quickly cross the blood-brain barrier to exert its effects. This accounts for the short effect-site equilibration time for these agents. The context-sensitive half-time of etomidate may be prolonged if repeated or continuous doses of the drug result in saturation of the inactive sites. Of the commonly used IV anesthetics, it has one of the shortest context-sensitive half-times for an infusion of given length (even shorter than propofol and markedly shorter than thiopental). However, it is rarely administered as an infusion out of concern for endocrine side effects. (117)

88. The mechanism by which etomidate exerts its effects is not completely understood, but it appears to act mainly through agonist effects at the $GABA_A$ receptor (similar to propofol, benzodiazepines, and barbiturates—although the specific binding sites most likely differ among these drug classes). (117)

89. Etomidate is a cerebral vasoconstrictor that decreases CBF, ICP, and $CMRO_2$. Etomidate has similar effects as barbiturates on the EEG as well, such that etomidate may be titrated to achieve EEG burst suppression and maximally decrease cerebral metabolic oxygen requirements. However, there is no evidence from either animal or human studies that etomidate provides neuroprotection. (117)

90. The administration of etomidate has been shown to increase the activity of seizure foci on an EEG. Etomidate is similar to methohexital in this regard. Its effects can be used intraoperatively to facilitate intraoperative mapping of seizure foci for surgical ablation. Etomidate produces myoclonus in over half of patients, and this may correlate with seizure-like activity on the EEG. (117)

91. Administration of an induction dose of etomidate results in minimal changes in heart rate, MAP, central venous pressure, stroke volume, or cardiac index. In hypovolemic patients, some decrease in blood pressure may still occur. The cardiovascular stability associated with etomidate sets it apart from the other induction agents and is the basis for its usefulness in patients with limited cardiac reserve. It is important to realize that etomidate does not have any analgesic effects. Supplemental agents must be administered to blunt the stimulatory effects of direct laryngoscopy, or hypertension and tachycardia may result. (117)

92. The administration of etomidate alone appears to result in less of a depressant effect on ventilation than propofol or thiopental. Respiratory depression may occur when etomidate is administered in combination with other anesthetics or opioids. (117)

93. Etomidate inhibits 11β-hydroxylase, a key enzyme in the cortisol synthesis pathway. Because of this effect, adrenocortical function is suppressed for at least 4 to 8 hours, and possibly up to 48 hours, after an induction dose of etomidate. This effect may render the adrenal cortex unresponsive to adrenocorticotropic hormone and unable to mount a desirable stress response during the perioperative period. There is great controversy over whether or not short-term adrenocortical suppression from etomidate leads to negative patient outcomes, particularly when used for critically ill patients. (117)

94. Compared with other IV anesthetics, induction doses of etomidate result in minimal decreases in SVR, myocardial contractility, and MAP. Patients who are particularly dependent on adequate SVR and diastolic blood pressure to maintain coronary perfusion, such as those with coronary artery disease or critical aortic stenosis, may be particularly suitable for etomidate induction.

Etomidate may provide superior hemodynamic stability in patients with hypovolemia, sepsis, or trauma, although the risks of adrenal suppression must be weighed carefully. Finally, etomidate is a frequent choice for rapid sequence induction of patients with head trauma, as it decreases ICP yet maintains MAP and CPP. Finally, etomidate is an excellent choice for electroconvulsive therapy as it allows for longer seizure duration than methohexital. (118)

95. Aside from adrenal suppression, potential negative effects associated with the administration of etomidate include pain during IV injection, superficial thrombophlebitis, involuntary myoclonic movements, and an increased incidence of PONV. (118)

DEXMEDETOMIDINE

96. Dexmedetomidine, the active S-enantiomer of medetomidine, is an imidazole. Dexmedetomidine undergoes rapid hepatic metabolism, and metabolites are excreted through the bile and urine. The context-sensitive half-time increases with increasing duration of administration. (118)

97. Dexmedetomidine is a highly selective α_2-adrenergic agonist and exerts its effects through activation of α_2-receptors in the CNS. The analgesic effects originate at the level of the spinal cord, and its hypnotic effects likely originate through receptor sites in the locus ceruleus. (118)

98. Through its activation of endogenous sleep pathways, sedation with dexmedetomidine produces a state that resembles physiologic sleep more than that produced by other IV anesthetics. At clinically useful doses, patients tend to be easily arousable and will wake up and follow commands with verbal or tactile stimulation. Sedative effects of dexmedetomidine are synergistic when combined with other sedative-hypnotics. (119)

99. Dexmedetomidine likely leads to a decrease in CBF without significant changes in ICP or $CMRO_2$. (119)

100. The EEG of patients receiving dexmedetomidine shares some features with physiologic sleep, such as spindles. Seizure foci are not suppressed by dexmedetomidine, making it a useful agent during epilepsy surgery with intraoperative mapping of seizure foci. (119)

101. Dexmedetomidine infusion decreases systemic blood pressure by moderate decreases in heart rate and SVR. Bradycardia associated with dexmedetomidine infusion may sometimes require treatment. Severe bradycardia, heart block, and asystole have been described. Elderly patients and those with low baseline blood pressure (MAP < 70 mm Hg) are at higher risk of hemodynamic instability with dexmedetomidine infusion. (119)

102. IV infusions of dexmedetomidine generally cause decreases in heart rate and blood pressure due to inhibition of sympathetic outflow from the CNS. By contrast, a bolus injection or rapid loading dose may produce transient increases in systemic blood pressure and pronounced decreases in heart rate, an effect that is probably mediated by vasoconstriction from peripheral α_2-adrenergic receptors. (119)

103. Dexmedetomidine has only minor effects on the respiratory system when compared with other IV anesthetics. These effects include small decreases in tidal volume without much change in the respiratory rate. The ventilatory response to carbon dioxide is unchanged, but the response to hypoxia is reduced to a similar degree as propofol. Upper airway obstruction as a result of sedation is possible and may be augmented when dexmedetomidine is combined with other sedative-hypnotics. (119)

104. When administered during general anesthesia, dexmedetomidine (0.5- to 1-μg/kg loading dose over a period of 10 to 15 minutes, followed by an infusion of 0.2 to 0.7 μg/kg/h) decreases the dose requirements for inhaled and injected anesthetics. (119)

105. Some common clinical uses for dexmedetomidine include infusion as an adjunct during general anesthesia in the operating room, sedation for procedures, sedation for airway management (i.e., awake fiberoptic intubation), and sedation of tracheally intubated patients in the ICU. (119)

9 OPIOIDS

Cynthia Newberry

BASIC PHARMACOLOGY

1. Which opioid was the first completely synthetic opioid?
2. In general terms, describe the acid-base status, protein-binding, and ionized state of the opioid class of drugs.
3. What is the mechanism of action of opioids?
4. Describe the locations and classes of opioid receptors.
5. How are opioids metabolized?
6. Which opioids have active metabolites?

CLINICAL PHARMACOLOGY

7. What are the four key pharmacokinetic behaviors of opioids?
8. What properties of an opioid affect its latency time to peak effect (i.e., bolus front-end kinetics) after a bolus injection?
9. How is remifentanil different from other opioids when used as a continuous infusion?
10. State a clinical example of how an opioid bolus latency time to peak effect would influence patient-controlled analgesia (PCA) dosing.
11. What is context-sensitive half-time (CSHT)? What are some clinical implications of the CSHT?
12. What are some therapeutic effects of opioids?
13. What are the effects of opioids on the cardiovascular system?
14. What are the effects of opioids on ventilation?
15. What are the effects of opioids on the central nervous system?
16. What are the effects of opioids on the thoracoabdominal muscles? How can they be treated?
17. What are the effects of opioids on the gastrointestinal system?
18. What are the effects of opioids on the genitourinary system?
19. What is the mechanism by which opioids are thought to cause nausea and vomiting?
20. How do opioids modulate immune function?
21. What is an example of a pharmacokinetic drug interaction of opioids?
22. What is an example of a pharmacodynamic drug interaction of opioids?
23. What are some considerations of using opioids in patients with hepatic failure?
24. What are some considerations of using opioids in patients with kidney failure?
25. Does gender have an influence on opioid pharmacology?
26. Does age have an influence on opioid pharmacology?
27. How should opioids be dosed in obese patients?
28. What is the active compound of codeine?
29. How does the onset time of morphine compare with the other opioids? What are some potential drawbacks of the administration of morphine?
30. How does fentanyl compare with morphine with regard to its effect-site equilibration time? What is the potency of fentanyl relative to morphine?

31. What are some routes for the administration of fentanyl?
32. How are the effects of fentanyl terminated? How does the CSHT of fentanyl compare with other opioids?
33. What are some systemic clinical effects associated with the administration of fentanyl?
34. What are some clinical uses of fentanyl in anesthesia practice?
35. What is the potency of sufentanil relative to morphine?
36. How does remifentanil compare with the other opioids with respect to its effect-site equilibration time and its CSHT?
37. What are some clinical uses of remifentanil?
38. By what mechanism do opioid agonist/antagonists work?
39. What are some clinical uses of opioid agonist/antagonists?
40. What specific risks does tramadol use carry based on its receptor affinity?
41. Why does preoperative buprenorphine use complicate perioperative pain management?
42. What role does the opioid antagonist naloxone play in clinical practice? What are some adverse effects of naloxone?
43. What role does the opioid antagonist naltrexone play in clinical practice?

CLINICAL APPLICATION

44. What are some common clinical indications for the use of opioids in anesthesia practice?
45. What is the basis of opioid selection in different clinical situations?

EMERGING DEVELOPMENTS

46. What are some concerns regarding opioid use and cancer recurrence?

ANSWERS*

BASIC PHARMACOLOGY

1. Meperidine was the first completely synthetic opioid. It is a basic phenylpiperidine structure, and the fentanyl congeners are more complex versions of this same skeleton. (123)
2. In general, opioids are highly soluble weak bases that are highly protein bound and largely ionized at physiologic pH. Physiochemical properties of opioids, such as protein binding, ionized fraction, and lipid solubility, affect their clinical behavior. (123)
3. Opioids exert their effects through their agonist actions at the opioid receptors. The main action of opioids appears to be through the interaction with G proteins, resulting in inhibition of the activity of adenylate cyclase and increasing potassium conductance. This ultimately results in hyperpolarization of the cell and leads to a suppression of synaptic transmission. (124)
4. Opioid receptors are located in various tissues throughout the central nervous system (CNS) and exert their therapeutic effects at multiple sites. They inhibit the release of substance P from primary sensory neurons in the dorsal horn of the spinal cord, mitigating the transfer of painful sensations to the brain. Opioid actions in the brainstem modulate nociceptive transmission in the dorsal horn of the spinal cord through descending inhibitory pathways. Three classical opioid receptors have been identified: μ, κ, and δ. More recently, a fourth opioid receptor ligand, ORL1 (also known as nociceptin opioid receptor [NOP]), has also been identified, but its function is quite different from that of the classical opioid receptors. Although the existence of opioid receptor subtypes (e.g., μ_1, μ_2) has been proposed, it is not clear from molecular biology techniques that distinct genes code for them. (124)

---

*Numbers in parentheses refer to pages, figures, boxes, or tables in Pardo MC, Miller RD, eds. *Basics of Anesthesia*. 7th ed. Philadelphia: Elsevier; 2018.

5. In general, opioids are metabolized by the liver, though some undergo hepatic conjugation and are renally excreted. (125)
6. Both meperidine and morphine have active metabolites that can accumulate in renal failure, and thus these drugs must be used with caution in this patient population. Genetic variations in codeine metabolism can also affect clinical drug effect. (125)

CLINICAL PHARMACOLOGY

7. The four key pharmacokinetic behaviors of opioids are (1) latency to peak effect site concentration after bolus injection (i.e., bolus front-end kinetics), (2) the time to clinically relevant decay of concentration after bolus injection (i.e., bolus back-end kinetics), (3) the time to steady-state concentration after starting a continuous infusion (i.e., infusion front-end kinetics), and (4) the time to clinically relevant decay in concentration after stopping a continuous infusion (i.e., infusion back-end kinetics). (125-126)
8. The latency time to peak effect (bolus front-end kinetics) of common intravenous opioids after administering a bolus is influenced by the opioid's ionization and lipid solubility. Opioids that are un-ionized, unbound, and have high lipid solubility rapidly equilibrate to the effect site. The time to peak effect is also influenced by the amount of drug administered in the initial bolus. (126)
9. Because remifentanil rapidly equilibrates to the effect site, it can be started as an infusion without a bolus and reach a steady-state effect-site concentration in an operative time period without continuing to increase in concentration. Infusions of other narcotics require a bolus to be administered to more quickly achieve near steady state, and concentrations may increase for hours with a continuous infusion. For this reason, remifentanil is often chosen for total intravenous anesthesia (TIVA). (127)
10. Front-end kinetics of fentanyl make it well suited for patient-controlled analgesia (PCA) use. In contrast to morphine, the peak effect of a fentanyl bolus is manifest before a typical PCA lockout period has elapsed, thus mitigating the "dose-stacking" problem. (127)
11. The context-sensitive half-time (CSHT) is defined as the time required for a 50% decrease in drug concentration after stopping a steady-state infusion. The CSHT predicts the termination of drug effect or "infusion back-end" kinetics. It has many clinical utilities. First, for most drugs, the CSHT changes with the length of time of the infusion. After a short duration of infusion, the predicted back-end kinetics for the various drugs do not differ much (remifentanil is an exception). But if the duration of infusion is increased, the CSHTs will vary for the different opioids. Second, clinically shorter- or longer-acting drugs should be chosen depending on the duration of opioid effect desired after discontinuing it. Finally, the shapes of these curves are not the same, such that there is a different degree of concentration decline—for example, a 20% or an 80% decrease in concentration. Of note, the CSHT does not account for active metabolites. (127)
12. Pain relief is the primary therapeutic effect of opioid analgesics. Acting at spinal and brain μ receptors, opioids attenuate nociceptive traffic from the periphery and alter central affective pain sensation. Additionally in the operative setting, opioid effects of drowsiness, decreased airway irritability, and attenuation of the cough reflex are considered therapeutic benefits. (128)
13. Opioids can alter cardiovascular physiology by several mechanisms. Compared to other anesthetics, however, opioids produce minimal cardiovascular effects. Fentanyl derivatives are known to cause increased vagal tone, which can lead to bradycardia. Opioid-induced depression of vasomotor centers in the brainstem and peripheral vessels can lead to decreased preload and afterload. Decreases in arterial blood pressure are more likely in patients relying on high sympathetic tone, such as patients in congestive heart failure. (129)

14. All the μ-receptor agonist opioids produce a dose-dependent depression of ventilation. This is reflected by an increase in the resting $Paco_2$, an increase in the apneic threshold, a decrease in the responsiveness to the ventilatory stimulant effects of carbon dioxide, and a decrease in the hypoxic ventilatory drive. The administration of opioids also affects the rate of breathing and the tidal volume. The respiratory rate is typically slowed and insufficiently compensated by an increase in the tidal volume. Consequently, the minute ventilation is decreased. The mechanism by which these effects of opioids on ventilation occur is thought to be through the direct depression of the medullary ventilatory centers. (130)

15. The administration of opioids results in several CNS effects. Opioids are unable to produce a dose-related general depression of the CNS typical of other general anesthetics. Instead, opioids have a ceiling effect that is not overcome by increasing the administered dose of opioids. Opioids do contribute to the minimum alveolar concentration (MAC) of anesthesia delivered and decrease the amount of volatile agent required to achieve a given anesthetic depth. Opioids are not considered to be true anesthetics, however, because of their inability to reliably produce unconsciousness even in high doses. Finally, the administration of opioids causes miosis through its cortical stimulation of the Edinger-Westphal nucleus of the oculomotor nerve. There is little tolerance to the miosis produced by opioids, which makes it a useful clinical indicator of opioid exposure. (130)

16. The administration of opioids can result in increased thoracoabdominal muscle tone, which may result in chest wall stiffness. This "stiff-chest" syndrome can interfere with ventilation. Although the exact mechanism for this muscle rigidity is not known, it appears to occur most frequently when rapid, large boluses of fentanyl congeners are initially administered. This rigidity can make bag and mask ventilation during induction of anesthesia impossible because of concurrent vocal cord rigidity and closure. Termination of the rigidity to allow for ventilation can be accomplished through the administration of a neuromuscular blocking drug or an opioid antagonist such as naloxone. Prophylaxis against this muscle rigidity can be achieved through the administration of a priming dose of a nondepolarizing neuromuscular blocking drug and the slow, intermittent administration of opioid. (130)

17. Among the several effects opioids have on the gastrointestinal system are effects on gastrointestinal motility, gastric emptying, and biliary smooth muscle tone. Opioid receptors are found in the entire enteric gastrointestinal plexus. Stimulation of these receptors causes tonic gastrointestinal contraction, decreases peristalsis, and leads to ileus. Opioids also delay gastric emptying, through both central and peripheral effects of the opioid. Centrally, this effect is mediated by the vagus nerve. Peripherally, binding of an opioid to the opioid receptors in the myenteric plexus and cholinergic nerve terminals inhibits the release of acetylcholine at these nerve terminals. Opioids also increase pyloric sphincter tone, further contributing to a delay in gastric emptying. Opioids can cause spasm of biliary smooth muscle, increasing biliary duct pressure. Opioids also increase the tone of the sphincter of Oddi. In patients receiving intraoperative cholangiograms, approximately 3% of patients who have been administered opioids have opioid-induced spasm of the sphincter of Oddi. The clinician can distinguish between opioid-induced biliary colic pain and myocardial ischemia through the administration of naloxone. Naloxone can relieve the pain of biliary colic, but it has no effect on the pain caused by myocardial ischemia. Glucagon also reverses biliary spasm from opioids. Nitroglycerin has resulted in pain relief in both circumstances, making diagnosis difficult. (130)

18. Opioids can decrease bladder detrusor tone and increase the tone of the urinary sphincter. This may lead to urinary retention in some patients, particularly in males and when the opioid is administered intrathecally or epidurally. When this occurs there may be the need to catheterize the patient's bladder to drain it. These effects are in part centrally mediated, although peripheral effects are also likely given the widespread presence of opioid receptors in the genitourinary tract. (130)

19. There are several mechanisms by which opioids are thought to cause nausea and vomiting. The primary mechanism appears to be through the direct stimulation of the chemoreceptor trigger zone in the area postrema on the floor of the fourth ventricle in the brain. In addition to this, opioids also increase gastrointestinal secretions, decrease gastrointestinal tract motility, and prolong gastric emptying time. (130)

20. Both administered and endogenous (e.g., endorphins) opioids depress cellular immunity. For example, opioids have been shown to inhibit the transcription of interleukin 2 in activated T cells. The different opioids may differ in the mechanism and extent of their immunomodulatory effects. Some possible adverse outcomes due to the impairment of cellular immunity may include impaired wound healing, perioperative infections, and cancer recurrence. These effects are not completely understood. (130)

21. A pharmacokinetic drug interaction is one in which the administration of a drug influences the concentration of another administered drug. An example of this occurs when opioids are administered concurrently with a continuous propofol infusion. Opioid concentrations may be higher when administered with a continuous propofol infusion than they are when the same dose is administered alone. This may be due in part to the hemodynamic changes induced by propofol. (130)

22. A pharmacodynamic drug interaction is one in which the administration of a drug influences the effect of another administered drug. The most common and most important pharmacodynamic drug interaction of opioids is their synergistic effect when administered with sedatives. Opioids also synergistically reduce the MAC when administered with volatile anesthetics. The reduction in the MAC of anesthesia can be substantial, by up to 75% or more. (130)

23. With the exception of remifentanil, the liver is the organ primarily responsible for the metabolism of opioids. The anhepatic phase of orthotopic liver transplantation is the only situation in which opioid concentrations may accumulate. Other than that, liver failure is usually not severe enough to have a major impact on opioid concentrations. Clinically, patients with severe liver disease, such as those with hepatic encephalopathy, may be more sensitive to the sedative effects of opioids. (131)

24. Kidney failure may have clinical effects on opioid administration, depending on the opioid. Kidney failure has major clinical relevance when administering morphine and meperidine. Two metabolites of morphine, morphine-3-glucuronide and morphine-6-glucuronide (M3G and M6G), are excreted via the kidney. M3G is inactive, but M6G is an analgesic whose potency approaches that of morphine. Life-threatening respiratory depression can develop in patients with renal failure administered morphine as a result of very high levels of M6G. Normeperidine is the main metabolite of meperidine and is excreted through the kidney. Normeperidine has analgesic and excitatory central nervous system (CNS) effects. Increasing levels of CNS toxicity of normeperidine include anxiety, tremulousness, myoclonus, and frank seizures. Therefore, normeperidine accumulation is of particular concern in patients with renal failure. For most other opioids, kidney failure has minimal clinical importance. Remifentanil, which is metabolized through ester hydrolysis, is not affected by kidney disease. (131)

25. Gender may have an influence on opioid pharmacology. Morphine is more potent in women but has a slower onset of action. (131)

26. Age has an important influence on opioid pharmacology. For example, fentanyl is more potent in the older patient. Pharmacokinetic changes, such as decreases in clearance and central volume of distribution in older patients, play a lesser role. Pharmacodynamic differences are primarily responsible for the decreased dose requirement in older patients (>65 years of age). Doses of opioids, including remifentanil, should be decreased by at least 50% or more in elderly patients. (131)

27. The clearance of opioids appears to be more closely related to lean body mass (LBM), such that obese patients do not require as high a dose as would be suggested by their total body weight (TBW). For this reason LBM should be used to calculate the dose of opioid administered. Pharmacokinetic simulations used to calculate the remifentanil dosage based on TBW or LBM in obese and lean patients showed dramatically higher concentrations of opioids when TBW was used in obese patients. (132)

28. Morphine is the active compound of codeine. The conversion of codeine to morphine is mediated in the liver by the gene *CYP2D6*. Interestingly, 10% of the Caucasian population lack this gene and do not exhibit a therapeutic effect from codeine. (132)

29. Morphine is the opioid to which other opioids are compared. Because of its low lipid solubility and almost completely ionized form at physiologic pH, morphine has a prolonged latency to peak effect, slow penetration of the CNS, and less initial respiratory depression than other opioids. Unfortunately, its pharmacology predisposes patients to delayed respiratory depression as well as potential dosestacking. Other potential drawbacks of morphine include histamine release and possible associated hypotension with its intravenous injection and the potential accumulation of the active metabolite M6G in patients with renal failure. (133)

30. Fentanyl administered intravenously has a more rapid onset and shorter duration of action than morphine. This reflects its greater lipid solubility. The effect-site equilibration time of fentanyl is about 6.5 minutes. Its shorter duration of action is reflective of its rapid redistribution to inactive tissue sites, leading to a rapid decrease in the plasma concentration of fentanyl. Fentanyl is 75 to 125 times more potent than morphine. (133)

31. Fentanyl can be administered numerous ways. In addition to the intravenous route, transdermal, transmucosal, transnasal, and transpulmonary routes are all effective for the administration of fentanyl. The oral transmucosal delivery of fentanyl citrate results in a faster achievement of higher peak levels than when the same dose is swallowed. (133)

32. The effects of fentanyl are terminated through its redistribution to inactive tissue sites followed by its metabolism by the liver. High intravenous doses of fentanyl or a continuous intravenous infusion can lead to saturation of the inactive tissue sites. This may result in prolonged redistribution, prolonged elimination, and prolonged pharmacologic effects of the drug. The cumulative drug effects during continuous intravenous infusions of fentanyl, sufentanil, alfentanil, and remifentanil have been compared. Alfentanil and remifentanil do not seem to produce clinically significant cumulative drug effects, and awakening appears to be prompt with minimal lingering side effects when compared with fentanyl. (133)

33. The administration of fentanyl is associated with a decrease in heart rate. The administration of fentanyl alone leads to little change in systemic blood pressure, whereas its administration after a benzodiazepine may lead to decreases in blood pressure. There are also synergistic effects between fentanyl and benzodiazepines on ventilatory depression and sedation. (133)

34. Clinical uses of fentanyl in anesthesia practice include perioperative analgesia, the induction and maintenance of anesthesia, the inhibition of the sympathetic nervous system response to direct laryngoscopy or surgical stimulation, and preemptive analgesia. Opioids are most commonly used during the maintenance of anesthesia as a supplement to inhaled anesthetics. Opioids used in this manner are often administered in small intravenous boluses or as a continuous infusion. High doses of a narcotic, especially fentanyl or sufentanil, may be used in patients who are unable to tolerate the effects of cardiac depression that inhaled anesthetics may produce. A disadvantage of an opioid-based anesthetic is the potential for patient awareness. (133)

35. Sufentanil is the most potent opioid currently in use in anesthesia practice. (133)

36. Remifentanil has a short effect-site equilibration time, and the CSHT of remifentanil is much shorter than that of the other opioids, approximately 5 minutes. This is independent of the duration of the continuous infusion, which is unique to remifentanil among the opioids. The basis for this is its structure, which has an ester link. The ester link allows for hydrolysis in the plasma to inactive metabolites. This accounts for its rapid titratability, noncumulative effects, and rapid recovery. (133)

37. The most common clinical application of remifentanil is for TIVA, when combined with propofol. It is also useful as a bolus injection when rapid effect and recovery are desired, in surgical cases that have rapidly fluctuating anesthetic requirements, when a "large-dose" opioid technique is advantageous but the patient won't be mechanically ventilated postoperatively, or during monitored anesthetic care for local infiltration. (134)

38. Opioid agonist/antagonists are partial μ-receptor agonists while simultaneously serving as competitive antagonists at μ receptors and other opioid receptors. (134)

39. Because of their mechanism, opioid agonist/antagonists are analgesics with lesser potency, a "ceiling effect," lesser potential for dependence, and more limited ventilatory depressive effects. They are used commonly for chronic pain and in opioid-addicted patient populations. (134)

40. Tramadol has weak μ-, κ-, and δ-receptor affinity but also inhibits the reuptake of serotonin and norepinephrine. Because of these effects, tramadol carries a risk of serotonin syndrome when used with other serotonergic medications, notably serotonin-specific reuptake inhibitors. Tramadol also has risks of CNS excitability and seizures. (134)

41. Buprenorphine is an opioid agonist/antagonist with 25 times the potency of morphine and 50 times the affinity for the μ receptor. When used in high doses for the treatment of chronic pain, its presence at the μ receptor can block the action of full agonists, making the management of acute perioperative pain difficult in the chronic buprenorphine user. (134)

42. Naloxone is an intravenous complete opioid antagonist used to emergently reverse opioid-induced ventilatory depression. Because of this action naloxone has been added to the World Health Organization essential medication list. In smaller doses naloxone can be used to during the emergence of anesthesia to restore adequate ventilatory effort. Another clinical use of naloxone is for the treatment of opioid-induced pruritus. Naloxone's duration of action is shorter than most opioids, so repeated use must be considered when treating an opioid overdose. Some adverse effects of naloxone include acute withdrawal syndrome, nausea, vomiting, tachycardia, hypertension, seizures, and pulmonary edema. (134)

43. Naltrexone is available orally as an additive to orally administered opioids. It undergoes extensive first-pass hepatic metabolism and is inactive when administered orally, but if oral opioids containing naltrexone are crushed and injected intravenously, the naltrexone will act as an antagonist. For this reason, naltrexone is used as a deterrent to opioid abuse. (134)

CLINICAL APPLICATION

44. Opioids have been used in various clinical areas of anesthesia. Their main and oldest indication is postoperative analgesia. To increase the safety of opioid use for postoperative pain control they can be delivered by a PCA machine. Opioids can be combined with other drugs and techniques to decrease pain as well. Another common indication of opioid use is for "balanced anesthesia." With this technique, the opioids are primarily used for their ability to decrease MAC, thereby minimizing the direct myocardial depression and other untoward hemodynamic effects of the volatile anesthetics. Cardioprotection against ischemia (preconditioning) is another possible beneficial indication of opioids. Total intravenous anesthesia can be achieved when opioids are administered in combination with propofol infusions. This is another recent indication of opioids during anesthesia that may result in postoperative euphoria and less nausea and vomiting. (135)

45. Pharmacokinetic differences between opioids are the main consideration in selecting them for appropriate purpose. All μ agonists are equally efficacious when given in equipotent doses. Among key elements when selecting an opioid for administration is the desired time of onset, the duration of effect, and potential side effects. Side effects for consideration include sedation and respiratory depression. (135)

EMERGING DEVELOPMENTS

46. There is concern regarding the demonstrated immunosuppressive effects of opioids, and this has led to retrospective studies comparing cancer recurrence rates in patients who had received standard opioid therapy after surgery compared to alternative therapy. Data from these retrospective studies have conflicting results. The influence of opioid therapy on cancer recurrence remains controversial. (136)

10 LOCAL ANESTHETICS

Charles B. Berde, Anjali Koka, and Kenneth Drasner

HISTORY

1. What was the first local anesthetic introduced into clinical practice? What is its structural class?
2. What was the first amino-amide local anesthetic introduced into clinical practice?
3. What are two differences between amino-ester and amino-amide local anesthetics that make classifying local anesthetics important?
4. Name seven amino-amide local anesthetics.
5. What distinguishes ropivacaine and levobupivacaine from the other local anesthetics?

NERVE CONDUCTION

6. What mediates nerve conduction when a nerve gets stimulated under normal circumstances?
7. What three characteristics are nerve fibers classified by? What are the three main nerve fiber types?
8. How does the diameter of a nerve influence nerve conduction velocity?
9. Which types of nerve fibers are myelinated? What is the function of myelin?

LOCAL ANESTHETIC ACTIONS ON SODIUM CHANNELS

10. What is the mechanism of action of local anesthetics?
11. Where is the major site of local anesthetic effect?
12. What is frequency-dependent blockade? How does frequency-dependent blockade relate to the activity of local anesthetics?
13. How does myelin affect the action of local anesthetics?
14. How many consecutive nodes of Ranvier must be blocked for the effective blockade of the nerve impulse by local anesthetic?
15. How is the resting membrane potential and the threshold potential altered in nerves that have been infiltrated by local anesthetic?
16. How is the effect of a local anesthetic on the nerve terminated?
17. What is the basic structure of local anesthetics?
18. Why are local anesthetics marketed as hydrochloride salts?
19. Is the pKa of local anesthetics more than or less than 7.4?
20. At physiologic pH, does most local anesthetic exist in the ionized or nonionized form? What form must the local anesthetic be in to cross nerve cell membranes?
21. Does local tissue acidosis create an environment for higher or lower quality local analgesia? Why?
22. What is the primary determinant of local anesthetic potency?

DIFFERENTIAL LOCAL ANESTHETIC BLOCKADE

23. Is nerve conduction blockade facilitated by increasing the concentration of local anesthetic or by increasing the length of nerve exposed to more dilute concentrations of local anesthetic?
24. What is meant by differential block?

SPREAD OF LOCAL ANESTHESIA AFTER INJECTION

25. How do local anesthetics diffuse through nerve fibers when deposited around a nerve? Which nerve fibers are blocked first?
26. How are the nerve fibers arranged from the mantle to the core in a peripheral nerve with respect to the innervation of proximal and distal structures? What is the clinical implication of this?
27. What is the temporal progression of the interruption of the transmission of neural impulses between the autonomic nervous system, motor system, and sensory system after the infiltration of a mixed peripheral nerve with local anesthetic?
28. Which two nerve fiber types primarily function to conduct sharp and dull pain impulses? Which of these two nerve fibers is more readily blocked by local anesthetic?
29. Which two nerve fiber types primarily function to conduct impulses that result in large motor and small motor activity?

PHARMACOKINETICS

30. What very fundamental difference exists between the local anesthetics and most systemically administered drugs with regard to drug efficacy and absorption?
31. After a local anesthetic has been absorbed from the tissues, what are the primary determinants of local anesthetic peak plasma concentrations?
32. What are some physicochemical properties of local anesthetics and of the target site of injection that influence the systemic uptake of an injected local anesthetic?
33. What is the clinical implication of the variability in local anesthetics to cause vasoconstriction?
34. How are amino-ester local anesthetics cleared?
35. How are the amino-amide local anesthetics metabolized?
36. What are two organs that influence the potential for local anesthetic systemic toxicity (LAST)?
37. What accounts for chloroprocaine's relatively low systemic toxicity?
38. Patients with atypical plasma cholinesterase are at an increased risk for what complication with regard to local anesthetics?
39. What is the correlation between the clearance of lidocaine from plasma and hepatic blood flow?
40. What percent of local anesthetic undergoes renal excretion unchanged?
41. How does the addition of epinephrine to a local anesthetic solution prepared for injection affect its systemic absorption?
42. How does the addition of epinephrine to a local anesthetic solution prepared for injection affect its duration of action?
43. How does the addition of epinephrine to a local anesthetic solution prepared for injection affect its potential for systemic toxicity?
44. How does the addition of epinephrine to a local anesthetic solution prepared for injection affect the rate of onset of anesthesia?
45. How does the addition of epinephrine to a local anesthetic solution prepared for injection affect local bleeding?
46. What are some potential negative effects of the addition of epinephrine to a local anesthetic solution prepared for injection?
47. Name some clinical situations in which the addition of epinephrine to a local anesthetic solution prepared for injection may not be recommended.
48. Other than epinephrine, what are some additives to local anesthetic solution that have been shown to prolong the duration of anesthesia?

ADVERSE EFFECTS

49. What are some potential negative side effects associated with the administration of local anesthetics?
50. What is the most common cause of LAST?
51. What are the factors that influence the magnitude of the systemic absorption of local anesthetic from the tissue injection site?
52. From highest to lowest, what is the relative order of peak plasma concentrations of local anesthetic associated with the following regional anesthetic procedures: brachial plexus, caudal, intercostal, epidural, sciatic/femoral?
53. Which two organ systems are most likely to be affected by excessive plasma concentrations of local anesthetic?
54. What are the initial and subsequent manifestations of central nervous system toxicity due to increasingly excessive plasma concentrations of local anesthetic?
55. What is a possible pathophysiologic mechanism for seizures that result from excessive plasma concentrations of local anesthetic?
56. What are some potential adverse effects of local anesthetic-induced seizures?
57. How should local anesthetic-induced seizures be treated?
58. What is the indication for, and disadvantage of, the administration of neuromuscular blocking drugs for the treatment of seizures?
59. Is the cardiovascular system more or less susceptible to local anesthetic toxicity than the central nervous system?
60. What are two mechanisms by which local anesthetics can produce hypotension?
61. What is the mechanism by which local anesthetics exert their cardiotoxic effects? How is this manifested on the electrocardiogram?
62. How is the relative cardiotoxicity between local anesthetic agents compared? What is the relative cardiotoxicity between lidocaine, bupivacaine, and ropivacaine?
63. What is the standard treatment of LAST?
64. What is the dose of lipid emulsion that should be used for LAST, according to the American Society of Regional Anesthesia and Pain Medicine (ASRA) guidelines?
65. What are some modifications to standard advanced cardiac life support (ACLS) protocols in the event of LAST leading to cardiovascular collapse, according to ASRA guidelines?
66. What are some factors that may contribute to local tissue toxicity from local anesthetic injection?
67. What is the allergic potential of local anesthetics?
68. What are the potential causes of a hypersensitivity reaction associated with the administration of local anesthetics?
69. Does cross-sensitivity exist between the classes of local anesthetics?

SPECIFIC LOCAL ANESTHETICS

70. What was the primary use of procaine during the early 1900s?
71. How does procaine compare to lidocaine with respect to stability and risks of hypersensitivity, transient neurologic symptoms (TNS), and nausea?
72. What is the principal use of tetracaine in current clinical practice? What is a potential adverse effect of tetracaine?
73. What properties of tetracaine limit its usefulness for use in epidural anesthesia or peripheral nerve blockade?
74. How does the rate of metabolism of tetracaine compare to the other amide-ester local anesthetics?
75. What is the nature of the neurotoxicity that has been reported in association with the use of epidural chloroprocaine? What is the mechanism by which this occurs?
76. What are some advantageous properties of chloroprocaine?
77. What are some uses of chloroprocaine in current clinical pediatric practice?
78. What are some uses of lidocaine in current clinical practice?

79. What are two adverse neurologic outcomes associated with lidocaine spinal anesthesia?
80. What is the mechanism by which spinal lidocaine has resulted in cauda equina syndrome?
81. What is TNS?
82. What are some risk factors for TNS?
83. What is the treatment for TNS?
84. How does mepivacaine compare with lidocaine with respect to its clinical use, duration of action, and incidence of TNS?
85. What is a potentially adverse effect of prilocaine that limits its use in clinical practice? What is the mechanism for this?
86. What are some uses of bupivacaine in current clinical practice?
87. How does bupivacaine compare to lidocaine when used for epidural anesthesia?
88. How does bupivacaine compare to lidocaine with respect to its cardiotoxic effects? What is the mechanism for this?
89. What is an enantiomer?
90. What is an advantage of ropivacaine and levobupivacaine over bupivacaine for epidural anesthesia?
91. What are some clinical uses and a potential risk of topical local anesthesia?
92. Which local anesthetics are in eutectic mixture of local anesthetics (EMLA) cream?
93. What are some clinical uses and a potential risk of tumescent local anesthesia?
94. After the administration of lidocaine tumescent anesthesia, when does the plasma concentration of lidocaine peak?
95. What are some clinical uses of systemic local anesthesia?

WHEN LOCAL ANESTHESIA FAILS

96. What are some potential causes of local anesthesia failure?
97. What are some techniques that can be used to confirm proper needle placement when administering local anesthetic for epidural anesthesia and peripheral nerve blocks?
98. What are some risk factors for developing tachyphylaxis to local anesthetics?
99. What is a potential adverse effect of developing tachyphylaxis to local anesthetics, and how can this be minimized?
100. What is the mechanism by which chronic pain alters the patient's response to local anesthetics?

ANSWERS*

HISTORY

1. The first local anesthetic introduced into clinical practice was cocaine in the 1880s. Cocaine's amino-ester structure was adapted to make benzocaine (topical), procaine, tetracaine, and chloroprocaine (injectable). (139)
2. The first amino-amide local anesthetic introduced into clinical practice was lidocaine in 1948. It was considered to be more stable and to have less allergic potential than the amino-ester local anesthetics. (139)
3. The metabolism and possibly the potential to produce allergic reactions differ between amino-ester and amino-amide local anesthetics, making this classification of local anesthetics important. (139)
4. The amino-amide local anesthetics include lidocaine, mepivacaine, bupivacaine, levobupivacaine, etidocaine, prilocaine, and ropivacaine. As a general rule, amino-ester local anesthetics will have only one "i" in their generic name, whereas the amino amides will have two. (139)

---

*Numbers in parentheses refer to pages, figures, boxes, or tables in Pardo MC, Miller RD (eds). *Basics of Anesthesia*. 7th ed. Philadelphia: Elsevier; 2018.

5. Ropivacaine and levobupivacaine are single enantiomers, rather than racemic mixtures, which characterizes the other local anesthetics. These were developed in an effort to reduce the potential for cardiac toxicity. (139)

NERVE CONDUCTION

6. Under normal circumstances, when a nerve gets stimulated there is an increase in the membrane permeability of sodium channels to sodium ions, which flow into the nerve. The membrane potential changes from negative to positive; when a critical potential is reached there is rapid influx of sodium ions propagating a wave of depolarization and an action potential. (140)

7. Fiber diameter, the presence or absence of myelin, and function are the three characteristics by which nerve fibers are classified. A, B, and C are the three main types of nerve fibers. (140)

8. A larger diameter of a nerve correlates with a more rapid nerve conduction velocity. (140)

9. The A and B nerve fiber types are myelinated, whereas in type C nerve fibers myelin is absent. Myelin is composed of plasma membranes of specialized Schwann cells that wrap around the axon during axonal growth. Myelin functions to insulate the axolemma, or nerve cell membrane, from the surrounding conducting media. It also forces the depolarizing current to flow through periodic interruptions in the myelin sheath called the *nodes of Ranvier*. The sodium channels that are instrumental in nerve pulse propagation and conduction are concentrated at these nodes of Ranvier. Myelin increases the speed of nerve conduction. (140)

LOCAL ANESTHETIC ACTIONS ON SODIUM CHANNELS

10. Local anesthetics act by producing a conduction blockade of neural impulses in the affected nerve. This is accomplished through the prevention of the passage of sodium ions through voltage-gated sodium channels in the nerve membranes. The inability of sodium ions to pass through their ion selective channels results in slowing of the rate of depolarization. As a result, the threshold potential is not reached, and an action potential is not propagated. (140)

11. Local anesthetics are thought to exert their predominant action on the nerve by binding to a specific receptor on the sodium ion channel. Binding changes the relative stability of the conformational states of the sodium channel. The location of the binding site appears to be within the inner vestibule of the sodium channel. (140)

12. According to the modulated receptor model, sodium ion channels alternate between several conformational states, and local anesthetics bind to these different conformational states with different affinities. During excitation, the sodium channel moves from a resting-closed state to an activated-open state, with passage of sodium ions and consequent depolarization. After depolarization, the channel assumes an inactivated-closed conformational state. Local anesthetics bind to the activated and inactivated states more readily than the resting state, attenuating conformational change. Drug dissociation from the inactivated conformational state is slower than from the resting state. Thus, repeated depolarization produces more effective anesthetic binding. The electrophysiologic consequence of this effect is progressive enhancement of conduction blockade with repetitive stimulation, an effect referred to as *use-dependent* or *frequency-dependent* block. For this reason, selective conduction blockade of nerve fibers by local anesthetics may in part be related to the characteristic frequency of activity of the nerve. (142)

13. Myelin makes the nerve membrane more susceptible to local anesthetic-induced conduction blockade. (142)

14. In general, three consecutive nodes of Ranvier must be exposed to adequate concentrations of local anesthetic for the effective blockade of nerve impulses to occur. (142)

15. Neither the resting membrane potential nor the threshold potential is appreciably altered by local anesthetics. (142)

16. The conduction blockade produced by a local anesthetic is normally completely reversible (i.e., reversal of the blockade is spontaneous, predictable, and complete). (142)

17. Local anesthetics consist of a lipophilic end and a hydrophilic end connected by a hydrocarbon chain. The lipophilic end is an aromatic ring, and the hydrophilic end is a tertiary amine and proton acceptor. The bond that links the hydrocarbon chain to the lipophilic end of the structure is either an amino ester (−CO−) or an amino amide (−HNC−). The local anesthetic is thus classified as either an amino-ester or an amino-amide local anesthetic. This allows for the local anesthetic to be soluble and diffuse through both hydrophilic (extracellular fluid) and hydrophobic (lipid bilayers of plasma membranes) environments. (142)

18. Local anesthetics are bases that are poorly water-soluble. For this reason, they are marketed as hydrochloride salts. The resulting solution is generally slightly acidic with a pH of about 6. (142)

19. The pKa of most local anesthetics is greater than 7.4 (benzocaine is a notable exception with a pKa of approximately 3.5). This means that the pH at which the cationic form and nonionized form will be equivalent is greater than 7.4 for almost all the clinically used anesthetics. (142)

20. Most local anesthetic molecules exist in the ionized, hydrophilic form at physiologic pH. However, local anesthetics must be in the nonionized, lipid-soluble form to cross the lipophilic nerve cell membranes. Bicarbonate is sometimes added to local anesthetic solutions before injection to increase the nonionized fraction and thus hasten the onset of anesthesia. (142)

21. Local tissue acidosis is associated with a lower quality analgesia. This is presumed to be due to an increase in the ionized fraction of the local anesthetic in an acidotic environment, with less of the neutral form available to penetrate the cell membrane. (142)

22. The primary determinant of the potency of a local anesthetic is its lipid solubility. (142)

DIFFERENTIAL LOCAL ANESTHETIC BLOCKADE

23. Nerve conduction blockade is facilitated both by increasing the concentration of local anesthetic and by increasing the length of nerve exposed to more dilute concentrations of local anesthetic. (143)

24. Differential block refers to the clinical observation that when using dilute concentrations of local anesthetic there is a block of autonomic or sensory nerves with relative sparing of motor function. (144)

SPREAD OF LOCAL ANESTHESIA AFTER INJECTION

25. Local anesthetics diffuse along a concentration gradient from the outer surface, or mantle, of the nerve toward the center, or core, of the nerve. As a result, the nerve fibers located in the mantle of the nerve are blocked before those in the core of the nerve. (144)

26. In a peripheral nerve, the nerve fibers in the mantle generally innervate more proximal anatomic structures. The distal anatomic structures are more frequently innervated by nerve fibers near the core of the nerve. This physiologic orientation of nerve fibers in a peripheral nerve explains the observed initial proximal analgesia with subsequent progressive distal spread as local anesthetics diffuse to reach more central core nerve fibers. (144)

27. After the infiltration of a mixed peripheral nerve with local anesthetic, the temporal progression of the interruption of the transmission of impulses is autonomic, sensory, and then motor nerve blockade. (144)

28. The nerve fiber type A-δ, which is myelinated, conducts sharp or fast/first pain impulses. The nerve fiber type C, which is unmyelinated, conducts dull burning pain impulses. The large-diameter type A-δ fiber appears to be more sensitive to blockade than the smaller diameter type C fiber. This lends support to the theory that myelination of nerves has a greater influence than nerve fiber diameter on the conduction blockade produced by local anesthetics. In clinical

practice the use of relatively high concentrations of local anesthetic will overcome this difference. (144)

29. The nerve fiber types A-α and A-β, which are both myelinated, conduct motor nerve impulses. The nerve fiber type A-α conducts large motor nerve impulses, and the nerve fiber type A-β conducts small motor nerve impulses. (144)

PHARMACOKINETICS

30. In contrast to most systemically administered drugs, local anesthetics are deposited at the target site. Systemic absorption competes with local anesthetic entry into the nerve. Systemic uptake from the injection site therefore diminishes, rather than increases, nerve blockade efficacy. (144)

31. The rate of systemic uptake and the rate of clearance of the drug are the two primary determinants of peak plasma concentrations of a local anesthetic after its absorption from tissue sites. (144)

32. Systemic uptake of a local anesthetic injected at the target site is delayed for local anesthetics with high lipophilicity and protein binding. Uptake is increased from areas of high local tissue blood flow. (144)

33. The variability in local anesthetics to cause vasoconstriction may explain differences in the risk of systemic toxicity; for example, inherent vasoconstrictive effects of a local anesthetic may decrease its incidence of systemic toxicity. A second clinical implication is the difference in the degree of prolongation of a local anesthetic's clinical effect with the addition of an additive vasoconstrictor. (144)

34. Amino-ester local anesthetics are cleared by hydrolysis by pseudocholinesterase enzymes in the plasma. (147)

35. Amino-amide local anesthetics undergo metabolism in the liver by hepatic microsomal enzymes. (147)

36. The lungs and the liver both influence the potential for local anesthetic systemic toxicity (LAST). The extent to which the lungs extract local anesthetics from the circulation—so-called first-pass pulmonary extraction—influences systemic toxicity by preventing the rapid accumulation of local anesthetics in the plasma. The liver also influences LAST, especially for the amino-amide local anesthetics that depend upon the liver for metabolism. (147)

37. The relatively rapid hydrolysis by plasma cholinesterase makes chloroprocaine less likely to produce sustained plasma concentrations. (147)

38. Patients with atypical plasma cholinesterase enzyme may be at increased risk for developing excessive plasma concentrations of amino-ester local anesthetics. Amino-ester local anesthetics rely on plasma hydrolysis for their metabolism, which may be limited or absent in these patients. (147)

39. Lidocaine, an amino-amide local anesthetic, is cleared by hepatic metabolism. The clearance of lidocaine from the plasma parallels hepatic blood flow. Liver disease or decreases in hepatic blood flow as can occur with congestive heart failure or general anesthesia can decrease the rate of metabolism of lidocaine. (147)

40. Less than 5% of the injected dose of local anesthetic undergoes renal excretion unchanged. The low water solubility of local anesthetics limits their renal excretion. (147)

41. The addition of epinephrine to a local anesthetic solution produces local tissue vasoconstriction. This results in a slowing of the rate of systemic absorption of the local anesthetic. (147)

42. The addition of epinephrine to a local anesthetic solution produces local tissue vasoconstriction. This results in a prolonged duration of action of the local anesthetic by keeping the anesthetic in contact with the nerve fibers for a longer period of time. (147)

43. The addition of epinephrine to a local anesthetic solution causes a slower rate of systemic absorption and a prolonged duration of action. This increases the likelihood that the rate of metabolism will match the rate of absorption, resulting in a decrease in the possibility of systemic toxicity. Inclusion of

epinephrine may also decrease the potential for toxicity by serving as a marker for misplaced intravascular injection, whereby the elevation of heart rate can serve as a warning of such misplacement, alerting the clinician to halt injection and thus prevent the administration of additional anesthetic. (147)

44. The addition of epinephrine to a local anesthetic solution has little effect on the rate of onset of anesthesia. (147)

45. The addition of epinephrine to a local anesthetic solution decreases bleeding in the area infiltrated owing to its vasoconstrictive properties. (147)

46. The systemic absorption of epinephrine from the local anesthetic solution may contribute to cardiac dysrhythmias or accentuate hypertension in vulnerable patients. (147)

47. The addition of epinephrine to a local anesthetic solution may not be recommended in patients with unstable angina, cardiac dysrhythmias, uncontrolled hypertension, or uteroplacental insufficiency. The addition of epinephrine to a local anesthetic solution is not recommended for intravenous anesthesia or for peripheral nerve block anesthesia in areas that may lack collateral blood flow, such as the digits. (147)

48. Clonidine and dexamethasone are both additives to local anesthetic solution that have been shown to prolong the duration of anesthesia. (147)

ADVERSE EFFECTS

49. Potential negative side effects associated with the administration of local anesthetics include systemic toxicity, neurotoxicity, and allergic reactions. (147)

50. LAST occurs as a result of excessive plasma concentrations of a local anesthetic drug. The most common cause of LAST is accidental intravascular injection of local anesthetic solution during the performance of a peripheral nerve block. (147)

51. The magnitude of the systemic absorption of local anesthetic from the tissue injection site is influenced by the pharmacologic profile of the local anesthetic, the total dose injected, the vascularity of the injection site, and the inclusion of a vasoconstrictor in the local anesthetic solution. (147)

52. The relative order from highest to lowest of peak plasma concentrations of local anesthetic associated with regional anesthesia procedures is intercostal, caudal, epidural, brachial plexus, and sciatic/femoral. (147)

53. The central nervous system and cardiovascular system are most likely to be affected by excessive plasma concentrations of local anesthetic. (147)

54. The initial manifestations of central nervous system toxicity due to increasingly excessive plasma concentrations of local anesthetic include circumoral numbness, facial tingling, restlessness, vertigo, tinnitus, and slurred speech. With progressively increasing concentrations of local anesthetic in the plasma, symptoms may progress to manifestations of central nervous system excitation, such as facial and extremity muscular twitching and tremors. Finally, tonic-clonic seizures, apnea, and death can follow. However, deviations from this classic progression are common. (147)

55. Local anesthetic drugs in excessive plasma concentrations sufficient to cause seizures are believed to initially depress inhibitory pathways in the cerebral cortex. This allows for the unopposed action of excitatory pathways in the central nervous system, which manifests as seizures. As the concentration of local anesthetic in the plasma increases, there is subsequent inhibition of both excitatory and inhibitory pathways in the brain. Ultimately this leads to generalized global central nervous system depression. (148)

56. Potential adverse effects of local anesthetic-induced seizures are arterial hypoxemia, metabolic acidosis, and pulmonary aspiration of gastric contents. (148)

57. The mainstay of treatment of local anesthetic-induced seizures, as with all seizures, is aimed toward supporting the patient while attempting to abort the seizure with anticonvulsant drugs. Supplemental oxygen should be administered. The patient's airway may need to be secured. Anticonvulsant

drugs that can be used to stop local anesthetic-induced seizures include benzodiazepines. Diazepam is the preferred agent; propofol should be used cautiously in small doses as seizures may portend cardiovascular toxicity that might be augmented by propofol's cardiovascular depression. (148)

58. The administration of paralyzing doses of a rapidly acting neuromuscular blocking drug may be necessary to facilitate intubation of the trachea during a seizure. The administration of a neuromuscular blocking drug with prolonged paralytic effects during a seizure may be indicated when benzodiazepines and barbiturates have not been effective in stopping the seizure activity. However, although the neuromuscular block aborts the peripheral seizure activity, it does not alter the abnormal cerebral electrical activity and therefore does not negate the need to adequately control underlying seizure activity with anticonvulsants. (148)

59. The cardiovascular system is generally less susceptible to local anesthetic toxicity than the central nervous system. That is, the dose of local anesthetic required to produce central nervous system toxicity is less than the dose of local anesthetic required to result in cardiac toxicity. (148)

60. Two mechanisms by which local anesthetics can produce hypotension include the relaxation of peripheral vascular smooth muscle and direct myocardial depression. (148)

61. Local anesthetics exert their cardiotoxic effects primarily through the blockade of sodium ion channels in the myocardium. This blockade results in an increase in the conduction time throughout the heart, manifested as a prolongation of the PR interval and widening of the QRS complex. Local anesthetics also produce a dose-dependent negative inotropic effect. Clinically, these effects may result in a decreased cardiac output. With extremely elevated serum levels of local anesthetic, bradycardia and sinus arrest can result. (148)

62. The relative cardiotoxicity of local anesthetic agents is made through a comparison of the dose (or serum concentration) required to produce cardiovascular collapse relative to central nervous system toxicity. Through the evaluation of these ratios, it has been determined that bupivacaine is roughly twice as cardiotoxic as lidocaine and that levobupivacaine and ropivacaine are intermediate. (148)

63. The standard treatment for LAST is the intravenous infusion of lipid emulsions. The mechanism by which lipid is effective is incompletely understood, but its predominant action is possibly related to its ability to extract bupivacaine (or other lipophilic drugs) from aqueous plasma or tissue targets, thus reducing their effective free concentration ("lipid sink"). Lipid rescue for LAST is important but is not 100% effective. (148)

64. According to the American Society of Regional Anesthesia and Pain Medicine (ASRA) guidelines, the initial bolus of lipid emulsion to treat LAST is 1.5 mL/kg (100 mg in adults). This should be followed by a continuous infusion at 0.25 mL/kg/min. (148)

65. ASRA guidelines recommend standard advanced cardiac life support (ACLS) modifications in the event of LAST, which include avoidance of vasopressin, calcium channel blockers, β-adrenergic blockers, and other local anesthetics (lidocaine, amiodarone). Incremental dosing of epinephrine should be decreased to less than 1 μg/kg. (148)

66. Toxicity to local tissues (nerves and muscles) from local anesthetic injection increases in incidence with increased local tissue concentration and duration of exposure. Other factors that may increase nerve vulnerability include preexisting nerve dysfunction, metabolic and inflammatory conditions, increased tissue pressure, and systemic hypotension. (148-149)

67. Less than 1% of all adverse reactions to local anesthetics are believed to be true allergic reactions. Confirmation by measuring increases of serum tryptase (a marker of mast cell degranulation) may have some value. When an allergic reaction to a local anesthetic is suspected to have occurred, full documentation

should be made in the chart regarding the dose and route of local anesthetic administered and the reaction that occurred. Intradermal testing may be useful to establish the local anesthetic as the offending antigen. (149)

68. A hypersensitivity reaction might result from exposure not only to the local anesthetic itself but also to one of its metabolites. Amino-ester local anesthetics have a proclivity to induce allergic reactions because of one of its breakdown products, para-aminobenzoic acid, making amino esters more likely than amino amides to cause allergic reactions. Hypersensitivity reactions may also be caused by another component of the anesthetic solution. For example, the preservative methylparaben, used in some commercial preparations of both amino amides and amino esters, appears to have significant antigenic potential. (149)

69. Cross-sensitivity has not been found to exist between the classes of local anesthetics. A patient found to be allergic to amino-ester local anesthetics would not be expected to be allergic to amino-amide local anesthetics. This is assuming the local anesthetic itself, and not a common preservative, is responsible for the initial allergic reaction. (149)

SPECIFIC LOCAL ANESTHETICS

70. The primary use of procaine during the early 1900s was as a spinal anesthetic. (149)

71. Compared to lidocaine, procaine has greater instability, risk of hypersensitivity, incidence of nausea, and only a small advantage with respect to the incidence of transient neurologic symptoms (TNS). (149)

72. Tetracaine is primarily used as a spinal anesthetic in current clinical practice, where its long duration of action, particularly if used with a vasoconstrictor, can at times be a useful attribute. When used with a vasoconstrictor, however, spinal tetracaine carries a high risk of TNS. (149)

73. Tetracaine is rarely used for epidural anesthesia or peripheral nerve block because of its slow onset, profound motor blockade, and potential toxicity when administered at high doses. (149)

74. The rate of metabolism of tetracaine is much slower when compared to the other amino-ester local anesthetics. It is one fourth that of procaine and one tenth that of chloroprocaine. (149)

75. The administration of epidural chloroprocaine has been associated with neurotoxic injury when administered at recommended doses for epidural anesthesia that appeared to have been inadvertently administered into the intrathecal space. Early studies suggested that this effect might have occurred owing to a combination of the low pH of the anesthetic solution (pH approximately 3.0) and the antioxidant sodium bisulfite, which resulted in the liberation of sulfur dioxide. However, this mechanism has been challenged by more recent studies, which implicate the high doses of chloroprocaine. Nevertheless, a formulation of chloroprocaine without preservatives and antioxidants is available. (149)

76. Advantageous properties of chloroprocaine that make it useful in clinical practice include its rapid onset and its rapid hydrolysis, which limits the risk of systemic toxicity. There are also encouraging reports of its potential for intrathecal use with limited risk of TNS, although this off-label use should be bisulfite-free, and the intrathecal dose should be limited to 60 mg. (149)

77. The rapid plasma clearance of chloroprocaine makes it useful in current clinical pediatric practice as a continuous epidural infusion in neonates and very young infants. It is also useful in patients with a postoperative epidural or peripheral perineural infusion who require a repeated loading dose because a repeated dose of another local anesthetic could potentially lead to toxic plasma concentrations of local anesthetic. (150)

78. Uses of lidocaine in current clinical practice include local, topical, regional, intravenous, peripheral nerve, spinal, and epidural anesthesia. (150)

79. The occurrence of major (cauda equina syndrome) and minor (TNS) sequelae occurring with lidocaine has resulted in near abandonment of this agent for spinal anesthesia. (150)

80. Cauda equina syndrome represents the clinical manifestation of injury to the nerve roots caudal to the conus. Symptoms may include perineal sensory loss, bowel and bladder dysfunction, and lower extremity motor weakness. In the past, a cluster of cases was reported in association with the use of lidocaine administered through microbore spinal catheters (also referred to as *small-bore* and defined as smaller than 27 gauge). It is believed that pooling of local anesthetic in the most dependent portion of the intrathecal space led to high concentrations of local anesthetic around the nerve roots of the cauda equina and subsequent irreversible neurotoxicity. Small-bore catheters for continuous spinal anesthesia are no longer marketed in the United States. However, risk remains because similar neurotoxic injury can occur with repetitive doses of any local anesthetic even if administered through a large-bore (e.g., epidural) catheter. In fact, this mechanism of neurotoxic injury has also been reported with repeat needle injection after a failed single-injection spinal anesthesia. (150)

81. TNS is a syndrome of pain/dysesthesia that can be quite severe in the lower back, posterior thighs, or buttocks. The onset of TNS generally occurs within 12 to 24 hours of recovery from a spinal anesthetic. Full recovery from the symptoms most often occurs within 3 days. Importantly, TNS is not associated with sensory loss, motor weakness, or bowel or bladder dysfunction. (150)

82. Risk factors for TNS following spinal anesthesia include the use of lidocaine, lithotomy position during surgery, and outpatient status. Indeed, when these three risk factors are combined, TNS may occur in up to one third of patients. Similar to lithotomy, positioning for knee arthroscopy appears to dramatically increase risk. (150)

83. The first-line treatment for TNS is nonsteroidal anti-inflammatory drugs, which can be very effective. Rarely, a patient will have to be rehospitalized for the control of pain caused by TNS. (150)

84. Mepivacaine has similar clinical uses as lidocaine except that it is not an effective topical anesthetic. The duration of action of mepivacaine is slightly longer than that of lidocaine, and it has a lower incidence of TNS than lidocaine. (150)

85. The administration of prilocaine has been associated with methemoglobinemia in a dose-dependent manner, with significant toxicity generally occurring with doses exceeding 600 mg. Methemoglobinemia results from the accumulation of ortho-toluidine, a metabolite of prilocaine. Ortho-toluidine is an oxidizing compound that oxidizes hemoglobin to methemoglobin, creating methemoglobinemia. Methemoglobinemia that occurs through the administration of prilocaine is spontaneously reversible. Alternatively, methylene blue (1 to 2 mg/kg over 5 minutes) may be administered intravenously to treat this condition. Methemoglobinemia can also be a significant clinical problem with benzocaine topically administered on mucosal surfaces. (150)

86. Uses of bupivacaine in current clinical practice include peripheral nerve blocks, spinal anesthesia, and epidural anesthesia. (150)

87. Bupivacaine has a longer duration of action than lidocaine. Bupivacaine also imparts greater high-quality sensory anesthesia relative to motor blockade than lidocaine, making it useful for epidural anesthesia for patients in labor or for postoperative pain management. (150)

88. Bupivacaine is more cardiotoxic than lidocaine per dose administered to achieve a given anesthetic effect. Accidental intravenous injection of 0.75% bupivacaine has resulted in refractory cardiac arrest. When electrophysiologic differences between anesthetics are compared, lidocaine is found to enter the sodium ion channel quickly and to leave quickly. In contrast, recovery from bupivacaine blockade during diastole is relatively prolonged, making it far more

potent with respect to depressing the maximum upstroke velocity of the cardiac action potential (Vmax) in ventricular cardiac muscle. As a result, bupivacaine has been labeled a "fast-in, slow-out" local anesthetic. This characteristic likely creates conditions favorable for unidirectional block and reentry. Other mechanisms may contribute to bupivacaine's cardiotoxicity, including disruption of atrioventricular nodal conduction, depression of myocardial contractility, and indirect effects mediated by the central nervous system. (151)

89. Isomers are different compounds that have the same molecular formula. Subsets of isomers that have atoms connected by the same sequence of bonds but that have different spatial orientations are called *stereoisomers*. Enantiomers are a particular class of stereoisomers that exist as mirror images. The term *chiral* is derived from the Greek word *cheir* for "hand," because the forms can be considered nonsuperimposable mirror images. Enantiomers have identical physical properties except for the direction of the rotation of the plane of polarized light. This property is used to classify the enantiomer as dextrorotatory (+) if the rotation is to the right or clockwise and as levorotatory (–) if it is to the left or counterclockwise. A racemic mixture is a mixture of equal parts of enantiomers and is optically inactive because the rotation caused by the molecules of one isomer is canceled by the opposite rotation of its enantiomer. Chiral compounds can also be classified on the basis of absolute configuration, generally designated as R (rectus) or S (sinister). Enantiomers may differ with respect to specific biologic activity. (151)

90. Ropivacaine and levobupivacaine differ from other local anesthetics because they are chiral compounds rather than racemic mixtures. Both are S(–) enantiomers and were marketed in response to the cardiotoxic effects of bupivacaine because they appear to cause modestly less myocardial depression and are modestly less arrhythmogenic than bupivacaine. Ropivacaine has the additional advantage that motor blockade is even less pronounced than the motor blockade produced by bupivacaine, although its lower lipid solubility also makes it less potent than bupivacaine. (151)

91. Clinical uses of topical local anesthesia include its use on cut skin to facilitate laceration repair and its use on intact skin for needle procedures, especially in children. A potential risk of topical local anesthesia is systemic toxicity due to rapid absorption through mucosal surfaces. This is a recognized problem with excessive dosing of local anesthetic sprays and gels from the oral, nasal, or tracheobronchial mucosa, especially in infants and children. (151)

92. Eutectic mixture of local anesthetics (EMLA) cream is a topical anesthetic cream that consists of lidocaine 2.5% and prilocaine 2.5%. This mixture has a lower melting point than either component, and it exists as an oil at room temperature that is capable of overcoming the barrier of the skin. EMLA cream is particularly useful in children for relieving pain associated with venipuncture or placement of an intravenous catheter, although it may take up to an hour before adequate topical anesthesia is produced. The prolonged onset time is due to the effectiveness of the barrier to the diffusion of topical anesthetics created by the keratinized layer of the skin. (152)

93. Tumescent local anesthesia is the subcutaneous infusion of large volumes of very dilute local anesthetic. Tumescent local anesthesia is used in a variety of plastic and cosmetic surgical procedures. A potential risk of tumescent local anesthesia is systemic toxicity because the total dose of local anesthetic is large when administered by this technique. (152)

94. After the administration of lidocaine tumescent anesthesia, plasma concentrations of lidocaine usually peak after 12 hours following injection. Plasma concentrations of lidocaine tumescent anesthesia generally stay in a safe range when adherence to guidelines are kept due to the pharmacokinetics of the drug. However, additional dosing of local anesthetics over the next day has resulted in toxic reactions. (152)

95. Some clinical uses for systemic local anesthesia include use as systemic analgesics and as adjuvant analgesics for postoperative pain management. For some patients with neuropathic pain, brief intravenous lidocaine infusions have produced remarkable and extended pain relief. The duration of the pain relief outlasts the pharmacologic duration of lidocaine, sometimes for days or weeks. The mechanism for this effect is poorly understood. (152)

WHEN LOCAL ANESTHESIA FAILS

96. Some potential causes of local anesthesia failure include technical failure with its administration (i.e., erroneous needle placement), clinician error regarding the relevant neuroanatomic basis of the pain, clinician underappreciation of biologic sources of pain variation, diminished effectiveness of local anesthetics in sites of infection and inflammation (local acidosis, edema, hyperemia), and rapidly developing tolerance termed *tachyphylaxis*. (152)

97. Techniques that can be used to confirm proper needle placement when administering local anesthetic for epidural anesthesia and peripheral nerve blocks include ultrasound guidance, Tusi's nerve stimulation for epidural catheter placement, transduction of epidural space pressure waves, and selective use of fluoroscopy. (152)

98. Repeated dosing and prolonged infusions are risk factors for developing tachyphylaxis to local anesthetics. (152)

99. Hyperalgesia is a potential adverse effect of developing tachyphylaxis to local anesthetics. This risk can be minimized by the coadministration of antihyperalgesic drugs or other analgesics with central actions. (152)

100. Chronic pain alters the patient's response to local anesthetics, often requiring higher volumes and concentrations of local anesthetic to achieve adequate analgesia. They often require coadministration of other analgesic or antihyperalgesic drugs as well. A possible mechanism for this effect is through alterations in the sodium channel in peripheral nerves. Nerve injury and inflammation change the expression of different sodium channel subtypes, altering sodium channel electrophysiology, and thereby altering local anesthetic responsiveness. (153)

11 NEUROMUSCULAR BLOCKING DRUGS

Ronald D. Miller and Tula Gourdin

1. Describe the physiologic effect of neuromuscular blocking drugs (NMBDs).

CLINICAL USES

2. What are some clinical situations in which NMBDs are used to produce skeletal muscle relaxation?
3. What analgesic effects do NMBDs have?
4. How does the clinician evaluate the intensity of the neuromuscular blockade?
5. What are some characteristics of NMBDs that may influence the choice of which drug is administered to a given patient?
6. What percentage of life-threatening anesthetic-related hypersensitivity reactions are caused by NMBDs?
7. Which NMBDs are the common offenders to triggering life-threatening anesthetic-related hypersensitivity reactions?
8. What is an antigenic component that is common to all NMBDs, resulting in possible allergic cross-reactivity of these drugs?
9. What is the most common hypersensitivity reaction to sugammadex?

NEUROMUSCULAR JUNCTION

10. What is the neuromuscular junction (NMJ)?
11. What events lead to the release of neurotransmitter at the NMJ? What is the neurotransmitter that is released?
12. What class of receptors is located at prejunctional and postjunctional sites?
13. What clinical effect results from the stimulation of postjunctional receptors?
14. How is the effect of acetylcholine on the postjunctional receptors terminated?
15. Where is acetylcholinesterase located in the NMJ?
16. With respect to the NMJ, what are the sites at which nicotinic cholinergic receptors are located?
17. What is the role of prejunctional receptors?
18. What is the structure of nicotinic cholinergic receptors?
19. Where are the binding sites for acetylcholine on the nicotinic cholinergic receptor?
20. What effect does acetylcholine binding have on the receptor?
21. What effect does the binding of a nondepolarizing NMBD have on the receptor?
22. What effect does the binding of a depolarizing NMBD have on the receptor?
23. What is the role of extrajunctional receptors?
24. How does the structure of extrajunctional nicotinic cholinergic receptors differ from the postjunctional receptors?
25. What is the potential clinical effect of the stimulation of extrajunctional receptors?

STRUCTURE-ACTIVITY RELATIONSHIPS

26. How does the chemical structure of NMBDs relate to their pharmacologic action?
27. How do the chemical structures of succinylcholine and nondepolarizing NMBDs compare to acetylcholine?

DEPOLARIZING NEUROMUSCULAR BLOCKING DRUGS

28. What are some characteristics of succinylcholine that makes it unique among the NMBDs?
29. What is the intubating dose of succinylcholine? What are its approximate time of onset and duration of action when administered at this dose?
30. How should the intubating dose of succinylcholine be altered if a subparalyzing dose of a nondepolarizing NMBD has been administered to blunt fasciculations?
31. What is the mechanism of action of succinylcholine?
32. What is phase I neuromuscular blockade?
33. What is phase II neuromuscular blockade? What is the mechanism by which it occurs?
34. When is phase II neuromuscular blockade most likely to occur clinically?
35. Why do skeletal muscle fasciculations occur with the administration of succinylcholine?
36. Why do plasma potassium concentrations increase with the administration of succinylcholine?
37. By how many milliequivalents (mEq) will the plasma potassium concentration increase with the administration of succinylcholine?
38. How is the effect of succinylcholine at the cholinergic receptor terminated?
39. How efficiently does plasma cholinesterase hydrolyze succinylcholine?
40. How is the duration of action of succinylcholine influenced by plasma cholinesterase?
41. Where is plasma cholinesterase produced?
42. What are some drugs, chemicals, or clinical diseases that may affect the activity of plasma cholinesterase?
43. What is atypical plasma cholinesterase? What is its clinical significance?
44. What is dibucaine? What is its clinical use?
45. What is a normal dibucaine number?
46. In the case of individuals heterozygous for atypical plasma cholinesterase, what is the associated dibucaine number, duration of action of an intubating dose of succinylcholine, and incidence in the population?
47. In the case of individuals homozygous for atypical plasma cholinesterase, what is the associated dibucaine number, duration of action of an intubating dose of succinylcholine, and incidence in the population?
48. What is the concern regarding the administration of succinylcholine to children?
49. What are some adverse cardiac dysrhythmias that may result from the administration of succinylcholine?
50. What is the mechanism of cardiac dysrhythmias associated with the administration of succinylcholine?
51. When are cardiac dysrhythmias associated with the administration of succinylcholine likely to occur?
52. How can the potential risk of adverse cardiac rhythms associated with the administration of succinylcholine be minimized?
53. What is the mechanism by which massive hyperkalemia may result from the administration of succinylcholine?
54. Which patients are especially at risk for massive hyperkalemia with the administration of succinylcholine?
55. Are renal failure patients at increased risk for hyperkalemia in response to the administration of succinylcholine?
56. What is the mechanism by which succinylcholine administration may cause postoperative myalgia?
57. Which muscles are typically affected by myalgia associated with the administration of succinylcholine?
58. Myalgia presenting after the administration of succinylcholine typically manifests in which skeletal muscles?
59. How might the fasciculations associated with the administration of succinylcholine be prevented?

60. What is the treatment for myalgia associated with the administration of succinylcholine?
61. What effect does the administration of succinylcholine have on intraocular pressure?
62. What is the clinical significance of the effect of succinylcholine on intraocular pressure?
63. What effect does the administration of succinylcholine have on intracranial pressure?
64. What is the clinical significance of the effect of succinylcholine on intracranial pressure?
65. What effect does the administration of succinylcholine have on intragastric pressure?
66. What is the clinical significance of the effect of succinylcholine on intragastric pressure?
67. What effect does the administration of succinylcholine have on masseter muscle tension?
68. What is the clinical significance of the effect of succinylcholine on masseter muscle tension?

NONDEPOLARIZING NEUROMUSCULAR BLOCKING DRUGS

69. What is the mechanism of action of nondepolarizing NMBDs?
70. How does the limited lipid solubility of nondepolarizing NMBDs affect their clinical effect?
71. What are some of the methods by which nondepolarizing NMBDs are cleared? How does this influence their duration of action?
72. What are some drugs and physiologic states that may enhance the neuromuscular blockade produced by nondepolarizing NMBDs?
73. What are some drugs and physiologic states that may diminish the neuromuscular blockade produced by nondepolarizing NMBDs?
74. What are some of the methods by which nondepolarizing NMBDs may exert cardiovascular effects?
75. What is the potential adverse effect of the prolonged administration of nondepolarizing NMBDs to patients in the intensive care unit?
76. Which patients are at risk for developing a myopathy in the intensive care unit?
77. What is the recommendation for the administration of nondepolarizing NMBDs to patients in the intensive care unit?

LONG-ACTING NONDEPOLARIZING NEUROMUSCULAR BLOCKING DRUGS

78. For pancuronium, what is the ED_{95} (95% effective dose), time of onset of action, and duration of action?
79. How is pancuronium cleared from the plasma?
80. How is clearance of pancuronium affected by renal disease?
81. What are the cardiovascular effects of pancuronium? What is the mechanism by which these effects occur?

INTERMEDIATE-ACTING NONDEPOLARIZING NEUROMUSCULAR BLOCKING DRUGS

82. Name some intermediate-acting nondepolarizing NMBDs.
83. How do the intermediate-acting nondepolarizing NMBDs compare to pancuronium?
84. For vecuronium, what is the ED_{95}, time of onset of action, and duration of action?
85. How is vecuronium excreted from the body?
86. How does renal failure affect the clearance of vecuronium?
87. What are the cardiovascular effects of vecuronium?
88. For rocuronium, what is the ED_{95}, time of onset of action, and duration of action?
89. How does the time of onset of rocuronium compare with the time of onset of succinylcholine?
90. How is rocuronium excreted from the body?

91. For atracurium, what is the ED_{95}, time of onset of action, and duration of action?
92. How is atracurium cleared from the plasma?
93. What is the major metabolite of atracurium and its potential physiologic effect?
94. What are the cardiovascular effects of atracurium?
95. For cisatracurium, what is the ED_{95}, time of onset of action, and duration of action?
96. What is the structural relationship between cisatracurium and atracurium?
97. How is cisatracurium cleared from the plasma?
98. What are the cardiovascular effects of cisatracurium?

SHORT-ACTING NONDEPOLARIZING NEUROMUSCULAR BLOCKING DRUGS

99. For mivacuronium, what is the ED_{95}, time of onset of action, and duration of action?
100. How is mivacurium cleared from the plasma?
101. How is the duration of action of mivacurium altered in patients with atypical plasma cholinesterase?

MONITORING THE EFFECTS OF NONDEPOLARIZING NEUROMUSCULAR BLOCKING DRUGS

102. What is the most reliable method for monitoring the effects of NMBDs during general anesthesia?
103. What are some uses of a peripheral nerve stimulator when administering NMBDs during general anesthesia?
104. Are there advantages to the routine monitoring of the effects of NMBDs during general anesthesia?
105. Which nerve and muscle are most commonly used to evaluate the neuromuscular blockade produced by NMBDs?
106. Which nerves may be used for the evaluation of the neuromuscular blockade produced by NMBDs through the use of a peripheral nerve stimulator when the arm is not available to the anesthesia provider?
107. How do the NMBDs vary with regard to their time of onset at the adductor pollicis muscle, orbicularis oculi muscle, laryngeal muscles, and diaphragm?
108. What are some of the mechanical responses evoked by a peripheral nerve stimulator that are used to monitor the effects of NMBDs?
109. What percentage of depression of a mechanically evoked single twitch response from its control height correlates with adequate neuromuscular blockade for the performance of intra-abdominal surgery?
110. What is the train-of-four stimulus delivered by a peripheral nerve stimulator?
111. What is the clinical use of a train-of-four stimulus delivered by a peripheral nerve stimulator?
112. What is the train-of-four ratio?
113. What is the clinical use of the train-of-four ratio?
114. What train-of-four ratio correlates with the complete return to control height of a single twitch response?
115. What train-of-four ratio reflects phase I neuromuscular blockade after the administration of succinylcholine?
116. What train-of-four ratio reflects phase II neuromuscular blockade after the administration of succinylcholine?
117. How accurate is the estimation of the train-of-four ratio by clinicians evaluating the response visually and manually?
118. What is the double burst stimulus delivered by a peripheral nerve stimulator?
119. What is the clinical use of the double burst stimulus?
120. What is tetanus? How is tetanus mechanically produced by a peripheral nerve stimulator?
121. What is the normal response to tetanus produced by a peripheral nerve stimulator?
122. How is the response to tetanus altered by the administration of a depolarizing NMBD?

123. How is the response to tetanus altered by the administration of a nondepolarizing NMBD?
124. What is post-tetanic facilitation?
125. What is the clinical use of post-tetanic facilitation?

ANTAGONISM OF NONDEPOLARIZING NEUROMUSCULAR BLOCKING DRUGS

126. Name some anticholinesterase drugs that are used for the antagonism of the effects of NMBDs.
127. What is the mechanism by which anticholinesterase drugs antagonize the neuromuscular blockade produced by nondepolarizing NMBDs?
128. How are the cardiac muscarinic effects of anticholinesterases attenuated?
129. If the response to peripheral nerve stimulation is normal, should one still give a small dose of neostigmine or sugammadex?

ADVERSE OUTCOMES FROM INADEQUATE ANTAGONISM OF NEUROMUSCULAR BLOCKADE

130. What are some potential complications in the postanesthesia care unit (PACU) that may be augmented by the presence of postoperative residual neuromuscular blockade?
131. Name some factors that influence the success of antagonism of NMBDs.
132. How can the adequacy of the recovery from the effects of neuromuscular blockade be evaluated?
133. When is the spontaneous recovery from NMBDs recommended?
134. What are some pharmacologic or physiologic factors that may interfere with the antagonism of the neuromuscular blockade produced by NMBDs?
135. What is sugammadex? What is the mechanism of action of sugammadex?
136. What are the major clinical differences between sugammadex and neostigmine?
137. What are some advantages of sugammadex for the antagonism of neuromuscular blockade?
138. What is the dose of sugammadex for the reversal of the effects of vecuronium or rocuronium?

ANSWERS*

1. Neuromuscular blocking drugs (NMBDs) interrupt the transmission of nerve impulses at the neuromuscular junction (NMJ) and thereby produce paresis or paralysis of skeletal muscles. (156)

CLINICAL USES

2. The most frequent clinical uses of NMBDs are to produce skeletal muscle relaxation to facilitate tracheal intubation and to provide optimal surgical working conditions. Other clinical situations in which NMBDs are used include during cardiopulmonary resuscitation and to facilitate mechanical ventilation of the lungs in emergency departments and in the intensive care unit. (157)
3. NMBDs do not have any anesthetic or analgesic effects. The potential exists for the patient to be rendered paralyzed without adequate anesthesia and subsequently experience awareness during anesthesia. (157)
4. Intraoperative clinical evaluation of the intensity of the neuromuscular blockade is by monitoring the mechanical response (twitch response) produced by electrical stimulation of a peripheral nerve delivered from a peripheral nerve stimulator. (157)
5. NMBDs vary in their mechanism of action, speed of onset, duration of action, route of elimination, and associated side effects. These characteristics of an NMBD may influence whether a specific NMBD is chosen for administration to a given patient. (157)

6. NMBDs are the cause of approximately 11% to 35% of life-threatening anesthetic-related hypersensitivity reactions. Antibiotics are the most common cause. (157)

7. The NMBDs rocuronium and succinylcholine are the most common offenders for triggering life-threatening anesthetic-related hypersensitivity reactions. (157)

8. The quaternary ammonium group is an antigenic component that is common to all NMBDs, resulting in possible allergic cross-reactivity of these drugs. (157)

9. The most common hypersensitivity reactions to sugammadex are nausea and urticaria. (157)

NEUROMUSCULAR JUNCTION

10. The NMJ is the location where the transmission of neural impulses at the motor nerve terminal becomes translated into skeletal muscle contraction at the motor end plate. The highly specialized NMJ consists of the prejunctional motor nerve ending separated from the highly folded postjunctional membrane of the skeletal muscle by a synaptic cleft. (158)

11. A nerve impulse conducted down the motor nerve fiber, or axon, ends in the prejunctional motor nerve ending. The resulting stimulation of the motor nerve terminal causes an influx of calcium into the nerve terminal, which leads to the release of the neurotransmitter acetylcholine into the synaptic cleft. This is why administration of calcium briefly improves neuromuscular function. The nerve synthesizes and stores acetylcholine in vesicles in the motor nerve terminals, which is available for release with the influx of calcium. Acetylcholine released into the synaptic cleft binds to receptors in the postjunctional skeletal muscle membrane, leading to skeletal muscle contraction. (158)

12. Nicotinic acetylcholine receptors are located at prejunctional and postjunctional sites. (158)

13. When acetylcholine binds to receptors (the ligand-gated channel) on postjunctional membranes, there is a change in membrane permeability to ions, principally to sodium and potassium. The resultant movement of these ions down their concentration gradients causes a decrease in the transmembrane potential from about -90 mV to -45 mV (threshold potential), at which point a propagated action potential spreads over the surfaces of skeletal muscle fibers and leads to muscular contraction. Thus, the clinical effect of stimulation of postjunctional receptors is skeletal muscle contraction. (158)

14. The effect of acetylcholine on the postjunctional receptors is through the hydrolysis of acetylcholine. Acetylcholine is rapidly hydrolyzed (within 15 ms) by the enzyme acetylcholinesterase, thus restoring membrane permeability (repolarization) and preventing sustained depolarization. (158)

15. Acetylcholinesterase is located in the folds of the motor end-plate region of the NMJ. This places acetylcholinesterase in close proximity to the site of action of acetylcholine. (158)

16. Nicotinic cholinergic receptors are located in three separate sites relative to the NMJ and are referred to by their varied locations: prejunctional, postjunctional, and extrajunctional. Prejunctional receptors are located at the motor nerve terminal. Postjunctional receptors are located just opposite the prejunctional receptors in the motor end plate and are the most important receptors for the action of NMBDs. Extrajunctional receptors are immature in form and are located throughout the skeletal muscles. (158-159)

17. Prejunctional receptors facilitate the replenishment of acetylcholine in the motor nerve terminal. The role of prejunctional receptors, i.e., replenishment of acetylcholine in the motor nerve terminal, is aided by calcium. (159)

18. Nicotinic cholinergic receptors are made up of glycoproteins divided into five subunits. There are two α-subunits and one each of β-, γ-, and δ-subunits. The subunits are arranged in such a way that they form a channel in the membrane. (159)

19. There are two binding sites for acetylcholine on the nicotinic cholinergic receptor, the two α-subunits. (159)
20. Acetylcholine must bind to both of the two α-subunits of the receptor to stimulate the receptor. When the receptor becomes stimulated by the binding of acetylcholine, the channel changes conformation such that it allows the flow of ions through the cell membrane along their concentration gradient. (159)
21. Nondepolarizing NMBDs also bind to the α-subunits of the receptor but only require that one α-subunit be bound to exert their pharmacologic effect. With the binding of a nondepolarizing NMBD to an α-subunit on the receptor, acetylcholine is unable to bind to the receptor, the flow of ions across the channel does not occur, and the physiologic effect of skeletal muscle contraction becomes blocked. (159)
22. The binding of a depolarizing NMBD requires that both α-subunits be bound before stimulating the receptor to change conformation and the resulting skeletal muscle contraction. Succinylcholine exerts its effect in this manner. The elimination of succinylcholine is through its clearance from the plasma and requires a few minutes to occur. This accounts for its prolonged binding period on the nicotinic cholinergic receptor and subsequent skeletal muscle paralysis for the minutes after its administration. (159)
23. Extrajunctional receptors are present throughout the skeletal muscles. They differ from the other two types of nicotinic cholinergic receptors both in their location and by their molecular structure. Under normal circumstances, the synthesis of extrajunctional receptors is suppressed by neural activity and has minimal contribution to skeletal muscle action. Extrajunctional receptors may proliferate under conditions of denervation, trauma, strokes, or burn injury. Conversely, when neuromuscular activity returns to normal, extrajunctional receptors quickly lose their activity. Extrajunctional receptors are stimulated more by lower concentrations of acetylcholine and depolarizing NMBDs than are prejunctional or postjunctional receptors. (159)
24. Extrajunctional receptors differ slightly from postjunctional nicotinic cholinergic receptors in that the γ- and δ-subunits of these receptors are altered from those of the postjunctional receptors. The two α-subunits, however, are identical. (159)
25. When activated, extrajunctional receptors remain open longer and permit more ions to flow across the skeletal muscle cell membrane. Clinically, this may manifest as an exaggerated hyperkalemic response when succinylcholine is administered to patients with denervation or burn injuries. (159)

STRUCTURE-ACTIVITY RELATIONSHIPS

26. Both depolarizing and nondepolarizing NMBDs have a chemical structure similar to that of acetylcholine, which explains the pharmacologic activity at the nicotinic cholinergic receptor. All NMBDs are quaternary ammonium compounds that have at least one positively charged nitrogen atom that binds to the α-subunit of postsynaptic cholinergic receptors. (159)
27. Succinylcholine is two acetylcholine molecules linked by methyl groups. The long, slender, flexible structure of succinylcholine allows it to bind to and activate cholinergic receptors. Nondepolarizing NMBDs are bulky rigid molecules that, though containing portions similar to acetylcholine, do not activate cholinergic receptors. (161)

DEPOLARIZING NEUROMUSCULAR BLOCKING DRUGS

28. Succinylcholine is the only nondepolarizing NMBD used in clinical practice. It is also unique among the NMBDs in its rapid onset and ultrashort duration. (161)
29. Although an intravenous dose of 0.5 to 1.5 mg/kg may be adequate, 1.0 to 1.5 mg/kg of succinylcholine is commonly administered to facilitate tracheal intubation. Complete muscle paralysis after the administration of succinylcholine is typically within 30 to 60 seconds, and the duration of action is usually 5 to 10 minutes. (161)

30. If a subparalyzing dose of a nondepolarizing NMBD has been administered to blunt fasciculations, the intubating dose of succinylcholine should be increased by about 70%. (161)

31. Succinylcholine acts at the nicotinic cholinergic receptor through a similar mechanism as acetylcholine. Succinylcholine attaches to the two α-subunits on the nicotinic cholinergic receptor and causes the ion channel in the muscle cell to open. This results in depolarization of the skeletal muscle cell. Unlike acetylcholine, succinylcholine is not hydrolyzed at the motor end plate but continues to attach to the cholinergic receptors until it is cleared from the plasma. The administration of succinylcholine therefore results in sustained depolarization of the motor end plate. The skeletal muscle paralysis associated with the administration of succinylcholine is due to the inability of the depolarized postjunctional membrane to respond to a subsequent release of acetylcholine. (161)

32. Phase I neuromuscular blockade, also known as depolarizing neuromuscular blockade, refers to the blockade of the transmission of neuromuscular impulses caused by succinylcholine with its initial administration. This neuromuscular blockade is due to succinylcholine remaining on the receptor and the sustained depolarization of skeletal muscle cells that results. The sustained depolarization prevents the muscle cell from being able to respond to a subsequent release of acetylcholine. (161)

33. Phase II neuromuscular blockade is present when the postjunctional membrane has become repolarized but still does not respond normally to acetylcholine (desensitization neuromuscular blockade). The mechanism of phase II blockade is unknown but may reflect the development of nonexcitable areas around the motor end plates that become repolarized but nevertheless prevent the spread of impulses initiated by the action of acetylcholine. Phase II neuromuscular blockade resembles the blockade produced by nondepolarizing NMBDs. (161)

34. Phase II neuromuscular blockade is most likely to occur when the NMJ is continuously exposed to a depolarizing NMBD. This may occur with a succinylcholine infusion, with the administration of a second dose of succinylcholine after the first, or when the intravenous dose of succinylcholine administered exceeds 3 to 5 mg/kg. (161)

35. When succinylcholine is administered there is a sustained depolarization, and subsequent sustained opening of the cholinergic receptor ion channel, that manifests clinically as skeletal muscle fasciculations. (161)

36. The sustained opening of the nicotinic cholinergic receptor ion channel that occurs with the administration of succinylcholine is associated with leakage of potassium from the interior of cells. This leads to an increase in plasma potassium concentrations. (162)

37. The potassium ion transfer associated with the administration of succinylcholine is sufficient to increase plasma concentrations of potassium by about 0.1 to 0.4 mEq/L. With proliferation of extrajunctional nicotinic cholinergic receptors and damaged muscle membranes, many more channels will leak potassium and can lead to greater increases in plasma potassium concentrations, making patients susceptible to hyperkalemia. (162)

38. The effect of succinylcholine at the cholinergic receptor is terminated by the diffusion of succinylcholine away from the NMJ and into the extracellular fluid. In the extracellular fluid succinylcholine is rapidly hydrolyzed by the enzyme plasma cholinesterase. The enzyme responsible for the hydrolysis of succinylcholine plasma cholinesterase is also referred to as pseudocholinesterase. This is in contrast to acetylcholinesterase, or true cholinesterase, the enzyme responsible for the hydrolysis of acetylcholine. (162)

39. Plasma cholinesterase hydrolyzes succinylcholine at a rapid rate and extremely efficiently, such that only a small fraction of the original intravenous succinylcholine dose reaches the NMJ. (162)

40. Plasma cholinesterase influences the duration of action of succinylcholine by controlling the amount of succinylcholine that is hydrolyzed before reaching the NMJ. (162)

41. Plasma cholinesterase is produced in the liver. (162)

42. Potent anticholinesterases often used in insecticides or for the treatment of myasthenia gravis, and certain chemotherapeutic drugs (e.g., nitrogen mustard, cyclophosphamide), can significantly decrease plasma cholinesterase activity such that prolonged skeletal muscle paralysis follows the administration of succinylcholine. Prolonged effects of succinylcholine lasting as long as 1 to 3 hours may occur. Liver disease may also result in a decrease in the amount of circulating plasma cholinesterase. The degree of liver disease must be severe before the synthesis of plasma cholinesterase is sufficiently decreased to result in prolonged skeletal muscle paralysis after the administration of succinylcholine. (162)

43. Atypical plasma cholinesterase is an abnormal genetic variant of the plasma cholinesterase enzyme that lacks the ability to hydrolyze ester bonds in drugs such as succinylcholine and mivacurium. Patients who are otherwise healthy may have atypical plasma cholinesterase enzyme. Its presence is often recognized only after an otherwise healthy patient experiences prolonged skeletal muscle paralysis (longer than 1 hour) after the administration of a conventional dose of succinylcholine or mivacurium. (162)

44. Dibucaine is an amide local anesthetic that inhibits normal plasma activity by about 80%, whereas the activity of atypical enzyme is inhibited by about 20%. This characteristic of dibucaine has led to an evaluation of the percent of inhibition of plasma cholinesterase activity by dibucaine, the result of which is referred to as the dibucaine number. The dibucaine number reflects the quality, and not the quantity, of plasma cholinesterase enzyme that is circulating in plasma. For example, decreases in plasma cholinesterase activity because of liver disease or anticholinesterases are often associated with a normal dibucaine number. (162)

45. The normal dibucaine number is 80. That is, normal plasma cholinesterase enzyme is inhibited by 80% in the presence of dibucaine. (162)

46. An individual heterozygous for atypical plasma cholinesterase would have a dibucaine number between 40 and 60. In these individuals a conventional dose of succinylcholine would lead to neuromuscular blockade that persisted for approximately 20 minutes. The incidence of individuals heterozygous for atypical plasma cholinesterase is about 1 in 480. (162)

47. An individual homozygous for atypical plasma cholinesterase would have a dibucaine number of about 20. In these individuals a conventional dose of succinylcholine would lead to neuromuscular blockade persisting for 60 to 180 minutes. The incidence of individuals homozygous for atypical plasma cholinesterase is about 1 in 3200. (162)

48. The Food and Drug Administration (FDA) has issued a warning against the use of succinylcholine in children except for emergency airway control. Administration of succinylcholine to apparently healthy boys with unrecognized muscular dystrophy has resulted in acute hyperkalemia and cardiac arrest. (163)

49. Adverse cardiac dysrhythmias that can result from the administration of succinylcholine include sinus bradycardia, junctional rhythms, and even sinus arrest. (163)

50. The mechanism of cardiac dysrhythmias associated with the administration of succinylcholine is likely due to the similarity of the chemical structures of succinylcholine and acetylcholine. In addition to stimulating nicotinic receptors, succinylcholine may stimulate cardiac postganglionic muscarinic receptors in the sinus node of the heart and mimic the normal effect of acetylcholine at these receptors. The effects of succinylcholine at autonomic nervous system ganglia also mimic the actions of the neurotransmitter

acetylcholine and may be manifested as a ganglionic stimulation with associated increases in systemic blood pressure and heart rate. (163)

51. Cardiac dysrhythmias associated with the administration of succinylcholine are most likely to occur when a second intravenous dose of succinylcholine is administered about 5 minutes after the first. (163)

52. The potential risk of adverse cardiac rhythms associated with the administration of succinylcholine may be minimized by pretreating patients. An effective pretreatment regimen is the intravenous administration of atropine 1 to 3 minutes before succinylcholine. Yet atropine administered intramuscularly with the preoperative medication does not reliably protect against succinylcholine-induced decreases in heart rate. (163)

53. Massive hyperkalemia (greater than 10 mEq/L in some patients) leading to serious cardiac arrhythmias and even cardiac arrest may result from the administration of succinylcholine. This occurs in susceptible patients secondary to a proliferation of extrajunctional receptors in the area of skeletal muscle after a denervation injury. These extrajunctional receptors are especially sensitive to succinylcholine. With the administration of succinylcholine to patients with a history of denervation injury there are more ion channels being opened and more sites for the leakage of potassium out of cells during depolarization. (163)

54. Patients at risk for massive hyperkalemia after succinylcholine administration include those with burns, trauma, and spinal cord or other neurologic damage. Patients may be susceptible to hyperkalemia 48 hours after injury, when there is prolonged skeletal muscle inactivity (such as immobile critical care patients) or when extensive muscle damage exists. When muscle returns to its normal state, hyperkalemia will not occur. However, the judgment of what is the "normal" state of the muscle is clinically difficult to estimate. The duration of susceptibility to the hyperkalemic effects of succinylcholine is unknown, but the risk is probably decreased 3 to 6 months after denervation injury. All factors considered, it is prudent to avoid the administration of succinylcholine to any patient more than 24 hours after a burn injury, extensive trauma, or spinal cord transection or who may become an intensive care patient. (163)

55. Even though patients with renal failure have increased potassium levels, they are not susceptible to an exaggerated release of potassium. Succinylcholine can be safely administered to patients with renal failure, unless they have uremic neuropathy. (163)

56. Postoperative myalgia after succinylcholine administration is thought to occur as a result of the transient, generalized, unsynchronized skeletal muscle fiber contractions, or fasciculations, that accompany its administration. (163)

57. Postoperative myalgia associated with the administration of succinylcholine is most often manifest in the muscles of the neck, back, and abdomen. Myalgias localized to the neck may be described as a sore throat by the patient and may be incorrectly attributed to tracheal intubation as the cause of the pain. (164)

58. Young adults undergoing minor surgical procedures that allow for early ambulation are most likely to complain about myalgia after the administration of succinylcholine. (164)

59. The fasciculations associated with the administration of succinylcholine may be prevented by the prior administration of subparalyzing doses of a nondepolarizing NMBD (pretreatment) or lidocaine. Prevention of fasciculations will decrease the incidence of, but not totally prevent, myalgia. Magnesium will also prevent fasciculations but not myalgia. (164)

60. Nonsteroidal anti-inflammatory drugs are effective in treating myalgia associated with the administration of succinylcholine. (164)

61. The administration of succinylcholine is associated with transient increases in intraocular pressure. The mechanism by which this occurs is unknown, although contraction of extraocular muscles with associated compression of the

globe may be involved. The transient increase in intraocular pressure peaks 2 to 4 minutes after the administration of succinylcholine and lasts 5 to 10 minutes. (164)

62. The clinical concern of the effect of succinylcholine on intraocular pressure is that the contraction of extraocular muscles could cause extrusion of intraocular contents in the presence of an open eye injury. This has resulted in the common clinical practice of avoiding the administration of succinylcholine to these patients. This theory has never been substantiated and is challenged by the report of patients with an open eye injury in whom the intravenous administration of succinylcholine did not cause extrusion of globe contents. Furthermore, there is evidence that contraction of extraocular muscles does not contribute to the increase in intraocular pressure that accompanies the administration of succinylcholine. (164)

63. The administration of succinylcholine causes increases in intracranial pressure. (164)

64. Increases in intracranial pressures associated with the administration of succinylcholine are of little or no clinical significance. (164)

65. The administration of succinylcholine causes unpredictable increases in intragastric pressure. When intragastric pressure does increase, it seems related to the intensity of fasciculations, thus emphasizing the potential value of preventing this skeletal muscle activity by prior administration of a subparalyzing dose of a nondepolarizing NMBD. (164)

66. An unproved hypothesis is that the increased intragastric pressure associated with the administration of succinylcholine may cause passage of gastric fluid and contents into the esophagus and pharynx and increase the risk for pulmonary aspiration. (164)

67. Succinylcholine administration can result in varying degrees of increased masseter muscle tension. For pediatric patients incomplete jaw relaxation with masseter jaw rigidity after a halothane-succinylcholine sequence is not uncommon. (164)

68. In extreme cases, the effect of succinylcholine on masseter muscle tension may be so severe that it can result in trismus and in difficulty opening the mouth for direct laryngoscopy and intubation of the trachea. A second clinical issue is the potential difficulty in separating the normal response to succinylcholine from the masseter rigidity that may be associated with malignant hyperthermia. Pediatric patients are especially at risk for this complication of succinylcholine administration, but because it is not recommended for use in children (except for emergency airway control), trismus in children is less of an issue. (164)

NONDEPOLARIZING NEUROMUSCULAR BLOCKING DRUGS

69. Nondepolarizing NMBDs act by competing with acetylcholine for α-subunits at the postjunctional nicotinic cholinergic receptors and preventing changes in ion permeability. As a result, depolarization cannot occur (hence the designation nondepolarizing neuromuscular blockade), and skeletal muscle paralysis develops. Fasciculations do not accompany the administration of nondepolarizing NMBDs. (164)

70. Nondepolarizing NMBDs have very limited lipid solubility. This is because of their quaternary ammonium groups, which are highly ionized, water-soluble compounds at physiologic pH. As a result, these drugs cannot easily cross lipid membrane barriers, such as the blood-brain barrier, renal tubular epithelium, gastrointestinal epithelium, or placenta. Therefore, nondepolarizing NMBDs do not produce central nervous system effects, undergo minimal renal tubular absorption, are ineffective when administered orally, and do not affect the fetus when administered to a parturient. (164)

71. Because of the hydrophilic nature of nondepolarizing NMBDs, all these NMBDs may be eliminated by glomerular filtration by the kidneys. When additional methods of clearance of the drugs are possible, the duration of action of the drug shortens. For example, the long-acting NMBDs, such as pancuronium,

undergo little hepatic metabolism and are primarily cleared by the kidneys. Yet intermediate-acting and short-acting nondepolarizing NMBDs are relatively independent of renal function for their clearance from the plasma. (164)

72. There are several drugs that are often administered in the perioperative period that may enhance the neuromuscular blockade produced by nondepolarizing NMBDs. These drugs include volatile anesthetics, aminoglycoside antibiotics, local anesthetics, cardiac antiarrhythmic drugs, dantrolene, magnesium, lithium, and tamoxifen. Hypothermia, hypokalemia, and decreases in pH may also prolong the action of nondepolarizing NMBDs. In addition, some neuromuscular diseases can be associated with altered pharmacodynamic responses to nondepolarizing NMBDs, for example, myasthenia gravis or Duchenne muscular dystrophy. (164)

73. Some drugs that may diminish the neuromuscular blockade produced by nondepolarizing NMBDs include calcium, corticosteroids, and some anticonvulsant drugs such as phenytoin. Burn injury and the skeletal muscles involved in a cerebrovascular accident are two examples of physiologic states that are associated with diminished responses to the effects of nondepolarizing NMBDs. (165)

74. Nondepolarizing NMBDs may exert minor cardiovascular effects through drug-induced release of histamine, effects on cardiac muscarinic receptors, or effects on nicotinic receptors at autonomic ganglia. The relative magnitude of the circulatory effects varies from patient to patient and depends on factors such as underlying autonomic nervous system activity, blood volume status, preoperative medication, drugs administered for maintenance of anesthesia, and concurrent drug therapy. (165)

75. Most patients receiving NMBDs for a prolonged period of time in the intensive care unit recover full muscle strength within a few hours of discontinuation of the drug. There have been reports of a subset of patients who, after receiving NMBDs for several days or weeks, have had persistent skeletal muscle weakness after the discontinuation of the NMBD. These patients exhibit moderate to severe quadriparesis with or without areflexia, but they usually retain normal sensory function. The time course of the weakness associated with the myopathy is unpredictable, and in some patients the weakness may progress and persist for weeks or months. (165)

76. The pathophysiology of developing a myopathy during intensive care unit care is not well understood. Risk factors include patients with asthma (receiving corticosteroids) or acutely injured patients with multiple organ system failure (including sepsis) requiring mechanical ventilation of the lungs for prolonged periods, usually more than 6 days. For patients who do develop myopathy, the administration of NMBDs can augment the severity of the condition. (166)

77. NMBDs should be administered to patients in the intensive care unit only after the use of analgesics, sedatives, and adjustments to ventilator settings have been maximized. Even so, NMBDs should only be administered for as short a duration as possible and for no longer than 2 days. (166)

LONG-ACTING NONDEPOLARIZING NEUROMUSCULAR BLOCKING DRUGS

78. For pancuronium, the ED_{95} (95% effective dose) is 70 μg/kg, the time of onset of action is 3 to 5 minutes, and the duration of action is 60 to 90 minutes. (166)

79. The principal route of clearance of pancuronium is by glomerular filtration. An estimated 80% of a single dose of pancuronium is eliminated unchanged in the urine. Between 10% and 40% of pancuronium undergoes hepatic metabolism. A metabolite of pancuronium, 3-desacetylpancuronium, possesses limited muscle relaxant properties. (166)

80. The clearance of pancuronium is greatly affected by renal disease; the plasma clearance of pancuronium in patients with renal failure is decreased by 30% to 50%. Patients with renal disease are therefore likely to exhibit prolonged neuromuscular blockade with the administration of conventional doses of pancuronium. (166)

81. The administration of pancuronium typically results in a modest 10% to 15% increase in heart rate, mean arterial pressure, and cardiac output. This effect of pancuronium is primarily due to selective blockade of the cardiac muscarinic receptors, (similar to atropine) primarily at the sinoatrial node. (166)

INTERMEDIATE-ACTING NONDEPOLARIZING NEUROMUSCULAR BLOCKING DRUGS

82. The intermediate-acting nondepolarizing NMBDs include rocuronium, vecuronium, atracurium, and cisatracurium. (166)

83. In contrast to the long-acting nondepolarizing NMBD pancuronium, the intermediate-acting nondepolarizing NMBDs possess efficient clearance mechanisms that create a shorter duration of action, approximately 20 to 35 minutes. When compared to pancuronium, these drugs have a similar onset of maximum neuromuscular blockade (with the exception of rocuronium), approximately one third the duration of action as pancuronium, and a 30% to 50% more rapid recovery rate. These drugs have minimal to absent cardiovascular effects, with the exception of atracurium. Neostigmine can be used for antagonism of the neuromuscular blockade; for rocuronium and vecuronium, sugammadex may also be used for antagonism of the neuromuscular blockade. (166)

84. For vecuronium, the ED_{95} is 50 µg/kg, the time of onset of action is 3 to 5 minutes, and the duration of action is 20 to 35 minutes. (166)

85. Vecuronium undergoes both hepatic and renal excretion, with only the 3-desacetylvecuronium metabolite having any significant neuromuscular blocking properties. Up to 60% of the injected dose of vecuronium, whether metabolized or unchanged, is excreted in the bile because of its increased lipid solubility as compared to pancuronium. Vecuronium is also partially cleared by the kidneys. (166)

86. Patients with renal failure may have impaired excretion of both vecuronium as well as its active metabolite. This may result in cumulative effects of vecuronium with the administration of large or repeated doses of vecuronium in renal failure patients. There are reports of prolonged neuromuscular blockade in renal failure patients in the intensive care unit who had been administered continuous infusions of vecuronium. (167)

87. Vecuronium administration does not have any cardiovascular effects. (167)

88. For rocuronium, the ED_{95} is 0.3 mg/kg, the time of onset of action is 1 to 2 minutes, and the duration of action is 20 to 35 minutes. (167)

89. Because rocuronium is a less potent NMBD than the other intermediate-acting NMBDs, a larger number of molecules must be administered to achieve a given effect. The larger number of molecules thus leads to a more rapid onset of action. The onset of maximum single twitch depression after the intravenous administration of rocuronium at 3 to 4 × ED_{95} (1.2 mg/kg) resembles the time of onset of succinylcholine after the intravenous administration of 1 mg/kg. However, the large doses of rocuronium (3 to 4 × ED_{95}) needed to mimic the onset time of succinylcholine produce a duration of action resembling that of pancuronium. (167)

90. Clearance of rocuronium is largely as an unchanged drug in the bile. Renal excretion of the drug may account for as much as 30% of the dose, and administration of this drug to patients in renal failure could result in a longer duration of action, especially with repeated doses or a prolonged intravenous infusion. (167)

91. For atracurium, the ED_{95} is 0.2 mg/kg, the time of onset of action is 3 to 5 minutes, and the duration of action is 20 to 35 minutes. (167)

92. Atracurium is cleared from the plasma by ester hydrolysis (two thirds) and Hofmann elimination (one third). The ester hydrolysis is by nonspecific plasma esterases and is therefore not affected in patients with atypical plasma cholinesterase. Hofmann elimination is spontaneous nonenzymatic degradation at normal body temperature and pH. Note that the clearance of atracurium from

the plasma is independent of renal or hepatic function, so its duration of action is unchanged in patients with renal failure. (167)

93. The major metabolite of atracurium is laudanosine. Laudanosine freely crosses the blood-brain barrier and can act as a central nervous system stimulant in high concentrations. Patients who have been administered prolonged continuous infusions of atracurium for several days, as in an intensive care unit setting, are especially at risk for the accumulation of the metabolite laudanosine and its central nervous system stimulatory effects. Laudanosine is primarily cleared through the liver. Patients with impaired hepatic function have a further risk of the adverse effects of laudanosine. (167)

94. Because of histamine release with larger doses, atracurium can cause hypotension and tachycardia. However, doses smaller than $2 \times ED_{95}$ rarely cause cardiovascular effects. (167)

95. For cisatracurium, the ED_{95} is 50 µg/kg, the time of onset of action is 3 to 5 minutes, and the duration of action is 20 to 35 minutes. (167)

96. Structurally, cisatracurium is an isolated form of one of the 10 stereoisomers of atracurium. (167)

97. Cisatracurium is cleared from the plasma primarily through Hofmann elimination. As with atracurium, the clearance of cisatracurium from the plasma is independent of renal or hepatic function. (167)

98. Cisatracurium administration is not associated with the release of histamine, and cisatracurium does not have any cardiovascular effects, even when administered at large doses. (167)

SHORT-ACTING NONDEPOLARIZING NEUROMUSCULAR BLOCKING DRUGS

99. For mivacurium, the ED_{95} is 80 µg/kg, the time of onset of action is 2 to 3 minutes, and the duration of action is 12 to 20 minutes. (167)

100. Mivacurium consists of three stereoisomers, with the two most active isomers undergoing hydrolysis by plasma cholinesterase. Hydrolysis of these two isomers is responsible for the short duration of action of mivacurium. (167)

101. In patients with atypical plasma cholinesterase, hydrolysis of mivacurium (as with succinylcholine) is decreased and its duration of action increased. Currently, mivacurium is not marketed in the United States and is not available for delivering anesthetic care. (168)

MONITORING THE EFFECTS OF NONDEPOLARIZING NEUROMUSCULAR BLOCKING DRUGS

102. The most reliable method for monitoring the effects of NMBDs during general anesthesia is through the use of a peripheral nerve stimulator. The peripheral nerve stimulator works by stimulating a motor nerve to conduct an impulse. A mechanically evoked muscle response is then evaluated by the clinician. The mechanical motor response of the muscle reflects the number of muscle fibers that are blocked and provides an indication to the clinician of the degree of neuromuscular blockade. (168)

103. A peripheral nerve stimulator is used when administering NMBDs during general anesthesia to titrate the NMBD to a desired pharmacologic effect, to judge spontaneous recovery from an NMBD-induced neuromuscular blockade, and to evaluate for effective antagonism by anticholinesterase drugs (e.g., neostigmine or sugammadex). (168)

104. Routine monitoring is strongly recommended by all experts in the field and supported by large epidemiologic studies and various safety organizations such as the Anesthesia Patient Safety Foundation. Only about 30% to 70% of anesthesia providers in the United States and Europe use a peripheral nerve stimulation as a monitor. The advantages are that monitoring allows NMBDs to be given in a more efficacious manner, provides a more precise guide for NMBD requirements intraoperatively, and allows for the effective antagonism by neostigmine and sugammadex. Most recently, complications in the PACU have been documented to be less frequent when monitoring is used. (168)

105. The ulnar nerve and adductor pollicis muscle are the nerve and muscle most commonly used for the evaluation of the neuromuscular blockade produced

by NMBDs through the use of a peripheral nerve stimulator. The adductor pollicis muscle is solely innervated by the ulnar nerve. This means that the only source for motor stimulation of the adductor pollicis muscle is through the mechanical stimulation of the ulnar nerve. Different muscle groups differ in their sensitivities to NMBDs. The adductor pollicis muscle is more sensitive to the effects of NMBDs than are the diaphragm or upper airway muscles. (168)

106. When the arm is not available to the anesthesia provider, the facial nerve on the lateral aspect of the face and observation of the orbicularis oculi muscle are often used for the evaluation of the neuromuscular blockade produced by NMBDs through the use of a peripheral nerve stimulator. Other nerves that may be used include the median, posterior tibial, and common peroneal nerves. (168)

107. In general, the administration of nondepolarizing MMBDs produces laryngeal muscle relaxation and conditions favorable for intubation of the trachea more rapidly than relaxation of the adductor pollicis muscle as measured by ulnar nerve stimulation. Facial nerve stimulation and measurement of neuromuscular blockade of the orbicularis oculi muscle more closely correlate with laryngeal muscle relaxation and vocal cord paralysis than ulnar nerve stimulation. An exception to the pattern of neuromuscular blockade onset in the various muscles is with the administration of succinylcholine. The administration of succinylcholine results in neuromuscular blockade at the adductor pollicis muscle and the laryngeal muscles at approximately the same time. Thus the measurement of neuromuscular blockade at the ulnar nerve provides a better indication of vocal cord paralysis when succinylcholine is administered. The diaphragm muscle appears to be resistant to the effects of NMBDs, such that larger doses of drug are required to produce relaxation of the diaphragm than doses required for relaxation of either the laryngeal muscles, orbicularis oculi, or adductor pollicis muscles. (168)

108. Mechanically evoked responses used for monitoring the effects of NMBDs include the single twitch response, train-of-four ratio, double burst stimulation, tetanus, and post-tetanic stimulations. The mechanically evoked response can be evaluated visually, manually by touch, or by recording. (168)

109. The depth of neuromuscular blockade may be defined as the percentage of inhibition of twitch response from control height. In fact, the ED_{95} of an NMBD is defined as the dose necessary to depress the twitch response 95%. Depression of the twitch response greater than 90%, or elimination of two to three twitches of the train-of-four, correlates with acceptable skeletal muscle relaxation for the performance of intra-abdominal surgery in the presence of an adequate concentration of volatile anesthetic. (168)

110. The train-of-four stimulus delivered by a peripheral nerve stimulator is four electrical stimulations at 2 Hz each delivered every 0.5 second. (169)

111. The train-of-four stimulus delivered by a peripheral nerve stimulator is useful for the evaluation of the degree of neuromuscular blockade based on the premise that each successive electrical stimulus will further deplete stores of acetylcholine in the nerve terminal. In the presence of neuromuscular blockade produced by nondepolarizing NMBDs, there will be a resultant decrease in the mechanically evoked muscle response with each stimulus. The amount of decrease in the mechanical muscle response correlates with the degree of neuromuscular blockade. Only four twitches are used in the train-of-four stimulus because any further stimulation of the nerve after the fourth does not result in any further depletion of acetylcholine stores at the nerve terminal. (170)

112. The train-of-four ratio is a calculation of the height of the fourth evoked twitch response divided by the height of the first evoked twitch response of a train-of-four stimulus. For example, if the height of the fourth twitch is one half the height of the first twitch, the train-of-four ratio would be 0.5. The control, or baseline, train-of-four ratio should be 1.0 before the administration of NMBDs. This corresponds to a height of the fourth mechanically evoked twitch response being equal to the height of the first evoked twitch response. (170)

113. Clinically, the train-of-four ratio is used to establish how much fade occurs with the stimulus, which correlates with the degree of neuromuscular blockade. (170)

114. A train-of-four ratio of 0.7 or greater correlates with the complete return to the control height of a single twitch response. That is, when the height of the fourth mechanically evoked twitch response is 70% of the height of the first evoked twitch response in a train-of-four stimulus, a single twitch response will have returned to its control height. (170)

115. Phase I neuromuscular blockade after the administration of succinylcholine would be reflected as a train-of-four ratio of 1.0 because the height of all four twitches would be similarly decreased. (170)

116. Phase II neuromuscular blockade after the administration of succinylcholine may be reflected as a train-of-four ratio less than 0.3. The train-of-four response thus shows some fade of the fourth twitch when compared with the first twitch of the train-of-four stimulus when phase II neuromuscular blockade is present. (170)

117. Accurate estimation of the train-of-four ratio is not reliable clinically by either visual or manual assessment. Difficulty estimating the train-of-four ratio may be due to the fact that the two middle twitch responses interfere with comparison of the first and last twitch response. (170)

118. The double burst stimulus delivered by a peripheral nerve stimulator is two bursts of three 50-Hz electrical stimulations separated by 750 ms between each burst, but it is perceived by the clinician as two separate twitches. (170)

119. Clinically, the double burst stimulus appears to make the estimation of the fade response easier for clinicians. It is thought that the estimation of the ratio between the two twitches is easier for clinicians because the middle two twitches of the train-of-four response are eliminated. A train-of-four ratio of 0.3 or less is most accurately detected by clinicians when using the double burst stimulus. Accuracy of the estimation of a train-of-four ratio greater than 0.7 is still poor, however. (170)

120. Tetanus is a skeletal muscle contraction that occurs secondary to continuous stimulation of the postjunctional receptors. Tetanus can be mechanically produced using the peripheral nerve stimulator by delivering a continuous electrical stimulus of 50 Hz for 5 seconds. (171)

121. The normal response to tetanus produced by a peripheral nerve stimulator is a sustained muscular contraction. (171)

122. Phase I neuromuscular blockade resulting from the administration of depolarizing NMBDs, such as succinylcholine, results in a mechanical muscle contraction in response to tetanus that is greatly decreased from the control response but does not fade. (171)

123. The administration of nondepolarizing NMBDs results in a mechanical muscular contraction in response to a tetanus that fades over time. (171)

124. Post-tetanic facilitation refers to the evaluation of a train-of-four response after a tetanic stimulus has been delivered. There is an increase in the available stores of acetylcholine in the motor nerve terminals after a tetanic stimulus, and this allows for a transient enhancement of the mechanical muscle response obtained when a train-of-four stimulus is delivered immediately after a tetanic stimulus. (171)

125. Clinically, the mechanical muscle response to a train-of-four stimulus after the delivery of a tetanic stimulus is useful during intense neuromuscular blockade when there is no evoked mechanical response to either a single twitch or a train-of-four stimulus. (171)

ANTAGONISM OF NONDEPOLARIZING NEUROMUSCULAR BLOCKING DRUGS

126. Anticholinesterase drugs that are used for the antagonism of the effects of NMBDs include neostigmine, edrophonium, and less frequently pyridostigmine. (171)

127. The antagonism of the neuromuscular blockade produced by nondepolarizing NMBDs can be achieved by the intravenous administration of an anticholinesterase drug. These drugs exert their effect by inhibiting the activity of acetylcholinesterase,

the enzyme that hydrolyzes acetylcholine in the NMJ. As a result of the inhibition of the hydrolysis of acetylcholine, acetylcholine accumulates in the NMJ. With more acetylcholine available at the NMJ, the competition between acetylcholine and the nondepolarizing NMBD is altered such that it is more likely that acetylcholine will be available to bind to the two α-subunits of the postjunctional receptor. In addition to increasing the amount of acetylcholine available in the NMJ to compete for sites on the postjunctional nicotinic cholinergic receptors, acetylcholine also accumulates at the muscarinic cholinergic receptor sites through the same mechanism. (171)

128. Anticholinesterases increase the concentration of acetylcholine available at the muscarinic cholinergic receptors as well as at the nicotinic cholinergic receptors. This can result in profound bradycardia through the stimulation of cardiac muscarinic cholinergic receptors. To attenuate the cardiac muscarinic effects of anticholinesterases, a peripheral-acting anticholinergic drug such as atropine or glycopyrrolate must be administered intravenously before or simultaneous with the intravenous administration of the anticholinesterase. (171)

129. Even if all tests of the adequacy of normal neuromuscular function are normal, 50% of the receptors at the NMJ may still be occupied by an NMBD. An excellent rule to follow is "When in doubt, it is better to have as many receptors free of the effects of neuromuscular blocking drugs as possible." Unequivocal clinical confirmation provides assurance of adequate recovery (spontaneous and drug assisted) from the effects of NMBDs. (172)

ADVERSE OUTCOMES FROM INADEQUATE ANTAGONISM OF NEUROMUSCULAR BLOCKADE

130. Some potential complications in the PACU that can be augmented by the presence of postoperative residual neuromuscular blockade include airway obstruction, inadequate ventilation, and hypoxia. In addition to residual neuromuscular blockade, obesity, the administration of opioids, long duration of surgery, and emergency and abdominal surgery are all risk factors for patients becoming hypoxic in the immediate postoperative period. For this reason, a dangerous time for perioperative anesthetic complications starts with the extubation of the trachea, transport to the PACU, and the first 30 minutes in the PACU. (172)

131. Factors influencing the success of antagonism of NMBDs include (1) the intensity of the neuromuscular blockade at the time that the pharmacologic antagonist is administered, (2) the choice of antagonist drug, (3) the dose of antagonist drug, (4) the rate of spontaneous recovery from the NMBD, and (5) the concentration of the inhaled anesthetic. (172)

132. The adequacy of the recovery from the effects of neuromuscular blockade should be confirmed prior to extubation of the patient's trachea at the conclusion of general anesthesia. Though a train-of-four ratio of at least 0.9 has been recommended, visual estimation of the train-of-four ratio is neither accurate nor reliable. More reliable clinical indicators include a sustained response to tetanus, the ability to maintain head lift for 5 to 10 seconds, or an evaluation of masseter muscle strength (the tongue depressor test). Grip strength is also a useful indicator of recovery from the effects of NMBDs. Although adequate ventilation may be indicated by a train-of-four ratio higher than 0.7, the pharyngeal musculature may still be weak, and upper airway obstruction remains a risk. In addition, diplopia, dysphagia, an increased risk of aspiration of gastric contents, and a decreased ventilator response to hypoxia are possible even in the presence of a train-of-four ratio more than 0.9, thus emphasizing the importance of using more sensitive clinical methods for assessing neuromuscular function. (172)

133. The spontaneous recovery from NMBDs without the aid of drug-assisted antagonism is not recommended unless there is compelling clinical evidence that there is no residual neuromuscular blockade. (172)

134. There are several pharmacologic and physiologic factors that may interfere with the antagonism of the neuromuscular blockade produced by NMBDs. Physiologic factors include abnormalities in the patient's temperature, acid-base status, electrolytes, or metabolism pathways, such as in the case of renal or liver disease. These may all interfere with the metabolism and clearance of the NMBD. Pharmacologic factors include the concurrent administration of aminoglycoside antibiotics, local anesthetics, volatile anesthetics, magnesium, dantrolene, lithium, tamoxifen, and cardiac antiarrhythmic drugs. Another cause of an apparent inability to antagonize the effects of NMBDs is not allowing sufficient time to pass for an anticholinesterase to begin exerting its effect. In the case of neostigmine, 15 to 30 minutes may need to pass before the maximal effect of neostigmine is realized. Finally, the lack of a mechanically evoked muscular response to a train-of-four stimulus is an indication that the antagonism of the neuromuscular blockade is not possible. (172)

135. Sugammadex is an NMBD antagonist that was recently approved by the FDA for use in the United States. It has been approved for use in Japan, Europe, and other countries. The mechanism of action of sugammadex is through encapsulation and inactivation of steroidal NMBDs, especially rocuronium and vecuronium. (173)

136. Sugammadex differs from neostigmine in several ways. First, it has no cardiovascular effects and does not require other drugs such as glycopyrrolate. Second, sugammadex, unlike neostigmine, can reverse a profound neuromuscular blockade. For example, if rocuronium 1.2 mg/kg has been given for a rapid sequence induction of anesthesia, its neuromuscular blockade can be completely reversed within minutes (e.g., 5 minutes). In this situation, neostigmine would be ineffective. Finally, the rate that it reliably reverses even profound neuromuscular blockade is rapid (2 to 3 minutes) and complete. (173)

137. Sugammadex confers several advantages for the antagonism of neuromuscular blockade. First, a rocuronium-sugammadex combination can be used for rapid sequence induction of anesthesia and subsequent reversal. Second, profound neuromuscular blockade can be achieved and maintained through the end of surgery and still have adequate reversal at the conclusion of surgery. Finally, the incidence of residual neuromuscular blockade can be reduced or eliminated. (173)

138. The dose of sugammadex for the reversal of the effects of vecuronium or rocuronium varies and is dependent on neuromuscular function monitoring with a peripheral nerve stimulator. For patients with two of the four twitches from a train-of-four stimulus, the dose of sugammadex is 2 mg/kg. For patients with no recovery of the twitch response from a train-of-four stimulus, and with one or two post-tetanic counts, the dose of sugammadex is 4 mg/kg. For patients who had been given rocuronium at a dose 1.2 mg/kg for a rapid sequence induction, neuromuscular blockade can be terminated with sugammadex at a dose of 16 mg/kg. (173)

12 ANESTHETIC NEUROTOXICITY

Sulpicio G. Soriano, II, and Mary Ellen McCann

INTRODUCTION

1. Is anesthetic neurotoxicity limited to pediatric patients?
2. Is the issue of anesthetic neurotoxicity a recent finding?
3. Has any regulatory agency commented on the issue of anesthetic neurotoxicity?

ANESTHETIC DRUGS AS A CAUSE FOR NEURO-DEGENERATION AND LONG-TERM NEUROCOGNITIVE DEFICITS

4. What are the primary receptors that are the targets of anesthetic drugs and the purported cellular intermediaries for the reported toxicity in preclinical reports?
5. What are the neurodevelopmental processes that are impaired with exposure to anesthetic drugs?
6. How does the developmental stage of the GABAergic neuron affect its excitatory state?
7. Does neuronal apoptosis always impair neurodevelopment?
8. Is there an age-dependent impact on dendritic development after exposure to anesthetic drugs?
9. What is the preclinical link between anesthesia and Alzheimer disease in older animal models?
10. Neonatal rat pups exposed to volatile anesthetics have been shown to develop learning deficits. Which interventions mitigate this adverse outcome?
11. What are the three factors that increase the development of neuronal cell death in neonatal laboratory animals exposed to anesthetic drugs?

CLINICAL EVIDENCE FOR NEUROTOXICITY

12. Recent retrospective reports detected neurocognitive deficits after exposure to surgery and anesthesia. What are the drawbacks of these investigations?
13. Are there any prospective reports that examine the impact of surgery and anesthetic at an early age on subsequent neurocognitive function?

INTRAOPERATIVE COURSE AND NEUROCOGNITIVE OUTCOMES

14. Are there any other perioperative factors that can impair subsequent neurocognitive function?
15. Parents are in your office for surgery and want to know the long-term risks of general anesthesia for their 6-month-old infant. They have concerns about the possible neurocognitive effects of general anesthesia and are contemplating a regional anesthetic rather than a general anesthetic. What is your advice to them?

ANSWERS*

INTRODUCTION

1. Preclinical reports clearly demonstrate a neurotoxic effect of anesthetic drugs at all stages of neurodevelopment. This effect spans from the fetus to the aged. (176)
2. Abnormal behavior has been reported in the 1950s in both children and the elderly after general anesthesia. Halothane was initially reported to be toxic to rodents in the 1960s. (176)
3. The Food and Drug Administration (FDA) held several open hearings and on December 14, 2016, published a cautionary perspective on the use of anesthetic drugs in patients under 3 years of age. The FDA warned that "repeated or lengthy use of general anesthetic and sedation drugs during surgeries or procedures in children younger than 3 years or in pregnant women during their third trimester may affect the development of children's brains." (176)

ANESTHETIC DRUGS AS A CAUSE FOR NEURO-DEGENERATION AND LONG-TERM NEUROCOGNITIVE DEFICITS

4. Most anesthetic and sedative drugs are either γ-aminobutyric acid (GABA) receptor agonists, N-methyl-D-aspartate (NMDA) glutamate receptor antagonists, or a combination of the two. General anesthesia and sedation can be achieved by inhalation or intravenous administration of specific drugs. Both GABA agonists and NMDA antagonists have been implicated in causing anesthetic-induced developmental neurotoxicity. (177)
5. Neurodevelopment progresses through several steps that include neurogenesis, neuronal morphogenesis, migration, synaptogenesis, and remodeling. Exposure to anesthetic drugs impaired these processes and has been implicated in the subsequent neurobehavioral deficits observed in laboratory animals. (177)
6. GABAergic general anesthetics act on the GABA receptor. Although GABA is inhibitory in the mature brain, it has been found in many preclinical studies to be an excitatory agent during early stages of brain development. The immature Na/K/2Cl transporter protein NKCCl produces a chloride influx leading to neuron depolarization. Therefore, GABA remains excitatory until the GABA neurons switch to the normal inhibitory mode when the mature chloride transporter, KCC2, is expressed and which actively transports chloride out of the neural cell. This switch begins around 15th postnatal week in term human infants but is not complete until about 1 year of age. (177)
7. The proliferative stage of neurogenesis produces an overabundance of progenitor cells that develop into neural and glial cells. Neural development is regulated by early elimination during embryonal and programmed cell death during postnatal modification of the central nervous system. Redundant neural progenitor cells and neurons that do not migrate properly or make synapses are physiologically pruned by apoptosis. (178)
8. Dendrites and axons extend from the cell body to form functional synapses with other neurons. Exposure to ketamine and isoflurane decreases synapse and spine density in very young infant rats. However, in slightly older rats, exposure to anesthetic drugs leads to an increase in dendritic spine formation. The implications of both the decrease in dendritic spine formation at a very young age and an increase in slightly older animals are unclear, but these different effects highlight the impact of specific developmental stages. (178-179)
9. Preclinical reports demonstrate expression of biological precursors of Alzheimer disease. Experimental surgery on mice increased β-amyloid accumulation in the hippocampus. Furthermore, exposure to isoflurane leads to increased tau and β-amyloid levels in cell culture and rodent brains. (179)

---

*Numbers in parentheses refer to pages, figures, boxes, or tables in Pardo MC, Miller RD, eds. *Basics of Anesthesia*. 7th ed. Philadelphia: Elsevier; 2018.

10. Anesthetic-induced cell death and neurobehavioral deficits in neonatal pups exposed to volatile anesthetics can be mitigated by concurrent exposure to an enriched environment, exercise, lithium, estrogen, erythropoietin, melatonin, and dexmedetomidine. (179–180)

11. The combination of high doses and prolonged exposure to anesthetic drugs and vulnerable age is directly related to neuronal cell death. (180)

CLINICAL EVIDENCE FOR NEUROTOXICITY

12. Most published reports implicating that general anesthesia is harmful to children are limited to retrospective epidemiologic analyses. This evidence may be confounded by the effects of surgery and the effects of the underlying comorbid conditions. Most of the studies have attempted to control for obvious confounders, but the retrospective nature of these investigations makes it impossible to control for all the known and unknown confounders. Large database clinical investigations from Canada and Sweden reveal that exposure to surgery and anesthesia at age greater than 2 to 4 years of age increased the odds ratio of cognitive deficits but not to the extent of previously published retrospective reports from smaller populations. Scrutiny of these large data sets reveals a lower percentage in academic achievement scores for toddlers undergoing ear, nose, and throat surgery. This finding suggests that early derangements in hearing and speech may have an impact on subsequent cognitive domains assessed by school performance. (180)

13. Two clinical reports that prospectively examined children receiving surgery and anesthesia (GAS and PANDA studies) did not demonstrate a decrement in cognitive function. The GAS study was an interim report of neurocognitive assessment after 2 years. A 5-year assessment is under way. A report on a smaller group of children exposed to anesthetic before 1 year showed deficits in measures of long-term recognition memory but no differences in familiarity, intelligence quotient, and Child Behavior Checklist scores. (181)

INTRAOPERATIVE COURSE AND NEUROCOGNITIVE OUTCOMES

14. The developing central nervous system is exquisitely sensitive to its internal milieu. Because critical periods of plasticity during brain development are modulated by the environmental milieu, perioperative conditions have the potential to influence brain development. Maternal deprivation, hypoglycemia, hypoxia, and hypotension and hypocarbia leading to cerebral ischemia during these critical periods of development may lead to neuronal injury and altered neurodevelopment. (181)

15. You advise them that they are correct to be concerned based on the animal and epidemiologic data, but the only published prospective randomized trial (GAS study) in children thus far did not show a neurocognitive difference between general and regional anesthesia. (181)

13 PREOPERATIVE EVALUATION AND MEDICATION

Rebecca M. Gerlach and Bobbie Jean Sweitzer

PREOPERATIVE ASSESSMENT: OVERVIEW

1. What is the purpose of preoperative evaluation?
2. What are the essential components of a complete preoperative evaluation?
3. How does the anesthesiologist classify a patient's physical status?
4. How is the patient's functional status determined?
5. Why is it important to assess the patient's functional status?
6. How much oxygen is consumed when performing one metabolic equivalent of task (MET) of activity?
7. Why is evaluation of the airway important?
8. What are the components of the airway examination?
9. Is "screening" preoperative testing indicated for every patient?
10. When should preoperative tests be ordered?
11. Should all patients of a certain age receive a preoperative electrocardiogram (ECG)?
12. What are the recommendations for obtaining a preoperative ECG?
13. How effective are ECG findings for predicting a major adverse cardiac event (MACE)?
14. Do all females of childbearing years require a β-human chorionic gonadotropin (β-hCG) assay prior to surgery?
15. Why might preoperative tests be useful when evaluating patients with severe comorbid conditions and undergoing intermediate- or high-risk procedures?
16. Which patient comorbid conditions when undergoing intermediate- or high-risk procedures may make preoperative albumin level testing useful?
17. Which patient comorbid conditions when undergoing intermediate- or high-risk procedures may make preoperative complete blood count (CBC) with platelets testing useful?
18. Which patient comorbid conditions when undergoing intermediate- or high-risk procedures may make preoperative creatinine level testing useful?
19. Which patient comorbid conditions when undergoing intermediate- or high-risk procedures may make obtaining a preoperative chest radiograph useful?
20. Which patient comorbid conditions when undergoing intermediate- or high-risk procedures may make obtaining a preoperative ECG useful?
21. Which patient comorbid conditions when undergoing intermediate- or high-risk procedures may make preoperative electrolyte testing useful?
22. Which patient comorbid conditions when undergoing intermediate- or high-risk procedures may make preoperative glucose level testing useful?
23. Which patient comorbid conditions when undergoing intermediate- or high-risk procedures may make preoperative liver function tests (LFTs) useful?
24. Which patient comorbid conditions when undergoing intermediate- or high-risk procedures may make preoperative platelet count testing useful?

25. Which patient comorbid conditions when undergoing intermediate- or high-risk procedures may make preoperative prothrombin time (PT) testing useful?
26. Which patient comorbid conditions when undergoing intermediate- or high-risk procedures may make preoperative partial thromboplastin time (PTT) testing useful?
27. Which patient comorbid conditions when undergoing intermediate or high-risk procedures may make preoperative thyroid function testing (TFT) useful?
28. Which patient comorbid conditions when undergoing intermediate- or high-risk procedures may make preoperative urinalysis useful?
29. Are any patient-specific baseline tests indicated before anesthesia?
30. What is the purpose of a preoperative consultation?
31. Is a consultation letter stating "cleared for surgery" or "low risk" adequate?

ANESTHETIC IMPLICATIONS OF COMMON COMORBID CONDITIONS

32. For which comorbid conditions are hypertensive patients at risk?
33. Should surgery be delayed because of elevated blood pressure (BP)? What is severe hypertension?
34. Is there a risk in normalizing BP in hypertensive patients?
35. How is a patient with known or risk factors for coronary artery disease evaluated prior to noncardiac surgery?
36. What is the Revised Cardiac Risk Index (RCRI)?
37. What are the six criteria that are incorporated in the RCRI?
38. How long should a patient wait after coronary revascularization before undergoing elective noncardiac surgery?
39. What are the current recommendations for use of perioperative β-blockade and statins for cardiovascular risk reduction?
40. What are the main types of heart failure? What are common causes of each type?
41. Should patients with advanced or decompensated heart failure undergo anesthesia?
42. When is a preoperative echocardiogram indicated in patients with heart failure?
43. Are all cardiac murmurs associated with valvular disease?
44. Which cardiac murmurs are always pathologic?
45. What are some clinical clues that suggest a patient may have valvular disease?
46. When is a preoperative echocardiogram indicated in a patient with a cardiac murmur?
47. Should patients with valvular disease undergo elective surgery?
48. For which patients is prophylaxis for infective endocarditis indicated? For which procedures?
49. What conditions typically prompt placement of a pacemaker or implantable cardioverter-defibrillator (ICD)?
50. What challenges does a cardiac implantable electronic device (CIED) present perioperatively? What are the potential risks to the patient?
51. What is the typical response to a magnet for an ICD? For a pacemaker? For an ICD in a patient who is also pacemaker dependent?
52. Are there any procedures for which electromagnetic interference of a CIED is not a concern?
53. What clinical conditions are predictors of postoperative pulmonary complications (PPCs)?
54. What methods are effective at reducing the rate of PPCs?
55. Are specific tests predictive of PPC risk?
56. What is obstructive sleep apnea (OSA)?
57. Which comorbid conditions are associated with OSA?
58. What components of the patient's history or physical examination can identify those at risk of OSA? Is there a questionnaire that predicts the diagnosis of OSA?

59. What impact does OSA have for anesthesia?
60. Should patients having anesthesia bring their continuous positive airway pressure (CPAP) devices to the hospital?
61. What are the American Society of Anesthesiologists (ASA) published recommendations for perioperative care of patients with OSA?
62. What body mass index (BMI) defines extreme obesity?
63. Which comorbid conditions are associated with obesity?
64. What physiologic effects can chronic hyperglycemia have on the organs?
65. What perioperative complications can result from chronic hyperglycemia?
66. If a diabetic patient has preoperative hyperglycemia, should the surgery be canceled? Is there benefit to acutely lowering the blood glucose?
67. What is the clinical significance of renal disease in the preoperative patient?
68. Is renal insufficiency a risk factor for perioperative complications?
69. When should a patient with end-stage renal disease receive dialysis before surgery?
70. Should surgery be canceled if a dialysis patient has a preoperative potassium level of 5.8 mEq/dL?
71. Does radiocontrast medium worsen renal function in normal patients?
72. Can the risk of renal injury be reduced in patients receiving radiocontrast medium?
73. Does anemia predict perioperative morbidity and mortality risks?
74. Does a patient with anemia require further evaluation to identify its cause before elective surgery?
75. What is the clinical significance of advanced age in the preoperative patient?
76. Are elderly patients at a higher risk for hospital admission after ambulatory surgery?
77. How does a patient's do-not-resuscitate (DNR) status transfer from the hospital ward to the operating room?

FORMULATION OF ANESTHETIC PLAN

78. What are some patient factors, procedural factors, and logistical factors the anesthesiologist considers when choosing an anesthetic technique?
79. What side effects of general anesthesia are commonly disclosed to patients?
80. What side effects of regional anesthesia are commonly disclosed to patients?
81. Why is an accurate assessment of risk important?
82. What risk assessment tools are available?
83. How is informed consent obtained?
84. Should all medications be continued perioperatively?
85. Should β-adrenergic blockers be continued preoperatively?
86. Should statins be continued preoperatively?
87. Should angiotensin-converting enzyme inhibitors (ACEIs) or angiotensin receptor blockers (ARBs) be continued preoperatively?
88. How is aspirin managed perioperatively? Should it always be withheld?
89. How are antiplatelet agents managed for regional or neuraxial anesthesia?
90. How are anticoagulants managed for regional or neuraxial anesthesia?
91. For which patients is bridging anticoagulation indicated?
92. If warfarin is being withheld before surgery, for how many days should it be stopped?
93. When should low-molecular-weight heparin (LMWH) be discontinued before surgery?
94. What should be done if the international normalized ratio (INR) is elevated near the day of surgery?
95. In which patients is LMWH contraindicated?
96. How should insulin dosing for type 1 and type 2 diabetics be managed preoperatively?
97. Should ultra-long-acting insulin such as glargine be continued on the day of surgery?

98. Does metformin need to be withheld on the day of surgery? Should surgery be canceled if a patient has taken metformin?
99. Should oral hypoglycemic drugs be withheld on the day of surgery?
100. Which medications should be continued on the day of surgery?
101. Which medications should be discontinued for surgery?
102. Which herbal medication should not be discontinued abruptly before surgery?
103. Is neuraxial anesthesia contraindicated in patients taking herbal medications?
104. Should psychiatric medications be continued preoperatively?
105. Should monoamine oxidase inhibitors (MAOIs) be discontinued before surgery?
106. Should narcotics, anxiolytics, or nicotine replacement be discontinued before surgery?
107. Should patients taking oral steroids take the steroid on the day of surgery?
108. How much cortisol does a patient typically produce a day?
109. Which patients are at risk for adrenal insufficiency?
110. What risks are associated with high-dose steroids?
111. How should perioperative glucocorticoids (e.g., "stress-dose" steroids) be dosed for a patient on chronic steroids?
112. What medications can be offered preoperatively to patients with a history of severe postoperative nausea and vomiting (PONV)?
113. Who is at risk for pulmonary aspiration, and how should these patients be premedicated?
114. What are the guidelines for food and fluid intake for adult patients before elective surgery?

ANSWERS*

PREOPERATIVE ASSESSMENT: OVERVIEW

1. The purpose of preoperative evaluation is to gather information to formulate an anesthetic plan, to assess perioperative risk of complications, to implement risk-reduction strategies to maximize the quality of postoperative recovery, and to order any tests or consultations that may be indicated. (189)
2. The preoperative evaluation includes a medical and anesthetic history, review of medications, and determination of the patient's functional capacity. The physical examination includes evaluation of the airway; vital signs; and cardiovascular, pulmonary and neurologic systems. Previous diagnostic tests, consultations, and laboratory results are reviewed and any further indicated tests are ordered. An anesthetic plan is formulated and discussed with the responsible adult before informed consent is obtained. Medical therapies are optimized, fasting instructions are provided, and preoperative medication recommendations are given. (189)
3. The American Society of Anesthesiologists (ASA) Physical Status Classification ranges from ASA 1 to ASA 6. A patient who is classified as ASA 1 is healthy, without disease (nonsmoking, no or minimal alcohol use). ASA 2 patients have mild systemic disease with no substantive functional limitation (current smoker, social alcohol drinker, pregnancy, obesity [BMI 30-40], well-controlled diabetes mellitus/hypertension, mild lung disease). ASA 3 patients have severe systemic disease causing substantive functional limitations (poorly controlled diabetes mellitus or hypertension, chronic obstructive pulmonary disease, morbid obesity [BMI >40], active hepatitis, alcohol dependence or abuse, implanted pacemaker, moderate reduction in ejection fraction, end-stage renal disease on regular dialysis, history [>3 months] of myocardial infarction, cerebrovascular accident,

---

*Numbers in parentheses refer to pages, figures, boxes, or tables in Pardo MC, Miller RD, eds. *Basics of Anesthesia.* 7th ed. Philadelphia: Elsevier, 2018.

transient ischemic attack, or coronary artery disease/stents). ASA 4 patients have severe systemic disease that is a constant threat to life and seriously limits daily activities (recent [<3 months] myocardial infarction, cerebrovascular accident, transient ischemic attack, or coronary artery disease/stents, ongoing cardiac ischemia or severe valvular disease, severe reduction in ejection fraction, sepsis, disseminated intravascular coagulation, acute respiratory distress syndrome, or end-stage renal disease not undergoing scheduled dialysis). ASA 5 refers to moribund patients not expected to survive without surgery (ruptured abdominal/thoracic aneurysm, massive trauma, intracranial bleed with mass effect, ischemic bowel in the setting of significant cardiac disease or multiple organ system dysfunction). ASA 6 is reserved for brain-dead patients who are organ donors. The letter E is added to a classification if the surgical procedure is an emergency. (190)

4. The patient's functional status is determined by assessing his or her functional capacity. The functional capacity is measured in metabolic equivalents of task (METs). A patient able to eat, get dressed, and work at a computer has a MET of 1. A patient who can walk one to two blocks has a MET of 3. Climbing one to two flights of stairs equals a MET of 5. A MET of 10 is achieved by running or jogging briskly. A MET of 12 is achieved with running rapidly for long distances. (190)

5. It is important to assess the patient's functional status because it predicts outcome and perioperative complications and guides the need for further evaluation. The ability to achieve a moderate (MET ≥ 4) level of activity predicts a low risk of perioperative complications. (190)

6. One MET of activity is equivalent to the consumption of 3.5 mL O_2/min per kilogram of the patient's body weight. (191)

7. Evaluation of the airway, both on history and physical examination, for factors predicting difficult endotracheal intubation or mask ventilation allows for necessary equipment to be set up and skilled personnel available for airway management. (191)

8. During the airway examination the following are assessed: the condition of the teeth; the ability of the patient to advance or protrude the mandibular incisors; the tongue size; visibility of the uvula, tonsils, soft palate, or hard palate only (Mallampati classification I-IV); the compliance of the mandibular or oral space; the presence of facial hair; the thyromental distance; and the length, thickness, and range of motion of the neck. (191)

9. "Screening" preoperative testing is never indicated. Preoperative "screening" tests ordered without specific clinical indications rarely result in changes in patient management and are not cost-effective. (191)

10. Preoperative tests are indicated to evaluate existing medical conditions or for the diagnosis of disease based on clinical risk factors. Tests should be ordered if the results will impact the decision to proceed with the planned procedure or alter the care plans. Preoperative testing may direct further testing or consultation, inform preoperative medication use, alter anesthetic or surgical technique, change postoperative disposition, or establish a perioperative risk profile. In addition, clinical evaluation of the patient may reveal new or worsening symptoms that warrant testing regardless of whether or not that patient is having an upcoming procedure. (191)

11. Age is not an indication for a preoperative electrocardiogram (ECG). Although ECG abnormalities are common in the elderly, they do not predict adverse events. A simplified algorithm can guide preoperative cardiovascular evaluation of patients having noncardiac surgery. (192)

12. A preoperative ECG may be indicated for assessment of suspected electrolyte abnormalities, arrhythmias, active cardiac conditions (dyspnea, new or worsening chest pain, heart failure), pulmonary hypertension, or use of digoxin. Preoperative resting 12-lead ECG is not indicated for low-risk surgery. Preoperative ECG is reasonable (class IIa recommendation) in patients with

significant coronary disease, peripheral arterial disease, cerebrovascular disease, or major structural heart disease if intermediate- or high-risk surgery is planned. (192)

13. Preoperative ECG findings have not been shown to predict major adverse cardiovascular events (MACE) beyond clinical risk factors and are not useful in determining further testing. (192)

14. Pregnancy testing should be offered to women of childbearing age. Some facilities make it mandatory before anesthesia; other facilities allow women to decline testing. The ASA practice advisory for preoperative evaluation states that current literature is not clear as to whether anesthesia causes harmful effects on early pregnancy, so testing should be offered if it will change management. (192)

15. Preoperative tests may be indicated in the assessment of severe disease to establish a diagnosis, predict risk, or guide therapy before intermediate- or high-risk surgery. (192-193)

16. Preoperative albumin level testing may be useful in patients undergoing intermediate- or high-risk procedures if the patient has anasarca, liver disease, malnutrition, or malabsorption. (192-193)

17. Preoperative complete blood count (CBC) with platelets testing may be useful in patients undergoing intermediate- or high-risk procedures if the patient has a history of alcohol abuse, anemia, dyspnea, hepatic or renal disease, malignancy, malnutrition, personal history of bleeding, poor exercise tolerance, or recent chemotherapy or radiation therapy. (192-193)

18. Preoperative creatinine level testing may be useful in patients undergoing intermediate- or high-risk procedures if the patient has renal disease or has risk factors for kidney disease. (192-193)

19. Preoperative chest radiograph analysis may be useful in patients undergoing intermediate- or high-risk procedures if the patient has an active, acute, or chronic pulmonary symptom such as a cough, dyspnea, abnormal unexplained physical findings on chest examination, decompensated heart failure, malignancy within the thorax, or radiation therapy (to chest, breasts, lungs, thorax). (192-193)

20. Preoperative ECG may be useful in patients undergoing intermediate- or high-risk procedures if the patient has a history of alcohol abuse, an active cardiac condition, an arrhythmia, an implantable cardioverter-defibrillator (ICD), obstructive sleep apnea (OSA), pacemaker, pulmonary hypertension, radiation therapy, severe obesity, syncope, or use of amiodarone or digoxin. (192-193)

21. Preoperative electrolyte testing may be useful in patients undergoing intermediate- or high-risk procedures if the patient has a history of alcohol abuse; cardiovascular, hepatic, renal, or thyroid disease; diabetes; malnutrition; or use of digoxin or diuretics. (192-193)

22. Preoperative glucose level testing may be useful in patients undergoing intermediate- or high-risk procedures if the patient has diabetes, is severely obese, or uses steroids. (192-193)

23. Preoperative liver function tests (LFTs) may be useful in patients undergoing intermediate- or high-risk procedures if the patient has a history of alcohol abuse, hepatic disease, recent hepatitis exposure, or an undiagnosed bleeding disorder. (192-193)

24. Preoperative platelet count testing may be useful in patients undergoing intermediate- or high-risk procedures if the patient has a history of alcohol abuse, hepatic disease, bleeding disorder, hematologic malignancy, recent chemotherapy or radiation therapy, or thrombocytopenia. (192-193)

25. Preoperative prothrombin time (PT) testing may be useful in patients undergoing intermediate- or high-risk procedures if the patient has a history of alcohol abuse, hepatic disease, malnutrition, bleeding disorder (personal or familial), or use of anticoagulants. (192-193)

26. Preoperative partial thromboplastin time (PTT) testing may be useful in patients undergoing intermediate- or high-risk procedures if the patient has a bleeding disorder (personal or familial), undiagnosed hypercoagulable state, or use of unfractionated heparin. (192-193)

27. Preoperative thyroid function testing (TFT) may be useful in patients undergoing intermediate- or high-risk procedures if the patient has a goiter, thyroid disease, unexplained dyspnea, fatigue, palpitations, or tachycardia. (192-193)

28. Preoperative urinalysis may be useful in patients undergoing intermediate- or high-risk procedures if a urinary tract infection is suspected. (192-193)

29. Certain patient-specific baseline tests prior to surgery may be indicated. A creatinine level should be checked within 3 months if a patient is to receive an injection of contrast dye. A hemoglobin/hematocrit should be checked if the surgery has the potential for significant blood loss, and a type and screen should be obtained if there is a likelihood of transfusion. On the day of surgery it may be useful to obtain a potassium level in a patient with end-stage renal disease, and a glucose determination in a patient with diabetes, although no absolute level of either potassium or glucose has been determined to preclude surgery and anesthesia. The benefits of the procedure must be balanced against the risk of proceeding in a patient with abnormal results. (192-193)

30. The purpose of a preoperative consultation is to diagnose, evaluate, or improve a new or poorly controlled condition. Consultation for the creation of a clinical risk profile helps guide the patient, anesthesiologist, and surgeon to make management decisions. (192-193)

31. A consultation letter stating "cleared for surgery" or "low risk" is not adequate. A request for consultation seeks specific advice to aid in safe anesthetic planning, not for "preoperative clearance," which is seldom helpful. A thorough consultation should summarize a patient's medical problems, condition, and the results of diagnostic tests and provide therapeutic recommendations to help the anesthesiologist provide a safe anesthetic. (192-193)

ANESTHETIC IMPLICATIONS OF COMMON COMORBID CONDITIONS

32. Hypertensive patients may develop end-organ damage depending on the severity and duration of hypertension. Ischemic heart disease, heart failure, renal insufficiency, and cerebrovascular disease are common in hypertensive patients. (193)

33. In patients with a baseline blood pressure (BP) less than 180/110 mm Hg, there is little evidence that delaying surgery improves outcome. However, severe preinduction hypertension (systolic BP greater than 200 mm Hg or diastolic BP greater than 110 mm Hg) is an independent risk factor for postoperative myocardial infarction (MI). Hypertensive patients are more likely to have arrhythmias, labile intraoperative BP, and myocardial ischemia. Surgery should be delayed for patients with severe hypertension when a true baseline blood pressure is obtained (consecutive measurements, low stress environment). If significant end-organ damage is present or intraoperative hypotensive techniques planned, preoperative optimization of BP over several weeks is recommended. (193)

34. If the BP of hypertensive patients is lowered rapidly and aggressively, a risk of cerebral or coronary ischemia exists. Extreme lowering of BP resulting in intraoperative hypotension is more dangerous than hypertension. It is recommended to maintain intraoperative BP within 20% of the patient's baseline BP for adequate organ perfusion. (194)

35. A guideline by the American College of Cardiology/American Heart Association (ACC/AHA) from 2014 directs preoperative testing and management of preoperative noncardiac surgery patients with coronary artery disease (CAD) based on validated risk stratification tools. A stepwise algorithm for patients with known or risk factors for CAD guides the decision to proceed with surgery. Patients with symptomatic heart failure, valvular heart disease, or significant arrhythmias are managed according to appropriate clinical practice guidelines.

Patients with heart failure or atrial fibrillation have a significantly higher risk of perioperative major adverse cardiovascular events (MACE) than patients with CAD alone. (194)

- Step 1 (emergency surgery): If the surgery is an emergency, the focus is on risk stratification and designing a safe anesthetic, not on delaying for further preoperative testing. Targeting therapies intraoperatively and postoperatively can lower risk of MACE. If the surgery is not emergent, continue to Step 2.
- Step 2 (acute coronary syndrome [ACS]): Patients with an ACS (unstable angina, non–ST-segment elevation myocardial infarction [NSTEMI], ST-segment elevation myocardial infarction [STEMI]) are managed according to appropriate practice management guidelines, and surgery is postponed. If no ACS, continue to Step 3.
- Step 3 (assessment of perioperative risk of MACE): Risk of MACE is calculated using an online risk calculator (http://www.surgicalriskcalculator.com) or using the Revised Cardiac Risk Index (RCRI). If the calculated risk of MACE is <1% or <2 RCRI criteria are present, proceed with surgery without further testing. If risk is elevated, proceed to Step 4.
- Step 4 (functional capacity): If the patient can achieve ≥4 METs of activity (refer to question 4) without symptoms, proceed to surgery without further testing. If not, proceed to Step 5.
- Step 5 (clinical impact of testing): Will further testing change clinical management? If yes, then proceed to Step 6. If no, then proceed to Step 7.
- Step 6 (pharmacologic stress testing): If a dobutamine stress echocardiogram or nuclear stress test is normal, proceed to Step 7. If stress testing is abnormal, coronary angiography or revascularization may be indicated. Revascularization is generally only beneficial if it would otherwise be indicated even if the patient were not having surgery. Coronary artery bypass grafting can lower perioperative risk and have long-term benefits in select patients, typically those with left main or three-vessel CAD. The role of percutaneous coronary intervention (PCI) preoperatively is very limited and can be associated with increased risk of noncardiac surgery. Then proceed to Step 7.
- Step 7 (management options): The most appropriate management option is selected. The patient may proceed with surgery, or alternative strategies may be pursued (noninvasive medical management, less invasive surgery, or palliation).

36. The RCRI is a tool for assessing the risk of MACE. (194)
37. The RCRI assesses the risk of MACE by the following six criteria: (1) presence of ischemic heart disease, (2) history of heart failure, (3) history of cerebrovascular disease, (4) diabetes mellitus treated with insulin, (5) creatinine ≥2 mg/dL, and (6) intrathoracic, intra-abdominal, or suprainguinal vascular procedures. The presence of 0, 1, 2, or ≥3 of these factors is associated with 0.5%, 1.3%, 4%, and 9% risk of MACE, respectively. (194)
38. The length of time a patient should wait after revascularization to undergo elective noncardiac surgery depends on the type of revascularization and the associated period of dual antiplatelet therapy (DAPT) to prevent thrombosis or restenosis. The recommendations for DAPT were updated by the ACC/AHA in 2016. After bare metal stent (BMS) placement, 1 month of DAPT is required. If a drug-eluting stent (DES) is placed for stable CAD, 6 months of DAPT is required; if DES is placed for an ACS or there are other high-risk features, 12 months is required. High-risk features include long, overlapping, or small stents or recent in-stent thrombosis. Early discontinuation of DAPT increases risk. For more urgent surgery 3-6 months after placement of a DES, the risk of discontinuation of DAPT is weighed against the risk of delayed surgery. If a patient with a stent requires a procedure that mandates the discontinuation of antiplatelet therapy, aspirin should be continued perioperatively and the second antiplatelet drug restarted as soon as possible. Evidence supports the continuation of low-dose aspirin (75-100 mg) in high-risk patients (secondary prevention or after coronary stenting) for most procedures despite the slightly increased risk of bleeding. During the preanesthetic visit,

the type of stent (DES or BMS) is identified and managed perioperatively with a cardiologist familiar with these stents, especially to prevent premature withdrawal of antiplatelet drugs. The patient should be made aware of the risks associated with premature discontinuation of the drugs, including stent thrombosis, MI, and death. If stent thrombosis does occur, it is best treated in the immediate postoperative period by percutaneous coronary intervention. During the high-risk period patients should only have surgery in facilities with immediate access to interventional cardiac care. (196)

39. Recommendations from the ACC/AHA advise that β-blockade be continued in patients who are on β-blockers chronically and should not be initiated on the day of surgery strictly to lower the risk of MACE. However, it may be reasonable to begin perioperative β-blockade in advance of surgery in high-risk patients (three or more RCRI criteria, intermediate- or high-risk myocardial ischemia on preoperative testing). β-Blockade therapy should always be guided by the clinical condition of the patient. Statins should be continued perioperatively, and it is reasonable to initiate statin therapy in patients having vascular surgery. In patients with clinical indications for statin use, perioperative initiation is considered. (196)

40. The two categories of heart failure are systolic dysfunction (decreased ejection fraction from decreased contractility) and diastolic dysfunction (increased filling pressures with abnormal relaxation but preserved contractility and ejection fraction). Patients may also have a combination of systolic and diastolic dysfunction. Systolic dysfunction is most commonly caused by ischemic heart disease; diastolic dysfunction is associated with hypertension and advanced age. (196)

41. Decompensated heart failure is a high-risk cardiac condition, and elective surgery should be postponed until it is controlled. Patients with class IV heart failure may undergo anesthesia, but the risks and benefits of proceeding should be discussed with a cardiologist and the lowest risk anesthetic technique planned. Patients with heart failure have an approximately 10% risk of MACE compared to approximately 3% risk of MACE in patients with CAD. (196)

42. For patients with heart failure, routine preoperative evaluation of left ventricular function with an echocardiogram is not recommended. If patients have new or worsening symptoms, a change in clinical condition within the past year, or have dyspnea of unknown origin, an echocardiogram is a reasonable investigation before surgery. Symptoms of recent weight gain, complaints of shortness of breath, fatigue, orthopnea, paroxysmal nocturnal dyspnea, nocturnal cough, peripheral edema, recent hospitalizations, or changes in medical management prompt echocardiographic evaluation. (196)

43. Not all cardiac murmurs are pathologic. Functional murmurs arise from turbulent flow across the aortic or pulmonary outflow tracts in high-output states, such as hyperthyroidism, pregnancy, or anemia. Functional murmurs are not associated with valvular abnormalities. It is difficult even for experienced cardiologists to differentiate functional from pathologic murmurs. (196)

44. Diastolic murmurs are always pathologic and require evaluation. (196)

45. Important factors for valvular disease include advanced age, CAD, a history of rheumatic fever, volume overload, pulmonary disease, cardiomegaly, an abnormal ECG, or a murmur. The same risk factors that predict CAD predict aortic sclerosis or stenosis. (196)

46. For patients with a cardiac murmur, a preoperative echocardiogram may be indicated if general or spinal anesthesia is planned, if a moderate or greater degree of valvular stenosis or regurgitation is suspected, and none has been done in the past year. It may also be indicated if there has been a significant change in clinical status. (196)

47. As long as the hemodynamic aspects of the valvular abnormality are taken into account, patients with moderate disease, asymptomatic severe aortic stenosis, asymptomatic severe mitral regurgitation, or asymptomatic severe aortic regurgitation with normal left ventricular function may undergo elective surgery. Appropriate intraoperative and postoperative monitoring is

recommended, as these patients are at elevated perioperative risk. If valvular intervention would otherwise be indicated based on either symptoms or disease severity, preoperative valvular intervention before elective noncardiac surgery is a class I recommendation for reducing perioperative risk. Replacement or repair may be indicated. (196)

48. Antibiotic prophylaxis for infective endocarditis is recommended for patients with prosthetic cardiac valves or prosthetic material for valve repair; patients with previous infective endocarditis; unrepaired cyanotic congenital heart disease, completely repaired defect with prosthetic material within the past 6 months, or repaired defect with residual disease; and cardiac transplant recipients with a structurally abnormal valve and regurgitation. In these patients, only a limited number of procedures require prophylaxis, including dental procedures involving manipulation of the gingiva or perforation of the oral mucosa. Nondental procedures may require prophylaxis only if manipulation of infected tissue is involved or for procedures on the respiratory tract. Genitourinary and gastrointestinal tract procedures do not routinely require antibiotic prophylaxis. (198)

49. Patients with heart failure, cardiomyopathies, or potentially lethal arrhythmias may have an ICD placed. Patients with bradyarrhythmias or heart block may require pacemakers. (198)

50. Electromagnetic interference (EMI) may interfere with the normal function of a cardiac implantable electronic device (CIED), both pacemakers and implantable cardioverter-defibrillators (ICD). EMI is caused most commonly by monopolar cautery ("Bovie"), external radiation, magnetism, or electrical stimulation. EMI may be oversensed by a pacemaker as electrical activity of the heart and cause the pacemaker to inappropriately suspend therapy. This can cause a pacemaker-dependent patient to have episodes of bradycardia and hemodynamic instability. EMI may be oversensed by an ICD as a malignant arrhythmia, causing the ICD to inappropriately discharge. Sudden unanticipated patient movement during critical moments of delicate surgery is potentially catastrophic, or the ICD may deliver inappropriate shocks to the myocardium. CIEDs must be set to "ignore" EMI (asynchronous mode for pacemakers and suspension of tachyarrhythmia therapies for ICDs) to avoid these complications. If a CIED is reprogrammed for a surgical procedure, the device must be re-interrogated and re-enabled before the patient leaves the monitored setting. (198)

51. A magnet will generally suspend the antitachycardia function of an ICD, and normal function is resumed once the magnet is removed. A magnet will generally place a pacemaker into an asynchronous mode at a set heart rate determined by the manufacturer of the device. A magnet will deactivate the ICD only but will have no effect on the pacing function of a CIED performing dual function. Therefore, a pacemaker-dependent patient with an CIED must have the device reprogrammed to an asynchronous pacing mode if EMI is anticipated and a magnet is used. Although usually true, these magnet modes may be altered in certain devices, and determination of the response to a magnet is best determined by an electrophysiology service. (198-199)

52. EMI is rarely caused by procedures below the umbilicus. If bipolar cautery is used, the risk is reduced. (199)

53. Predictors of postoperative pulmonary complications (PPCs) include advanced age, heart failure, chronic obstructive pulmonary disease, smoking, poor general health (impaired sensorium, functional dependency), and OSA. (199)

54. Risk of PPCs are reduced by maximizing airflow in obstructive disease (appropriate use of corticosteroids and β-adrenergic agonists), treating infections, treating heart failure, and postoperative use of incentive spirometry, deep breathing, positive end-expiratory pressure, and continuous positive airway pressure. Preoperative exercise regimens to increase functional capacity of patients may also reduce risk. (200)

55. Routine testing with pulmonary function testing, chest radiography, or arterial blood gases does not predict or lower PPCs. (200)

56. OSA is intermittent airway obstruction or significant desaturations during sleep. (200)

57. OSA is associated with increased rates of diabetes, hypertension, atrial fibrillation, bradyarrythmias, ventricular ectopy, stroke, heart failure, pulmonary hypertension, dilated cardiomyopathy, and CAD. (200)

58. The STOP-BANG questionnaire can be used to identify patients at risk for OSA. The questions address snoring, daytime fatigue, observed apneas during sleep, treatment for high blood pressure, BMI of 35 or more, age of 50 or over, neck circumference greater than 15.7 inches (40 cm), and male gender. Patients are at high risk for OSA if they answer yes to three or more items. (201)

59. Ventilation by mask, direct laryngoscopy, endotracheal intubation, and fiberoptic visualization of the airway are more difficult in patients with OSA. Patients with OSA may have perioperative airway obstruction, hypoxemia, atelectasis, ischemia, pneumonia, need for postoperative reintubation, and prolonged hospitalizations. (201)

60. If CPAP is used at home, the patient should bring the home CPAP device on the day of the procedure for perioperative use. (201)

61. The ASA recommends that patients with OSA have preoperative diagnosis and treatment. The appropriateness of ambulatory surgery should be reviewed since patients with OSA are at a higher risk for perioperative complications and prolonged hospitalization than are patients without OSA. (201)

62. A BMI greater than 40 defines extreme obesity. (201)

63. Obesity is associated with OSA, heart failure, diabetes, hypertension, pulmonary hypertension, difficult airway management, and decreased arterial oxygenation. (201)

64. Chronic hyperglycemia can result in renal insufficiency, strokes, peripheral neuropathies, visual impairment, and cardiovascular disease. (201)

65. Chronic hyperglycemia contributes to impaired wound healing, surgical site infections, and bloodstream infections. (201)

66. Provided the patient is not showing signs of ketosis or dehydration, there is no evidence to support the cancellation of surgery of a patient with a preoperative hyperglycemia. Targeting tight glucose control in the immediate perioperative period is not likely to substantially impact outcomes in diabetics having surgery. No data support cancellation of procedures for any increased level of blood glucose. However, optimal preoperative control of blood sugar should be the goal for elective higher risk surgery. Poorly controlled diabetes is associated with increased perioperative infections and poor wound healing. Measuring HbA_{1c} is an accurate way to assess long-term control and predicts perioperative blood glucose levels. Avoiding perioperative hypoglycemia is critical. (201)

67. Renal disease is associated with hypertension, cardiovascular disease, intravascular volume overload, electrolyte abnormalities, metabolic acidosis, and often the need to alter the types or amounts of anesthetic drugs administered. (201)

68. Renal insufficiency with a creatinine level above 2 mg/dL is an RCRI criterion for risk of MACE. (201)

69. Dialysis is best performed within 24 hours of surgery but not immediately prior to surgery to avoid acute volume depletion and electrolyte alterations. (201)

70. Patients with chronic elevations in potassium tolerate slight hyperkalemia. If the potassium level is less than 6 mEq/dL and within the range of a patient's established levels, then chronic hyperkalemia does not need to be corrected. (201)

71. Radiocontrast medium transiently decreases the glomerular filtration rate (GFR) in most patients, but patients with diabetes or renal insufficiency are at highest risk. (201)

72. The risk of renal injury from radiocontrast medium may be reduced by simple hydration in patients with a GFR less than 60 mL/kg/min and maintenance of adequate mean arterial pressure. (201)

73. Anemia is a marker for an increased risk of perioperative death. Both anemia and blood transfusions predict perioperative morbidity and mortality risks. (202)

74. For an elective procedure, anemia should be evaluated preoperatively. Efforts should be directed at correcting anemia to avoid transfusions. Erythropoietin administration is indicated in certain patients (e.g., renal insufficiency, anemia of chronic disease, refusal of transfusion) if significant blood loss is anticipated. If a patient is asymptomatic with chronic anemia and is undergoing a low-risk procedure, then transfusion is not warranted unless the hemoglobin is less than 6 g/dL. If a patient has CAD or significant blood loss is anticipated, transfusion to a higher hemoglobin level may be indicated. If the cause of the anemia is unknown, an evaluation is indicated. A patient with sickle cell disease should be evaluated by a hematologist perioperatively to guide therapy. (202)

75. Patients with advanced age are more likely to have comorbid conditions including arthritis, hypertension, cardiovascular diseases, diabetes, and renal insufficiency. They may also respond differently to medications, and dosing of medicines may need to be altered. (202)

76. Patients older than 85 years with a history of hospital admission within the previous 6 months are at risk for postoperative admission after ambulatory surgery. (202)

77. A patient has the right to self-determination in the perioperative period. DNR policies should be reviewed with the patient or the patient's surrogate before surgery and modified as needed to uphold the patient's wishes. There are three parts to the perioperative DNR. Choice A is full attempt at resuscitation. This choice requests full suspension of existing directives during the anesthetic and immediate postoperative period, thereby consenting to the use of any resuscitation procedures to treat clinical events during this time. Choice B is a limited attempt at resuscitation defined with regard to specific procedures, which may apply or reject certain specific resuscitation measures (e.g., chest compressions, defibrillation, tracheal intubation). Choice C is a limited attempt at resuscitation defined with regard to the patient's goals. This choice allows the anesthesiologist and surgical team to use clinical judgment in determining which resuscitation procedures are appropriate in the context of the situation and the patient's stated goals. (202)

FORMULATION OF ANESTHETIC PLAN

78. Many factors influence an anesthesiologist's choice of the optimal anesthetic technique. Patient factors include the patient's coexisting diseases, risk of aspiration, age, patient cooperation, anticipated ease of airway management, coagulation status, previous response to anesthesia, and expressed preferences of the patient. Factors related to the procedure include the site of surgery, operative technique, position of the patient during surgery, and anticipated duration of surgery. Logistical factors include the postoperative disposition, analgesia plan, and equipment availability for the desired technique. (202)

79. With general anesthesia, side effects that occur frequently but have minimal consequences include oral or dental damage, sore throat, hoarseness, postoperative nausea/vomiting, drowsiness/confusion, and urinary retention. Side effects of general anesthesia that occur infrequently but have severe consequences include intraoperative awareness, visual loss, aspiration, organ failure, malignant hyperthermia, drug reactions, failure to wake up/recover, and death. (202)

80. With regional anesthesia, side effects that occur frequently but with minimal impact include prolonged numbness/weakness, post–dural puncture headache, and failure of technique. Side effects of regional anesthesia that occur infrequently but with severe consequences include bleeding, infection, nerve damage/ paralysis, persistent numbness/weakness, seizures, coma, and death. (202)

81. An accurate assessment of risk provides a common language for communication with both patient and surgeon, especially in making a recommendation to delay or cancel a procedure. Risk assessment helps in comparing outcomes, allocating resources, and compensation. It is also essential to obtaining informed consent from the patient. (202)

82. The ASA physical status is a robust and simple method to risk-stratify patients, although it does not account for risk inherent to the procedure. The American College of Surgeons (ACS) National Surgical Quality Improvement (NSQIP) tool, which is easily accessed online at www.riskcalculator.facs.org, provides a comprehensive estimate of patient and procedural risk. (202)

83. Informed consent is obtained when a patient agrees to proceed after hearing and understanding the indications for treatment as well as alternatives. Both risks and benefits of options for treatment are discussed in terms a layperson will understand. As patients are often under considerable stress immediately before a procedure, a calm and reassuring demeanor will help allay anxiety, which can impede the informed consent process. (202)

84. Perioperative medications should be evaluated on a case-by-case basis. Patient comorbid conditions and the nature of the procedure should be considered. Generally, cardiac medications, antihypertensive drugs, and non-loop diuretics when taken for hypertension are continued preoperatively. If angiotensin-converting enzyme inhibitors (ACEIs) or angiotensin receptor blockers (ARBs) are continued, doses of induction and other anesthetic drugs may be altered, and vasopressors should be available to prevent or mitigate hypotension. (202)

85. There are class I recommendations that β-blockers should be continued preoperatively in patients who take them to treat angina, symptomatic arrhythmias, or hypertension. (202)

86. Statins should be continued preoperatively as they have been shown to reduce length of hospital stay and the risk of stroke, renal dysfunction, MI, and even death. Terminating statin administration is associated with an increased risk. (202)

87. Continuing ACEIs or ARBs prior to surgery may contribute to hypotension under anesthesia, though no harm from these events has been established. Patients with heart failure or CAD may be at increased risk with discontinuation of ACEIs or ARBs. These medications may be discontinued 12 to 24 hours before surgery if taken only for hypertension and the surgical procedure will be lengthy, there will be significant blood loss or fluid shifts, or there is planned administration of general anesthesia. (202)

88. The perioperative management of aspirin is determined according to the risk of bleeding versus the risk of thrombotic complications with discontinuation. Generally, if aspirin is taken for primary prevention (no history of stroke, stents, or MI), it can safely be discontinued 5 to 7 days before surgery. In high-risk patients (history of stents or vascular disease), aspirin is continued unless the risk of bleeding into an enclosed space with surgery is too high (intracranial, intraspinal). (204)

89. The management of antiplatelet agents for regional/neuraxial anesthesia is guided by recommendations from the American Society of Regional Anesthesia (ASRA). In 2015, the guidelines were updated to stratify procedures by risk of bleeding including low risk (e.g., peripheral nerve blocks), intermediate risk (e.g., paravertebral blocks), and high risk (e.g., epidural instrumentation). Although nonsteroidal anti-inflammatory drugs (NSAIDs) are withheld for 5 half-lives of the drug for high-risk procedures only, clopidogrel is withheld for 7 days for intermediate- and high-risk procedures. Aspirin, if for primary prevention, is withheld for 6 days in high-risk procedures only. (204-206)

90. The management of anticoagulants for regional/neuraxial anesthesia is guided by ASRA guidelines. Intravenous heparin is held for 4 hours before any

procedure, and subcutaneous heparin is held for 8 to 10 hours. Low-molecular-weight heparin (LMWH) is held for 12 hours for prophylactic doses and 24 hours for therapeutic dosing. Warfarin is held for 5 days before intermediate- or high-risk procedures. Newer anticoagulants, such as dabigatran (4-5 days), rivaroxaban (3 days), and apixaban (3-5 days), are discontinued before intermediate- or high-risk procedures. (207-209)

91. Bridging anticoagulation with LMWH is indicated for patients at high risk (>10% annually) of thrombotic complications. This group includes patients with specific mechanical heart valves (mitral prosthesis, caged-ball or tilting disk valve, and stroke/TIA within past 6 months); atrial fibrillation and a CHADS$_2$ score of 5 or 6, stroke/TIA within the past 3 months, rheumatic valvular disease; venous thromboembolism in the past 3 months or severe thrombophilia (e.g., protein C or S deficiency, antithrombin deficiency, antiphospholipid antibodies). Bridging is not recommended for low-risk patients. (207-209)

92. If the INR is 2 to 3, warfarin administration is stopped 5 days before most surgeries (unless the procedure is minor such as cataract surgery) to allow the INR to decrease to less than 1.5. (207-209)

93. LMWH is discontinued 12 hours if prophylactic dosing 0.5 mg/kg/day or 24 hours if therapeutic dosing 1 mg/kg/day before procedures with a risk of bleeding or planned neuraxial anesthesia. (207-209)

94. If the INR is measured a day or two before surgery and is greater than 1.8, a small dose of vitamin K (1-5 mg orally or subcutaneously) can reverse anticoagulation. (207-209)

95. LMWH is typically contraindicated in patients with creatinine clearance less than 40 mL/min, body weight greater than 150 kg, porcine allergy, heparin-induced thrombocytopenia, or a history of bleeding complications while on LMWH. (207-209)

96. Type 1 diabetics have an absolute insulin deficiency and require insulin to prevent ketoacidosis even if they are not hyperglycemic. Type 2 diabetics are often insulin resistant and prone to extreme hyperglycemia. Both type 1 and type 2 diabetics should discontinue intermittent short-acting regular insulin with the exception of the insulin pump. The insulin pump should be continued at the lowest basal rate, which is generally the nighttime dose. Insulin is discontinued if the blood sugar level is less than 100 mg/dL. Type 1 diabetics should take half of their usual intermediate- to long-acting morning insulin (lente or NPH) the day of surgery to avoid ketoacidosis. Type 2 diabetics should take none or up to a half-dose of intermediate- to long-acting insulin (lente or NPH) or a combination of a 70/30 preparation insulin on the day of surgery. (207-209)

97. An ultra-long-acting insulin such as glargine is continued on the day of surgery, but the dose should not exceed 1 unit/kg or more. (207-209)

98. Metformin is held on the day of surgery. However, it will not cause hypoglycemia during fasting periods of 1 to 2 days, and there is no risk of lactic acidosis with metformin in patients with functioning liver and kidneys, so surgery does not need to be canceled if a patient has taken metformin. (207-209)

99. To avoid potential hypoglycemia in fasting patients from some oral agents, oral hypoglycemics are generally withheld on the day of surgery. (209)

100. On the day of surgery patients should continue asthma medications, birth control pills, cardiac medications, triamterine and hydrochlorothiazide if used for hypertension (while loop diuretics are typically withheld), eye drops, gastrointestinal reflux medications, seizure medications, steroids (oral or inhaled), thyroid medications, and autoimmune medications such as methotrexate. Entanercept, infliximab, and adalimumab are generally discontinued, but one should check with the prescribers and surgeon. Patients may continue estrogen compounds when used for birth control or cancer therapy and narcotics for pain or addiction. (209)

101. Herbal and nonvitamin supplements are discontinued 7 to 14 days before surgery. The administration of NSAIDs should be stopped 48 hours before surgery unless neuraxial anesthesia is planned, for which stopping NSAIDs for at least 5 half-lives is recommended. Topical creams, ointments, and erectile dysfunction medications are discontinued 24 hours before surgery. Sildenafil should only be continued perioperatively if taken for right-sided heart failure or pulmonary hypertension. Vitamins, minerals, and iron should not be taken on the day of surgery. (209)

102. Valerian is a central nervous system depressant, which may cause a benzodiazepine-like withdrawal when abruptly discontinued. It is safest to taper this medication. (209)

103. Herbal therapy alone is not an absolute contraindication to neuraxial or regional anesthesia per ASRA guidelines. However, for elective procedures that are at high risk of bleeding, discontinuation of agents known to potentiate bleeding is recommended for 7 days (garlic, dong quai, danshen, ginkgo biloba, ginseng). The same recommendations are followed for low- or medium-risk procedures in patients who have other risk factors (advanced age, renal/hepatic dysfunction, history of major bleeding with procedures). (209)

104. Antidepressant, antianxiety, and psychiatric medications including monoamine oxidase inhibitors (MAOIs) are continued preoperatively. Anesthesia management may need to be altered for patients taking MAOIs. (209)

105. MAOIs have a long duration of action, approximately 3 weeks. Discontinuation of MAOIs may produce severe depression or result in suicide. The safest alternative is to continue MAOIs and adjust the anesthetic plan. (209)

106. Patients may continue narcotic pain medications to prevent withdrawal symptoms and discomfort. Anxiolytics are continued as well. Drugs used to treat addiction, such as methadone or nicotine-replacement therapies, are also continued. (209)

107. Patients taking oral steroids should take their usual dose on the day of surgery. (209)

108. A normal daily adrenal output of cortisol is 30 mg, which is equivalent to 5 to 7.5 mg of prednisone. (209)

109. The hypothalamic-pituitary axis (HPA) may be suppressed in patients taking 5 to 20 mg/day of prednisone or its equivalent for more than 3 weeks. The HPA is usually suppressed with more than 20 mg/day of prednisone for more than 3 weeks. The risk of adrenal insufficiency remains for up to 1 year after the cessation of high-dose steroids. A patient with a suppressed HPA may need supplemental perioperative steroids if his or her HPA cannot increase the output of glucocorticoids during the period of surgery, trauma, or infection. (209)

110. High-dose steroids are associated with infections, psychosis, poor wound healing, and hyperglycemia. (209)

111. Patients on chronic steroids should have their perioperative glucocorticoid dosing guided by the stress and duration of the surgery. For a minor procedure (e.g., inguinal herniorrhaphy), the target hydrocortisone equivalent is 25 mg/day, so additional supplementation is not necessary and the patient should just take the usual daily dose of steroid. For a moderate-stress surgical procedure (colon resection, total joint replacement, lower extremity revascularization) the target hydrocortisone equivalent is 50 to 75 mg/day for 1 to 2 days. The patient takes the usual daily dose of steroid, receives 50 mg hydrocortisone intraoperatively, then 20 mg hydrocortisone every 8 hours through postoperative day 1, and then resumes home dosing of steroid. If a major surgery is planned (pancreatoduodenectomy, esophagectomy), then the target hydrocortisone equivalent is 100 to 150 mg/day for 2 to 3 days. The patient should take the usual daily dose of steroid, receive 50 mg hydrocortisone intraoperatively, and continue with 50 mg hydrocortisone every 8 hours through postoperative day 2. After postoperative day 2, the patient resumes the home dose of steroid. (209)

112. Patients at risk for PONV may be prescribed a scopolamine patch to be placed 2 to 4 hours preoperatively. Scopolamine is contraindicated in patients with angle-closure glaucoma. (209)

113. Patients at increased risk for pulmonary aspiration include laboring parturients, those with intra-abdominal masses, nonfasting individuals, and patients with an incompetent lower esophageal sphincter with reflux, symptomatic hiatal hernia, diabetes mellitus, gastric motility disorders, anticipated difficult airway, bowel obstruction, and ascites. Alteration of gastric contents to increase pH and limit the severity of potential pulmonary aspiration can be achieved with histamine-2 (H_2) antagonists, proton pump inhibitors, and nonparticulate antacids. Gastric emptying can be stimulated with prokinetic agents. (209)

114. The ASA has released practice guidelines for preoperative fasting. Up to 8 hours prior to surgery, any food or fluid may be consumed. For patients without risk factors for pulmonary aspiration the following applies: up to 6 hours before surgery, the patient may have a light meal (toast and clear liquids), infant formula, or nonhuman milk; up to 4 hours before surgery, breast milk may be consumed; up to 2 hours before surgery, the patient may take clear liquids without milk, pulp, or alcohol. During the 2 hours before surgery, no solids or liquids may be taken orally. If the patient has risk factors for pulmonary aspiration, no food or fluid should be consumed within 8 hours of the surgery. Preoperative consumption of clear liquids with carbohydrates has advantages and should be strongly encouraged in individuals at low risk for aspiration. (209)

14 CHOICE OF ANESTHESIA TECHNIQUE

Elizabeth L. Whitlock

TYPES OF ANESTHESIA

1. What are the three major categories of anesthetic technique?
2. What four components are part of the clinically accepted definition of general anesthesia?
3. What are the four levels on the continuum of sedation, as defined by the American Society of Anesthesiologists? Describe them in terms of patient responsiveness, ability to maintain a patent airway and spontaneous ventilation, and ability to maintain cardiovascular homeostasis.
4. Which of the four levels on the sedation continuum might an anesthesia provider encounter during monitored anesthesia care?

CHOOSING AN APPROPRIATE ANESTHETIC TECHNIQUE

5. What major factors go into the choice of anesthetic technique?
6. What are some perioperative roles of peripheral nerve blockade and neuraxial anesthesia besides surgical analgesia?
7. How is "preventive analgesia" defined?

PRACTICAL ASPECTS OF ANESTHESIA CHOICE

8. What is preoxygenation? Why is it performed prior to anesthesia induction?
9. By what drug administration routes may induction of general anesthesia occur?
10. What is the most common high-potency volatile anesthetic gas used for inhaled induction of anesthesia, and why?
11. When is a rapid sequence induction (RSI) technique used? What differentiates an RSI from a standard intravenous induction?
12. Why is mask ventilation not performed in a true RSI? What defines a modified RSI?
13. How is cricoid pressure achieved? How efficacious is cricoid pressure?
14. What airway management technique is considered safest in a cooperative patient at high risk for difficult or impossible intubation?
15. What technique is used to achieve endotracheal intubation in a patient at risk for both aspiration of gastric contents and difficult or impossible intubation?
16. What advantages do potent volatile anesthetics offer as a maintenance drug?
17. What are the drawbacks of potent volatile anesthetics?
18. What differentiates nitrous oxide from the potent volatile anesthetics?
19. What are the advantages and disadvantages of propofol as an anesthetic maintenance drug, compared with potent volatile anesthetics?
20. Name some procedural and patient requirements for successful regional anesthesia as the sole anesthetic technique.
21. Why might regional or neuraxial anesthesia be particularly desirable for patients with severe systemic disease?
22. What are some options available to the anesthesiologist in the event that a peripheral nerve block is attempted but surgical anesthesia is not accomplished?

23. List some pharmacologic and nonpharmacologic methods of providing sedation and anxiolysis during monitored anesthesia care (MAC).
24. What are common manifestations of respiratory depression from oversedation?

25. What is the atmospheric impact of potent volatile anesthetics and nitrous oxide?
26. What are techniques to minimize the environmental impact of inhaled anesthetics?

ANSWERS*

TYPES OF ANESTHESIA

1. Anesthetic technique is often grouped into three major categories: general anesthesia, regional anesthesia, and monitored anesthesia care (MAC). A surgical procedure (e.g., extremity surgery) may be amenable to more than one type of anesthesia. (213)
2. The four components of general anesthesia include immobility, amnesia, analgesia, and patient lack of harm. The concept of lack of harm was developed because of the potentially dangerous effects of general anesthetics, such as respiratory depression and hypotension. The modern approach to general anesthesia involves administration of several medications, often targeted to a specific component of general anesthesia (e.g., fentanyl for analgesia). (213)
3. The American Society of Anesthesiologists (ASA) defines the following four levels on the continuum of sedation:
   Minimal sedation: A patient responds briskly to verbal stimulus, and airway and cardiovascular function are unaffected.
   Moderate sedation: A patient responds purposefully to verbal or tactile stimuli, and airway and cardiovascular function are usually maintained.
   Deep sedation: Repeated or painful stimulus is required for the patient to respond. Spontaneous ventilation may be inadequate, and airway intervention may be required. Cardiovascular function is usually maintained.
   General anesthesia: The hallmark of general anesthesia is absence of patient responsiveness, even with a painful stimulus. Airway intervention is typically required, as spontaneous ventilation is usually inadequate. Cardiovascular homeostasis may be impaired by the medications required to induce general anesthesia. (214)
4. When caring for a patient receiving MAC, an anesthesia provider must be prepared for all degrees of sedation, from minimal sedation to an "unplanned" general anesthetic if the surgical procedure cannot be accomplished safely with sedation. The appropriate medications and airway equipment for general anesthesia should be available for a patient receiving MAC. (214)

CHOOSING AN APPROPRIATE ANESTHETIC TECHNIQUE

5. The anesthesia provider must weigh several factors when deciding anesthetic technique, including the demands of the type of surgical procedure, the patient's coexisting diseases, and patient preferences. Reconciling the requirements and risks inherent to the surgical procedure and pathology it is intended to treat (e.g., acute appendicitis, presenting for laparoscopic appendectomy) with the patient in whom the disease occurs (e.g., a 5-year-old with no current intravenous access) and designing a safe and effective anesthetic plan is one of the most important challenges for the anesthesia professional. (214)
6. Peripheral nerve blockade or neuraxial anesthesia may be used in combination with general anesthesia to provide postoperative analgesia, reduce rates of postoperative chronic pain, and perhaps even reduce intraoperative blood loss.

*Numbers in parentheses refer to pages, figures, boxes, or tables in Pardo MC, Miller RD, eds. *Basics of Anesthesia.* 7th ed. Philadelphia: Elsevier; 2018.

For example, consider the development of "enhanced recovery after surgery" care pathways (e.g., for elective laparoscopic bowel resection), which emphasize the use of partial neuraxial analgesia via an epidural catheter both intraoperatively and postoperatively. In this situation an epidural catheter may be used despite the requirement for deep neuromuscular blockade and controlled ventilation to facilitate laparoscopic surgery, which necessitates general anesthesia during the surgical procedure itself. (215)

7. Preventive analgesia is defined as analgesia lasting longer than 5.5 half-lives of an analgesic drug. (215)

PRACTICAL ASPECTS OF ANESTHESIA CHOICE

8. Performed prior to induction of anesthesia for a general anesthetic, preoxygenation–also called denitrogenation–is the replacement of nitrogen in the patient's functional residual capacity by the inhalation of 100% oxygen by face mask. Adequate preoxygenation can reduce or eliminate hypoxemia occurring between induction of anesthesia and institution of controlled ventilation. It does this by providing a reservoir of oxygen in the lungs, which is gradually absorbed even during periods of apnea. There are two regimens that typically achieve replacement of 80% of the functional residual capacity with oxygen:
   - Allow the patient to take eight vital capacity breaths of 100% oxygen over 60 seconds.
   - Allow normal tidal breathing of 100% oxygen for 3 minutes. (216)

9. Induction of anesthesia may be accomplished by an inhaled technique using volatile anesthetic gases or by an intravenous technique. In some cases, both techniques are used simultaneously. For example, a common method of inducing anesthesia in a pediatric patient is to perform an inhaled induction with the goal of immobility (deep sedation or general anesthesia) while an intravenous line is placed; then, to ensure adequate depth of anesthesia for intubation, an additional dose of intravenous hypnotic (e.g., propofol) is given prior to instrumenting the airway. (216)

10. For inhaled anesthesia induction, sevoflurane is most commonly used because of its high potency, low pungency, and relatively low lipid solubility, resulting in desirable rapidity of onset. Desflurane is very pungent and causes airway irritability manifested as coughing, bronchospasm, or laryngospasm; it is poorly tolerated as an agent for inhaled induction. Isoflurane is less pungent than desflurane, but because of its high lipid solubility it cannot be used to induce general anesthesia rapidly as a sole agent. (216)

11. Rapid sequence induction (RSI) is used for patients at risk for aspiration of gastric contents. This group includes patients with a known full stomach, an unknown fasting time, clinically significant gastroesophageal reflux disease, or delayed gastric emptying. The goal of RSI is to minimize the time between onset of unconsciousness and tracheal intubation. The hallmark of RSI is the administration of a rapid-onset neuromuscular blocking drug in "rapid sequence" with a hypnotic of choice. After preoxygenation, an intubating dose of a hypnotic is administered, followed immediately by an intubating dose of neuromuscular blocking drug. Tracheal intubation occurs as soon as intubating conditions are achieved, without the use of mask ventilation. If cricoid pressure is used, it is applied immediately upon loss of responsiveness and only released upon confirmation of correct endotracheal tube placement. (217)

12. During RSI, mask ventilation is generally avoided because it can result in gastric insufflation, increasing the risk of aspiration of gastric contents. In a "modified" RSI, gentle positive-pressure ventilation using pressures less than 20 cm H_2O may be judiciously attempted. Theoretically, low-pressure positive-pressure ventilation reduces the risk of gastric insufflation compared with standard mask ventilation and may be used to reduce the risk of hypoxemia prior to tracheal intubation. (217)

13. Cricoid pressure is achieved by applying a force of 30 newtons (about 7 pounds) of pressure on the cricoid cartilage. This is thought to occlude the esophagus

beneath and decrease the risk of the aspiration of gastric contents. Although the application of cricoid pressure for RSI has been the standard of care for decades, a recent meta-analysis did not demonstrate that its use has had a measurable impact on clinical outcomes during RSI. (217)

14. Awake fiberoptic intubation is typically performed for patients at high risk of a "cannot intubate, cannot ventilate" situation. The hallmark of this technique is the maintenance of consciousness, and therefore a patent airway with adequate spontaneous ventilation, until endotracheal tube placement is confirmed. Induction hypnotics are administered until after endotracheal intubation. (217)

15. Awake fiberoptic intubation may be selected for a patient at high risk for both aspiration and difficult or impossible intubation. The RSI technique relies on rapid endotracheal intubation to avoid hypoxemia, which may progress to cardiac arrest if assisted ventilation cannot be provided. Thus, an awake fiberoptic endotracheal intubation may be performed to (1) maintain a patient's conscious ability to clear regurgitated gastric contents away from the lungs and (2) maintain a patent airway and spontaneous ventilation until endotracheal tube placement is confirmed. (217)

16. Potent volatile anesthetics have several advantages for maintenance of anesthesia. They are easy to titrate, suppress the autonomic response to noxious stimulation, and provide a modest degree of muscle relaxation at clinically relevant doses, which can facilitate surgical exposure. Monitoring the end-tidal anesthetic gas concentration provides a surrogate measure for depth of hypnosis, which is as effective at preventing intraoperative awareness as purpose-built processed electroencephalogram monitors. (217)

17. There are drawbacks to the potent volatile anesthetics for anesthesia maintenance. They increase the risk for nausea and vomiting. Emergence from anesthesia is associated with a paradoxical hyperreactivity state, which can clinically be manifested as airway hyperreactivity (bronchospasm, laryngospasm) and coughing. Volatile anesthetics also depress cardiac contractility and cause peripheral vasodilation, which may be manifested as clinically significant hypotension. (217)

18. There are key differences between nitrous oxide and the potent volatile anesthetics. Nitrous oxide provides relatively less vasodilation and cardiac depression than potent volatile anesthetics. It also has analgesic properties, and due to its low blood solubility also has rapid onset and offset. However, the minimum alveolar concentration required to suppress movement to a painful stimulus is greater than can be delivered at atmospheric pressure, so it cannot be used as a sole agent to ensure hypnosis. (217)

19. Propofol has distinct advantages and disadvantages compared to volatile anesthetics. Propofol reduces postoperative nausea and vomiting rates, and emergence is associated with less coughing and laryngospasm risk. Delivery does not rely on controlled ventilation, so it may be more favorable for open-airway procedures (e.g., bronchoscopy, laryngeal surgery with intraoperative jet ventilation). Propofol does not suppress somatosensory and motor evoked potential signals as severely as volatile anesthetics and thus may facilitate intraoperative neurologic monitoring. However, propofol requires a reliable site of intravenous administration, there is no clinically available way to measure serum propofol concentrations, and the drug may be associated with higher rates of intraoperative awareness due to inadvertent interruption of intravenous administration. Depth of hypnosis monitoring using electroencephalography or auditory evoked potentials may protect against intraoperative awareness, particularly if neuromuscular blockade is concurrently used. (217)

20. In order to provide successful regional anesthesia, there are important procedural and patient requirements to consider, including the following:
    Procedural: The location of the procedure must be amenable to regional anesthesia; for example, the distal extremities in the case of peripheral nerve block or the lower trunk and legs in the case of neuraxial anesthesia. Systemic neuromuscular blockade and controlled ventilation must not be required.

Patient: A cooperative patient who provides informed consent for any planned interventions is required for successful regional anesthesia. (218)

21. For a patient with severe systemic disease, there are unique aspects of regional anesthesia techniques that may be of benefit for the patient. Surgical anesthesia can theoretically be achieved without systemic sedation, assuming appropriate procedure selection. This avoids potential complications of deep sedation and general anesthesia including cardiac depression in patients with marginal cardiac function, difficult or impossible liberation from controlled ventilation in patients with severe underlying lung disease, or unpredictable or undesirable pharmacokinetic effects of organ failure (renal, hepatic) by systemic medications. (218)

22. If surgical anesthesia is not achieved with a peripheral nerve block, either because it was difficult or the resultant block inadequate, several options are available to the anesthesiologist depending on the clinical situation. The block can be supplemented with local anesthetic infiltration, intravenous analgesics and/or sedatives can be administered, surgery can be postponed and the block reattempted at a later time, or general anesthesia can be administered. (218)

23. Although many think first of medications as the means of providing sedation and anxiolysis during monitored anesthetic care, nonpharmacologic methods also have an important role in ensuring patient safety and comfort. Commonly used pharmacologic options include propofol, opioids, and hypnotic medications (most commonly benzodiazepines). Potential nonpharmacologic methods include video or audio distraction and verbal reassurance. Nonpharmacologic methods avoid undesirable side effects (e.g., respiratory depression, paradoxical agitation, or a duration of action longer than required for the procedure). These methods may provide sufficient comfort for well-selected patients who wish to avoid medications. (218)

24. Respiratory depression is common with deep sedation. The respiratory effects of oversedation may be manifested as upper airway obstruction (snoring, obstructive apnea), hypoventilation, and hypoxemia. These risks require that the anesthesia provider be prepared to assist or take over ventilation as the clinical situation indicates. Sedatives that are less likely to cause hypoventilation include ketamine and dexmedetomidine, but these drugs have other side effects and may have synergistic sedative effects with other hypnotic medications. (218)

ENVIRONMENTAL IMPACT

25. Waste anesthetic gases are typically scavenged by a suction mechanism from the operating room to limit occupational exposure for operating room personnel; however, scavenged gas is often vented outside the facility, into the environment. Potent volatile anesthetics and nitrous oxide are ozone-depleting greenhouse gases. Although the global warming potential by volume is greatest for desflurane, nitrous oxide is the most important inhaled anesthetic cause of atmospheric harm because it is used in relatively high concentrations (e.g., 50% to 70% by volume). (219)

26. Environmental impact is minimized by using the lowest total amount of inhaled anesthetic, either by eliminating its use entirely (and providing anesthetic maintenance using total intravenous anesthesia) or by reducing fresh gas flow in the context of low-flow or closed-circuit anesthesia. Choosing the lowest impact volatile anesthetic gas—sevoflurane or isoflurane, depending on acceptable fresh gas flow rates, and avoiding nitrous oxide—also minimizes impact. There exist collection systems for waste (scavenged) gases that are intended to capture anesthetic gases prior to atmospheric release and then potentially reprocess them for human reuse; however, none is yet widely used. As nitrous oxide (from all sources, including anesthetic) is likely to be the most significant ozone-depleting emission for the 21st century, the selection of an anesthetic regimen that takes environmental impact into account—while adding an extra layer of complexity to the choice of anesthetic technique—provides a sophisticated acknowledgment by the anesthesia provider that, as professionals, we have a duty not just to the patient before us but to future patients as well. (219)

Chapter

15 ANESTHESIA DELIVERY SYSTEMS

Patricia Roth

ANESTHESIA WORKSTATION

1. What are some components of an anesthesia workstation?
2. What is the purpose of the fail-safe valve? What triggers the fail-safe valve on the anesthesia machine?
3. Can a hypoxic mixture be delivered from the anesthesia machine with an intact fail-safe valve? Explain.
4. How are oxygen, nitrous oxide, and air gases that are used in anesthesia typically delivered to the anesthesia machine? At what pressure must these gases be delivered for proper function of the anesthesia machine?
5. How is the delivery of erroneous gases to the anesthesia machine minimized?
6. What is the purpose of the cylinders of oxygen and nitrous oxide that are found on the back of the anesthesia machine?
7. How is an erroneous hookup of a gas cylinder to the anesthesia machine minimized?
8. Please complete the following table illustrating the characteristics of compressed gases stored in E-sized cylinders:

Characteristics	Oxygen	Nitrous Oxide	Carbon Dioxide	Air
Cylinder color				
Physical state in cylinder (gas/liquid)				
Cylinder contents (liters)				
Cylinder pressure full (psi)				

9. How is the pressure of oxygen related to the volume of oxygen in an oxygen gas cylinder? What does this mean with regard to calculating the volume of oxygen remaining in a used oxygen cylinder?
10. How is the pressure of nitrous oxide related to the volume of nitrous oxide in a nitrous oxide gas cylinder?
11. Why does atmospheric water vapor accumulate as frost on the outside surface of oxygen tanks and nitrous oxide tanks in use? Does internal icing occur?
12. What is the purpose of flowmeters on an anesthesia machine?
13. How do flowmeters on an anesthesia machine work?
14. Are flowmeters for various gases interchangeable?
15. Why is the oxygen flowmeter the last flowmeter in a series on the anesthesia machine with respect to the direction in which the gas flows?
16. What is the purpose of the oxygen flush valve?

17. What is the flow of oxygen delivered to the patient when the oxygen flush valve is depressed?
18. What is the risk of activating the oxygen flush valve during a mechanically delivered inspiration?

VAPORIZERS

19. Why do volatile anesthetics require placement in a vaporizer for their inhaled delivery to patients via the anesthesia machine?
20. What is the heat of vaporization?
21. What is vapor pressure? What influence does temperature have on vapor pressure?
22. Describe how contemporary vaporizers for volatile anesthetics are classified.
23. Why are contemporary vaporizers unsuitable for use with desflurane?
24. What does the term agent-specific refer to?
25. What do the terms variable-bypass and flow-over refer to?
26. What does the term temperature-compensated refer to? Between what temperatures is vaporizer output reliably constant?
27. What does the term out of circuit refer to?
28. How does tipping of a vaporizer affect vaporizer output?
29. How is the delivery of two different volatile anesthetics to the same patient via the same anesthesia machine prevented?
30. How is the potential risk of filling the agent-specific vaporizer with the erroneous volatile anesthetic minimized?

ANESTHETIC BREATHING SYSTEMS

31. What is the function of anesthetic breathing systems?
32. How do anesthetic breathing systems impart resistance to the spontaneously ventilating patient?
33. What are some features of anesthetic breathing systems that enable them to be classified as either open, semiopen, closed, or semiclosed?
34. What are the most commonly used anesthetic breathing systems?
35. What characterizes the Mapleson systems?
36. Describe the Mapleson F anesthetic breathing system. What is another name for this anesthetic breathing system?
37. When is the Mapleson F system commonly used?
38. What are some advantages of the Mapleson F anesthetic breathing system?
39. What are some disadvantages of the Mapleson F anesthetic breathing system?
40. Describe the Bain circuit anesthetic breathing system.
41. What are some advantages of the Bain circuit anesthetic breathing system?
42. What are some disadvantages of the Bain circuit anesthetic breathing system?
43. How does the circle anesthetic breathing system get its name?
44. How does the circle system prevent rebreathing of carbon dioxide?
45. What are the classifications of a circle system, and on what feature does this classification depend?
46. What is the most commonly used circle system approach?
47. What are some advantages of the semiclosed and closed circle systems?
48. What are some disadvantages of the circle anesthetic breathing system?
49. What is the impact of the rebreathing of anesthetic gases in a semiclosed circle system?
50. What are the components of a circle system?
51. What is the purpose of unidirectional valves in the circle system? What would occur if one of the unidirectional valves should become incompetent?
52. Where is the dead space in the circle system?
53. What is advantageous about the corrugated tubing in the circle system?
54. What is disadvantageous about the corrugated tubing in the circle system?
55. Describe the Y-piece connector in the circle system circuit.
56. What are other names for the adjustable pressure-limiting (APL) valve?
57. Describe the function of the APL valve when the bag/vent selector switch is set to bag.

58. What are the advantages of the reservoir bag on the circle system?
59. Describe a closed anesthetic breathing system. What is the inflow volume of fresh gases in a closed anesthetic breathing system?
60. What are some advantages to the closed circle anesthetic breathing system?
61. What is a disadvantage to the closed circle anesthetic breathing system?
62. What are the dangers of the closed circle anesthetic breathing system?
63. Are inspired concentrations of oxygen more or less predictable when nitrous oxide is also being delivered in a closed circle anesthetic breathing system? Why?
64. How can the potential problem of the inadequate delivery of oxygen using a closed circle anesthetic breathing system be minimized?
65. In a closed circle anesthetic breathing system, to what extent is the inhaled concentration of anesthetic dependent on the exhaled concentration of anesthetic? What is the potential problem with this? How can this problem be partially offset?

ANESTHESIA MACHINE VENTILATORS

66. What parts of a circle system are eliminated in anesthesia machine ventilators when the "bag/vent" selector switch is set to "vent"?
67. What are two different ways in which anesthesia machine ventilators are powered?
68. Describe the mechanics of a conventional anesthesia machine ventilator during inspiration.
69. Why is oxygen preferred over air as the ventilator driving gas?
70. Describe the mechanics of a conventional anesthesia machine ventilator during exhalation.
71. Describe the mechanically driven piston-type of ventilators found on some newer anesthesia machines.
72. Why are standing or ascending bellows preferred over hanging or descending bellows?
73. How are inhaled gases normally humidified in awake patients breathing through their native airway?
74. What effect does tracheal intubation or the use of a laryngeal mask airway have on airway humidification? What are the negative consequences of this?
75. Describe anesthetic breathing system humidification. What effect does chemical neutralization of carbon dioxide have on this process?
76. What are three types of humidifiers used for anesthesia and in the intensive care unit?
77. Describe heat and moisture exchanger (HME) humidifiers. What is the difference between an HME and an HMEF?
78. What are the advantages of HME humidifiers over other types of humidifiers?
79. What are the disadvantages of HME humidifiers?
80. What is the advantage of heated water vaporizers and humidifiers over HME humidifiers? When are they used most frequently?
81. What are the risks of heated water vaporizers and humidifiers?
82. Describe nebulizer humidifiers used for anesthesia and in the intensive care unit.

POLLUTION OF THE ATMOSPHERE WITH ANESTHETIC GASES

83. In the operating room, what are the Occupational Safety and Health Administration (OSHA) recommendations for the maximum concentrations of nitrous oxide and volatile anesthetics in parts per million?
84. What is required to control pollution of the atmosphere with anesthetic gases?
85. Describe operating room scavenging.
86. Describe the two types of scavenging systems used in the operating room.
87. What are the advantages of active scavenging with a waste gas receiver mounted on the side of the anesthesia machine?
88. What are the potential hazards of scavenging systems?
89. What two features do scavenging systems have to minimize their potential hazards?

90. Where might be the source of a high-pressure leak of nitrous oxide?
91. Where might be the source of a low-pressure leak of nitrous oxide?
92. What anesthetic techniques can lead to operating room pollution?
93. How often should the air in the operating room be exchanged?

ELIMINATION OF CARBON DIOXIDE

94. How is carbon dioxide eliminated in open and semiopen breathing systems?
95. How is carbon dioxide eliminated in a semiclosed or closed anesthetic breathing system?
96. What three components are common to all carbon dioxide absorbents?
97. What do all carbon dioxide absorbents use as the neutralizing base for carbon dioxide produced during respiration?
98. Why is water a necessary component of carbon dioxide absorbents?
99. How does the type of catalyst contained in the carbon dioxide absorbent influence the differences between the absorbents?
100. Name three individual carbon dioxide absorbents. Which are traditional and which are new generation?
101. What do soda lime granules consist of?
102. Why is silica added to soda lime?
103. Describe the neutralization of carbon dioxide by soda lime.
104. Why is the water in the soda lime carbon dioxide absorbent canister hazardous?
105. Can soda lime lead to degradation of sevoflurane to compound A? What is responsible for this?
106. Can soda lime lead to significant concentrations of carbon monoxide? What is responsible for this?
107. What are the compositional differences between the new generation carbon dioxide absorbents Amsorb Plus and Litholyme versus traditional soda lime?
108. Can Amsorb Plus or Litholyme lead to degradation of sevoflurane to compound A? Why or why not?
109. Can Amsorb Plus or Litholyme lead to degradation of inhaled anesthetics to carbon monoxide? Why or why not?
110. Describe the neutralization of carbon dioxide by Amsorb Plus or Litholyme.
111. Why is the water formed by the neutralization of carbon dioxide by all carbon dioxide absorbents useful? What if the carbon dioxide absorbent canister fails to become warm during use?
112. What two factors influence the efficiency of carbon dioxide neutralization?
113. How does the size of the carbon dioxide absorbent granules affect the efficiency of carbon dioxide neutralization?
114. What is the optimal carbon dioxide absorbent granule size? How is this sizing system defined?
115. What does channeling in the carbon dioxide absorbent granule-containing canister refer to? How does channeling in the canister affect the efficiency of carbon dioxide neutralization?
116. What is the most frequent cause of channeling in the carbon dioxide absorbent granule-containing canister? How can it be minimized?
117. Define carbon dioxide absorbent absorptive capacity. What can cause a decrease in absorptive capacity?
118. Why do the carbon dioxide absorbent granules change color?
119. Contrast the color change of soda lime granules with those of Amsorb Plus and Litholyme.
120. Contrast the degradation of inhaled anesthetics to toxic compounds by carbon dioxide absorbents. What is the impact of desiccation on the degradation process?
121. What factors lead to increased compound A production with carbon dioxide absorbents? What is the clinical effect of this?
122. Why is carbon monoxide (CO) poisonous?
123. What factors lead to increased carbon monoxide production with carbon dioxide absorbents? Are the concentrations of carbon dioxide produced significant?

124. Why do most instances of increased blood concentrations of carboxyhemoglobin occur in anesthetized patients on a Monday?

125. What causes the development of fire and extreme heat in the breathing system? How can this be avoided?

126. Complete the following table:

Feature	Soda Lime	Amsorb Plus
Mesh size		
Generation of compound A with sevoflurane		
Generation of carbon monoxide with inhaled anesthetics		
Risk of exothermic reactions and fire in the presence of sevoflurane		

CHECKING THE ANESTHESIA MACHINE AND CIRCLE SYSTEM FUNCTION

127. What are the current recommendations for pre-anesthesia checkout procedures? How do these apply to newer machines with automated checkout procedures?

128. How often should these checkout procedures be performed?

129. What are the most important preoperative checks?

130. Does the presence of a Jackson-Rees circuit along with a full oxygen E-cylinder mounted on the back of the anesthesia machine comply with the current checkout recommendations?

131. What does a leak check of the machine's low-pressure system evaluate? Why is this so important?

132. Why is calibration of the oxygen monitor so important?

133. Does a manual positive-pressure leak test check the integrity of the unidirectional valves?

ANSWERS*

ANESTHESIA WORKSTATION

1. Components of the anesthesia workstation include what was previously recognized as the anesthesia machine (the pressure-regulating and gas-mixing components), vaporizers, anesthesia breathing circuit, ventilator, scavenging system, and respiratory and physiologic monitoring systems (electrocardiogram, arterial blood pressure, temperature, pulse oximeter, and inhaled and exhaled concentrations of oxygen, carbon dioxide, anesthetic gases, and vapors). (220)

2. The fail-safe valve is designed to protect against delivery of hypoxic gas mixtures from the anesthesia machine in the event of failure of the oxygen supply. The fail-safe valve is triggered when the pressure in the oxygen delivery line decreases to less than 30 psi. When the fail-safe valve is triggered, it either shuts off or proportionally decreases the flow of all gases. Note that it is only the pressure of oxygen that triggers the fail-safe valve. (221)

3. An intact fail-safe valve is actually only a pressure-sensor valve. A hypoxic mixture may still be delivered to the patient if the fail-safe valve is sensing an adequate gas pressure in the circuit of the anesthesia machine when the oxygen flow is zero. This confirms the importance of the oxygen analyzer on the

*Numbers in parentheses refer to pages, figures, boxes, or tables in Pardo MC, Miller RD, eds. *Basics of Anesthesia*. 7th ed. Philadelphia: Elsevier; 2018.

anesthesia machine. Far superior to the fail-safe valve or an oxygen analyzer is the continuous presence of a vigilant anesthesia provider. (221)

4. The oxygen, nitrous oxide, and air gases that are used in anesthesia are most often delivered to the anesthesia machine as compressed gases from a central supply source located in the hospital. These hospital-supplied gases enter the operating room from a central source through pipelines to color-coded wall outlets. Pressure hoses then connect the wall outlets to the anesthesia machine. These gases must be delivered at a pressure of about 50 psi for the anesthesia machine to function properly. (221)

5. The delivery of erroneous gases from the central supply source to the pipeline inlet connections on the anesthesia machine is minimized in two ways. First, the wall outlets and pressure hoses are color-coded. Second, and more important, the pressure hoses are connected to the wall outlets and anesthesia machine by fittings that are noninterchangeable (*diameter index* safety system [DISS] or Quick Connects), which are designed to prevent misconnections of pipeline gases. (221)

6. The purpose of the cylinders of oxygen and nitrous oxide that are found on the back of the anesthesia machine is for the delivery of those gases should the central gas supply fail. (222)

7. An erroneous hookup of a gas cylinder to the anesthesia machine is minimized in two ways. First, the cylinders are color-coded. Second, and more important, the color-coded cylinders are attached to the anesthesia machine by a hanger yoke assembly, which consists of two metal pins that correspond to holes in the valve casing of the gas cylinder. This *pin index* safety system (PISS) is designed to make it impossible to attach an oxygen cylinder to any yoke on the anesthesia machine other than that designed for oxygen. Otherwise, a cylinder containing nitrous oxide could be attached to the oxygen yoke, which would result in the delivery of nitrous oxide when the oxygen flowmeter was activated. (222)

8.

Characteristics	Oxygen	Nitrous Oxide	Carbon Dioxide	Air
Cylinder color	Green	Blue	Gray	Yellow
Physical state in cylinder (gas/liquid)	Gas	Liquid and gas	Liquid and gas	Gas
Cylinder contents (liters)	625	1590	1590	625
Cylinder pressure full (psi)	2000	750	838	1800

(223)

9. The pressure in an oxygen cylinder is directly proportional to the volume of oxygen in the cylinder. For example, a full oxygen cylinder is evidenced by a pressure of approximately 2000 psi, which contains about 625 L of oxygen. If the pressure gauge on an oxygen cylinder were to read 500 psi, one fourth of the initial pressure, it can be estimated that only one fourth of the volume remains in the oxygen cylinder. The volume in the cylinder could be estimated to be $\frac{625}{4}$, or about 156 L. (223)

10. In contrast to oxygen, the pressure gauge for nitrous oxide does not indicate the amount of gas remaining in the cylinder because the pressure in the gas cylinder remains at 750 psi as long as any liquid nitrous oxide is present. When nitrous oxide leaves the cylinder as a vapor, additional liquid is vaporized to maintain an unchanging pressure in the cylinder. After all the liquid nitrous oxide is vaporized, the pressure begins to decrease, and it can be assumed that

about 75% of the contents of the gas cylinder have been exhausted. Because a full nitrous oxide cylinder (E-size) contains about 1590 L, approximately 400 L of nitrous oxide remains when the pressure gauge begins to decrease from its previously constant value of 750 psi. (223)

11. Vaporization of a liquefied gas (nitrous oxide), as well as expansion of a compressed gas (oxygen), absorbs heat, which is extracted from the metal cylinder and the surrounding atmosphere. For this reason, atmospheric water vapor often accumulates as frost on gas cylinders and in valves, particularly during high gas flow from these tanks. Internal icing does not occur because compressed gases are free of water vapor. (223)

12. Flowmeters on the anesthesia machine precisely control and measure gas flow to the common gas inlet. (223)

13. Measurement of the flow of gases is based on the principle that flow past a resistance is proportional to pressure. Typically, gas flow enters the bottom of a vertically positioned and tapered (the cross-sectional area increases upward from site of gas entry) glass flow tube. Gas flow into the flowmeter tube raises a bobbin or ball-shaped float. The float comes to rest when gravity is balanced by the decrease in pressure caused by the float. The upper end of the bobbin or the equator of the ball indicates the gas flow in milliliters or liters per minute. (223)

14. Proportionality between pressure and flow is determined by the shape of the tube (resistance) and the physical properties (density and viscosity) of the gas. The flowmeters are initially calibrated for the indicated gas at the factory. Because few gases have the same density and viscosity, flowmeters are not interchangeable with other gases. (223)

15. The oxygen flowmeter should be the last in the sequence of flowmeters, and thus oxygen should be the last gas added to the manifold (mixing chamber). This arrangement reduces the possibility that leaks in the apparatus proximal to oxygen inflow can diminish the delivered oxygen concentration, whereas leaks distal to that point result in loss of volume without a qualitative change in the mixture. Nevertheless, an oxygen flowmeter tube leak can produce a hypoxic mixture regardless of the flowmeter tube arrangement. (223)

16. The purpose of the oxygen flush valve is to provide a large volume of oxygen to the patient quickly. Oxygen delivered to the patient when the oxygen flush valve is depressed bypasses the flowmeters and manifold. (223-224)

17. The flow of oxygen that is delivered to the patient via the oxygen flush valve is 35 to 75 L/min. (224)

18. Activation of the oxygen flush valve during a mechanically delivered inspiration from the anesthesia machine ventilator permits the transmission of high airway pressure to the patient's lungs, with the possibility of barotrauma. (224)

VAPORIZERS

19. Volatile anesthetics are liquids at room temperature and atmospheric pressure. Vaporization, which is the conversion of a liquid to a vapor, takes place in a closed container, referred to as a vaporizer. The inhaled delivery of volatile anesthetics requires that they be vaporized. The vapor concentration resulting from vaporization of a volatile liquid anesthetic must be delivered to the patient with the same accuracy and predictability as other gases (oxygen, nitrous oxide). (224)

20. The heat of vaporization of a liquid is the number of calories required at a specific temperature to convert 1 g of a liquid into a vapor. (224)

21. Vaporization in the closed confines of a vaporizer ceases when equilibrium is reached between the liquid and vapor phases such that the number of molecules leaving the liquid phase is the same as the number reentering. The molecules in the vapor phase collide with each other and the walls of the container, thereby creating pressure. This pressure is termed vapor pressure and is unique for each volatile anesthetic. Vapor pressure is

temperature dependent, such that a decrease in the temperature of the liquid is associated with a lower vapor pressure and fewer molecules in the vapor phase. Cooling of the liquid anesthetic reflects a loss of heat (heat of vaporization) necessary to provide energy for vaporization. This cooling is undesirable because it lowers the vapor pressure and limits the attainable vapor concentration. (224)

22. Contemporary vaporizers are classified as agent-specific, variable-bypass, flow-over, temperature-compensated, and out of circuit. (224)

23. Desflurane has a vapor pressure near 1 atm (664 mm Hg) at 20° C. For this reason, a desflurane vaporizer is electrically heated to 23° C to 25° C and pressurized with a backpressure regulator to 1500 mm Hg to create an environment in which the anesthetic has a relatively lower, but predictable, volatility. (224)

24. Agent-specific refers to the fact that vaporizers are calibrated to accommodate a single volatile anesthetic. (224)

25. Variable-bypass describes dividing (splitting) the total fresh gas flow through the vaporizer into two portions. The first portion of the fresh gas flow (20% or less) passes into the vaporizing chamber of the vaporizer, where it becomes saturated (flow-over) with the vapor of the liquid anesthetic. The second portion of the fresh gas flow passes through the bypass chamber of the vaporizer. Both portions of the fresh gas flow mix at the patient outlet side of the anesthesia machine. The proportion of fresh gas flow diverted through the vaporizing chamber, and thus the concentration (in volume percent) of volatile anesthetic delivered to the patient, is determined by the concentration control dial. (224)

26. As the vaporizer temperature changes, a temperature-sensitive bimetallic strip or an expansion element inside the vaporizer influences proportioning of total gas flow between the vaporizing and bypass chambers. For example, as the temperature of the liquid anesthetic in the vaporizer chamber decreases, the temperature-sensing elements allow increased gas inflow into this chamber to offset the effect of decreased anesthetic liquid vapor pressure. Vaporizers are often constructed of metals with high thermal conductivity (copper, bronze) to further minimize heat loss. As a result, vaporizer output is nearly linear between 20° C and 35° C. (225)

27. Out of circuit describes the fact that vaporizers are isolated from the anesthetic breathing system. (225)

28. Tipping of vaporizers can cause liquid anesthetic to spill from the vaporizing chamber into the bypass chamber, with a resultant increased vapor concentration exiting from the vaporizer. (225)

29. A safety interlock mechanism ensures that only one vaporizer at a time can be turned on, thereby preventing the delivery of two different volatile anesthetics to the same patient. (225)

30. Use of an anesthetic-specific keyed filler device prevents placement of a liquid anesthetic into the vaporizing chamber that is different from the anesthetic for which the vaporizer was calibrated. This is uniquely important for desflurane because its vapor pressure is near 1 atm, and accidental placement of desflurane in a contemporary vaporizer could result in an anesthetic overdose. (225)

ANESTHETIC BREATHING SYSTEMS

31. The function of anesthetic breathing systems is to deliver oxygen and anesthetic gases to the patient and to eliminate carbon dioxide. (225)

32. Anesthetic breathing systems can add considerable resistance to inhalation because peak flows as high as 60 L/min are reached during spontaneous inspiration. This resistance is influenced by unidirectional valves and connectors. The components of the breathing system, particularly the tracheal tube connector, should have the largest possible lumen to minimize this resistance to breathing. Right-angle connectors should be replaced with curved connectors to minimize resistance. Substituting controlled ventilation of the patient's lungs for spontaneous breathing

can offset the increased resistance to inhalation imparted by anesthetic breathing systems. (225)

33. Anesthetic breathing systems are classified as open, semiopen, semiclosed, and closed according to the presence or absence of (1) a gas reservoir bag in the circuit, (2) rebreathing of exhaled gases, (3) means to chemically neutralize exhaled carbon dioxide, and (4) unidirectional valves. (226)

34. The most commonly used anesthetic breathing systems are the (1) Mapleson F (Jackson-Rees) system, (2) Bain circuit, and (3) circle system. (226)

35. The Mapleson systems are characterized by the absence of valves to direct gases to or from the patient and the absence of chemical carbon dioxide neutralization. (226)

36. The Mapleson F system is a T-piece arrangement with a reservoir bag and an adjustable pressure-limiting overflow valve on the distal end of the gas reservoir bag. Another name for this anesthetic breathing system is the Jackson-Rees circuit. (226)

37. The Mapleson F system is commonly used for controlled ventilation during transport of tracheally intubated patients. (226)

38. Advantages of the Mapleson F anesthetic breathing system include its minimal dead space and resistance. This makes this system ideal for pediatric anesthesia. It is also inexpensive, is lightweight, can be repositioned easily, and can be used with a face mask or endotracheal tube. (226-227)

39. Disadvantages of the Mapleson F system include (1) the need for high fresh gas inflow to prevent rebreathing, (2) the possibility of high airway pressure and barotrauma should the overflow valve become occluded, and (3) the lack of humidification. The degree of rebreathing is influenced by both the method of ventilation (spontaneous versus controlled) and the adjustment of the pressure-limiting overflow valve to allow for venting. When the patient is breathing spontaneously, fresh gas flow equal to two to three times the patient's minute ventilation is recommended to prevent rebreathing. Lack of humidification can be offset by allowing the fresh gas to pass through an in-line heated humidifier. (227)

40. The Bain circuit is a coaxial version of the Mapleson D system in which the fresh gas supply tube runs coaxially inside the corrugated expiratory tubing. The fresh gas tube enters the circuit near the reservoir bag, but the fresh gas is actually delivered at the patient end of the circuit. The exhaled gases are vented through the overflow valve near the reservoir bag. (227)

41. Advantages of the Bain circuit include (1) warming of the fresh gas inflow by the surrounding exhaled gases in the corrugated expiratory tube, (2) conservation of moisture as a result of partial rebreathing, and (3) ease of scavenging waste anesthetic gases from the overflow valve. It is lightweight, easily sterilized, reusable, and useful when access to the patient is limited, such as during head and neck surgery. (227)

42. Hazards of the Bain circuit include unrecognized disconnection or kinking of the inner fresh gas tube. The outer expiratory tube should be transparent to allow inspection of the inner tube. (227)

43. The essential components of a circle anesthetic breathing system are arranged in a circular manner. (227)

44. The circle system prevents rebreathing of carbon dioxide by chemical neutralization of carbon dioxide with carbon dioxide absorbents. (227-228)

45. A circle system can be classified as semiopen, semiclosed, or closed, depending on the amount of fresh gas inflow. In a semiopen system, very high fresh gas flow is used to eliminate rebreathing of gases. A semiclosed system is associated with rebreathing of gases, and in a closed system the fresh gas inflow exactly matches that being consumed by the patient. (228)

46. A semiclosed system is associated with rebreathing of gases and is the most commonly used approach. (228)

47. The semiclosed and closed circle system are both advantageous in that they allow for the rebreathing of exhaled gases. The rebreathing of exhaled gases results in (1) some conservation of airway moisture and body heat and (2) decreased pollution of the surrounding atmosphere with anesthetic gases when the fresh gas inflow rate is set at less than the patient's minute ventilation. (228)

48. Disadvantages of the circle system include (1) increased resistance to breathing because of the presence of unidirectional valves and carbon dioxide absorbent, (2) bulkiness with loss of portability, and (3) enhanced opportunity for malfunction because of the complexity of the apparatus. (228)

49. The rebreathing of exhaled gases in a semiclosed circle system influences the inhaled anesthetic concentrations of these gases. For example, when uptake of the anesthetic gas is high, as during induction of anesthesia, rebreathing of exhaled gases depleted of anesthetic greatly dilutes the concentration of anesthetic in the fresh gas inflow. This dilutional effect of uptake is offset clinically by increasing the delivered concentration of anesthetic. As uptake of anesthetic diminishes, the impact of dilution on the inspired concentration produced by rebreathing of exhaled gases is lessened. (228)

50. The circle system consists of (1) a fresh gas inlet, (2) inspiratory and expiratory unidirectional check valves, (3) inspiratory and expiratory corrugated tubing, (4) a Y-piece connector, (5) an adjustable pressure-limiting (APL) valve, also referred to as an overflow or "pop-off" valve, (6) a reservoir bag, (7) a canister containing carbon dioxide absorbent, (8) a bag/vent selector switch, and (9) a mechanical anesthesia ventilator. (229)

51. Two unidirectional valves are situated in different limbs of the corrugated tubing in a circle system such that one functions for inhalation and the other for exhalation. These valves (1) permit positive-pressure breathing and (2) prevent the rebreathing of exhaled gases until they have passed through the carbon dioxide absorbent canister and have had their oxygen content replenished. Rebreathing and hypercapnia can occur if the unidirectional valves stick in the open position, and total occlusion of the circuit can occur if they are stuck in the closed position. If the expiratory valve is stuck in the closed position, breath stacking and barotrauma can occur. (229)

52. Dead space in the circle system is between the Y-piece and the patient. (229)

53. The inspiratory and expiratory corrugated tubes serve as conduits for delivery of gases to and from the patient. Their large bore provides minimal resistance, and the corrugations provide flexibility, resist kinking, and promote turbulent instead of laminar flow. (229)

54. During positive-pressure ventilation, some of the delivered gas distends the corrugated tubing and some is compressed within the circuit, which leads to a smaller delivered tidal volume. (229)

55. The Y-piece connector at the patient end of the circuit has (1) a curved elbow, (2) an outer diameter of 22 mm to fit inside a face mask, and (3) an inner diameter of 15 mm to fit onto an endotracheal tube connector. (229)

56. The APL valve is also known as the overflow or "pop-off" valve. (229)

57. When the bag/vent selector switch is set to bag, the APL (overflow or "pop-off") valve (1) allows venting of excess gas from the breathing system into the waste gas scavenging system and (2) can be adjusted to allow the anesthesia provider to provide assisted or controlled ventilation of the patient's lungs by manual compression of the gas reservoir bag. The APL valve should be fully open during spontaneous ventilation so that circuit pressure remains negligible throughout inspiration and expiration. (229)

58. When the bag/vent selector switch is set to bag, the gas reservoir bag maintains an available reserve volume of gas to satisfy the patient's spontaneous inspiratory flow rate (up to 60 L/min), which greatly exceeds conventional fresh gas flows (commonly 3 to 5 L/min) from the anesthesia

machine. The bag also serves as a safety device because its distensibility limits pressure in the breathing circuit to less than 60 cm H_2O, even when the APL valve is closed. (229)

59. In a closed anesthetic breathing system, there is total rebreathing of exhaled gases after absorption of carbon dioxide, and the APL valve or relief valve of the ventilator is closed. A closed system is present when the fresh gas inflow into the circle system (150 to 500 mL/min) satisfies the patient's metabolic oxygen requirements (150 to 250 mL/min during anesthesia) and replaces anesthetic gases lost by virtue of tissue uptake. If sidestream gas analyzers are used, the analyzed gas exiting the analyzer must be returned to the breathing system to maintain a closed system. (229)

60. Advantages of a closed circle anesthetic breathing system over a semiclosed circle anesthetic breathing system include (1) maximal humidification and warming of inhaled gases, (2) less pollution of the surrounding atmosphere with anesthetic gases, and (3) economy in the use of anesthetics. (229-230)

61. A disadvantage of a closed circle anesthetic breathing system is an inability to rapidly change the delivered concentration of anesthetic gases and oxygen because of the low fresh gas inflow. (230)

62. The principal dangers of a closed anesthetic breathing system are delivery of (1) unpredictable and possibly insufficient concentrations of oxygen and (2) unknown and possibly excessive concentrations of potent anesthetic gases. (230)

63. Unpredictable and possibly insufficient delivered concentrations of oxygen when using a closed anesthetic breathing system are more likely if nitrous oxide is included in the fresh gas inflow. For example, decreased tissue uptake of nitrous oxide with time in the presence of unchanged uptake of oxygen can result in a decreased concentration of oxygen in the alveoli. (230)

64. The potential problem of the inadequate delivery of oxygen using a closed circle anesthetic breathing system can be minimized by the use of an oxygen analyzer placed on the inspiratory or expiratory limb of the closed circle system. (230)

65. Exhaled gases, devoid of carbon dioxide, form a major part of the inhaled gases when a closed anesthetic breathing system is used. This means that the composition of the inhaled gases is influenced by the concentration present in the exhaled gases. The concentration of anesthetic in exhaled gases reflects tissue uptake of the anesthetic. Initially, tissue uptake is maximal, and the concentration of anesthetic in the exhaled gases is minimal. Subsequent rebreathing of these exhaled gases dilutes the inhaled concentration of anesthetic delivered to the patient. Therefore, high inflow concentrations of anesthetic are necessary to offset maximal tissue uptake. Conversely, only small amounts of anesthetic need to be added to the inflow gases when tissue uptake has decreased. The unknown impact of tissue uptake on the concentration of anesthetic in exhaled gases makes it difficult to estimate the inhaled concentration delivered to the patient through a closed anesthetic breathing system. This disadvantage can be partially offset by administering higher fresh gas inflow (3 L/min) for about 15 minutes before instituting the use of a closed anesthetic breathing system. This approach permits elimination of nitrogen from the lungs and corresponds to the time of greatest tissue uptake of anesthetic. (230)

ANESTHESIA MACHINE VENTILATORS

66. When the anesthesia machine ventilator bag/vent selector switch is set to vent, the gas reservoir bag and APL valve are eliminated from the circle anesthetic system, and the patient's ventilation is delivered from the mechanical anesthesia ventilator. (230)

67. Anesthesia ventilators are powered by compressed gas, electricity, or both. (230)

68. Most conventional anesthesia machine ventilators are pneumatically driven by oxygen or air that is pressurized and, during the inspiratory phase, routed to the space inside the ventilator casing between the compressible bellows and the

rigid casing. Pressurized air or oxygen entering this space forces the bellows to empty its contents into the patient's lungs through the inspiratory limb of the breathing circuit. This pressurized air or oxygen also causes the ventilator relief valve to close, thereby preventing inspiratory anesthetic gas from escaping into the scavenging system. (230)

69. Oxygen is preferable to air as the ventilator driving gas because if there is a leak in the bellows, the fraction of inspired oxygen will be increased. If there is a leak in the bellows in a ventilator driven by 50 psi oxygen or air, the peak inspiratory pressure will rise. (230)

70. During exhalation, the driving gas is either vented into the room or directed to the scavenging system, and the bellows refills as the patient exhales. (230)

71. Some newer anesthesia machines have mechanically driven piston-type of ventilators. The piston operates much like the plunger of a syringe to deliver the desired tidal volume or airway pressure to the patient. (230)

72. Ventilators with bellows that rises during exhalation (standing or ascending bellows) are preferred because the bellows will not rise (fill) if there is a leak in the anesthesia breathing system or the system becomes accidentally disconnected. Ventilators with a bellows that descends during exhalation (hanging or descending bellows) are potentially dangerous because the bellows will continue to rise and fall during a disconnection. Whenever a ventilator is used, a disconnect alarm must be activated and audible. (230-231)

73. The upper respiratory tract (especially the nose) functions as the principal heat and moisture exchanger (HME) to bring inspired gas to body temperature and 100% relative humidity in its passage to the alveoli. (231)

74. Water is removed from medical gases (cylinders or piped) to prevent corrosion and condensation. Tracheal intubation or the use of a laryngeal mask airway bypasses the upper airway and thus leaves the tracheobronchial mucosa the burden of heating and humidifying inspired gases. Humidification of inspired gases by the lower respiratory tract in intubated patients can lead to dehydration of the mucosa, impaired ciliary function, impaired surfactant function, inspissation of secretions, atelectasis, and a rise in the alveolar-to-arterial gradient. Breathing of dry and room temperature gases in intubated patients is associated with water and heat loss from the patient. Heat loss is more important than water loss, and the most important reason to provide heated humidification for intubated patients is to decrease heat loss and reduce associated decreases in body temperature. This is especially true in infants and children, who are rendered poikilothermic by general anesthesia. (231-232)

75. Humidification is a form of vaporization in which water vapor (moisture) is added to the gases delivered by the anesthetic breathing system to minimize water and heat loss. The water formed and the heat generated by chemical neutralization of carbon dioxide help humidify and heat the gases in the breathing circuit. (232)

76. Humidifiers used for anesthesia and in the intensive care unit include (1) heat and moisture exchanger (HME) humidifiers, (2) heated water vaporizers and humidifiers, and (3) nebulizers. (232)

77. HME humidifiers are devices that, when placed between the endotracheal tube and Y-piece of the circle system, conserve some of the exhaled water and heat and return it to the inspired gases. They contain a porous hydrophobic or hygroscopic membrane that traps exhaled humidified gases and returns them to the patient on inspiration. Bacterial and viral filters can be incorporated in HME humidifiers to convert them into heat and moisture exchanger filters (HMEFs). (232)

78. The advantages of HME humidifiers over other types of humidifiers are that they are (1) simple and easy to use, (2) lightweight, (3) not dependent on an external power source, (4) disposable, and (5) low cost. (232)

79. The disadvantages of HME humidifiers are that they (1) are not as effective as heated water vaporizers and humidifiers in maintaining patient temperature, (2)

add resistance and increase the work of breathing and therefore should be used with caution in spontaneously ventilating patients, (3) can become clogged with patient secretions or blood, and (4) can increase dead space, which can cause significant rebreathing in pediatric patients. Special low-volume HME humidifiers are available for pediatric patients. (232)

80. Heated water vaporizers and humidifiers are used to deliver a relative humidity higher than that delivered by HME humidifiers. Heated water vaporizers are more frequently used in pediatric anesthesia and intensive care unit patients. (232)

81. Risks from heated water vaporizers and humidifiers include (1) thermal injury, (2) nosocomial infection, (3) increased work of breathing, and (4) increased risk of malfunction due to the complexity of these systems. (232)

82. Nebulizers produce a mist of microdroplets of water suspended in a gaseous medium. The quantity of water droplets delivered is not limited by the temperature of the carrier gas. In addition to water, nebulizers can deliver medications to peripheral airways. (232)

POLLUTION OF THE ATMOSPHERE WITH ANESTHETIC GASES

83. In the operating room, OSHA recommends that the concentration of nitrous oxide not exceed 25 ppm and exposure concentrations of volatile anesthetics not exceed 2 ppm. (232)

84. Control of pollution of the atmosphere with anesthetic gases requires (1) scavenging of waste anesthetic gases, (2) periodic preventive maintenance of anesthesia equipment, (3) attention to the anesthetic technique, and (4) adequate ventilation of the operating rooms. (232)

85. Scavenging is the collection and subsequent removal of vented gases from the operating room. The amount of delivered gas used to anesthetize a patient commonly far exceeds the patient's needs. The excess gas comes from either the APL valve if the bag/vent selector switch is set to bag or from the ventilator relief valve if the bag/vent selector switch is set to vent. All excess gas from the patient exits the breathing system through these valves. In addition, when the bag/vent selector switch is set to vent, some anesthetic breathing systems direct the drive gas inside the bellows canister to the scavenging system. If sidestream gas analyzers are used, the analyzed gas exiting the analyzer must be directed to the scavenging system or returned to the breathing system. (233)

86. Scavenging systems may be characterized as active or passive. An active system is connected to the hospital's vacuum system, and gases are drawn from the machine by a vacuum. A passive system is connected to the hospital's ventilation duct and waste gases flow out of the machine on their own. (233)

87. Many anesthesia machines provide active scavenging with a waste gas receiver mounted on the side of the anesthesia machine. Advantages of this system include (1) a needle valve that allows the clinician to manually adjust the amount of vacuum flow through the scavenging system, (2) a needle valve that can be adjusted such that the 3-L reservoir bag will be slightly inflated and appear to "breathe" with the patient, and (3) unlike other active scavenging systems, a waste gas receiver that does not require a strong vacuum to operate. (233)

88. Hazards of scavenging systems include (1) obstruction of the scavenging pathways, which can result in excessive positive pressure in the breathing circuit and possible barotrauma, and (2) excessive vacuum applied to the scavenging system, which can cause negative pressures in the breathing system. (233)

89. Scavenging systems contain two relief valves to minimize their potential hazards. If gas accumulates in the scavenging system and cannot leave the anesthesia machine properly, the positive-pressure scavenge relief valve opens when the pressure reaches 10 cm H_2O to allow the gas to escape into the room. If negative pressure is applied to the scavenging system, the negative-pressure

scavenge relief valve opens and allows room air to be drawn in (instead of drawing gas from the patient). Additionally, if the amount of fresh gas flow exceeds the capacity of the scavenging system, the excess waste anesthetic gas exits the scavenging system through the positive-pressure relief valve and pollutes the operating room. (233)

90. High-pressure leakage of nitrous oxide can occur as a result of faulty yokes attaching the nitrous oxide tank to the anesthesia machine or faulty connections from the central nitrous oxide gas supply to the anesthesia machine. (233)

91. Low-pressure leakage of anesthetic gases can occur because of leaks inside the anesthesia machine and leaks between the machine and patient. (233)

92. Anesthetic techniques that can lead to operating room pollution include (1) poorly fitting face masks, (2) flushing the anesthetic delivery circuit, (3) filling anesthetic vaporizers, (4) the use of uncuffed endotracheal tubes, (5) failure to turn off the nitrous oxide flow or vaporizers at the end of the anesthetic, and (6) the use of semiopen breathing circuits such as the Jackson-Rees, which are difficult to scavenge. (233)

93. The air in the operating room should be exchanged at least 15 times per hour by the operating room ventilation system. This rate should be checked periodically by the hospital's clinical engineering department. (233)

ELIMINATION OF CARBON DIOXIDE

94. Open and semiopen breathing systems eliminate carbon dioxide by venting all exhaled gases to the atmosphere. (233)

95. Semiclosed and closed breathing systems eliminate carbon dioxide by chemical neutralization. Chemical neutralization is accomplished by directing the exhaled gases through a carbon dioxide absorber, which consists of a canister containing carbon dioxide absorbent granules. (233)

96. The three components common to all carbon dioxide absorbents are the neutralizing base, water, and catalysts. (233)

97. All carbon dioxide absorbents use calcium hydroxide ($Ca(OH)_2$) as the neutralizing base for carbon dioxide produced during respiration. (233)

98. Water is an essential ingredient common to all carbon dioxide absorbents, and it is necessary for efficient and safe carbon dioxide absorption. (233)

99. The catalysts contained in carbon dioxide absorbents are responsible for the differences in absorptive properties and safety profiles between individual absorbents. (234)

100. Soda lime is a traditional carbon dioxide absorbent. Amsorb Plus and Litholyme are new generation absorbents. (234)

101. Soda lime granules consist of calcium hydroxide, water, and small amounts of the strong bases sodium and potassium hydroxide that serve as catalysts for carbon dioxide absorption. (234)

102. Soda lime granules fragment easily and produce alkaline dust, which can lead to bronchospasm if inhaled. Silica is added to the granules to provide hardness and minimize alkaline dust formation. (234)

103. Neutralization of carbon dioxide with soda lime begins with reaction of carbon dioxide with water present in the soda lime granules and the subsequent formation of carbonic acid. Carbonic acid then reacts with the hydroxides present in the soda lime granules to form carbonates (with bicarbonates as intermediates), water, and heat. (234)

104. The water formed from the neutralization of carbon dioxide, the water present in the soda lime granules, and the water condensed from the patient's exhaled gases leach the alkaline bases from the soda lime granules and produce a slurry containing NaOH and KOH in the bottom of the canister. These monovalent bases can be corrosive to the skin. (234)

105. The strong base sodium hydroxide and potassium hydroxide catalysts in soda lime can lead to degradation of sevoflurane to compound A. (234)

106. The strong base sodium hydroxide and potassium hydroxide catalysts in soda lime can lead to degradation of inhaled anesthetics to clinically significant concentrations of carbon monoxide. (234)

107. Amsorb Plus and Litholyme are new-generation carbon dioxide absorbents that consist of calcium hydroxide and water, but unlike soda lime, they do not contain the strong bases sodium hydroxide or potassium hydroxide. Instead they contain catalysts that are chemically inert. (234)

108. Unlike soda lime, Amsorb Plus and Litholyme do not contain the strong bases sodium hydroxide or potassium hydroxide. Instead they contain catalysts that are chemically inert and do not degrade sevoflurane to compound A. (234)

109. Unlike soda lime, Amsorb Plus and Litholyme do not contain the strong bases sodium hydroxide or potassium hydroxide. Instead they contain catalysts that are chemically inert and do not degrade inhaled anesthetics to carbon monoxide. (234)

110. Neutralization of carbon dioxide with Amsorb Plus or Litholyme begins with the reaction of carbon dioxide with water present in the granules and the subsequent formation of carbonic acid. Carbonic acid then reacts with the calcium hydroxide present in the granules to form calcium carbonate, water, and heat. (234)

111. The water formed by the neutralization of carbon dioxide with soda lime, Amsorb Plus, and Litholyme is useful for humidifying the gases and for dissipating some of the heat generated in these exothermic reactions. The heat generated during the neutralization of carbon dioxide can be detected by the warmness of the canister. Failure of the canister to become warm should alert the anesthesia provider to the possibility that chemical neutralization of carbon dioxide is not taking place. (234)

112. The efficiency of carbon dioxide neutralization is influenced by the size of the carbon dioxide granules and the presence or absence of channeling in the carbon dioxide canister. (234)

113. The optimal absorbent granule size represents a compromise between absorptive efficiency and resistance to airflow through the carbon dioxide absorbent canister. Absorbent efficiency increases as absorbent granule size decreases because the total surface area coming in contact with carbon dioxide increases. The smaller the absorbent granules, however, the smaller the interstices through which gas must flow and the greater the resistance to flow. (235)

114. Absorbent granule size is designated as mesh size, which refers to the number of openings per linear inch in a sieve through which the granular particles can pass. The granular size of carbon dioxide absorbents in anesthesia practice is between 4 and 10 mesh, a size at which absorbent efficiency is maximal with minimal resistance. A 4-mesh screen means that there are four quarter-inch openings per linear inch. A 10-mesh screen has ten tenth-inch openings per linear inch. (235)

115. Channeling is the preferential passage of exhaled gases through the carbon dioxide absorber canister via pathways of low resistance such that the bulk of the carbon dioxide absorbent granules are bypassed. This can result in decreased efficiency of carbon dioxide neutralization. (235)

116. Channeling results from loose packing of absorbent granules and can be minimized by gently shaking the canister before use to ensure firm packing of the absorbent granules. Carbon dioxide absorbent canisters are designed to facilitate uniform dispersion of exhaled gas flow through the absorbent granules. (235)

117. Absorptive capacity is determined by the maximum amount of carbon dioxide that can be absorbed by 100 g of carbon dioxide absorbent. Channeling of exhaled gases through the absorbent granules can substantially decrease their efficiency. Carbon dioxide absorber canister design also influences the absorptive capacity of the carbon dioxide absorbent. (235)

118. Carbon dioxide absorbents contain a pH-sensitive indicator dye that changes color when the carbon dioxide absorbent granules are exhausted. When the absorptive components of the granules are exhausted, carbonic acid accumulates and produces a change in the pH and thus in the indicator dye color. (235)

119. The indicator dye in soda lime changes granule color from white to purple when exhausted. However, over time, exhausted soda lime granules may revert to their original white color even though absorptive capacity does not recover with time. On reuse, the dye quickly produces the purple color change again. In contrast, Amsorb Plus and Litholyme each contain an indicator dye that changes granule color from white to purple when exhausted and, once changed, does not revert to its original color. (235)

120. Soda lime, whether moist and containing a normal water complement or dry, degrades sevoflurane to nephrotoxic compounds (compound A). Desiccated soda lime may degrade desflurane, enflurane, or isoflurane to carbon monoxide. In contrast, Amsorb Plus and Litholyme, whether desiccated or moist, do not degrade inhaled anesthetics. (235)

121. Degradation of sevoflurane by soda lime can result in the production of compound A, which is a dose- and time-dependent nephrotoxin. Production of compound A with soda lime increases with (1) low fresh gas flows, (2) higher concentrations of sevoflurane, and (3) higher absorbent temperatures. To date, no clinically significant renal toxicity has been associated with the use of sevoflurane. In contrast, Amsorb Plus and Litholyme do not degrade sevoflurane to compound A. (235)

122. Carbon monoxide (CO) is an odorless, colorless gas that is poisonous because it displaces oxygen from hemoglobin in blood and thereby leads to the formation of carboxyhemoglobin. (235)

123. Soda lime degrades inhaled anesthetics to carbon monoxide. In contrast, Amsorb Plus and Litholyme do not degrade inhaled anesthetics to carbon monoxide. Degradation of inhaled anesthetics by desiccated soda lime can lead to significant concentrations of carbon monoxide that can produce carboxyhemoglobin concentrations reaching 30% or higher. Production of carbon monoxide and carboxyhemoglobin increases with (1) the inhaled anesthetic used (desflurane = enflurane > isoflurane >> halothane = sevoflurane), (2) low fresh gas flows, (3) higher concentrations of inhaled anesthetics, (4) higher absorbent temperatures, and most important, (5) the degree of dryness of the absorbent (desiccation). (235)

124. Desiccation of soda lime increases the degradation of inhaled anesthetics to carbon monoxide. Desiccation requires a prolonged period (usually 48 hours) of high dry gas flow between cases. Desiccation is worsened if the breathing bag is left off the circuit. In this circumstance the inspiratory valve produces resistance to forward flow, and the fresh gas takes the retrograde path of least resistance through the bottom to the top of the absorbent canister and out the 22 mm breathing bag mount. Accordingly, most instances of increased blood concentrations of carboxyhemoglobin occur in patients anesthetized on a Monday after continuous flow of oxygen (flowmeter accidentally left on) through the soda lime carbon dioxide absorbent over the weekend. (235)

125. Desiccation of the carbon dioxide absorbent Baralyme (no longer clinically available) can lead to fire within the circle system with sevoflurane use. A poorly characterized chemical reaction between sevoflurane and Baralyme can produce sufficient heat and combustible degradation products to lead to the spontaneous generation of fires within the carbon dioxide absorber canister and breathing circuit. Cases of extreme heat without fire associated with desiccated soda lime have been reported in Europe. To avoid this problem, anesthesia providers should make every effort to not use desiccated carbon dioxide absorbents. (236)

126.

Feature	Soda Lime *	Amsorb Plus	Litholyme
Contents			
$Ca(OH)_2$ (%)	76-81	>80	>75
Water (%)	14-19	13-18	12-19
NaOH (%)	4	0	0
KOH (%)	1	0	0
$CaCl_2$ (%)	0	4	0
LiCl (%)	0	0	3
Mesh size	4-8	4-8	4-10
Generation of compound A with sevoflurane	Yes	No	No
Generation of carbon monoxide with inhaled anesthetics	Yes	No	No
Risk of exothermic reactions and fire in the presence of sevoflurane	No	No	No

(236)

CHECKING THE ANESTHESIA MACHINE AND CIRCLE SYSTEM FUNCTION

127. In 2008 the American Society of Anesthesiologists developed new Recommendations for Pre-Anesthesia Checkout (PAC) Procedures in order to provide guidelines applicable to all anesthesia delivery systems. This allows individual departments to develop a PAC specific to the anesthesia delivery systems currently used at their facilities that can be performed consistently and expeditiously. Specifically, for newer anesthesia delivery systems that incorporate automated checkout features, items that are not evaluated by the automated checkout need to be identified, and supplemental manual checkout procedures should be included as needed. (236)

128. A complete anesthesia machine and circle system function checkout procedure should be performed each day before the first case. An abbreviated checkout should be performed before each subsequent use that day. (236)

129. The most important preoperative checks are (1) verification that an auxiliary oxygen cylinder and self-inflating manual ventilation device (Ambu bag) are available and functioning, (2) a leak check of the machine's low-pressure system, (3) calibration of the oxygen monitor, and (4) a positive-pressure leak check of the breathing system. (236)

130. Failure to ventilate is a major cause of morbidity and death related to anesthesia care. Because equipment failure with resulting inability to ventilate the patient can occur at any time, a self-inflating manual ventilation device (e.g., Ambu bag) should be present at every anesthetizing location for every case and should be checked for proper function. In addition, a source of oxygen separate from the anesthesia machine and pipeline supply, specifically an oxygen cylinder with a regulator and a means to open the cylinder valve, should be immediately available and checked. (236)

131. A leak check of the machine's low-pressure system is performed to confirm the integrity of the anesthesia machine from the flowmeters to the common gas outlet. It evaluates the portion of the anesthesia machine that is downstream from all safety devices, except the oxygen monitor. The low-pressure circuit is the most vulnerable part of the anesthesia machine because the components

located within this area are the ones most subject to breakage and leaks. The machine's low-pressure system must be checked because leaks in this circuit can lead to hypoxia or patient awareness, or both. (236)

132. The oxygen monitor is the only machine safety device that detects problems downstream from the flowmeters. The other machine safety devices (the fail-safe valve, the oxygen supply failure alarm, and the proportioning system) are all upstream from the flowmeters. (237)

133. A positive-pressure leak check of the breathing system must be performed before every procedure. This test does not check the integrity of the unidirectional valves because a breathing system will pass the leak check even if the unidirectional valves are incompetent or stuck shut. (237)

16 AIRWAY MANAGEMENT

Kerry Klinger and Andrew Infosino

ANATOMY AND PHYSIOLOGY OF THE UPPER AIRWAY

1. How does resistance to airflow through the nasal passages compare to that through the mouth?
2. What nerves provide sensory innervation to the nasal cavity?
3. What nerves provide sensory innervation to the hard and soft palate?
4. What nerve provides sensory innervation to the anterior two thirds of the tongue?
5. What nerve innervates the posterior third of the tongue, the soft palate, and the oropharynx?
6. What are the three components of the pharynx?
7. What nerves innervate the pharynx?
8. What are the three unpaired cartilages that are located in the larynx?
9. What are the three paired cartilages that are located in the larynx?
10. What is different about the cricoid cartilage compared with the other tracheal cartilages?
11. Where is the narrowest part of the adult airway?
12. What two nerves provide the motor innervation to the larynx?
13. Damage to what nerve would cause paralysis to the principal abductors of the vocal cords, the posterior cricoarytenoid muscles?
14. Which nerve provides motor function to one of the tensors of the vocal cords, the cricothyroid muscle?

AIRWAY ASSESSMENT

15. How should the patient's airway be assessed prior to airway management for a procedure?
16. What is the purpose of the Mallampati classification system?
17. Describe the observer/patient position during Mallampati classification.
18. Describe the Mallampati classes.
19. Why are decreased submandibular space and compliance associated with difficult intubation?
20. What are some clinical conditions associated with decreased submandibular compliance?
21. What is the purpose of the upper lip bite test (ULBT)?
22. Describe the ULBT classes.
23. What is the concern with a patient with a short thyromental distance?
24. What three axes must be aligned to obtain a line of vision during direct laryngoscopy? How is this accomplished? What is this final position called?
25. What position is associated with improved alignment of the three axes to obtain a line of vision during laryngoscopy in obese patients?
26. What maneuver facilitates identification of the cricoid cartilage in patients who do not have a prominent thyroid cartilage?

AIRWAY MANAGEMENT TECHNIQUES

27. List variables associated with difficult face mask ventilation.
28. What are the causes of difficult or inadequate mask ventilation?
29. Describe preoxygenation prior to the induction of anesthesia. What is its value?
30. How is preoxygenation accomplished?
31. What are the two factors that influence the duration of apnea without desaturation?
32. Why is it important to limit ventilation pressure to less than 20 cm H_2O during face mask ventilation?
33. What is an advantage of nasal airways over oral airways in a lightly anesthetized patient? What are some contraindications to nasal airway placement?

SUPRAGLOTTIC AIRWAY DEVICES

34. What are the advantages of supraglottic airway devices over endotracheal intubation in elective airway management?
35. List variables associated with difficult supraglottic airway placement.
36. What are some potential contraindications to supraglottic airway placement?
37. What are some reported complications of laryngeal mask airway use in difficult airway patients?
38. Describe features of the second generation supraglottic airways, such as LMA Fastrach, LMA ProSeal or Supreme, Air-Q Masked Laryngeal Airways, and I-gel, that make them different from LMA Classic.
39. Describe advantages of the esophageal tracheal Combitube (ETC) and King Laryngeal Tube (King LT).

ENDOTRACHEAL INTUBATION

40. What is the best way to position the patient for direct laryngoscopy and endotracheal intubation?
41. What are some indications for intubation?
42. What is the purpose of the Cormack and Lehane score?
43. Describe the Cormack and Lehane grades.
44. What are four management principles to consider for intubation of a patient with a history of or an examination concerning for a difficult airway?
45. How can thyroid cartilage maneuvers facilitate visualization of the glottic opening during direct laryngoscopy?
46. What are the advantages of curved (Macintosh) laryngoscope blades and the straight (Miller) laryngoscope blades?
47. Describe the proper placement of the tip of a curved (Macintosh) laryngoscope blade versus that of a straight (Miller) laryngoscope blade for exposure of the glottic opening during direct laryngoscopy.
48. What is the main advantage of video laryngoscopes over direct laryngoscopy?
49. Describe why an angulated video laryngoscope blade is advantageous when intubating a patient with a suspected or known difficult airway and the technique for insertion.
50. Describe how a channeled differs from a nonchanneled video laryngoscope and how a channeled video laryngoscope blade is used.
51. Explain the difference between endotracheal tube stylets, introducers, and airway exchange catheters.
52. Name some uses of endotracheal tube stylets, introducers, and airway exchange catheters.
53. What are some complications of endotracheal tube stylets, introducers, and airway exchange catheters?
54. Explain how to exchange a supraglottic airway for an endotracheal tube using an Aintree intubation catheter.

FLEXIBLE FIBEROPTIC ENDOTRACHEAL INTUBATION

55. What are some indications for fiberoptic endotracheal intubation?
56. What are disadvantages to fiberoptic endotracheal intubations?
57. Why is fiberoptic endotracheal intubation recommended for patients with unstable cervical spines?

58. Why is fiberoptic endotracheal intubation recommended for patients who have sustained an injury to the upper airway from either blunt or penetrating trauma?
59. When is an awake fiberoptic endotracheal intubation indicated?
60. What are some advantages and disadvantages of nasal fiberoptic endotracheal intubation?
61. Why should an antisialagogue be given before fiberoptic endotracheal intubation?
62. What are the advantages of topical anesthesia over nerve blocks for airway anesthesia?
63. Why is lidocaine the preferred topical local anesthetic for the airway?
64. Describe preparation of the tongue and oropharynx for nasal or oral fiberoptic endotracheal intubation.
65. Describe preparation of the nose and nasopharynx for nasal fiberoptic endotracheal intubation.
66. Why is nebulization of local anesthetic more effective at providing topical anesthesia to the trachea than spraying?
67. Name two blocks that can be performed to provide topical anesthesia for the larynx and trachea.
68. How can the risks of mucosal trauma/bleeding or submucosal tunneling with nasal endotracheal intubation be minimized?
69. What is the utility of oral intubating airways during oral fiberoptic endotracheal tracheal intubation?
70. What are the advantages of inflating the endotracheal tube cuff during fiberoptic intubation?
71. How is endotracheal tube depth verified during fiberoptic intubation?
72. What are possible causes of resistance when advancing the fiberoptic bronchoscope?
73. What are possible causes of resistance when removing the fiberoptic bronchoscope?
74. Why is visualization more difficult during fiberoptic endotracheal intubation in an asleep patient?

BLIND NASOTRACHEAL INTUBATION

75. Describe the blind nasal endotracheal intubation technique.

ENDOTRACHEAL TUBE SIZES

76. How are endotracheal tubes sized?
77. Why are endotracheal tubes radiopaque and transparent?
78. Why are low-pressure, high-volume cuffs on endotracheal tubes preferred?
79. What are some serious complications attributable to excessive endotracheal cuff pressures?

CONFIRMATION OF ENDOTRACHEAL TUBE PLACEMENT

80. What are some methods to confirm the correct placement of an endotracheal tube?
81. Describe endotracheal tube movement during head flexion and extension.

SPECIAL SITUATIONS

82. What is the purpose of cricoid pressure and when should it be used?
83. How is cricoid pressure performed?
84. What are some possible complications of cricoid pressure?

TRANSTRACHEAL TECHNIQUES

85. In what situations are transtracheal techniques most commonly used? What are different transtracheal techniques that can be used?
86. What are predictors of difficult access through the cricothyroid membrane?
87. What is a cricothyrotomy, and when is it usually performed?
88. Describe a percutaneous cricothyroidotomy.
89. Describe a surgical cricothyroidotomy.
90. What are the possible complications of cricothyroidotomy?
91. Describe how access for transtracheal jet ventilation is obtained.
92. What are the possible complications of transtracheal jet ventilation?
93. Describe how a retrograde endotracheal intubation is performed.

ENDOTRACHEAL EXTUBATION

94. What are the steps of tracheal extubation?
95. Why is tracheal extubation during a light level of anesthesia dangerous?
96. What is laryngospasm? When is it most likely to occur?
97. What are the benefits, indications, and contraindications to extubation before the return of protective airway reflexes (deep extubation)?

COMPLICATIONS OF TRACHEAL INTUBATION

98. What are some possible complications of endotracheal intubation?
99. What are the causes of major airway-related adverse events after tracheal extubation?
100. How should laryngospasm be treated?
101. What is the major complication of prolonged tracheal intubation, and how can it be potentially prevented?

AIRWAY MANAGEMENT IN INFANTS AND CHILDREN

102. What are some differences between the infant and the adult airway? At what age does the pediatric upper airway take on more adult-like characteristics?
103. At what level in the neck is the larynx located in infants as compared to adults? What effect does this have on the tongue?
104. Is the infant's tongue, in proportion to the size of the mouth, larger or smaller than an adult's tongue? What are the consequences of this?
105. How does an infant's epiglottis differ from an adult's epiglottis?
106. What is the narrowest portion of an infant's airway?
107. Describe the best head and neck positioning of an infant during direct laryngoscopy.
108. What is different about an infant's nares compared to an adult's? Why is this important?
109. How does oxygen consumption per kilogram compare between infants and adults? Why is this important?
110. What are some questions for the parents regarding the pediatric patient's history that are important for airway management?
111. Why is premedication useful in pediatric anesthesia?
112. What is the premedication dose of oral midazolam for infants or children?
113. If a child is uncooperative with taking oral midazolam as a premedication, what other options are available?
114. Describe an inhaled induction in a child. When should nitrous oxide be discontinued?
115. Describe maneuvers to overcome airway obstruction during mask induction in infants and children.
116. What determines the appropriate size of an laryngeal mask airway (LMA) for use in infants and children?
117. Describe the difference between the cuff pressure and the leak pressure in a supraglottic airway device.
118. What advantage does the Air-Q intubating laryngeal airway (ILA) have over an LMA in pediatric patients?
119. What formula is often used to estimate the appropriate size of an endotracheal tube for infants and children? Is this formula for cuffed or uncuffed endotracheal tubes?
120. How is the formula used to estimate the appropriate size of an endotracheal tube for infants and children adapted for cuffed endotracheal tubes?
121. What are the advantages of cuffed versus uncuffed endotracheal tubes in infants and children? What are the disadvantages?
122. What are the potential complications of using too large an uncuffed endotracheal tube or an overinflated cuffed endotracheal tube?
123. Are cuffed endotracheal tubes associated with a higher incidence of postextubation croup than uncuffed endotracheal tubes?
124. What is the appropriate leak pressure when using uncuffed endotracheal tubes in infants and children?

125. What is the appropriate cuff pressure for endotracheal tubes in infants and children? What is the best way to measure the cuff pressure?
126. What three advantages do Microcuff endotracheal tubes have over conventional pediatric cuffed endotracheal tubes?
127. What are the advantages and disadvantages of straight laryngoscope blades over curved laryngoscope blades when intubating infants or small children?
128. Describe the most useful sizes of laryngoscope blades according to age.
129. What are the advantages of video laryngoscopes over direct laryngoscopy in infants and children? What are the disadvantages?
130. Describe the different GlideScope sizes and models according to age and weight.
131. Describe the limitations of flexible fiberoptic bronchoscopes used in infants and children.
132. Is an awake fiberoptic endotracheal intubation usually an option in managing an expected difficult airway in infants and children?
133. What is the safest vasoconstrictor to apply to the nasal mucosa when performing a nasal fiberoptic endotracheal intubation in infants or children?
134. What is the most important first step when an unexpected difficult airway occurs in pediatric patients?
135. In a difficult pediatric intubation situation, why should repeated attempts at direct laryngoscopy be avoided? What should be done instead?
136. What personnel and equipment should be in the operating room before induction of anesthesia in a pediatric patient with an expected difficult airway?
137. Why is tracheal extubation in infants and children riskier than in that of adults?
138. What is the most common reason for postextubation croup in infants and children? What are other risk factors for postextubation croup in infants and children?
139. What are the clinical manifestations of postextubation croup?
140. How is postextubation croup treated in infants and children?
141. What are pediatric patients with obstructive sleep apnea at risk for in the postoperative period?
142. Describe tracheal extubation and postoperative monitoring for infants and children with obstructive sleep apnea.
143. When does laryngospasm typically occur in infants and children?
144. How should laryngospasm be treated in infants and children?
145. How should extubation after a difficult intubation be handled in infants and children?

ANSWERS*

ANATOMY AND PHYSIOLOGY OF THE UPPER AIRWAY

1. Resistance to airflow through the nasal passages is twice that through the mouth and accounts for approximately 50% to 75% of total airway resistance. (241)
2. The majority of the sensory innervation of the nasal cavity is derived from the ethmoidal branch of the ophthalmic nerve and branches of the maxillary division of the trigeminal nerve from the sphenopalatine ganglion. (241)
3. The greater and lesser palatine nerves branch from the sphenopalatine ganglion to innervate the hard and soft palate. (241)
4. The mandibular division (V_3) of the trigeminal nerve (cranial nerve V) forms the lingual nerve, which provides sensation to the anterior two-thirds of the tongue. (241)
5. The posterior third of the tongue, the soft palate, and the oropharynx are innervated by the glossopharyngeal nerve (cranial nerve IX). (241)

---

*Numbers in parentheses refer to pages, figures, boxes, or tables in Pardo MC, Miller RD, eds. *Basics of Anesthesia.* 7th ed. Philadelphia: Elsevier; 2018.

6. The three components of the pharynx are the nasopharynx, the oropharynx, and the hypopharynx. (241)
7. The pharynx is innervated by cranial nerves IX (glossopharyngeal) and X (vagus). (241)
8. The three unpaired cartilages located in the larynx are the epiglottis, thyroid, and cricoid cartilages. (242)
9. The three paired cartilages located in the larynx are the arytenoids, corniculates, and cuneiform cartilages. (242)
10. The cricoid cartilage is the most cephalad tracheal cartilage and is the only one that has a full ring structure. It is shaped like a signet ring, wider in the cephalocaudal dimension posteriorly. (242)
11. The vocal cords are the narrowest portion of the adult airway. (242)
12. The superior laryngeal nerve, external division, and the recurrent laryngeal nerve provide motor innervation to the larynx. (242)
13. Damage to the recurrent laryngeal nerve would cause paralysis of the cricoarytenoid muscles. These muscles are the principal abductors of the vocal cords. (242)
14. The superior laryngeal nerve, external division, innervates the cricothyroid muscle. This is the only laryngeal muscle innervated by the superior laryngeal nerve, external branch. (242)

AIRWAY ASSESSMENT

15. Assessment of the patient's airway prior to airway management includes history gathering and a physical examination. Aspects of the history may include a history of the patient's airway experiences, review of previous anesthetic and medical records, and the gathering of information that may be pertinent such as congenital defects, disease states, and gastrointestinal disorders. The physical examination should evaluate for features to predict the potential for difficult airway management. (242)
16. Mallampati proposed a classification system (Mallampati score) to correlate the oropharyngeal space with the predicted ease of direct laryngoscopy and tracheal intubation. (243)
17. With the observer at eye level, the patient holds the head in a neutral position, opens the mouth maximally, and protrudes the tongue without phonating. (243)
18. The Mallampati classes are as follows:
    Class I: The soft palate, fauces, uvula, and tonsillar pillars are visible.
    Class II: The soft palate, fauces, and uvula are visible.
    Class III: The soft palate and base of the uvula are visible.
    Class IV: The soft palate is not visible. (243)
19. Decreased submandibular space and compliance correlate with poor laryngoscopic view. The submandibular space is the area into which the soft tissues of the pharynx must be displaced to obtain a line of vision during direct laryngoscopy. Anything that limits the size of this space or compliance of the tissue will decrease the amount of anterior displacement that can be achieved. (243)
20. Ludwig angina, tumors or masses, radiation scarring, burns, and previous neck surgery are conditions that can decrease submandibular compliance. (243)
21. The upper lip bite test (ULBT) assesses the ability to prognath the mandible, which correlates with visualization of glottic structures on direct laryngoscopy. (243)
22. The classes of the ULBT are as follows:
    Class I: Lower incisors can bite above the vermilion border of the upper lip.
    Class II: Lower incisors cannot reach vermilion border.
    Class III: Lower incisors cannot bite upper lip. (243)
23. A thyromental distance (mentum to thyroid cartilage) less than 6 to 7 cm correlates with a poor laryngoscopic view. This is typically seen in patients with a receding mandible or short neck. Three ordinary fingerbreadths approximate this distance. (243)

24. The laryngeal, pharyngeal, and oral axes must be aligned to obtain a line of vision during direct laryngoscopy. Flexion of the neck, by elevating the head approximately 10 cm, aligns the laryngeal and pharyngeal axes. Extension of the head on the atlanto-occipital joint aligns the oral and pharyngeal axes. These maneuvers place the head in the "sniffing" position and bring the three axes into optimal alignment. (245)

25. Obesity is associated with difficulty in airway management. To increase the likelihood of successful endotracheal intubation, a wedge-shaped bolster placed behind the obese patient's shoulders and back results in a more optimal sniffing position. (245)

26. In patients who do not have a prominent thyroid cartilage, identification of the cricoid cartilage can be achieved by palpating the neck at the sternal notch and sliding the fingers up the neck until a tracheal cartilage that is wider and higher (cricoid cartilage) than those below is felt. (246)

AIRWAY MANAGEMENT TECHNIQUES

27. Independent variables associated with difficult face mask ventilation are (1) age older than 55 years, (2) increased body mass index (BMI), (3) a beard, (4) lack of teeth, (5) a history of snoring or obstructive sleep apnea, (6) Mallampati class III to IV, (7) history of neck radiation, (8) male gender, (9) limited ability to protrude the mandible, and (10) history of an airway mass or tumor. Difficult face mask ventilation can also develop after multiple laryngoscopy attempts. (246)

28. Inadequate face mask ventilation may be due to one or more of the following problems: inadequate mask or supraglottic airway seal, excessive gas leak, or excessive resistance to the ingress or egress of gas. (246)

29. "Preoxygenation" describes the administration of oxygen to patients prior to the induction of anesthesia resulting in apnea. The goal is to achieve an end-tidal oxygen level of about 90%. Preoxygenation increases the duration of apnea without oxygen desaturation by filling the functional residual capacity with oxygen, thus increasing the patient's reserve of oxygen while apneic. (247)

30. Methods by which to preoxygenate a patient prior to the induction of anesthesia include having the patient breathe 100% oxygen for 3 minutes or take eight deep breaths in 60 seconds. Although it was previously believed that having a patient take four deep breaths was sufficient for preoxygenation, this has been since proved not to be as effective as the other two methods. In obese patients, adequate preoxygenation may take longer. Having the obese patient sit in an upright position and applying continuous positive airway pressure may facilitate preoxygenation in this population. (247)

31. The two factors that influence the duration of apnea without desaturation are oxygen consumption and the volume of the functional residual capacity. (247)

32. Ventilating pressure during face mask ventilation should be less than 20 cm H_2O to avoid insufflation of the stomach. (248)

33. Nasal airways are advantageous over oral airways in that they are tolerated at lower levels of anesthesia. Oral airways are more likely to generate a gag reflex or cause laryngospasm in a lightly anesthetized patient. Nasal airways are relatively contraindicated in patients who have coagulation or platelet abnormalities, are pregnant, or have basilar skull fractures. (248)

SUPRAGLOTTIC AIRWAY DEVICES

34. For elective airway management, advantages of supraglottic airway devices over endotracheal intubation include placement quickly and without the use of laryngoscope, less hemodynamic changes with insertion and removal, less coughing and bucking with removal, no need for muscle relaxants, preserved laryngeal competence and mucociliary function, and less laryngeal trauma. (248)

35. Difficult supraglottic airway placement or failure has been associated with small mouth opening, supra- or extraglottic pathology, fixed cervical spine deformity, use of cricoid pressure, poor dentition or large incisors, male sex, surgical table rotation, and increased BMI. (248)

36. Some potential contraindications for using supraglottic airway devices are patients at risk for regurgitation of gastric contents, nonsupine position, obesity, pregnant patients, long surgical time, and intra-abdominal or airway procedures. There are clinical situations when supraglottic airway placement may be acceptable despite a relative contraindication, but one must consider the risk versus benefit in these situations. (248)

37. Reported complications of laryngeal mask airway use in difficult airway patients include bronchospasm, postoperative swallowing difficulties, respiratory obstruction, laryngeal nerve injury, edema, and hypoglossal nerve paralysis. (248)

38. The second generation supraglottic airways such as the LMA Fastrach, LMA ProSeal or Supreme, Air-Q, and I-gel supraglottic airways have one or more of the following features: (1) improved airway seal to allow for ventilation with higher airway pressures, (2) a second lumen that acts as an esophageal vent to keep gases and fluid separate from the airway and facilitate placement of an orogastric tube, (3) an airway channel that can be used as a conduit for intubation, and (4) a bite block that is present in the airway shaft. (249)

39. The esophageal tracheal Combitube (ETC) and King Laryngeal Tube (King LT) devices are inserted blindly, require minimal training, and need no movement of the head or neck. These airway devices are primarily used in prehospital settings for emergency airway control when esophageal intubation cannot be achieved. (250)

ENDOTRACHEAL INTUBATION

40. The best way to position the patient for direct laryngoscopy and endotracheal intubation is to elevate the patient's head 8 to 10 cm with pads under the occiput (shoulders remaining on the table) and to extend the head at the atlanto-occipital joint. This maximally aligns the oral, pharyngeal, and laryngeal axes to create a line of vision from the lips to the glottic opening. The height of the operating table should be adjusted such that the patient's face is near the level of the standing anesthesia provider's xiphoid cartilage. (250)

41. Indications for endotracheal intubation include (1) the need to provide a patent airway, (2) prevention of inhalation (aspiration) of gastric contents, (3) need for frequent suctioning, (4) facilitating positive-pressure ventilation of the lungs, (5) operative position other than supine, (6) operative site near or involving the upper airway, (7) operative conditions requiring neuromuscular blockade, and (8) difficult airway maintenance by mask. (250)

42. The Cormack and Lehane score grades the glottic view that is obtained with direct laryngoscopy and can be a predictor of a difficult airway. (251)

43. The Cormack and Lehane score grades the direct laryngoscopic view as follows:
Grade I: Most of the glottis is visible.
Grade II: Only the posterior portion of the glottis is visible.
Grade III: The epiglottis, but no part of the glottis, can be seen.
Grade IV: No airway structures are visualized. (251)

44. In patients with anticipated or history of a difficult airway, the following management principles should be considered: (1) awake intubation versus intubation after the induction of general anesthesia, (2) initial intubation method via noninvasive versus invasive techniques, (3) video laryngoscopy as an initial approach to intubation, and (4) maintaining versus ablating spontaneous ventilation. (251)

45. Backward upward rightward pressure (BURP) on the thyroid cartilage with the laryngoscopist's right hand may facilitate visualization of the glottic opening during direct laryngoscopy. (251)

46. The advantages of the curved (Macintosh) blade include less trauma to teeth, more room for passage of the endotracheal tube, larger flange size improves the ability to sweep the tongue, and less bruising of the epiglottis because the tip of the blade does not directly lift this structure. The advantages of the straight (Miller) blade are better exposure of the glottic opening and a smaller profile, which can be beneficial in patients with smaller mouth opening. (252)

47. During laryngoscopy with a Macintosh blade, the distal end of the curved blade is advanced into the space between the base of the tongue and the pharyngeal surface of the epiglottis. During laryngoscopy with a Miller blade, the distal end of the straight blade is advanced beneath the laryngeal surface of the epiglottis. The epiglottis is then elevated by the blade to expose the glottic opening. (252)

48. Video laryngoscopes can help obtain a view of the larynx by providing indirect visualization of the glottic opening without alignment of the oral, pharyngeal, and tracheal axes, and enable tracheal intubation in patients who have conditions (limited mouth opening, inability to flex the neck) that can make traditional laryngoscopy difficult or impossible. There is also a slightly improved view of the larynx because the camera is located more distally on the blade, providing for a wider visual field. (252)

49. Angulated video laryngoscope blades allow for a more anteriorly oriented view that can be obtained with minimal flexion or extension of the patient's head and neck. They are usually inserted midline in the mouth, and the tip of the video laryngoscope blade may be placed in the vallecula or be used to lift the epiglottis directly. A preshaped stylet that matches the curvature of the blade is usually required. (253)

50. Channeled video laryngoscope blades (Airtraq and King Vision) have a guide channel that directs an endotracheal tube toward the glottic opening via blades that are more angulated than traditional Macintosh blades. The endotracheal tube is preloaded into the guide channel, and the video laryngoscope is inserted midline in the mouth until the epiglottis is visualized. Nonchanneled video laryngoscopes (GlideScope, C-MAC, McGrath) require that an endotracheal tube (usually with a preshaped stylet) is advanced into the mouth under direct visualization until it can be viewed on the monitor and advanced into the trachea. When using nonchanneled video laryngoscopes advancement of the endotracheal tube blindly without direct visualization can result in tonsillar and pharyngeal injuries. (253)

51. Malleable metal stylets are used to stiffen and provide curvature to an endotracheal tube to help facilitate laryngoscopy and tracheal intubation. A bougie or an introducer is used when there is a poor laryngoscopic view and difficulty passing an endotracheal tube. They are shaped with a curve near the distal tip, which facilitates placement into the airway. An endotracheal tube can be advanced over the bougie or introducer into the airway. Airway exchange catheters are designed for exchange of endotracheal tubes. When placed prior to extubation, they can also be left in the airway as a conduit for reintubation in the case of failed extubation. (255)

52. Endotracheal tube stylets, introducers, and airway exchange catheters can be used to facilitate difficult endotracheal intubation, endotracheal tube exchange, and supraglottic airway exchange for an endotracheal tube. (255)

53. Complications of intubating endotracheal tube stylets include bleeding, sore throat, and tracheal trauma. Complications of endotracheal tube exchangers include tracheal/bronchial laceration and gastric perforation. If placed deeper there is a risk of bronchial perforation and pneumothorax. The use of high-pressure jet ventilation through the endotracheal tube exchanger can lead to other serious complications. (255)

54. To exchange a supraglottic airway for an endotracheal tube, the airway exchange catheter (AIC) is threaded onto a fiberoptic bronchoscope. The distal end of the fiberoptic bronchoscope is not covered by the AIC to allow for manipulation. The AIC and fiberoptic bronchoscope are then placed in the lumen of the supraglottic airway and advanced as a unit through the vocal cords into the trachea. The fiberoptic bronchoscope is then removed while the AIC remains in the trachea. The supraglottic airway is removed over the AIC, and an endotracheal tube is then placed over the AIC into the trachea. Finally, the AIC is removed. (255)

FLEXIBLE FIBEROPTIC ENDOTRACHEAL INTUBATION

55. Indications for fiberoptic endotracheal intubation include patients with predicted difficult airway, patients with unstable cervical spines, and patients who have sustained an injury to the upper airway from either blunt or penetrating trauma. (256)

56. Disadvantages of fiberoptic endotracheal intubation are that it requires time to set up and prepare the patient's airway. Therefore, if immediate airway management is required, another technique should be used. Also, the fiberoptic bronchoscope needs space to pass through. Anything that impinges on upper airway size (edema of the pharynx or tongue, infection, hematoma, infiltrating masses) will make fiberoptic intubation more difficult. Blood and secretions in the upper airway can obscure optics of the fiberoptic bronchoscope, making visualization difficult. A relative contraindication to fiberoptic intubation is the presence of a pharyngeal abscess, which could be disrupted as the endotracheal tube is advanced and result in aspiration of purulent material. (256)

57. Fiberoptic endotracheal intubation does not require movement of the patient's neck and can be performed awake, before induction of general anesthesia, thereby allowing for evaluation of the patient's neurologic function after tracheal intubation and surgical positioning. (256)

58. Patients who have sustained an injury to the upper airway from either blunt or penetrating trauma are at risk for the endotracheal tube creating a false passage by exiting the airway through the disrupted tissue during direct laryngoscopy. By performing a fiberoptic intubation, not only can the injury be assessed, but also the tracheal tube can be placed beyond the level of the injury. This eliminates the risk of causing subcutaneous emphysema, which could compress and further compromise the airway. (256)

59. Awake fiberoptic endotracheal intubation is most frequently chosen when a difficult tracheal intubation by direct laryngoscopy is anticipated in a patient who is able to cooperate with the procedure. By intubating before induction of general anesthesia, the patient maintains upper airway patency and spontaneous respirations and can eliminate the risk of failed ventilation and failed tracheal intubation. The technique also does not require movement of the patient's neck, thereby maintaining cervical spine immobility in patients with unstable cervical spines, and allows for evaluation of the patient's neurologic function after tracheal intubation or surgical positioning. (256)

60. In general, the nasal route is easier than the oral route for fiberoptic endotracheal intubation because the angle of curvature of the endotracheal tube naturally approximates that of the patient's upper airway. Additionally, nasal fiberoptic endotracheal intubation tends to be less of a stimulus for the gag reflex. A disadvantage of nasal fiberoptic endotracheal intubation is that the risk of inducing bleeding is higher when the nasal route is used. Therefore, the nasal route is relatively contraindicated in patients with platelet abnormalities or coagulation disorders. (257)

61. An antisialagogue (glycopyrrolate, 0.2 mg IV) should be administered before fiberoptic endotracheal intubation to inhibit the formation of secretions that can obscure fiberoptic visualization. (257)

62. Topical anesthesia for airway anesthesia is less invasive and better tolerated in awake patients than nerve blocks. Topical anesthesia can be as effective as nerve blocks for airway anesthesia but has a higher risk of local anesthetic toxicity. (257)

63. Lidocaine is the preferred topical local anesthetic for the airway because of its broad therapeutic window. Benzocaine can cause methemoglobinemia even in therapeutic doses. Tetracaine has a very narrow therapeutic window, and the maximum allowable dose can easily be exceeded. Cetacaine is a mixture of benzocaine and tetracaine and has the disadvantages of each local anesthetic. Cocaine can cause sympathomimetic effects, such as tachycardia and hypertension, and central nervous system stimulation, and it can have abuse potential. (257)

64. Topical anesthesia of the tongue and oropharynx may be achieved by spraying or direct application or by bilateral blocks of the glossopharyngeal nerve. For a glossopharyngeal nerve block, approximately 2 mL of 2% lidocaine is injected at a depth of 0.5 cm (after first confirming negative aspiration) at the base of each anterior tonsillar pillar. (257)

65. Anesthetizing the nasal mucosa can be achieved by spraying (atomizing or nebulizing) or direct application (ointment, gels, or gargling solutions) of local anesthetics onto the nasal mucosa. Local anesthetic solutions can also be applied by placing soaked cotton-tipped swabs or pledgets into the nares. When a nasal intubation is performed, vasoconstriction is also necessary. Vasoconstriction with 0.05% oxymetazoline HCL spray is recommended. (257)

66. Nebulization of local anesthetic is more effective at providing topical anesthesia to ("topicalizing") the trachea than spraying because the small particle size of local anesthetic created by a nebulizer is carried more effectively into the trachea. It does, however, also travel into the smaller airways, where the anesthetic is not needed, and undergoes more rapid systemic absorption. The larger local anesthetic particle size of a spray causes it to be deposited in the pharynx, with only a small proportion reaching the trachea. (257)

67. Two blocks that can be performed for topical anesthesia of the larynx and trachea include the superior laryngeal nerve block and the transtracheal block. The transtracheal block is designed to block the sensory distribution of the recurrent laryngeal nerve. (257)

68. Softening the endotracheal tube in warm water and lubricating it before use make it less likely to cause mucosal trauma/bleeding or submucosal tunneling during nasal endotracheal intubation. (257)

69. Use of an oral intubating airway facilitates directing the bronchoscope in midline and creating space during oral fiberoptic endotracheal intubation. (257)

70. Inflation of the endotracheal tube cuff during advancement with the fiberoptic bronchoscope in the pharynx serves to create an enlarged pharyngeal space. Because secretions tend to adhere to the pharyngeal walls, endotracheal tube cuff inflation also helps keep the optics of the fiberoptic bronchoscope from being obscured. The inflated cuff further aims the tip of the endotracheal tube anteriorly. (257)

71. The appropriate depth of endotracheal tube placement can be verified by observing the distance between the carina and the tip of the endotracheal tube as the fiberoptic bronchoscope is withdrawn. (257)

72. Resistance to advancement of the endotracheal tube often means the endotracheal tube is impacted on an arytenoid. If this occurs, rotation of the endotracheal tube may be helpful. Forcing advancement of the endotracheal tube may result in kinking of the endotracheal tube, advancement into the esophagus, and damage to the fiberoptic bronchoscope. (258)

73. If there is any resistance when removing the fiberoptic bronchoscope, the scope is either through the Murphy eye or kinked in the pharynx. In both instances, the endotracheal tube and the scope must be withdrawn together to prevent damaging the fiberoptic bronchoscope. (258)

74. An important difference in performing fiberoptic laryngoscopy in an anesthetized patient is that the soft tissues of the pharynx, in contrast to the awake state, tend to relax and limit space for visualization with the fiberoptic bronchoscope. Using jaw thrust, using specialized oral airways, expanding the endotracheal tube cuff in the pharynx, or applying traction on the tongue may overcome this problem. It is advisable to have a second person trained in anesthesia delivery assisting when a fiberoptic endotracheal intubation is performed under general anesthesia because it is difficult to maintain the patient's airway, be attentive to the monitors, and perform the fiberoptic intubation alone. (258)

BLIND NASOTRACHEAL INTUBATION

75. Blind nasotracheal intubation involves advancing an endotracheal tube blindly from the nose into the trachea while listening to breath sounds or attaching the endotracheal tube to an anesthesia circuit and observing end-tidal CO_2. However, this technique is rarely used for difficult airway management, as there are now numerous other devices available for management of the difficult airway. (258)

ENDOTRACHEAL TUBE SIZES

76. Endotracheal tubes are sized according to their internal diameter (ID), which is marked on each tube. They are available in 0.5 mm ID increments. (258)

77. Endotracheal tubes are radiopaque to ascertain radiographically the position of the distal tip relative to the carina. They are transparent to permit visualization of secretions or airflow as evidenced by condensation of water vapor in the lumen of the tube ("breath fogging") during exhalation. (258)

78. Pressure on the tracheal wall is minimized through the use of a low-pressure, high-volume endotracheal tube cuff. The cuff needs to be inflated to facilitate positive-pressure ventilation of the lungs and to decrease the risk of the aspiration of gastric contents. Using the minimum volume of air in the cuff that prevents air leaks during positive ventilation pressure (20 to 30 cm H_2O) also minimizes the likelihood of mucosal ischemia resulting from prolonged pressure on the tracheal wall. (258)

79. Serious complications attributable to excessive endotracheal tube cuff pressures include tracheal stenosis, tracheal rupture, tracheoesophageal fistula, tracheocarotid fistula, and tracheoinnominate artery fistula. (258)

CONFIRMATION OF ENDOTRACHEAL TUBE PLACEMENT

80. Confirmation of placement of the endotracheal tube in the trachea is verified by identification of carbon dioxide in the patient's exhaled tidal volume and by physical examination. The presence of carbon dioxide in the exhaled gases from the endotracheal tube as detected by capnography (end-tidal P_{CO_2} >30 mm Hg for three to five consecutive breaths) should be immediate and sustained. Symmetric chest rise with manual ventilation, bilateral breath sounds, and absence of breath sounds over the epigastrium are confirmed after tracheal intubation. Palpation or balloting of the endotracheal tube cuff in the suprasternal notch can help determine endotracheal versus endobronchial intubation. (258)

81. Flexion of the patient's head may advance and convert tracheal placement of an endotracheal tube into an endobronchial intubation, especially in children. Conversely, extension of the head can withdraw the tube and result in pharyngeal placement and extubation from the trachea. (259)

SPECIAL SITUATIONS

82. Cricoid pressure (Sellick maneuver) is thought to prevent spillage of gastric contents into the pharynx during the period from induction of anesthesia (unconsciousness) to successful placement of a cuffed endotracheal tube. The use of cricoid pressure remains controversial. It should probably be considered in selected patients at high risk for regurgitation during induction but should be released if it impedes oxygenation, ventilation, or view of glottic structures. (259)

83. An assistant should exert downward external pressure with the thumb and index finger on the cricoid cartilage to displace the cartilaginous cricothyroid ring posteriorly and thus compress the underlying upper esophagus against the cervical vertebrae. The recommended magnitude of downward external pressure is 30 newtons, but this pressure is difficult to judge. (259)

84. Possible complications of cricoid pressure include increasing the difficulty of mask ventilation or worsening laryngoscopic view, nausea, vomiting, and esophageal rupture. (259)

85. In situations when ventilation and intubation are unsuccessful despite use of a supraglottic airway, emergency invasive access should be used. Invasive emergency access consists of percutaneous or surgical airway, jet ventilation, and retrograde intubation. (259)

86. Predictors of difficult access through the cricothyroid membrane include increased neck circumference, overlying neck pathology, and a fixed cervical spine flexion deformity. (259)

87. A cricothyrotomy involves the placement of an endotracheal tube through the cricothyroid membrane. It can be done using a percutaneous or surgical technique. Cricothyrotomy can be a lifesaving procedure in a "cannot intubate, cannot ventilate" situation or can be used as a first-line technique to secure an airway when using a less invasive technique is not possible owing to factors such as facial trauma, upper airway bleeding, or upper airway obstruction. (259)

88. The percutaneous cricothyrotomy uses a Seldinger technique in which a needle is advanced at a 90-degree angle through the cricothyroid membrane while aspirating with an attached syringe. A change in resistance is felt as a pop when the needle enters the trachea and air is aspirated. The needle should be then angled at a 30- to 45-degree angle and directed caudally. A guidewire is then advanced through the needle, followed by removal of the needle and placement of a combined dilator and airway of adequate caliber (>4 mm). Finally, the wire and dilator are removed, leaving the airway in place. (260)

89. The surgical cricothyrotomy technique involves a vertical or horizontal skin incision, followed by a horizontal incision through the cricothyroid membrane through which a standard endotracheal tube or tracheostomy tube is placed. A tracheal hook, dilator, airway exchange catheter, or bougie can assist in placement of the airway. (260)

90. Possible complications of a cricothyrotomy include bleeding, laryngeal or tracheal injury, infection, and subglottic stenosis. (260)

91. Transtracheal jet ventilation is achieved by placement of an over-the-needle catheter in the trachea through the cricothyroid membrane. The cricothyroid membrane should be identified, and a catheter over a needle connected to a syringe should puncture the membrane at a 90-degree angle until air is aspirated. The catheter should be advanced off the needle into the trachea at a 30- to 45-degree angle caudally. After reconfirming correct placement by aspiration of air, the catheter should be connected to a high-pressure oxygen source. (260)

92. Possible complications of transtracheal jet ventilation include pneumothorax, pneumomediastinum, bleeding, infection, and subcutaneous emphysema. Transtracheal jet ventilation should not be performed when there is upper airway obstruction or any disruption of the airway. (260)

93. Retrograde endotracheal intubation allows intubation without identification of the glottic inlet. The cricothyroid membrane is punctured with a needle at a 90-degree angle while aspirating with an attached syringe. Once in the trachea, the syringe is detached and a guide (usually a wire or catheter) is threaded through the needle in a cephalad direction. It is then retrieved from the mouth or nose. An endotracheal tube, with or without a fiberoptic laryngoscope, is threaded over the wire until it stops on impact with the anterior wall of the trachea. Tension on the guide can be relaxed to allow the endotracheal tube to pass farther into the trachea before removing the wire. Retrograde endotracheal intubation should not be performed in patients with anterior neck pathology (tumors, infection) or coagulopathy. (260)

ENDOTRACHEAL EXTUBATION

94. Before extubation, patients should be placed on 100% oxygen and any residual neuromuscular blockade should be reversed. Routine extubation criteria such as spontaneous respirations with adequate minute ventilation, satisfactory oxygenation and acid-base status, and hemodynamic stability should be met. The oropharynx is suctioned, and a bite block should be placed to prevent

occlusion of the endotracheal tube, if not already present. For deep extubation, adequate anesthesia should be confirmed, and awake patients should be able to follow commands. Then the endotracheal tube can removed by deflating the endotracheal tube cuff and rapidly removing the endotracheal tube from the patient's trachea and upper airway while a positive-pressure breath is delivered to help expel any secretions. After tracheal extubation, 100% oxygen is delivered by face mask. Adequate airway patency, ventilation, and oxygenation are then confirmed. (260)

95. Tracheal extubation after general anesthesia must be performed when the patient is either deeply anesthetized or fully awake. Tracheal extubation during a light level of anesthesia (disconjugate gaze, breath holding or coughing, and not responsive to command) increases the risk for laryngospasm. (260)

96. Laryngospasm is an involuntary spasm/closure of the vocal cords that may present as stridor or attempts to breathe without air exchange. Laryngospasm is likely to occur during tracheal extubation, particularly under a light level of anesthesia when the vocal cords are stimulated by mucus, blood, or other substances. (260)

97. Tracheal extubation before the return of protective airway reflexes (deep tracheal extubation) is generally associated with less coughing and attenuated hemodynamic effects on emergence. This may be preferred in patients at risk from adverse effects of increased intracranial or intraocular pressure, bleeding into the surgical wound, or wound dehiscence. Previous difficult face mask ventilation or difficult endotracheal intubation, high risk of aspiration, restricted access to the airway, obstructive sleep apnea or obesity, and a surgical procedure that may have resulted in airway edema, bleeding or increased irritability are relative contraindications to deep tracheal extubation. (260)

COMPLICATIONS OF TRACHEAL INTUBATION

98. Possible complications of endotracheal intubation can be divided into those incurred during laryngoscopy and tracheal intubation, those that occur while the tracheal tube is in place, and those that can occur after extubation of the trachea. Risks of direct laryngoscopy and endotracheal intubation include dental damage, oral or pharyngeal injury, lip lacerations and bruises, and laryngeal, arytenoid, esophageal, or tracheal damage. Systemic hypertension, tachycardia, increases in intracranial pressure, and aspiration of gastric contents may also occur during this time. During tracheal intubation possible complications include obstruction, accidental endobronchial intubation, accidental extubation, and tracheal tube cuff leak. Complications that can occur after extubation of the trachea include edema, laryngospasm, bronchospasm, aspiration of gastric contents, pharyngitis, laryngitis, tracheal stenosis, vocal cord paralysis, and arytenoid cartilage dislocation. (261)

99. After tracheal extubation, major airway-related adverse events are often due to airway obstruction from laryngeal edema, laryngospasm, or bronchospasm. (261)

100. If laryngospasm occurs, oxygen delivered with positive pressure through a face mask and jaw thrust may be sufficient treatment. Administration of succinylcholine or an anesthetic drug, such as propofol, is indicated if laryngospasm persists. (261–262)

101. The major complication of prolonged tracheal intubation (>48 hours) is damage to the tracheal mucosa, which may progress to destruction of cartilaginous rings and subsequent fibrous scar formation and tracheal stenosis. Using high-volume, low-pressure cuffs and keeping cuff pressures less than 25 cm H_2O can help prevent this complication. (262)

AIRWAY MANAGEMENT IN INFANTS AND CHILDREN

102. Differences between the infant and adult airway include positioning of the larynx in the neck, tongue size, epiglottis size, size of the head relative to the body, neck length, nares size, and location of the narrowest point. Usually by the time the child is about 10 years old the upper airway has taken on more adult-like characteristics. (262)

103. The infant larynx is located higher in the neck at the level of C3-C4. In adults the larynx is at the level of C4-C5. In infants the larynx at this level causes the tongue to shift more superiorly, closer to the palate. The tongue more easily opposes the palate, which can cause airway obstruction in situations such as during the inhalation induction of anesthesia. (263)

104. An infant's tongue is larger in proportion to the size of the mouth than an adult's. The relatively large size of the tongue makes direct laryngoscopy more difficult and can contribute to obstruction of the upper airway during sedation, inhalation induction of anesthesia, or emergence from anesthesia. (263)

105. The epiglottis in an infant's airway is often described as relatively larger, stiffer, and more omega-shaped than an adult epiglottis. More important, an infant's epiglottis is typically angled in a more posterior position, thereby blocking visualization of the vocal cords during direct laryngoscopy. During direct laryngoscopy in infants and small children it may be necessary to lift the epiglottis with the tip of the laryngoscope blade to visualize the vocal cords. (263)

106. The narrowest portion of an infant's airway is at the cricoid cartilage, whereas the narrowest portion of an adult's airway is at the vocal cords. (263)

107. An infant's head and occiput are relatively larger than an adult's. The proper position for direct laryngoscopy and tracheal intubation in an adult is often described as the sniffing position with the head elevated and the neck flexed at C6-C7 and extended at C1-C2. An infant, on the other hand, requires a shoulder roll or neck roll to establish an optimal position for face mask ventilation and direct laryngoscopy. (263)

108. An infant's nares are relatively smaller than an adult's. This can offer significant resistance to airflow and increase the work of breathing, especially when secretions, edema, or bleeding narrow them. (263)

109. Oxygen consumption per kilogram is much higher in infants than in adults. The clinical importance of this is that even after preoxygenation there is less allowable time for endotracheal intubation before the infant desaturates. (263)

110. Questions for the parents regarding the pediatric patient's history that are important for airway management include asking about history of previous airway issues and if there are any syndromes associated with difficult airway management. The parents should be asked if there is a history of snoring. Snoring in infants or children should prompt additional questioning about whether the child has obstructive sleep apnea and should alert the anesthesia provider that respiratory obstruction may develop during the induction and emergence phases of anesthesia, as well as in the postoperative period. This is of particular concern if opioids are given for pain management. The parents should also be asked whether the child has any loose teeth. It may be beneficial to remove very loose teeth prior to proceeding with airway management to prevent the possibility of dislodgement and aspiration. (263)

111. Preanesthetic medication can facilitate separation of the infant or child from the parents before the induction of anesthesia. Preanesthetic medication can also facilitate the inhalational induction of anesthesia in infants and children. Preanesthetic medication is often not necessary in infants younger than 6 months because stranger anxiety does not usually develop until 6 to 9 months of age. (263)

112. For infants or children premedication with midazolam syrup (2 mg/mL) can be given orally in a dose of 0.5 mg/kg up to a maximum dose of about 20 mg. (264)

113. If the child is uncooperative with taking oral midazolam and preanesthetic medication is essential, midazolam can also be given intranasally, intramuscularly, or rectally. If necessary, ketamine can be given intramuscularly in a dose of about 3 mg/kg. (264)

114. In a child without an intravenous catheter in place, the induction of anesthesia with the odorless mixture of nitrous oxide and oxygen through a face mask and then slowly increasing the concentration of sevoflurane is the best approach in a cooperative child. When the infant or child becomes unconscious, the nitrous oxide should be turned off to administer 100% oxygen. (264)

115. There are several maneuvers to relieve airway obstruction during mask induction in infants and children. The first step is to open the mouth, extend the neck, and provide anterior pressure to the angle of the mandible. An oral airway or a nasal airway may need to be inserted. Occasionally, a supraglottic airway may need to be inserted. (264)

116. The weight of the infant or child determines the appropriate size of the laryngeal mask airway (LMA). (265)

117. The cuff pressure is the actual pressure of the cuff of the supraglottic airway and is measured with a manometer in cm H_2O. The leak pressure is measured by slowly closing the APL valve to slowly increase the level of positive pressure that is delivered via the anesthesia circuit. The leak pressure is the pressure at which one first hears air leakage around the cuff of the supraglottic airway device. With supraglottic airway devices it is common for the cuff pressures to be higher than the leak pressures. (265)

118. The major advantage of the Air-Q ILA over an LMA is a design that facilitates endotracheal intubation with standard oral endotracheal tubes. The airway tube has a larger diameter than the LMA, allowing for intubation with a larger endotracheal tube than the correspondingly sized LMA. In addition, the Air-Q ILA can be used with a specially designed ILA removal stylet that stabilizes the endotracheal tube and allows controlled removal of the ILA without dislodging the tube from the trachea. (265)

119. The appropriately sized endotracheal tube for infants and children can be estimated by using the following formula: (age + 16)/4 = endotracheal tube size. This formula is for uncuffed endotracheal tubes. (265)

120. When using a cuffed endotracheal tube in infants and children, the formula used to estimate the appropriately sized uncuffed endotracheal tube must be adapted. To adapt the formula it is necessary to subtract half a size from the calculated size to estimate the appropriate size of a cuffed endotracheal tube. (266)

121. The advantages of cuffed endotracheal tubes in infants and children are that they (1) minimize the need for repeated laryngoscopy, (2) allow for lower fresh gas flows, (3) decrease the amount of inhalational agent used, and (4) decrease the concentrations of anesthetic gases detectable in operating rooms. The disadvantage of a cuffed endotracheal tube as compared to an uncuffed endotracheal tube is that a smaller cuffed than uncuffed tube is required and can increase resistance through the endotracheal tube and the work of breathing. (266)

122. If too large an uncuffed endotracheal tube or an overinflated cuffed endotracheal tube is utilized, the tracheal mucosa will be compressed causing subglottic edema either at the level of the cricoid cartilage or below. This complication can result in postextubation croup in mild cases and tracheal stenosis in more severe cases involving prolonged tracheal intubation. (266)

123. Using cuffed endotracheal tubes does not increase the incidence of postextubation croup as compared to using uncuffed endotracheal tubes. (266)

124. The leak pressure when using uncuffed endotracheal tubes in infants and children should be 20 to 25 cm H_2O. If the leak pressure is too high, a smaller endotracheal tube should be used, and if the leak pressure is too low, a larger endotracheal tube should be used. (266)

125. The cuff pressure should be 20 to 25 cm H_2O when using cuffed endotracheal tubes in infants and children and should be measured with a manometer. (266)

126. The new Microcuff pediatric endotracheal tubes appear to offer several distinct advantages over conventional cuffed pediatric endotracheal tubes. The Microcuff endotracheal tubes have a cuff that is made from a microthin polyurethane membrane that is stronger than conventional cuffs and seals the airway at lower cuff pressures than conventional endotracheal tubes. This reduces the potential for mucosal edema and postextubation croup. The cuff on the Microcuff endotracheal tube is also shorter and placed closer to the tip

of the endotracheal tube, increasing the chances that the endotracheal tube is correctly placed. The Microcuff endotracheal tube also has an intubation depth mark, which indicates the correct depth for insertion and also increases the ability for correct placement. (267)

127. The advantages of straight laryngoscope blades when intubating infants and small children are as follows: (1) they have a smaller profile that fits more easily into the smaller mouths of infants and children, and (2) they have a smaller tip that more effectively lifts the epiglottis to provide a better view of the vocal cords. The disadvantage of a straight blade is that it does not retract the tongue as well to the left side of the mouth. A curved blade has a larger flange that retracts the tongue to the left more effectively and may be useful in certain patient populations in which the tongue is larger than normal. (267)

128. In infants younger than 1 year, a Miller 1 straight laryngoscope blade is most useful. In children between 1 and 3 years of age, a 1½ straight laryngoscope blade, such as a Wis-Hipple, is often useful. A longer straight laryngoscope blade such as a Miller 2 is appropriate for most children between 3 and 10 years of age. The tracheas of children older than 11 years are often more easily intubated with a curved laryngoscope blade such as a Macintosh 3. Both straight and curved laryngoscope blades of various sizes should always be available. (267)

129. The advantages of video laryngoscopes over direct laryngoscopy in infants and children include (1) the ability to see the glottis opening and vocal cords without aligning the oral, pharyngeal, and laryngeal axes; (2) improved ability to visualize the glottis opening and vocal cords in patients with limited neck extension, hypoplastic mandibles, or anterior airways; and (3) the ability to teach as both the student and teacher can view the monitor at the same time. Disadvantages include the requirement of adequate mouth opening and the potential need for increased time to intubate. (267)

130. The different GlideScope sizes and models according to the patient's age and weight are as follows: GVL 0 is designed for infants weighing less than 2.5 kg, the GVL 1 for infants from 2.5 to 5.0 kg, the GVL 2 for infants from 5 to 15 kg, and the GVL 2.5 for children from 15 to 30 kg. The Glidescope Titanium S3 or T3 is recommended for children and teenagers from 30 to 70 kg, and the Titanium S4 or T4 for teenagers more than 70 kg. (268)

131. The limitations of the smaller flexible fiberoptic bronchoscopes used in infants and small children include (1) limited field of vision, (2) view that is easily obscured by secretions or bleeding, (3) inferior optics compared to larger adult bronchoscopes because of fewer fiberoptic bundles, and (4) no suction channel. (268)

132. It is unlikely that infants and children will cooperate with procedures such as an awake fiberoptic endotracheal intubation, so it is usually necessary to induce anesthesia and manage the difficult airway in these patients while they are asleep. (268)

133. The safest vasoconstrictor to apply to the nasal mucosa when performing a nasal fiberoptic endotracheal intubation in infants or children is oxymetazoline HCl 0.05% nasal spray. Phenylephrine applied to the nasal mucosa in infants and children has been associated with cases of phenylephrine toxicity. (268-269)

134. When an unexpected difficult airway appears in pediatric patients, the most important first step is to call for an additional anesthesia colleague to help. (269)

135. In a difficult pediatric intubation situation, it is critical to not persist with repeated attempts at direct laryngoscopy, which can result in trauma to the upper airway, edema, and bleeding. In most situations, a supraglottic airway should be inserted to provide an airway to oxygenate and ventilate the patient and allow time to obtain additional personnel and airway equipment. A supraglottic airway may be the only way to maintain an airway until the patient wakes up or a surgical airway is established. A supraglottic airway is also an excellent conduit for fiberoptic intubation. (269)

136. For expected difficult airway in the pediatric patient, an additional anesthesia colleague should be available for help during the induction of anesthesia, inserting an intravenous line, and securing the airway. A surgeon capable of establishing a surgical airway and emergency airway equipment should be in the operating room before beginning the induction of anesthesia. (269)

137. Infants and small children are at a higher risk than adults for croup, stridor, and laryngospasm after tracheal extubation. (270)

138. Croup occurs most commonly when either an uncuffed endotracheal tube that is too large or an overinflated cuffed endotracheal tube is used. The resulting mechanical pressure on the tracheal mucosa causes venous congestion and edema, and in severe cases can even compromise the arterial blood supply, causing mucosal ischemia. The resulting edema can narrow the tracheal lumen, especially in infants and small children. Because resistance to flow in an endotracheal tube is inversely proportional to the radius of the lumen to the fourth power, 1 mm of edema in an infant airway is much more significant than 1 mm of edema in an adult airway. Other risk factors for postextubation croup include multiple tracheal intubation attempts, unusual positioning of the head during surgery, increased duration of surgery, and procedures involving the upper airway, such as rigid bronchoscopy. (270)

139. An infant or child with postextubation croup usually has respiratory distress in the postanesthesia care unit. Nasal flaring, retractions, an increased respiratory rate, audible stridor, and decreased oxygen saturation are common clinical findings. (270)

140. Treatment of postextubation croup or stridor in infants and children depends on the degree of respiratory distress. Mild symptoms can be managed with humidified oxygen and prolonged observation in the postanesthesia care unit. More severe cases may require aerosolized racemic epinephrine and postoperative observation in an intensive care unit. Patients whose respiratory distress is severe and not relieved with these measures may need to be reintubated with an endotracheal tube smaller than the one previously used. Steroids administered intravenously for preventing upper airway edema are more beneficial when given before the airway is instrumented and should be administered before procedures such as rigid bronchoscopy. (270)

141. Infants and children with obstructive sleep apnea are at significant risk for airway obstruction, respiratory distress, and the potential for apnea in the postoperative period. At baseline these infants and children hypoventilate, which results in hypercapnia and often arterial hypoxemia while asleep. Residual inhaled anesthetics or residual neuromuscular blockade can depress airway reflexes, skeletal muscle tone and strength, and respiratory drive and result in significant airway compromise in infants and children with obstructive sleep apnea. (270)

142. Tracheal extubation in patients with obstructive sleep apnea should be considered only when these infants and children are fully awake. All infants and children with obstructive sleep apnea should be monitored postoperatively with pulse oximetry and apnea monitoring. High-risk patients should be monitored postoperatively in an intensive care unit setting. Opioids must be very carefully titrated both intraoperatively and postoperatively because they can depress the ventilatory drive and contribute to significant hypercapnia and arterial hypoxemia in these infants and children. (270)

143. Laryngospasm most commonly occurs in infants and children during either inhalational induction of anesthesia or the emergence from anesthesia often after extubation or removal of a supraglottic airway device. (270)

144. The majority of laryngospasm episodes in pediatric patients can be treated successfully with continuous positive-pressure ventilation via face mask with 100% oxygen, while applying a chin lift and jaw thrust. The positive pressure may have to be as high as 50 cm H_2O to successfully break the laryngospasm. If positive pressure is not successful and the infant or child is desaturating or

bradycardic, further intervention is necessary. If there is intravenous access, laryngospasm should be treated with approximately 0.6 to 1.0 mg/kg of intravenous propofol and, if necessary, 0.2 to 0.3 mg/kg of intravenous rocuronium. If there is no intravenous access, laryngospasm should be treated with 0.6 to 1.0 mg/kg of intramuscular rocuronium or 1.5 to 2.0 mg/kg of intramuscular succinylcholine. (270)

145. Tracheal extubation of an infant or child after a difficult intubation is considered carefully because reintubation can be more difficult than the initial intubation. The tracheas of infants and children with difficult airways should be extubated only when they are fully awake and there is no residual neuromuscular blockade. An infant or child with a difficult airway should be extubated only when appropriate equipment and personnel are available for urgent reintubation. (270)

17 SPINAL, EPIDURAL, AND CAUDAL ANESTHESIA

Alan J.R. Macfarlane, Richard Brull,
Kenneth Drasner, and Vincent W.S. Chan

ANATOMY	1. What is the clinical significance of the curvatures of the spinal canal with respect to spinal and epidural anesthesia?
	2. What are the rostral and caudal limitations of the spinal cord? What accounts for the disparity between the vertebral level and the spinal cord level?
	3. What is the cauda equina, and what characteristic features are relevant to spinal anesthesia?
	4. What are the three meningeal layers surrounding the spinal cord?
	5. Where is cerebrospinal fluid (CSF) relative to the meningeal layers? What are two interchangeable terms for this space?
	6. What structures form the boundaries of the epidural space?
	7. What structures are contained within the epidural space?
	8. What is the number of each type of vertebra composing the vertebral column?
	9. What are the different characteristic features of the spinous processes and laminae of the thoracic and lumbar vertebrae? How does this impact on the clinical performance of neuraxial blocks?
	10. How are the laminae of adjacent vertebrae connected?
	11. How are the tips of the spinous processes of adjacent vertebrae connected?
	12. What passes through the intervertebral foramina?
	13. As the nerves pass through the intervertebral foramen they become encased by the dura, arachnoid, and pia, forming what three components of a peripheral nerve?
	14. Where do the preganglionic nerves of the sympathetic nervous system originate, and what is their course of travel after leaving the spinal cord?
	15. Describe the blood supply of the spinal cord. Which area of the cord is most vulnerable to ischemic insult?
	16. What is the artery of Adamkiewicz?
	17. Describe venous drainage of the spinal cord.
MECHANISM OF ACTION AND PHYSIOLOGY	18. What types of nerves fibers are blocked in neuraxial anesthesia, and in what temporal order does this occur?
	19. What is differential sensory block?
	20. What is the level of sympathetic nerve blockade compared to sensory nerve blockade in each spinal and epidural anesthesia?
	21. What is the effect of neuraxial anesthesia on systemic vascular resistance, and why?
	22. In healthy, normovolemic patients, what percent decrease in systemic vascular resistance is typically seen after neuraxial blockade if a normal cardiac output is maintained?
	23. What is the effect of neuraxial anesthesia on cardiac output, and why?

24. What is the effect of neuraxial anesthesia on coronary blood flow, and why?
25. What is the effect of neuraxial anesthesia on the respiratory system, and why?
26. What is the effect of neuraxial anesthesia on the gastrointestinal tract, and why?
27. What is the effect of neuraxial anesthesia on the renal system, and why?

INDICATIONS AND CONTRAINDICATIONS

28. What are the common indications for spinal anesthesia?
29. What are the common indications for epidural anesthesia?
30. How do the hemodynamic effects of epidural anesthesia compare with those of spinal anesthesia?
31. What are the absolute contraindications to neuraxial anesthesia?
32. Does chronic back pain preclude performance of a neuraxial anesthetic?
33. Does spinal stenosis preclude performance of a neuraxial anesthetic?
34. Does previous spine surgery preclude performance of a neuraxial anesthetic?
35. Does multiple sclerosis preclude performance of a neuraxial anesthetic?
36. Does spina bifida preclude performance of a neuraxial anesthetic?
37. Does aortic stenosis preclude performance of a neuraxial anesthetic?
38. Do coagulation abnormalities preclude performance of a neuraxial anesthetic?
39. Does infection preclude performance of a neuraxial anesthetic?

SPINAL ANESTHESIA

40. What surface landmarks are used to determine the approximate level of spinal anesthesia?
41. What are the three adjustable factors that most influence the distribution of the local anesthetic solution in CSF after its administration into the subarachnoid space?
42. How is the baricity of a local anesthetic solution to be administered into the subarachnoid space defined? Why is this clinically important?
43. What is added to local anesthetics for spinal anesthesia to make the solution hyperbaric? What is the principal advantage of hyperbaric solutions?
44. What is added to local anesthetics for spinal anesthesia to make the solution hypobaric? What is the principal advantage of hypobaric solutions?
45. What role does the contour of the vertebral canal play in hyperbaric spinal anesthetic distribution and, hence, level of spinal block?
46. What is a "saddle block"?
47. What situations might warrant use of a hypobaric solution?
48. How do the patient factors of height, weight, and age affect the spread of spinal anesthesia and thus the spinal levels that are anesthetized (block height)?
49. How long after the administration of intrathecal local anesthetic does patient position affect block height?
50. How do spinal needle type, needle orientation, level of injection, injection rate, and barbotage (repeated aspiration and reinjection of CSF) affect block height of isobaric and hyperbaric solutions?
51. What are the factors that most influence the duration of a spinal anesthetic?
52. How are local anesthetics for spinal anesthesia most commonly classified? What are the common anesthetics in each group?
53. What is the concern regarding the use of lidocaine for spinal anesthesia?
54. Which local anesthetics may be suitable for day case spinal anesthesia?
55. Which local anesthetics may be suitable for long duration (1-3 hours) surgical procedures?
56. What are the potentially useful effects derived from adding an opioid to the local anesthetic used for spinal anesthesia? What is their mechanism of action?
57. What is the purpose of adding a vasoconstrictor to the local anesthetic solution used for spinal anesthesia? What is their mechanism of action?
58. Which drugs other than vasoconstrictors may prolong spinal anesthesia?
59. How are spinal needles classified?
60. Which characteristics of a spinal needle will result in the lowest incidence of post–dural puncture headache?

61. What is the advantage of performing spinal anesthesia in an awake patient?
62. What are the common positions patients are placed in for administration of a spinal anesthetic?
63. What are some advantages and disadvantages of the sitting position during performance of a spinal anesthetic compared to lateral decubitus?
64. What is the reason for placing a spinal anesthetic at a level below the L2 vertebra?
65. What vertebral level is crossed by a line drawn across the patient's back at the level of the top of the iliac crests? What interspaces are located directly above and below this line?
66. What are the tissue planes that will be traversed as the needle is advanced toward the subarachnoid space in the midline?
67. What accounts for the "pop" the anesthetist may feel when advancing a spinal needle into the subarachnoid space?
68. How is subarachnoid placement of the spinal needle confirmed?
69. After the syringe containing the local anesthetic solution for administration into the subarachnoid space is attached to the spinal needle, how can continued subarachnoid placement of the spinal needle be confirmed?
70. How does the paramedian approach compare to the midline approach for spinal anesthesia? What are their relative advantages and disadvantages?
71. What are some advantages and disadvantages of a continuous spinal technique?
72. What was the likely mechanism of cauda equina syndrome after continuous spinal techniques?
73. After the intrathecal injection of local anesthetic, which sensation is tested for an early indication of the level of spinal anesthesia?
74. What is the Bromage scale?
75. How do spinal anesthetics regress during the recovery from spinal anesthesia?

EPIDURAL ANESTHESIA

76. What drug factors affect the spread of epidural anesthesia?
77. What patient factors affect the spread of epidural anesthesia?
78. What procedural factors affect the spread of epidural anesthesia?
79. What is the major site of action of local anesthetics administered epidurally?
80. Why are procaine and tetracaine rarely used for epidural anesthesia?
81. What are the characteristics of epidural prilocaine when administered in lower concentrations and when administered in large doses?
82. How do chloroprocaine, lidocaine, and mepivacaine compare in their onset time and duration of action after epidural administration?
83. Does epidural lidocaine cause transient neurologic symptoms (TNS)?
84. How are bupivacaine and ropivacaine similar and different after epidural administration?
85. What are some potential advantages of adding epinephrine to the local anesthetic solution used for epidural anesthesia?
86. What are some potential advantages of adding opioids to the local anesthetic solution used for epidural anesthesia?
87. How does the lipophilic nature of an opioid affect its mechanism of action when administered in the epidural space?
88. What are some potential advantages of adding clonidine or dexmedetomidine to the local anesthetic solution used for epidural anesthesia?
89. What are some potential advantages of adding bicarbonate to the local anesthetic solution used for epidural anesthesia?
90. What surface landmarks can be used to identify specific spinal process interspaces and guide placement of an epidural needle?
91. What are the advantages and disadvantages of epidural catheters with multiple side orifices near the tip instead of a single end hole at the tip?
92. Is it acceptable to place an epidural injection after the induction of general anesthesia?

93. What is the "loss-of-resistance" technique?
94. What are the advantages of using air or saline during the loss-of-resistance technique?
95. What is the "hanging-drop" technique?
96. What is the technique used for placement of a catheter following identification of the epidural space?
97. How does the Tsui test help confirm epidural catheter tip location?
98. When might the paramedian epidural approach be beneficial over the midline approach?
99. What is the purpose of a "test dose" for an epidural catheter?
100. What is "combined spinal-epidural" anesthesia, and what is its clinical use? What is epidural volume extension?

CAUDAL ANESTHESIA

101. What are some indications for caudal anesthesia?
102. How does the approach to caudal anesthesia compare to that of epidural anesthesia with respect local anesthetic dose, position, and technique?
103. How is the sacral hiatus identified?
104. Describe the technique for caudal anesthesia.
105. Where does the dural sac end?

COMPLICATIONS

106. What are the potential complications that should be discussed with the patient before proceeding with a spinal or epidural anesthetic?
107. What are factors associated with paraplegia following neuraxial anesthesia?
108. What are factors associated with cauda equina syndrome following neuraxial anesthesia?
109. What are risk factors associated with epidural hematoma following neuraxial anesthesia?
110. What are some signs and symptoms of an epidural hematoma?
111. What are factors associated with nerve injury following neuraxial anesthesia?
112. What are factors associated with post–dural puncture headache following neuraxial anesthesia?
113. What is the cause and typical onset of a post–dural puncture headache?
114. What are the signs and symptoms of a post–dural puncture headache?
115. What are the treatment options for a post–dural puncture headache?
116. What are transient neurologic symptoms (TNS)? What are factors associated with TNS following neuraxial anesthesia?
117. What are factors associated with hypotension following neuraxial anesthesia?
118. What are factors associated with bradycardia following neuraxial anesthesia?
119. What are factors associated with cardiac arrest following neuraxial anesthesia?
120. What are factors associated with respiratory depression following neuraxial anesthesia?
121. What are some infections that can occur following neuraxial anesthesia, and what are some associated factors?
122. What is the association between backache and epidural anesthesia in parturients?
123. What are factors associated with nausea and vomiting following neuraxial anesthesia?
124. What is the cause of urinary retention following neuraxial anesthesia?
125. How can pruritus following neuraxial anesthesia be treated?
126. How can the risk of shivering following neuraxial anesthesia be reduced?
127. How can the risk of unintentional intravascular injection of local anesthetic during epidural anesthesia be reduced?
128. What are the clinical characteristics of unintentional subdural injection during epidural anesthesia?

ANSWERS*

ANATOMY

1. On a lateral view, the vertebral canal exhibits four curvatures, of which the thoracic convexity (kyphosis) and the lumbar concavity (lordosis) are of major importance to the distribution of local anesthetic solution in the subarachnoid space. In contrast, these curves have little effect on the spread of local anesthetic solutions in the epidural space. Scoliosis is of less importance to local anesthetic spread but can make needle insertion more awkward. (273–275)

2. The spinal cord is continuous with the medulla oblongata. In the fetus the spinal cord extends the entire length of the vertebral canal. However, because of disproportionate growth of neural tissue and the vertebral canal, the spinal cord generally terminates around the L3 vertebra at birth and at the lower border of the L1 vertebra in adults. As a further consequence of this differential growth, the spinal nerves become progressively longer and more closely aligned with the longitudinal axis of the vertebral canal. (274)

3. The cauda equina—so named because of its resemblance to a horse's tail—is the collection of lumbar and sacral nerves that extend beyond the end of the spinal cord in the spinal canal. Each pair of spinal nerves exits via the intervertebral foramina at its respective vertebral column levels. The nerve roots of the cauda equina move relatively freely within the CSF, a fortunate arrangement that results in their being more likely to be displaced rather than pierced by an advancing needle. (274)

4. The outermost meningeal layer surrounding the spinal cord, the dura mater, is a tough fibroelastic membrane that provides structural support. It originates at the foramen magnum and continues caudally to terminate between S1 and S4. Closely adherent to the inner surface of the dura lies the arachnoid membrane. Though far more delicate than the dura, the arachnoid serves as the major pharmacologic barrier preventing movement of the drug from the epidural to the subarachnoid space. The innermost layer of the spinal meninges, the pia, is a highly vascular structure closely applied to the cord that forms the inner border of the subarachnoid space. (274)

5. CSF is contained between the pia and arachnoid meningeal layers. This space is consequently referred to as the *subarachnoid space,* but another term for this compartment is the *intrathecal space.* (274)

6. The epidural space is bounded cranially by the foramen magnum, caudally by the sacrococcygeal ligament, anteriorly by the posterior longitudinal ligament, laterally by the vertebral pedicles, and posteriorly by both the ligamentum flavum and vertebral lamina. (274)

7. The epidural space is an irregular column containing spinal nerves, fat, lymphatics, and blood vessels. It is not a closed space but communicates with the paravertebral spaces by way of the intervertebral foramina. (274)

8. The vertebral column is composed of 7 cervical vertebrae, 12 thoracic vertebrae, and 5 lumbar vertebrae, as well as the 5 fused sacral and 4 fused coccygeal vertebrae. (275)

9. The spinous processes in the thoracic area are angled more downward, which defines the angle required for placement and advancement of a needle intended to access the vertebral canal. The interlaminar space in the lumbar spine is wide, reflecting the fact that the lamina occupies only about half the space between adjacent vertebrae. In contrast, the interlaminar space is just a few millimeters wide at the level of the thoracic vertebrae. Again this offers less space to insert a needle to the epidural space, making thoracic needle placement more challenging. (275)

---

*Numbers in parentheses refer to pages, figures, boxes, or tables in Pardo MC, Miller RD, eds. *Basics of Anesthesia.* 7th ed. Philadelphia: Elsevier; 2018.

10. The laminae of adjacent vertebrae are connected by the ligamentum flavum. The ligamentum flavum thickness, distance to the dura, and skin-to-dura distance vary with the area of the vertebral canal. (275)

11. The tips of the spinous processes of adjacent vertebrae are connected by the supraspinous ligaments. (275)

12. The spinal nerves pass through the intervertebral foramina and supply a specific dermatome/osteotome/myotome. (275)

13. The dura, arachnoid, and pia encasement of the peripheral nerve are the origins of the epineurium, perineurium, and endoneurium, respectively. (275)

14. Preganglionic nerves of the sympathetic nervous system originate from the spinal cord at the T1 to L2 levels. From there they travel with the spinal nerves before separating to form the sympathetic chain at more distant sites such as the celiac plexus. (275)

15. The blood supply of the spinal cord arises from a single anterior and two paired posterior spinal arteries. The posterior spinal arteries emerge from the cranial vault and supply the dorsal (sensory) portion of the spinal cord. Because they are paired and have rich collateral anastomotic links from the subclavian and intercostal arteries, this area of the spinal cord is relatively protected from ischemic damage. This is not the case with the single anterior spinal artery that originates from the vertebral artery and supplies the ventral (motor) portion of the spinal cord. Ischemia affecting the anterior spinal artery may result in "anterior spinal artery syndrome," characterized by motor paralysis and loss of pain and temperature sensation below the level affected. Ischemia can result from profound hypotension, mechanical obstruction, vasculopathy, hemorrhage, or any combination of these factors. (276)

16. The anterior spinal artery receives branches from the intercostal and iliac arteries, but these branches are variable in number and location. The largest anastomotic link, the artery of Adamkiewicz, arises from the aorta between the T7 and L4 region. The vessel is highly variable but, most commonly, is on the left and enters the vertebral canal through the L1 intervertebral foramen. The artery of Adamkiewicz is critical to the blood supply of the lower two thirds of the spinal cord, and damage to it will produce anterior spinal artery syndrome as described earlier. (276)

17. There are communicating longitudinal and segmental radicular veins in the anterior and posterior spinal cord. These veins drain into the internal vertebral plexus in the medial and lateral components of the epidural space. They then drain into the azygous system. (276)

MECHANISM OF ACTION AND PHYSIOLOGY

18. The speed of neural blockade depends on the size, surface area, and degree of myelination of the nerve fibers exposed to the local anesthetic. The small preganglionic sympathetic fibers (B fibers, 1 to 3 μm, minimally myelinated) are most sensitive to local anesthetic blockade. The C fibers (0.3 to 1 μm, unmyelinated), which conduct cold temperature sensation, are blocked more readily than the A-delta pinprick sensation fibers (1 to 4 μm, myelinated). The A-beta fibers (5 to 12 μm, myelinated), which conduct touch sensation, are the last sensory fibers to be affected. The A-alpha motor fibers (12 to 20 μm, myelinated) are the most resistant to local anesthetic blockade. Regression of neural blockade follows the reverse order. (277)

19. Differential sensory block describes how maximum block height in neuraxial anesthesia varies according to the sensory modality. The loss of sensation to cold (approximates sympathetic blockade) is 1 to 2 segments higher than the loss of sensation to pinprick, which is higher still than loss of sensation to touch. (278)

20. The sympathectomy from neuraxial blockade is typically 2 to 6 dermatomes above the sensory block level with spinal anesthesia but is at the same level with epidural anesthesia. (278)

21. Neuraxial anesthesia commonly causes a decrease in systemic vascular resistance due to blockade of peripheral (T1-L2) sympathetic fibers as well as decreases in adrenal medullary catecholamine secretion. The degree of the vasodilatory change and corresponding hemodynamic change depends on both baseline sympathetic tone (higher sympathetic tone in elderly patients results in a greater hemodynamic change) and the extent of the sympathectomy (height of the block). (279)

22. In healthy, normovolemic patients, systemic vascular resistance typically decreases by about 15% to 18% after neuraxial blockade if a normal cardiac output is maintained. (279)

23. Cardiac output is the product of heart rate and stroke volume. It is usually maintained but may decrease during neuraxial anesthesia. The heart rate does not change significantly in most patients during neuraxial anesthesia. However, in an estimated 10% to 15% of patients, significant bradycardia occurs. As with hypotension, the risk for bradycardia increases with increasing sensory levels of anesthesia. Speculated mechanisms for such bradycardia include the block of cardioaccelerator fibers originating from T1 through T4 and decreased venous return (Bezold-Jarisch reflex), especially in the presence of hypovolemia. (279)

24. Coronary blood flow decreases when mean arterial pressure decreases. However, patients with ischemic heart disease may benefit from a high thoracic block with improvement in global and regional myocardial function and reversal of ischemic changes. This is likely due to decreased myocardial oxygen demand and left ventricular afterload. (279)

25. Neuraxial anesthesia has little, if any, effect on resting alveolar ventilation (arterial blood gases unchanged). Expiratory reserve volume decreases slightly, resulting in a decrease in vital capacity. High levels of motor anesthesia can produce paralysis of abdominal and intercostal muscles and lead to a decreased ability to cough and expel secretions. These changes are more marked in patients with respiratory disease or who are obese. Hypoperfusion of the respiratory centers due to severe hypotension and low cardiac output can result in respiratory arrest, but this situation is rare and reverses when hemodynamics are restored. (279)

26. Neuraxial blockade from T6 to L1 inhibits sympathetic nervous system innervation to the gastrointestinal tract. This results in contracted intestines, hyperperistalsis, and relaxed sphincters due to unopposed parasympathetic nervous system activity. Nausea and vomiting may occur in as many as 20% of patients and can be treated with atropine if the level of blockade is high (T5). (279)

27. Neuraxial anesthesia may decrease renal blood flow, but this is of little physiologic importance. (279)

INDICATIONS AND CONTRAINDICATIONS

28. Spinal anesthesia is commonly used for surgical procedures of a known duration involving the lower abdominal area, perineum, and lower extremities. It may also be indicated when the risks of general anesthesia are increased, such as in the presence of severe respiratory disease. (280)

29. Epidural anesthesia, like spinal anesthesia, can be used as the primary anesthetic for surgeries involving the lower abdomen or lower extremities, particularly if prolonged anesthesia is required. Epidural analgesia is more frequently used as a supplement to general anesthesia for thoracic and abdominal procedures where significant benefit derives from the ability to provide continuous postoperative analgesia. Similarly, continuous epidural anesthesia is very effective and widely used for the control of labor pain. (280)

30. Because the onset of sympathetic nervous system block is more gradual in epidural versus spinal anesthesia, the hemodynamic effects of epidural anesthesia are usually less marked. Incremental dosing of an epidural block may lessen some of the hemodynamic changes associated with neuraxial anesthesia. (280)

31. Absolute contraindications to neuraxial anesthesia include patient refusal, infection at the site of planned needle puncture, allergy to any of the drugs to be administered, and elevated intracranial pressure. (280)

32. Chronic back pain does not preclude performance of a neuraxial anesthetic. A neuraxial anesthetic may be avoided in these patients if they perceive a relationship between postoperative exacerbation of back pain and the block, even though they are not causally related. (280)

33. Spinal stenosis does not preclude performance of a neuraxial anesthetic, although there is an association between the presence of spinal stenosis and nerve injury following neuraxial techniques. The contribution of surgical factors and natural history of the spinal disease in these cases is unknown. (280)

34. Previous spine surgery does not preclude performance of a neuraxial anesthetic, although performance of the neuraxial block may be technically more difficult. In addition, spread of local anesthetic may be unpredictable or incomplete. (280)

35. Multiple sclerosis does not preclude performance of a neuraxial anesthetic, although these patients may be more sensitive to neuraxial local anesthetics and exhibit prolonged motor and sensory blockade. (280)

36. Spina bifida does not preclude performance of a neuraxial anesthetic, although the potential for needle injury to the spinal cord may be increased. In addition, the spread of local anesthetic may be markedly variable. (280)

37. Aortic stenosis does not preclude performance of a neuraxial anesthetic, although patients with a fixed cardiac output due to mitral stenosis, idiopathic hypertrophic subaortic stenosis, and aortic stenosis are intolerant of significant decreases in systemic vascular resistance commonly associated with neuraxial anesthesia. Though not an absolute contraindication, neuraxial blocks should not routinely be used in such cases, and patients should be evaluated on a case-by-case basis. (280)

38. A spinal hematoma can be catastrophic, and has occurred in patients on low-molecular-weight heparin. The decision to insert a needle into the intrathecal or epidural space for a neuraxial block in patients with abnormal coagulation, either endogenous or produced by the administration of anticoagulants, must be based on a risk-benefit assessment and include discussion with the patient and the surgical team. Guidelines developed by the American Society of Regional Anesthesia (www.asra.com) are updated periodically based on evolving literature and changes in clinical practices. (281)

39. Infection does not preclude performance of a neuraxial anesthetic, although there is concern that an epidural abscess or meningitis might result from iatrogenic seeding during the procedure. Institution of appropriate antibiotic therapy and a demonstrated response before the block may decrease the risk for infection. Neuraxial techniques in patients with significant bacteremia or septic shock should be avoided. (281)

SPINAL ANESTHESIA

40. The surface landmarks and their respective dermatomal levels most often used clinically are as follows: nipple, T4-T5; tip of xiphoid, T7; umbilicus, T10; and inguinal ligament, T12. (281)

41. Drug, patient, and procedural factors affect block height, but not all are controllable by the anesthesiologist. The three adjustable factors that most influence the distribution of local anesthetic solution in the subarachnoid space are the dose, baricity of the solution, and position of the patient during, and for the first few minutes after, its administration. (281)

42. Baricity is defined as the ratio of density of a local anesthetic solution relative to the density of CSF (conventionally measured at 37° C because density varies with temperature). Local anesthetics are therefore classified as hypobaric, isobaric, and hyperbaric relative to CSF. Baricity is clinically important because, in conjunction with patient positioning and vertebral curvatures, it determines the direction that local anesthetic solution will move after injection into the CSF. (281)

43. Local anesthetic solutions are made hyperbaric for spinal anesthesia by the addition of dextrose. The principal advantage of hyperbaric solutions is the more predictable spread, moving to dependent regions of the spinal canal. Hyperbaric local anesthetics injected in the supine position result in a higher level of block than isobaric or hypobaric solutions. (281)

44. Local anesthetic solutions are made hypobaric for spinal anesthesia by the addition of sterile water. The principal advantage of hypobaric solutions is their spread to nondependent regions of the spinal canal. (281)

45. The contour of the vertebral canal is critical to the subarachnoid distribution of hyperbaric local anesthetic solutions. For example, in the supine horizontal position, the patient's thoracic kyphosis will be dependent relative to the peak created by the lumbar lordosis. Anesthetic delivered cephalad to this peak will thus move toward the thoracic kyphosis, which is normally around T6-T8. Placing the patient in a head-down (Trendelenburg) position will generally accentuate this cephalad spread of local anesthetic solution. (281)

46. A saddle block involves the intrathecal injection of a low dose of hyperbaric local anesthetic solution with the patient seated, and this upright seated position is maintained for up to 30 minutes to deliberately restrict spread. This results in sacral anesthesia, referred to as a "saddle block," reflecting sensory anesthesia of the area that would be in contact with a saddle. (284)

47. Hypobaric local anesthetics are less commonly used in clinical practice. They may find use in patients undergoing perineal procedures in the "prone jackknife" position, or more commonly in patients undergoing elective or emergency hip surgery where anesthetic can "float up" to the nondependent operative site. In the case of a fractured neck of femur, this means the patient does not need to lie on the painful fracture during insertion of a spinal needle in the lateral decubitus position. Plain bupivacaine at room temperature is actually slightly hypobaric. (284)

48. In the normal range of the adult patient's height the spinal levels of anesthesia are not influenced by the patient's height. CSF volume may be decreased in patients who are obese with increased abdominal mass, and this may increase the resultant block height. Advanced age is associated with increased block height as well as increased nerve root sensitivity to local anesthetics. (284)

49. The spread of local anesthetic after its intrathecal injection appears to stop after 20 to 25 minutes. Patient position during this time can affect block height but in particular in the first few minutes after intrathecal injection. (284)

50. Spinal needle type, needle orientation, injection rate, and barbotage (repeated aspiration and reinjection of CSF) of isobaric and hyperbaric solutions do not appear to affect block height. Spinal needle type and orientation may affect block quality, however. The level of injection does not affect block height with hyperbaric solutions, but with isobaric solutions the block height is generally higher the more cephalad the injection. (284)

51. The factors that most influence the duration of a spinal anesthetic are the local anesthetic selected, the dose, and the use of additives. (284)

52. Although local anesthetics may be classified by pharmacologic structure (i.e., ester or amide), it is the duration of action that is most commonly used as a means of classification. Short- and intermediate-acting local anesthetics include lidocaine, chloroprocaine, prilocaine, and mepivacaine. Long-acting local anesthetics include bupivacaine and ropivacaine. (285)

53. Lidocaine has been linked to permanent nerve injury and, in up to one third of patients receiving this anesthetic for spinal anesthesia, the development of transient neurologic symptoms (TNS) (pain or dysesthesia in the back, buttocks, and lower extremities). The use of lidocaine for spinal anesthesia has declined. (285)

54. Chloroprocaine is an ultra-short-acting ester that is rapidly metabolized by pseudocholinesterase with minimal systemic or fetal effects. TNS can occur but at a lesser rate than with lidocaine. Prilocaine is short acting and is rarely associated with TNS, but in large doses can cause methemoglobinemia. Mepivacaine is also of intermediate duration, and TNS are less frequent with the isobaric compared to the hyperbaric preparation. Lower doses of bupivacaine may be used in "selective" or "unilateral" spinal anesthesia. By utilizing baricity and patient positioning a low dose of bupivacaine can be used to provide shorter duration anesthesia, with more rapid recovery and time to mobilization. (285)

55. Bupivacaine, ropivacaine, and tetracaine (with an additive) can all be used for spinal anesthesia for longer duration surgical procedures. Bupivacaine is similar to ropivacaine in its slow onset and 2.5- to 3-hour duration of action, and it is rarely associated with TNS. Ropivacaine has less motor block than bupivacaine, has earlier recovery, and is less cardiotoxic. (286)

56. Opioids are commonly added to intrathecal local anesthetic solutions to enhance the duration and quality of surgical anesthesia and provide postoperative analgesia. Intrathecal opioids primarily exert their effect at the dorsal horn of the spinal cord. Opioid lipid solubility affects onset, duration of action, and uptake into blood vessels. Lipophilic opioids in particular, such as fentanyl, are also taken up rapidly into blood vessels with a resultant systemic effect. The onset time of intrathecal fentanyl is 10 to 20 minutes, and duration of action is 4 to 6 hours. Fentanyl is used for short surgical procedures, and its administration does not preclude discharge home on the same day. More hydrophilic drugs such as preservative-free morphine have less systemic uptake and therefore spread further within the CSF. Preservative-free morphine can provide effective control of postoperative pain for approximately 24 hours, but rostral spread within the CSF toward the brainstem necessitates in-hospital monitoring for late respiratory depression. (286)

57. Vasoconstrictors added to spinal anesthetic solutions can increase the duration of spinal anesthesia. This is most commonly achieved by the addition of epinephrine or phenylephrine. Increased duration of anesthesia is believed to result from α_1-adrenergic–mediated vasoconstriction, which decreases local anesthetic uptake. Epinephrine itself may also contribute directly to analgesia via α_2-adrenergic receptor activation. Phenylephrine is associated with TNS. (286)

58. Intrathecal clonidine and dexmedetomidine act on prejunctional and postjunctional α_2-receptors in the dorsal horn of the spinal cord. Clonidine prolongs sensory and motor blockade by approximately 1 hour and improves analgesia with less urinary retention than morphine. However, clonidine can cause hypotension and sedation lasting up to 8 hours. Dexmedetomidine is about 10 times more α_2-selective than clonidine and can prolong motor and sensory block without hemodynamic compromise. (287)

59. Spinal anesthesia needles are classified by their size in gauge and the shape of their tip. The two basic needle tip designs are either (1) an open-ended (beveled or cutting) needle or (2) a closed tapered-tip pencil-point needle with a side port. (287)

60. The incidence of post–dural puncture headache reduces as the size of the needle becomes smaller. The incidence is also lower when a pencil-point (Whitacre or Sprotte) rather than a beveled-tip (Quincke) needle is used, because the pencil-point needle is believed to spread the dura rather than cut it. Consequently, 25- to 27-gauge pencil-point needles are usually selected when spinal anesthesia is performed. (287)

61. The advantage of performing spinal anesthesia in an awake patient is that an awake patient can provide feedback if the needle may be in close proximity to nerve tissue by reporting pain or paresthesia. The current consensus guidelines state that neuraxial blocks should be performed with the patient awake, except where the risk outweighs the benefit. (288)

62. Spinal anesthesia can be performed with the patient in the lateral decubitus, sitting, or rarely, prone position. If possible, the spine should be flexed by having the patient bend at the waist and bring the chin toward the chest to open the interspinous space. The position chosen should optimize spread of the local anesthetic solution to provide anesthesia to the operative site. (288)

63. The sitting position for spinal anesthesia facilitates recognition of the midline, which can be particularly helpful in an obese patient. The lateral decubitus position may be more comfortable and better suited for the ill or frail. The lateral position also facilitates the administration of sedation. Vasovagal syncope and hypotension may be more likely in the sitting position. (288)

64. The caudal limitation of the spinal cord in an adult usually lies between the L1 and L2 vertebrae. For this reason, spinal anesthesia is not ordinarily performed above the L2-L3 interspace. Nevertheless, some risk remains because the spinal cord extends to the third lumbar vertebra in approximately 2% of adults. Furthermore, the cauda equina nerves are also still present in the dural sac below the L2 level. (288)

65. A line drawn across the patient's back at the level of the top of the iliac crests is generally considered to identify the L4 vertebral level. The interspace palpated directly above this line would be L3-L4, and the interspace palpated directly below this line would be L4-L5. However, this may vary, and not uncommonly use of this conceptual line will result in estimates that are inaccurate by as much as two interspaces. (288)

66. As the spinal needle progresses toward the subarachnoid space, it passes through the skin, subcutaneous tissue, supraspinous ligament, interspinous ligament, ligamentum flavum, and the epidural space to reach and pierce the dura/arachnoid. (288)

67. The anesthetist may feel a characteristic "pop" just before accessing the subarachnoid space as the spinal needle is being advanced. This "pop" is produced by the spinal needle passing through the dura mater. (288)

68. Subarachnoid placement of the spinal needle is confirmed by the appearance of clear CSF in the hub of the spinal needle. (288)

69. After the syringe containing the local anesthetic solution for administration into the subarachnoid space is attached to the spinal needle, the anesthetist typically aspirates back on the syringe to confirm continued subarachnoid placement of the spinal needle tip. Confirmation is made by the characteristic swirl in the syringe as CSF enters the syringe and mixes with the local anesthetic solution. The local anesthetic solution can then be deposited into the subarachnoid space at approximately 0.2 mL/sec. After completion of the deposition of the local anesthetic solution into the subarachnoid space, CSF can again be aspirated to verify delivery of the anesthetic. The spinal needle and syringe should be removed together as a single unit. (288)

70. Spinal anesthesia can be accomplished using a midline or a paramedian approach. The midline approach is technically easier, and the needle passes through less sensitive structures, thus requiring less local anesthetic infiltration to ensure patient comfort. However, the paramedian approach is better suited to challenging circumstances when there is narrowing of the interspace, difficulty in flexion of the spine, or calcified interspinous ligaments. In the paramedian approach the spinal introducer and needle are angled 10 to 15 degrees off the sagittal plane and "walked up" the lamina. With this approach the needle is not passing through the supraspinous and interspinous ligaments. (288)

71. Inserting a catheter into the subarachnoid space (continuous spinal technique) permits incremental dosing and possibly greater hemodynamic stability than a higher dose, single-injection technique. A catheter also allows repeated drug administration and anesthesia for prolonged operations. The use of large-bore epidural needles and catheters for continuous spinal anesthesia poses significant risk of post–dural puncture headache. Microcatheters are available, but they may be more difficult to insert and have unfortunately been associated with the development of cauda equina syndrome. (288)

72. It is likely that the injury associated with the use of high-resistance, low-flow microcatheters resulted from maldistribution of local anesthetic solution due to pooling in the dependent sacral sac. The resultant high local anesthetic concentration in the sacral sac can lead to neurotoxicity of the cauda equina. (288)

73. After intrathecal injection of local anesthetic, loss of cold sensation usually occurs first and can be tested by using ice or alcohol. Loss of pinprick sensation follows, and then loss of sensation to touch, and finally loss of strength. The dermatomal order of blockade produced by a spinal anesthetic, from highest to lowest, is sympathetic, sensory, then motor. (289)

74. The Bromage scale can be used to test the extent of motor block of the lumbosacral fibers. In this scale, the intensity of motor block is assessed by the patient's ability to move the lower extremities. (289)

75. Regression of the spinal anesthetic is from the highest dermatome in a caudad direction. Furthermore, motor fibers recover first, followed by sensory. (289)

EPIDURAL ANESTHESIA

76. Drug factors, patient factors, and procedural factors all affect spread of epidural local anesthetic. The major drug factors affecting the spread of epidural anesthesia are the dose and volume of the local anesthetic solution administered (dose = volume × concentration). Volume is important because an equivalent dose at lower concentration (i.e., greater volume) may foster greater spread. As a general principle, 1 to 2 mL of solution should be injected per segment to be blocked. Local anesthetic additives and baricity do not affect epidural anesthetic spread. (289)

77. The distribution of local anesthetic within the epidural space is enhanced in patients when the epidural space is of small caliber and with reduced compliance. Spread is also enhanced when there is, decreased local anesthetic leakage through the intervertebral foramina (e.g., elderly and spinal stenosis), and increased epidural space pressure (e.g., pregnancy). Body height only seems important at the extremes of the range, and weight does not correlate well with block height. (290)

78. The level of injection of epidural anesthetic is the most important procedural-related factor that affects epidural block height. Lumbar epidural injections produce preferential cephalad spread, possibly because of negative intrathoracic pressure transmitted to the epidural space combined with resistance to caudad spread created by narrowing of the epidural space at the lumbosacral junction. In contrast, midthoracic injections tend to produce symmetric anesthesia and also may result in greater dermatomal spread for a given dose of local anesthetic. This latter effect results in part from the smaller volume of the thoracic epidural space. In the upper cervical region, local anesthetic spreads mostly caudal to the injection site. The level at which the local anesthetic solution is injected into the epidural space also defines the area of peak anesthetic effect, which decreases with increasing distance from the injection site. Patient position during performance of an epidural block is less important than with a spinal block, but the dependent portion of the body may still manifest more intense anesthesia than the nondependent side. This is less true in sitting or supine positions. Needle bevel direction and speed of injection do not affect epidural spread. (290)

79. The major site of action of local anesthetic solutions placed in the epidural space is the spinal nerve roots, where the dura is relatively thin. (290)

80. Procaine is rarely used for epidural anesthesia because the block can be unreliable and of poor quality. Tetracaine is also unreliable and toxic in larger doses. (290)

81. Epidural prilocaine, when administered in lower concentrations (2% solution), produces a sensory block with minimal motor block. In larger doses, prilocaine is associated with methemoglobinemia. (290)

82. After epidural administration, chloroprocaine has a short onset time and a short duration of action. Mepivacaine and lidocaine have similar short onset time and intermediate duration of action. (290)

83. Unlike lidocaine for spinal anesthesia, epidural lidocaine does not cause TNS. (290)

84. After epidural administration bupivacaine and ropivacaine have similar onset time and duration of action. Ropivacaine differs from bupivacaine in that it provides less motor block, a higher seizure threshold, and less cardiotoxicity. (290)

85. Advantages of adding epinephrine to the local anesthetic solution used for epidural anesthesia include decreased vascular absorption and prolonged anesthesia and analgesia, most notably with short- and intermediate-acting local anesthetics. Epinephrine may also serve as a marker of intravascular injection that can occur with cannulation of an epidural vein. Finally, epinephrine may have some direct analgesic effects via dorsal horn α_2-receptor activation. Phenylephrine is less effective than epinephrine in prolonging the epidural anesthetic effect and is not as widely used. (291)

86. Advantages of adding opioids to the local anesthetic solution used for epidural anesthesia include synergistic enhancement of analgesic effects without prolonging motor block and a reduction in dose-related adverse effects of both the opioid and local anesthetic. A bolus injection can lead to an analgesic effect that exceeds the duration of the epidural block. (291)

87. Epidural opioids cross the dura and arachnoid membrane to reach the CSF and the spinal cord dorsal horn. Lipophilic opioids, such as fentanyl and sufentanil, partition into epidural fat more readily and are more rapidly absorbed into the systemic circulation (which may be a principal mechanism of action). Hydrophilic opioids, such as morphine and hydromorphone, are poorly absorbed into fat and remain largely within the epidural space and have a longer duration of action. (291)

88. Advantages of adding clonidine to the local anesthetic solution used for epidural anesthesia include prolongation of sensory over motor block and a reduction in requirements for epidural local anesthetics and opioids. Clonidine may also decrease immune stress and cytokine response. Side effects of epidural clonidine include hypotension, bradycardia, dry mouth, and sedation. Advantages of adding dexmedetomidine to the local anesthetic solution include reduction of requirements for local anesthetic and opioids, improved postoperative analgesia, and prolongation of both motor and sensory block. (291)

89. The addition of bicarbonate to the local anesthetic solution used for epidural anesthesia increases the solution pH and therefore the nonionized free-base portion of the local anesthetic. Data suggest no clinical advantage in the speed of onset or quality of the block, however. (292)

90. Surface landmarks are used to help estimate the level of spinal interspaces. The intercristal line generally traverses the L4-L5 interspace. The C7 spinous process (vertebra prominens) can be appreciated as a bony knob at the lower end of the neck, and a line drawn between the lower limits of the scapulae correlates approximately with the vertebral body of T7. (292)

91. The tip of an epidural catheter may have either a single end hole at the tip or multiple side orifices near the tip. Multiple orifice catheters tend to produce more uniform distribution of local anesthetic solution and improve analgesia, but can increase the risk of epidural vein cannulation in parturients. (292)

92. Although the experience of paresthesia during awake needle placement is neither sensitive nor specific for nerve injury, there clearly is no opportunity for an asleep patient to recognize or report any adverse symptoms during the procedure. Current consensus guidelines on neurologic injury therefore state that, as with spinal anesthesia, epidural injections in adults should be performed awake unless the physician feels that the benefits of anesthesia or heavy sedation outweigh the risks. There is also no evidence that epidural

anesthesia in the lumbar or thoracic area is any more or less safe in an anesthetized patient. The same considerations do not apply to pediatric anesthesia, where a conscious patient would probably impart no benefit but instead add substantial risk. (292)

93. With the "loss-of-resistance" technique, a syringe containing saline, air, or both is attached to the needle, and the needle is slowly advanced while resistance to injection is assessed. Once the needle tip reaches and is properly seated in the ligamentum flavum, it becomes difficult to inject the saline or the air bubble, and the plunger of the syringe will "spring back" to its original position. Upon advancing further, an abrupt loss of resistance to injection signals passage through the ligamentum flavum and into the epidural space, at which point the contents of the syringe may be delivered without resistance. (293)

94. Air is reportedly less reliable than saline in identifying the epidural space when using the loss-of-resistance technique. This can result in a higher likelihood of incomplete block and may cause both pneumocephalus and even venous air embolism in rare cases. Fluid inserted through the epidural needle before catheter insertion can also reduce the risk of epidural vein cannulation by the catheter. One disadvantage of saline is that it may make it more difficult to detect an accidental dural puncture. (293)

95. The "hanging-drop" technique is an alternative method for identifying the epidural space. With this technique, a small drop of saline is placed at the hub of the epidural needle. As the needle passes through the ligamentum flavum into the epidural space, the saline drop is "sucked" into the needle by the negative pressure in the epidural space. (293)

96. Following identification of the epidural space, the catheter is gently advanced 4 to 6 cm beyond the tip of the needle positioned in the epidural space. Further advancement increases the risk that the catheter might enter an epidural vein, exit an intervertebral foramen, or wrap around a nerve root. Less than 4 cm may increase the risk of dislodgment. The epidural needle is withdrawn over the catheter, with care taken to not move the catheter. (293)

97. The Tsui test helps confirm epidural catheter tip location through the use of a special electrically conducting catheter. A low electric current stimulates spinal nerve roots via the catheter, and tip localization is determined by evaluating which muscles have a twitch response. (293)

98. In the thoracic region the spinous processes are more steeply angulated and closely approximated, which can make the midline approach challenging. The paramedian approach can be useful in the thoracic area, either when the midline approach fails or as the primary approach. The paramedian approach to lumbar epidural anesthesia may also be useful in patients who cannot tolerate or are not able to maintain a sitting position. (293)

99. The test dose is a small amount of local anesthetic administered via the epidural catheter to exclude accidental intrathecal or intravascular catheter placement. Epinephrine is sometimes included in the test dose, as an increase in heart rate may signal accidental intravascular injection. Unfortunately, this is not a reliable test for intravascular catheter placement, and therefore the patient must still always be monitored for symptoms and signs of intravascular local anesthetic toxicity. If after several minutes there is no significant sensory or motor block near the level of the catheter insertion and no signs of local anesthetic toxicity, the remaining planned dose of local anesthetic may be injected incrementally. (294)

100. Combined spinal-epidural anesthesia is a technique in which a spinal anesthetic and an epidural catheter are placed concurrently. This approach capitalizes on the rapid onset and intense sensory anesthesia of a spinal anesthetic and the ability to supplement and extend the duration of the block afforded by an epidural catheter. The technique is commonly used in obstetric anesthesia, or any case when it is anticipated the duration of surgery may

last longer than an average spinal anesthetic (2.5 to 3 hours). Using a low-dose spinal anesthetic and subsequently increasing the block height gradually through incremental epidural boluses of local anesthetic or saline can offer more hemodynamic stability in high-risk patients and decrease the required dose of spinal local anesthetic. This sequential technique is termed *epidural volume extension*. (294)

CAUDAL ANESTHESIA

101. Caudal anesthesia is most popular in pediatric anesthesia because the spread of caudal local anesthetic in adults is unpredictable. For adults, caudal anesthesia is most commonly used in chronic pain and cancer pain management but may also be used when the lumbar approach is not possible. (295)

102. The approach to caudal anesthesia is similar to that of epidural anesthesia. The same local anesthetics are used, although twice the lumbar dose may be necessary in caudal anesthesia to achieve a similar block. Patient position can be lateral or even prone with knee to chest. Loss of resistance technique is used to confirm entry into the epidural space, and a test dose should be administered prior to dosing with local anesthetic to exclude intrathecal or intravascular placement of the needle. (295)

103. The sacral hiatus, the opening between the unfused lamina of the fourth and fifth sacral vertebrae, can be identified by palpation. The sacrococcygeal ligament, an extension of the ligamentum flavum hiatus, overlies the sacral hiatus between the two sacral cornua. (295)

104. After sterile preparation and local infiltration above the hiatus, the needle is introduced at an angle of 45 degrees to the sacrum and advanced through skin, then the sacrococcygeal ligament (generally felt as a rather distinct pop), and then further until the sacrum is contacted. The needle is then slightly withdrawn, the angle reduced, and the needle readvanced no more than 1 to 2 cm into the caudal epidural canal. Proper positioning of the needle tip is confirmed by injecting 5 mL of air or saline through the needle while palpating the skin over the caudal canal. Subcutaneous crepitus or midline swelling indicates that the needle is positioned posterior to the bony sacrum and requires replacement. Subarachnoid injection may occur if the needle is advanced too far cephalad in the sacral canal. (296)

105. The dural sac normally ends at the level of S2, but it extends beyond S2 in approximately 10% of individuals. (296)

COMPLICATIONS

106. Complications that should be discussed with the patient before proceeding with a spinal or epidural anesthetic include (1) those that are rare but serious, including nerve damage, bleeding, and infection, and (2) those that are common but of lesser consequence, such as a post–dural puncture headache and nausea and vomiting. The possibility of a failed block should also be discussed, and patients should be reassured that in such circumstances, alternative anesthetic techniques will be provided to ensure their comfort. (296)

107. Paraplegia is an extremely rare but serious complication of neuraxial anesthesia. Direct injury may occur from needle trauma, but the injectate can also be neurotoxic. Preservatives in local anesthetics or additives have been thought to be responsible in the past for adhesive arachnoiditis and cauda equina syndrome. Profound hypotension causing anterior spinal artery syndrome can also result in paralysis. An epidural hematoma can cause ischemic compression of the spinal cord. (296)

108. Cauda equina syndrome following neuraxial anesthesia has been associated with direct exposure of large doses of local anesthetic, whether as a single highly concentrated injection (e.g., 5% lidocaine) or through prolonged exposure to local anesthetic through a continuous small-gauge catheter. (296)

109. Risk factors associated with an epidural hematoma following neuraxial anesthesia include difficult or traumatic needle or catheter insertion, coagulopathy, elderly age, and female gender. (296)

110. Signs and symptoms of an epidural hematoma include radicular back pain, unexpected prolonged motor blockade, and bladder or bowel dysfunction. The space-occupying lesion within the vertebral canal can causes ischemic compression of the spinal cord and lead to permanent neurologic deficit if not evacuated expeditiously. These features should prompt magnetic resonance imaging on an emergent basis. (296)

111. Factors associated with nerve injury following neuraxial anesthesia include radicular pain or paresthesia occurring during the procedure and epidural or combined spinal and epidural anesthesia for the purpose of perioperative anesthesia or analgesia. (296)

112. Post–dural puncture headache is relatively common (around 1% incidence) and is a direct consequence of the hole made in the dura during spinal anesthesia or accidental dural puncture during epidural needle placement. The patient factors that increase the risk of post–dural puncture headache are age, sex, and pregnancy. Risk slowly declines with advancing age. Female sex and pregnancy are independent risk factors. Procedural factors include needle diameter, bevel direction during dural puncture, multiple dural punctures, and the shape of the hole created by the needle. Noncutting, pencil-point needle tips (e.g., Whitaker, Sprotte), which spread the dural and arachnoid fibers, reduce the risk of a post–dural puncture headache. (296)

113. Post–dural puncture headache is caused by CSF leakage through the dura, which results in downward displacement of the brain with a resultant traction on pain-sensitive supporting structures. Symptoms of a post–dural puncture headache usually begin within 3 days of dural puncture, with about 66% within the first 48 hours. (296)

114. The hallmark of a post–dural puncture headache is its frontal or occipital location and its postural component; it worsens with upright or seated posture and is partially or completely relieved by lying supine. Associated symptoms can include nausea, vomiting, neck pain, dizziness, tinnitus, diplopia, hearing loss, cortical blindness, cranial nerve palsies, and even seizures. (297)

115. Initial treatment of post–dural puncture headache is usually conservative and consists of bed rest, hydration, caffeine, and oral analgesics. Spontaneous resolution occurs within 7 days in the majority of cases. If conservative measures are ineffective, a blood patch can be performed in which up to 20 mL of the patient's blood is aseptically injected into the epidural space. Persistent resolution of symptoms occurs in over 60% of patients following an epidural blood patch. A second epidural blood patch may be performed in 24 to 48 hours if the first is ineffective. Of note, prophylactic epidural blood patching is not efficacious. (297)

116. TNS is characterized by mild or sometimes severe bilateral or unilateral pain in the buttocks, commonly radiating to the legs, and no neurologic deficits. The symptoms usually occur within 24 hours of resolution of a spinal anesthetic and usually resolve spontaneously in less than a week. TNS are more common with intrathecal injection of concentrated lidocaine or mepivacaine, the addition of dextrose or phenylephrine, and solution osmolarity. The lithotomy position also increases risk. (297)

117. Factors associated with hypotension following neuraxial anesthesia include peak block height at T5 or higher, age of 40 years or older, baseline systolic blood pressure less than 120 mm Hg, combined spinal and general anesthesia, spinal puncture at or above the L2-L3 interspace, and the addition of phenylephrine to the local anesthetic. Hypotension is also independently associated with alcoholism, history of hypertension, increased BMI, and urgency of surgery. (298)

118. Factors associated with bradycardia following neuraxial anesthesia include baseline heart rate less than 60 beats/min, age younger than 37 years, male gender, nonemergency status, β-adrenergic blockade, and prolonged duration of surgery. (298)

119. Factors associated with cardiac arrest (which is rare) following neuraxial anesthesia include hypoxemia and oversedation. Cardiac arrest is more likely with spinal than epidural anesthesia. (298)

120. Factors associated with respiratory depression following neuraxial anesthesia include (dose-dependent) use of neuraxial opioids. Respiratory depression can occur for the first 24 hours following the administration of intrathecal or epidural opioids, mediated by its rostral spread within the CSF to the respiratory centers in the brainstem. Risk increases with increased age and with the coadministration of systemic sedatives. (298)

121. Infections following neuraxial anesthesia include bacterial meningitis and epidural abscess. Fortunately both are rare but they can be catastrophic. Staphylococcal infections arising from the patient's skin are one of the most common epidural-related infections, whereas oral bacteria such as *Streptococcus viridans* are a common cause of infection after spinal anesthesia. Factors associated with infection following neuraxial anesthesia include the presence of a concomitant systemic infection, diabetes, immunocompromised states, and prolonged maintenance of an epidural (or spinal) catheter. Infection is twice as common after epidural compared to spinal techniques. (298)

122. There is no association between new-onset back pain and epidural anesthesia in patients up to 6 months postpartum. (298)

123. Factors associated with nausea and vomiting following neuraxial anesthesia include direct exposure of the chemoreceptor trigger zone in the brain to opiates, hypotension, and gastrointestinal hyperperistalsis secondary to unopposed parasympathetic activity. Other factors include peak spinal anesthesia block height of T5 or higher, baseline heart rate greater than 60 beats/min, and history of motion sickness. Intrathecal morphine carries a higher risk of nausea than intrathecal fentanyl, although the risk of nausea with either is dose dependent. (298)

124. Urinary retention following neuraxial anesthesia can occur in as many as one third of patients through blockade of the S2, S3, and S4 nerve roots and weakening of the detrusor muscle and sensation of urgency. Factors associated with urinary retention include male gender, advanced age, and intrathecal morphine. (298)

125. Pruritus is a side effect related to the intrathecal injection of opioids. It can be treated with naloxone, naltrexone, or the partial opioid agonist nalbuphine. Ondansetron and propofol may also be effective. (299)

126. The risk of shivering following neuraxial anesthesia can be reduced through the addition of neuraxial opioids (especially fentanyl and meperidine) to the local anesthetic solution, prewarming the patient with a forced air warmer, and avoiding the administration of cold epidural and intravenous fluids. (299)

127. Unintentional intravascular injection of local anesthetic during epidural anesthesia can result in local anesthetic toxicity, which usually presents as seizures. Unintentional intravascular injection usually occurs in an epidural vein and is more likely to occur in the obstetric patient in whom these vessels are relatively dilated. The frequency of puncture of an epidural vein or catheter can be as high as 10%. The risk of unintentional intravascular injection can be reduced in the obstetric population by placing the patient in the lateral position during needle and catheter insertion, administering fluid through the epidural needle before catheter insertion, using a single-orifice epidural catheter, advancing the catheter less than 6 cm into the epidural space, aspiration of the catheter prior to dosing, and the incremental administration of local anesthetic. (299)

128. A subdural injection occurs when the local anesthetic is inadvertently injected between the potential space between the dura and the arachnoid. It is relatively uncommon (<1% of epidural injections) and is characterized by block height that is higher than expected but with less motor block relative to sensory block. (299)

18 PERIPHERAL NERVE BLOCKS

Edward N. Yap and Andrew T. Gray

INTRODUCTION

1. Name some peripheral nerve blocks. What is their clinical use?
2. Besides ultrasound-guided nerve blocks, what are other ways to perform peripheral nerve blocks?
3. What can continuous peripheral nerve catheters be used for?
4. What knowledge is needed to perform a safe and effective peripheral nerve block?
5. What should be reviewed preoperatively prior to deciding to provide a peripheral nerve block?
6. Where should a peripheral nerve block be performed?
7. What are the expected onset times and durations of some commonly used local anesthetics?
8. What are some advantages to adding epinephrine to the local anesthetic for a peripheral nerve block?
9. What are the necessary equipment and supplies needed for performing a safe peripheral nerve block?
10. What should be included in a regional block checklist?
11. What are ways to prevent infections during peripheral nerve blocks?
12. What are the risks of developing a hematoma, and how can that risk be reduced?
13. What is local anesthetic systemic toxicity (LAST), and what are the risks? How is it treated and prevented?
14. How can nerve injury occur, and how can you minimize the risk of nerve injury?
15. How can a wrong-sided block be prevented?

ULTRASOUND BASICS

16. What are piezoelectric crystals?
17. What is acoustic impedance?
18. How does changing the frequency change the ultrasound image?
19. How do nerves appear on ultrasound images?
20. How can ergonomics be improved when performing peripheral nerve blocks?
21. What are the five basic ultrasound transducer manipulation techniques?
22. What are some of the approaches to peripheral nerve blocks?

CERVICAL PLEXUS BLOCK

23. What nerves make up the cervical plexus?
24. At what location is the cervical plexus block performed?
25. What anesthesia does the cervical plexus provide?

UPPER EXTREMITY BLOCKS

26. What nerves compose the brachial plexus?
27. How do you decide where along the brachial plexus a peripheral nerve block should be performed?
28. Where is the interscalene block performed?
29. What surgeries are suited for the interscalene block?
30. What is the "stop-light" appearance seen during an interscalene block?
31. What are the potential risks and side effects of the interscalene block?
32. Where is the supraclavicular block performed?
33. What are the advantages of the supraclavicular block?
34. What are the risks of the supraclavicular block?
35. What is the target of the infraclavicular block, and where is it performed?
36. What is the goal of local anesthetic spread for an infraclavicular block?
37. What are the advantages of the infraclavicular block?
38. What are the targets of the axillary block?
39. What are the advantages and disadvantages of the axillary block?
40. What is the most common indication for an intercostobrachial nerve block?

LOWER EXTREMITY BLOCKS

41. What nerves and plexuses provide sensation to the lower extremity?
42. What nerves compose the femoral nerve?
43. What does the femoral nerve innervate?
44. What surgeries will a femoral nerve block help with analgesia?
45. What are important structures to identify on ultrasound when performing a femoral nerve block?
46. What are the advantages and disadvantages of the femoral nerve block?
47. What are the advantages of an adductor canal block?
48. Where is an adductor canal block performed?
49. What are some options for the approach to a saphenous nerve block?
50. What nerves compose the sciatic nerve?
51. What is the function of the sciatic nerve?
52. What are the three main approaches to the sciatic nerve block?
53. What are the advantages and disadvantages of the sciatic nerve block?
54. Where is the popliteal block performed?
55. What surgeries is the popliteal nerve block used for?
56. Where is the sciatic nerve in relation to the popliteal artery and vein?
57. What five peripheral nerves need to be blocked for total analgesia of the ankle?
58. What are the sensory innervations of each of the five peripheral nerves for an ankle block?

CHEST AND ABDOMEN BLOCKS

59. What are benefits of peripheral nerve blocks of the chest and abdomen?
60. What is the target of the intercostal nerve block?
61. What are the benefits of intercostal nerve blocks?
62. What are the disadvantages of intercostal nerve blocks?
63. What are the targets of the transversus abdominis plane (TAP) block?
64. What surgeries may a TAP block help with?
65. What are some disadvantages of the TAP block?

INTRAVENOUS REGIONAL ANESTHESIA OR BIER BLOCK

66. When is it appropriate to use intravenous regional anesthesia or a Bier block?
67. Describe the technique of the Bier block.
68. What are the contraindications to a Bier block?
69. What are the benefits of a double tourniquet?
70. What are common local anesthetics used in Bier blocks?
71. What are some advantages of a Bier block?
72. What are the risks of a Bier block?

ANSWERS*

INTRODUCTION

1. Examples of peripheral nerve blocks include blocks of the cervical plexus, brachial plexus, median nerve, ulnar nerve, radial nerve, sciatic nerve, femoral nerve, saphenous nerve, and ankle block. The two most common uses for peripheral nerve blocks is for surgical anesthesia and for postoperative pain relief (Table 18-1). (304)

2. Paresthetic technique, nerve stimulation technique, and a combination of ultrasound and nerve stimulation technique can be used to localize nerves for nerve blocks. (303)

3. Continuous peripheral nerve catheters can be used in both the inpatient and outpatient settings. They can be used to facilitate vigorous early joint mobilization after orthopedic surgery, as well as provide potent analgesia for outpatient surgery. (303)

4. To perform safe and effective peripheral nerve blocks, an understanding of peripheral neuroanatomy, ultrasound technology, local anesthetic pharmacology, and risks associated with peripheral nerve blocks is needed. (303)

5. A thorough preoperative review of the patient's medical history, including any comorbid diseases, allergies, prior neuropathy, and concurrent anticoagulation medications, must be performed to rule out any contraindications in providing a peripheral nerve block. (303)

6. Peripheral nerve blocks that are not performed in the operating room should be performed in a block room or area with the appropriate monitors, drugs, equipment, and oxygen should their use become urgently necessary. (303)

7. The choice of local anesthetic agent for peripheral nerve blockade depends on a number of factors, including the desired onset, duration, and degree of conduction block. Lidocaine and mepivacaine, 1% to 1.5%, produce surgical anesthesia in 10 to 20 minutes that lasts 2 to 3 hours. Ropivacaine, 0.5%, and bupivacaine, 0.375% to 0.5%, have a slower onset and produce less motor blockade, but the effect lasts for at least 6 to 8 hours (see Chapter 10). (304)

8. The addition of epinephrine (1:200,000) to the local anesthetic for a peripheral nerve block allows for a marker for intravascular injection, increases the duration of the conduction block, and decreases the rate of systemic absorption. This can help decrease peak plasma levels of local anesthetic and thus the potential risk for local anesthetic systemic toxicity (LAST). (304)

9. Peripheral nerve blocks can be performed preoperatively in a dedicated block room or area or in the operating room. The patient must have a functional peripheral intravenous line in case of any needed administration of emergency medications. Monitoring devices including pulse oximetry, electrocardiograph, and noninvasive blood pressure should be placed on the patient prior to performing the nerve block. Supplemental oxygen as well as emergency medications and airway equipment must be accessible. A functioning ultrasound machine and options for needles and local anesthetics should be available as well. Lipid emulsion (20% or 30%, 100 mL) should be available. (304)

10. The regional block checklist should include surgical consent and site marking, allergies and anticoagulation status, proposed peripheral nerve block and local anesthetic dose, side of the block, monitors implemented, emergency equipment available, and sedation plan. (304)

11. Performing proper hand hygiene, using maximal barriers during the peripheral nerve block, and cleaning the area of the site insertion with antiseptic solution can decrease the rate of infection. (304)

---

*Numbers in parentheses refer to pages, figures, boxes, or tables in Pardo MC, Miller RD, eds. *Basics of Anesthesia*. 7th ed. Philadelphia: Elsevier; 2018.

12. The risk of developing a hematoma is reliant on the location of the peripheral nerve block being performed, the proximity to vascular structures, and their compressibility. Patients receiving anticoagulants or who have coagulopathy are at higher risk of developing a hematoma. The risks can be reduced by the use of ultrasound and by applying pressure to the site. (304)

13. LAST is the sequela of local anesthetic absorption into the body that reaches levels at which side effects can occur, ranging from mild symptoms to major neurologic or cardiovascular toxicity. Lipid emulsion resuscitation remains the cornerstone to therapy to treat patients with LAST, as well as supportive care. There is no single measure to prevent LAST; however, using the lowest effective dose, incremental injection, and aspiration prior to injection; using an intravascular marker (i.e., epinephrine); and performing peripheral nerve blocks using ultrasound guidance may decrease the risk of LAST. (304)

14. Nerve injury may result from direct needle trauma to the nerve, inadvertent intraneural injection of local anesthetic, and drug neurotoxicity. The use of ultrasound to identify nerves, limiting injection pressure, and patient feedback may potentially help decrease the rate of nerve injury. (305)

15. Having a universal protocol that utilizes a checklist to ensure the correct patient, proper surgical site, and laterality and confirming the proposed peripheral nerve block may reduce the risk of wrong-sided block. (305)

ULTRASOUND BASICS

16. Piezoelectric crystals are used in ultrasound transducers to convert electric currents into mechanical sound waves and vice versa. These electric currents are then processed in an ultrasound computer to produce images. (305)

17. Acoustic impedance depends on the density of the tissue and changes of the propagation of ultrasound waves. Solid tissues have dense particles with high acoustic impedance that will reflect ultrasound waves and be displayed as bright or hyperechoic structures. Less dense tissues do not reflect ultrasound waves and are displayed as darker or hypoechoic structures. Tissues that do not reflect ultrasound are anechoic. (305)

18. Increasing the frequency of the ultrasound will improve the resolution of an image; however, it will decrease the penetration of the ultrasound waves. Decreasing the frequency will lower the resolution, but it will improve the penetration of the ultrasound. (305)

19. Peripheral nerves can be recognized by their fascicular echotexture. Nerves that are close to the spine have fewer fascicles and can be recognized by their monofascicular or oligofascicular appearance on ultrasound scans. More peripheral nerves can be seen as polyfascicular and look like a collection of small round hypoechoic dots surrounded by hyperechoic connective tissue. (305)

20. Optimizing provider posture and position, patient position, bed height, and position of the ultrasound machine are ways to improve ergonomics when performing peripheral nerve blocks. (306)

21. The five basic transducer manipulation techniques to help optimize the ultrasound image are sliding, tilting, rocking, rotation, and compression. (306)

22. There are multiple approaches to peripheral nerve blocks. Nerves can be viewed in the short or long axis of their course. The needle approach can be in-plane (within the same plane of the ultrasound image) or out-of-plane (crossing the plane of ultrasound imaging). (306)

CERVICAL PLEXUS BLOCK

23. The cervical plexus is formed by the second, third, and fourth cervical nerves. (307)

24. The cervical plexus block is performed at the posterior lateral border of the sternocleidomastoid muscle. Local anesthetic is infiltrated deep to the platysma and investing fascia of the neck. (307)

25. The anesthesia produced by a cervical plexus block includes the area from the inferior surface of the mandible to the level of the clavicle. Cervical plexus blocks are used most often in patients undergoing carotid endarterectomy. (307)

26. The brachial plexus is a network of nerves composed of five nerve roots: C5, C6, C7, C8, and T1. The nerves provide both motor and sensory input for the upper extremity. (307)

27. The location of the surgery, experience of the provider, and patient factors help determine where along the brachial plexus a peripheral nerve block should be performed. (307)

28. The interscalene block targets the ventral rami of the brachial plexus and is traditionally performed near the C6 vertebral level, where the plexus emerges between the anterior and middle scalene muscles. (307)

29. The interscalene block is suited for surgeries that involve the distal clavicle, shoulder, and upper arm. The interscalene block can spare the inferior trunk, and therefore, it is not always suitable for distal forearm and hand surgeries. (307)

30. The "stop-light" appearance of the brachial plexus refers to the C5, C6, and C7 ventral rami aligned in parallel fashion in the interscalene groove. (307)

31. The interscalene block has the potential risk of Horner syndrome, recurrent laryngeal nerve block, epidural and subarachnoid injection, vertebral artery injection, pneumothorax, and phrenic nerve block. (307)

32. The supraclavicular block is performed at the site where the brachial plexus is tightly bundled and adjacent to the subclavian artery and cephalad to the clavicle. (309)

33. The supraclavicular block provides rapid onset and ability to perform the block with the arm in any position. The supraclavicular block should provide anesthesia of the upper extremity from the shoulder down to the fingers (except for the innervation of the intercostobrachial nerve). (309)

34. Pneumothorax is the most serious complication of a supraclavicular block and can be manifested as cough, dyspnea, or pleuritic chest pain. Block of the phrenic nerve also occurs frequently but generally causes no significant symptoms. (309)

35. The infraclavicular block targets the medial, lateral, and posterior cords of the brachial plexus. The block is performed caudad to the clavicle. The block is suitable for surgeries of the arm below the shoulder. (310)

36. The goal of the infraclavicular block is to spread local anesthetic around the axillary artery in a U-shaped manner. This approach will assure blockade of all three cords of the brachial plexus. (310)

37. The infraclavicular block has consistent anatomy and is a stable site for placement of a continuous peripheral nerve catheter. Arm tourniquets are well tolerated after infraclavicular blocks. (310)

38. The axillary block targets the terminal branches of the brachial plexus in the axilla: the median, ulnar, radial, and musculocutaneous nerves. The axillary block is suitable for surgeries of the elbow, forearm, wrist, and hand. (310)

39. The advantages of the axillary block include lower risk of complications compared to other brachial plexus blocks, such as pneumothorax or phrenic nerve block. The superficial nature of the block also makes it a simpler block to perform. However, given the proximity to the axillary artery and vein, there is a higher risk of intravascular injection and hematoma. The location is a poor candidate for a peripheral nerve catheter given that the divisions of the terminal branches are circumferential to the artery. (310)

40. The intercostobrachial nerve, which provides cutaneous innervation to the medial half of the arm, is most commonly blocked to improve surgical conditions for proximal arm surgery or for increased patient tolerance of an arm tourniquet. It is typically done in conjunction with a brachial plexus block. (310)

LOWER EXTREMITY BLOCKS

41. The lower extremity innervation originates from the lumbar (L1-L4) and sacral (S1-S4, with contribution from L4-L5) plexuses. The nerves that branch from these plexuses are the lateral femoral cutaneous, femoral, obturator, and sciatic nerves. (310)

42. The femoral nerve is the largest branch of the lumbar plexus and is derived from the ventral rami of L2 to L4. (310)

43. The femoral nerve provides motor function to the quadriceps and sensation from the anterior thigh and medial leg. Other motor innervation includes the sartorius and pectineus muscles. With high volumes of local anesthetic, branches to the iliopsoas muscle can also be blocked. (310)

44. A femoral nerve block will help with surgeries of the anterior thigh, hip, femur, and knee. (313)

45. When performing a femoral nerve block it is important to image the femoral artery, femoral vein, femoral nerve, the sartorius and iliopsoas muscles and the fascia lata and fascia iliaca. (313)

46. The femoral nerve block is reliable in providing analgesia to the anterior thigh and medial leg. It is a good location for a peripheral nerve catheter and is a relatively easy block to perform. The femoral nerve block causes quadriceps weakness that may impede early mobilization and increase the risk of falls postoperatively. (313)

47. The adductor canal blocks the femoral nerve as it travels deep to the sartorius muscle. The advantage is that the block provides analgesia for knee surgery with minimal quadriceps weakness. (313)

48. The adductor canal block is performed mid-thigh where the superficial femoral artery is near the middle of the undersurface of the sartorius muscle belly. The adductor canal's borders consist of sartorius (anterior), vastus medialis (lateral), and adductor longus (medial and posterior) muscles. The nerves may be visible lateral to the superficial femoral artery; however, the nerves may be difficult to discern. (313)

49. The saphenous nerve, a terminal branch of the femoral nerve, carries sensory nerve fibers from the medial aspect of the leg, ankle, and foot. The saphenous nerve can be blocked anywhere along its course depending on the location of the desired blockade. Alternatively, many practitioners use the adductor canal block to block the saphenous nerve. (314)

50. The sciatic nerve is the largest branch of the sacral plexus and consists of the L4, L5, and S1 to S4 spinal nerves. (314)

51. The sciatic nerve provides motor innervation to the posterior thigh and lower leg and provides sensation of the posterior thigh and most of the lower leg (except for the saphenous distribution from the femoral nerve). (314)

52. The approaches to the sciatic nerve block include the anterior, the transgluteal, and the subgluteal approaches. (314)

53. The advantages of the sciatic nerve block include its reliability of posterior thigh and leg analgesia for surgeries of the posterior thigh, lower leg, foot, and ankle, and it provides some analgesia for knee surgery. The location is away from the thigh tourniquet if a peripheral nerve catheter is used. The disadvantages of the sciatic nerve block include hamstring weakness as well as procedural discomfort and difficulty owing to the increased depth of the block. (315)

54. The popliteal block targets the sciatic nerve as it travels through the popliteal fossa, at which point the nerve divides into its common peroneal and tibial nerve components. (316)

55. The popliteal block is commonly used for foot and ankle surgery. The block is usually combined with a saphenous nerve block to cover the medial aspect of the leg. (316)

56. The sciatic nerve is located posterior to the popliteal artery and vein. (316)

57. The five peripheral nerves that supply the foot are the tibial, sural, saphenous, superficial, and deep peroneal nerves. (317)

58. The tibial nerve provides sensation to the sole of the foot. The sural nerve innervates the lateral side of the foot. The saphenous nerve innervates the medial aspect of the foot. The deep peroneal nerve innervates the webbing between the first and second toes. The superficial peroneal nerve innervates the dorsum of the foot. (317)

CHEST AND ABDOMEN BLOCKS

59. Peripheral nerve blocks of the chest and abdomen can provide intraoperative and postoperative analgesia, reduce systemic pain medications, improve patient satisfaction, and improve patient discharge times. (317)

60. The intercostal nerve block targets the ventral rami of the thoracic spinal nerve. The intercostal nerves travel inferior to the associated rib within the subcostal groove. The intercostal vein and artery travel superior to the inercostal nerve within the subcostal groove. (317)

61. Intercostal nerve blocks are beneficial for thoracic and upper abdominal surgery, as well as following chest wall trauma. (317)

62. Because of the close proximity of the pleura, there is risk of pneumothorax with intercostal nerve blocks. LAST is also possible owing to the high peak plasma levels after injection. Because of overlapping dermatomes, multiple levels may need to be blocked to provide adequate analgesia of a surgical incision. (317)

63. The transversus abdominis plane (TAP) block is an abdominal wall field block that targets the ventral rami of the thoracic and lumbar spinal nerves as they travel in the plane between the transversus abdominis and internal oblique muscles. (318)

64. The TAP block provides analgesia for lower abdominal surgery and may help with laparoscopic surgery. (318)

65. Because the TAP block relies on a large volume of local anesthetic for appropriate spread, there is risk of LAST. There is also a small potential for intraperitoneal and intrahepatic injection. (318)

INTRAVENOUS REGIONAL ANESTHESIA OR BIER BLOCK

66. Intravenous regional anesthesia or a Bier block is a method to provide anesthesia to the arm or leg for surgeries that have minimal postoperative pain and a duration of 2 hours or less. (318)

67. To perform the Bier block, a small peripheral intravenous catheter is placed in the distal portion of the extremity to be blocked. The extremity is exsanguinated by wrapping it with an Esmarch bandage from distal to proximal, and a tourniquet is inflated at least 100 mm Hg above the patient's systolic blood pressure. Plain local anesthetic solution (usually 40 to 50 mL for an arm tourniquet) is injected through the intravenous catheter and the catheter is removed. (318)

68. Contraindications to a Bier block include contraindications to a tourniquet (sickle cell disease, ischemic vascular disease, infection to the extremity) and lacerations on the surgical extremity that may cause escape of local anesthetic. (318)

69. A double tourniquet allows for a second tourniquet option for the pain patients may begin experiencing at the initial tourniquet site. Once the patient begins feeling pain, the distal cuff is inflated and the proximal cuff is then deflated. (318)

70. Commonly used local anesthetics for Bier blocks include 0.5% lidocaine or chloroprocaine plain (without epinephrine) preservative-free solutions. (319)

71. Advantages of a Bier block include its rapid onset of anesthesia, its duration being dependent on the duration of the tourniquet, its relative technical ease and speed to perform, and its applicability to all age groups, including pediatric patients. (319)

72. The risks of a Bier block include LAST, especially when the tourniquet is deflated and large amounts of local anesthetic solution enter the systemic circulation. For this reason racemic bupivacaine is avoided for this type of block. Other complications may include hematoma, engorgement of the extremity, thrombophlebitis, and subcutaneous hemorrhage. (319)

19 PATIENT POSITIONING AND ASSOCIATED RISKS

Kristine E.W. Breyer

PHYSIOLOGIC ASPECTS OF POSITIONING

1. What are the cardiovascular and hemodynamic changes that occur in the awake patient reclining from an upright to a supine position?
2. What are the physiologic pulmonary changes that occur in the awake patient reclining from an upright to a supine position?

GENERAL POSITIOINING

3. Who is responsible for checking patient positioning in the operating room?
4. Why is patient positioning under anesthesia so important?

SPECIFIC POSITIONS

5. What is the most common patient position for surgery?
6. How should the patient's arms be placed during supine positioning?
7. How can brachial plexus injury occur secondary to improper supine positioning?
8. How can ulnar nerve injury occur secondary to improper supine positioning?
9. What are some advantages of the lawn-chair position over the supine position?
10. How can hip dislocation occur secondary to improper frog-leg positioning?
11. What are some common indications for Trendelenburg positioning?
12. How does the Trendelenburg position affect a patient's cardiovascular system?
13. How does the Trendelenburg position affect a patient's pulmonary system?
14. How does the Trendelenburg position affect intraocular pressure (IOP) and intracranial pressure (ICP)?
15. How can brachial plexus injury occur secondary to improper Trendelenburg positioning?
16. How does the reverse Trendelenburg position affect a patient's hemodynamics?
17. At what patient level should invasive arterial blood pressure monitors be zeroed when a patient is in the reverse Trendelenburg position?
18. Why might a patient wake up with a backache after supine positioning for surgery?
19. What is the concern for positioning an obese patient supine in the reverse axis on the operating table?
20. Why do a patient's legs need to be raised and lowered simultaneously during lithotomy positioning?
21. Which lower extremity nerve is particularly at risk for injury during lithotomy positioning?
22. How can finger injuries occur during lithotomy positioning?
23. What are the cardiopulmonary changes that occur when placing the patient in the lithotomy position?
24. How can lower extremity compartment syndrome occur secondary to lithotomy positioning?
25. What are the risk factors for positioning-related compartment syndrome?

26. How should the patient's extremities be placed when in the lateral decubitus position?
27. When the patient is in the lateral decubitus position, where should an axillary roll be placed and what is its purpose?
28. Which arm is the best choice for placement of invasive arterial monitors in the lateral decubitus position and why?
29. What are some head and neck concerns when placing a patient in the lateral decubitus position?
30. How can injury to the brachial plexus occur secondary to improper lateral decubitus positioning?
31. What are the pulmonary changes associated with lateral decubitus positioning?
32. What are some concerns when turning a patient from the supine to prone position?
33. What parts of the face are at risk for injury during prone positioning?
34. How should the extremities be placed when in the prone position?
35. What is the ideal placement of bolsters beneath the patient in the prone position and why?
36. What are the cardiopulmonary changes that occur with prone positioning?
37. For which surgical procedures might the patient be placed in the sitting position?
38. How should the extremities be placed in the sitting position?
39. What are some complications that can occur as a result of placing the patient in the sitting position?
40. How can an intraoperative venous air embolus be detected?
41. What are some other complications that can occur as a result of a venous air embolus?
42. What is the concern regarding the patient with an anatomic intracardiac shunt scheduled for surgery in the sitting position?
43. What is the risk of pneumocephalus in the sitting position?
44. What are some symptoms of clinically significant postoperative pneumocephalus?
45. What is a concern regarding excessive head flexion in the sitting position?

SPECIAL CIRCUMSTANCES

46. What unique positioning challenges does robotic surgery pose?
47. What are the consequences of docking the robot?
48. What physiologic changes occur during robotic surgery?

INJURIES

49. In what time course can a pressure injury occur?
50. In what time course do pressure injuries present after surgery?
51. What tissue is at risk in pressure injuries?
52. What body areas are at risk of pressure injuries in each of the supine, prone, and sitting positions?
53. In which surgical procedures are patients most likely to incur pressure injuries?
54. Which subset of patients are most at risk for self-inflicted bite injuries during general anesthesia?
55. What is the most common neuropathy represented by claims to the American Society of Anesthesia (ASA) database?
56. What are the possible causes of peripheral nerve injuries?
57. What is the best way to prevent perioperative neuropathies?
58. What have retrospective studies of ASA closed claims shown to be risk factors for ulnar nerve injuries?
59. What positions or surgeries are associated with brachial plexus injury?
60. How common are injuries to the radial or median nerves?
61. What patient position is most likely to lead to common peroneal or sciatic nerve injury?
62. What are some potential causes of obturator nerve injury?
63. How should a postoperative nerve deficit be evaluated and treated?

64. What is the typical time course to recovery from sensory and motor neuropathies?
65. What is the value of electrophysiologic evaluation of an intraoperative nerve injury?
66. What are the risk factors for corneal abrasion under general anesthesia?
67. What are the symptoms of a corneal abrasion?
68. What are some precautions that can be taken to minimize the risk of corneal abrasion?
69. What is the cause of postoperative vision loss due to central retinal artery occlusion?
70. What are the surgical and patient risk factors for postoperative vision loss due to ischemic optic neuropathy (ION)?

ANSWERS*

PHYSIOLOGIC ASPECTS OF POSITIONING

1. When the awake patient reclines from an upright to a supine position venous return to the heart increases, which increases preload, stroke volume, and cardiac output. Briefly arterial blood pressure increases until this effect is countered by parasympathetic impulses to the sinoatrial node and myocardium. The parasympathetic outflow is mediated by baroreceptors in response to the increase in arterial blood pressure. The net result is that systemic arterial blood pressure is maintained within a narrow range during postural changes in the awake patient. (321)
2. When the awake patient reclines from an upright to a supine position the functional residual capacity (FRC) decreases from the diaphragm shifting upward. Under general anesthesia the decrease in FRC is more pronounced and often FRC can exceed closing capacity, leading to increases in ventilation-perfusion mismatching and hypoxemia. (322)

GENERAL POSITIOINING

3. Anesthesia providers, operating room nurses, and surgeons all share responsibility for checking patient positioning for safety. Anesthesia providers should document positioning checks throughout the procedure and particularly following positioning changes. (322)
4. Even while asleep people normally change positions in order to protect themselves from pressure injury and excessive stretch. Under general anesthesia patients lose the ability to change position, and sometimes patients remain in one position for long periods of time. This puts skin, soft tissue, and nerves at risk of compression, stretch, and potential injury. (322)

SPECIFIC POSITIONS

5. The supine position is the most common patient position for surgery. (322)
6. While in the supine position the patient's arms can be abducted or adducted. If the arms are abducted the angle should not exceed 90 degrees to prevent brachial plexus injury. The hands and forearms should be placed in a neutral position, either supinated or with the palms toward the body, to limit external pressure on the ulnar nerve. (322)
7. Brachial plexus injury can occur in the supine position if the arm is abducted at an angle greater than 90 degrees and the head of the humerus pushes into the axilla. (322)
8. Ulnar nerve injury can occur secondary to improper supine positioning if there is external pressure on the ulnar nerve. (322)

---

*Numbers in parentheses refer to pages, figures, boxes, or tables in Pardo MC, Miller RD, eds. *Basics of Anesthesia*. 7th ed. Philadelphia: Elsevier; 2018.

9. Advantages of the lawn-chair position over the supine position include facilitated venous drainage from the elevated position of the legs; reduced stress on the back, hips, and knees; and reduced tension on the abdominal musculature. and the position is better tolerated in patients who are awake or undergoing monitored anesthesia care. (322)

10. Hip dislocation can occur secondary to improper frog-leg positioning if the knees are not adequately supported and there is external pressure placed on the leg. (322)

11. Common indications for Trendelenburg positioning include increased venous return during hypotension, improved surgical exposure during abdominal and laparoscopic surgeries, and prevention of air emboli during central line placement or removal. (322)

12. The Trendelenburg position causes an autotransfusion from the legs, resulting in about a 9% increase in cardiac output in 1 minute and sustained for about 10 minutes. After about 10 minutes the cardiovascular effects of the Trendelenburg position revert to the patient's baseline. (322)

13. The Trendelenburg position decreases both functional residual capacity (FRC) and pulmonary compliance from the abdominal contents, displacing the diaphragm upward. (322)

14. The Trendelenburg position increases both intraocular pressure (IOP) and intracranial pressure (ICP). (323)

15. Brachial plexus injury can occur secondary to improper Trendelenburg positioning in two ways. If the patient slides downward, there could be stretch on the brachial plexus, or if shoulder braces are used, there could be external compression on the brachial plexus. (323)

16. The reverse Trendelenburg position causes a decrease in venous return and could cause hypotension, particularly in patients who are hypovolemic. (323)

17. When a patient is in the reverse Trendelenburg position the invasive arterial blood pressure monitors must be zeroed at the level of the external auditory meatus to optimize cerebral perfusion. (323)

18. A patient may wake up with a backache after supine positioning for surgery because of the loss of normal lumbar lordotic curvature during general anesthesia or neuraxial blockade. Extra padding or slight flexion of the hip and knee may be helpful to reduce back pain. (323)

19. When positioning an obese patient supine in the reverse axis on the operating table the torso, and thus the heaviest part of the patient's body, is at the head of the table and opposite the weighted base. If sufficient weight is placed on the head portion, particularly if in the Trendelenburg position, the operating table can tilt and tip over. Attention must be paid to the weight limits of the operating table. (324)

20. A patient's legs must be raised and lowered simultaneously during lithotomy positioning in order to prevent spine torsion or injury. (324)

21. The common peroneal nerve, which wraps arounds the head of the fibula on the lateral leg, is particularly at risk for injury during lithotomy positioning. (324)

22. Finger crush injuries can occur during lithotomy positioning when the foot portion of the bed is raised or reattached at the end of surgery if the fingers are alongside the patient and get caught in the hinge of the operating table. (325)

23. When placing the patient in the lithotomy position elevation of the legs leads to a transient increase in venous return and cardiac output, and abdominal contents displace the diaphragm upward, decreasing lung compliance. (325)

24. Lower extremity compartment syndrome can occur in the lithotomy position owing to inadequate arterial blood flow from leg elevation or obstructed venous outflow from compression or excessive hip flexion. (325)

25. Based on retrospective studies the risk factors for positioning-related compartment syndrome are lithotomy or lateral decubitus position and long surgical time (greater than 5 hours in high lithotomy position). (325)

26. When in the lateral decubitus position, the patient's dependent leg should be flexed and a pillow or padding placed between the knees. The dependent arm should be placed in front of the patient on a padded arm board and the non-dependent arm supported by pillows or blankets or with a padded arm rest. (325)

27. When the patient is in the lateral decubitus position an axillary roll should be placed underneath the patient caudal to the axilla and not in the axilla. The purpose of the axillary roll is to prevent compression injury to the brachial plexus and axillary vascular structure on the dependent side. (325)

28. Invasive arterial monitors should ideally be placed in the dependent arm during lateral decubitus positioning in order to detect neurovascular compression in the axilla. (325)

29. Head and neck concerns when placing a patient in the lateral decubitus position include maintaining the head and neck in the neutral position, preventing folding or excessive pressure on the dependent ear, and avoiding external compression on the dependent eye. (325)

30. Injury to the brachial plexus can occur in the lateral decubitus position if there is lateral rotation of the neck and stretch of the brachial plexus or if an arm is abducted greater than 90 degrees, causing injury to the brachial plexus from the humeral head. (325)

31. In the lateral decubitus position, the lateral weight of the mediastinum and cephalad pressure on the diaphragm decrease lung compliance of the dependent lung. (325)

32. When turning a patient from the supine to prone position care must be taken to prevent dislodgment of all intravenous and arterial lines, as well as the endotracheal tube. The turn should be coordinated such that the head, neck, and spine are maintained in a neutral position. (325)

33. The bony prominences of the face, forehead, malar regions, and chin are at risk of compression or pressure injury during prone positioning. Additionally, there should not be pressure on the eyes, nose, or mouth. (325-326)

34. When in the prone position the legs should be padded and flexed slightly at the hips and knees. The arms can be positioned tucked at the patient's side or placed on arm boards next to the patient's head. The arms should not be abducted greater than 90 degrees. (326)

35. The ideal placement of bolsters beneath the prone patient is from the clavicle to the iliac crest. This helps reduce abdominal compression and its effects on the lungs and inferior vena cava, minimizing decreases in pulmonary compliance and venous return. Bolsters should not go beyond the iliac crests in order to protect the genitalia and femoral vessels. The abdomen and breasts should be placed medial to the bolsters in order to be free of compression. (328)

36. Hemodynamics are well maintained and pulmonary function is improved with prone positioning of the patient. The FRC is improved, leading to improved oxygenation in the prone position compared to the supine position. (328)

37. The sitting position is most advantageous for surgical procedures involving the superior cervical spine and the posterior fossa. A modified sitting position, or beach-chair position, is often used for shoulder surgery. (328)

38. In the sitting position the arms should rest at the patient's sides and should be well padded and supported. The shoulders should be even or slightly elevated in order to minimize stretch injury between the neck and shoulders. The knees should be supported and padded in a slightly flexed position to reduce stretching of the sciatic nerve. (328)

39. Complications that can occur as a result of placing the patient in the sitting position include venous air embolism, pneumocephalus, hypotension, cerebral hypoperfusion, and macroglossia. (328)

40. An intraoperative venous air embolus can be detected through the use of an intraoperative TEE or precordial Doppler ultrasound in the patient with adequate intravascular volume. (329)

41. Complications that can occur as a result of a venous air embolus include paradoxical air embolism, arrhythmias, acute pulmonary hypertension, and circulatory collapse. (329)

42. A patient with an anatomic intracardiac shunt is at risk for a paradoxical air embolism and subsequent stroke or myocardial infarction should a venous air embolus occur. Because some studies have shown that up to 100% of patients undergoing neurosurgery in the sitting position have some degree of venous air entrainment, patients should be evaluated to rule out an intracardiac shunt prior to planned surgery in the sitting position. Preoperative diagnosis of an intracardiac shunt is a contraindication to surgery in the sitting position. (329)

43. Pneumocephalus occurs in almost all patients undergoing cervical spine or posterior fossa surgery in the sitting position, although clinically significant pneumocephalus is rare. (329)

44. Symptoms of clinically significant postoperative pneumocephalus include headache, confusion, seizures, and even temporary hemiparesis. Patients with these symptoms must have the diagnosis of stroke excluded. (329)

45. Excessive head flexion in the sitting position can impede cerebral venous outflow and cerebral arterial inflow and cause brain hypoperfusion. Macroglossia can also occur, especially if TEE monitoring is combined with neck flexion. A minimum of two fingerbreadths between the mandible and the sternum is recommended for normal-sized adults to prevent these complications. (329)

SPECIAL CIRCUMSTANCES

46. Robotic surgery usually requires steep Trendelenburg positioning and that the patient be very well secured to the operating room table. Often a bean-bag or nonslip mattress is used in addition to strapping. Caution must be exercised if shoulder braces are used in order to minimize stretch between the neck and shoulders. Laryngeal edema and optic neuropathy can result from the steep Trendelenburg positioning that may be required for robotic surgery. (329)

47. Docking the robot limits direct access to the patient. Often the patient's head is located farther away from the anesthesia provider than normal and the patient's arms are tucked bilaterally. A metal tray or table may be placed above the patient's face to provide protection from laparoscopic equipment. (329)

48. Physiologic changes during robotic surgery occur from the combination of laparoscopic insufflation and also from the Trendelenburg position. FRC and pulmonary compliance are decreased. (329)

INJURIES

49. Pressure injuries are due to prolonged pressure that inhibits capillary flow over a bony prominence. Animal studies reveal that pressure injuries can develop in as little as 2 hours with 70-mm Hg force. (330)

50. Pressure injuries are typically noted within 72 hours after surgery. (330)

51. Pressure injuries can vary from nonblanchable erythema to full-thickness tissue loss. Skin, soft tissue, and muscle are all at risk of injury from pressure. Interestingly, muscle damage occurs before skin and subcutaneous tissue damage, likely because of the increased oxygen requirement of muscle. (330)

52. In the supine position the sacrum, heels, and occiput are areas at risk of pressure injury. In the prone position the chest and knees are most at risk of pressure injuries, while in the sitting position the ischial tuberosities are most at risk. (330)

53. Surgeries in which patients are most likely to incur pressure injuries include cardiac, thoracic, orthopedic, and vascular surgeries. The longer the surgery, the greater the risk. (330)

54. Patients undergoing surgery that involves monitoring with transcranial motor evoked potentials (Tc-MEPs) are known to be at risk of a bite injury from the contraction of the temporalis and masseter muscles during the Tc-MEP. The tongue is most frequently injured, but lip and even tooth injuries have occurred. (330)

55. Claims to the ASA database reveal that ulnar neuropathy (28%) is the most common peripheral nerve injury, followed by brachial plexus (20%), lumbosacral

nerve root (16%), and spinal cord (12%). The distribution of nerve injury claims has changed over time, with a decrease in ulnar nerve injury and an increase in spinal cord injury. Spinal cord injury and lumbosacral nerve root neuropathy are predominantly associated with regional anesthesia. (330)

56. Possible causes of peripheral nerve injuries include stretch, compression, ischemia, metabolic derangement, and direct trauma/laceration during surgery. (330)

57. There is no clear evidence for prevention of perioperative neuropathies. Most neuropathies occur in the presence of good positioning and padding. However, maintaining neutral position, avoiding excessive extension or flexion, and adequate padding are all essential. (330)

58. Risk factors for ulnar nerve injuries include diabetes, alcoholism, cigarette smoking, and cancer in retrospective studies of ASA closed claims. (333)

59. Positions and surgeries associated with brachial plexus injury include arm abduction greater than 90 degrees, lateral rotation of the head, asymmetric resection of the sternum for internal mammary dissection during cardiac surgery, and direct trauma. (333)

60. Fortunately, injuries to the radial or median nerves are rare. (333)

61. The lithotomy position is most likely to lead to common peroneal or sciatic nerve injury. The sciatic nerve can be injured with stretch and external rotation of the leg, as well as from hyperflexion at the hip. (333)

62. Obturator nerve injury can occur during difficult forceps delivery, by excessive flexion of the thigh to the groin, or by lithotomy position. (333)

63. A postoperative nerve deficit should be evaluated and the extent of sensory and motor deficits documented. A neurologic consultation can help to localize the lesion and determine severity. Most nerve injuries resolve spontaneously over time, but patient reassurance and follow-up are recommended. (333)

64. Sensory neuropathies are generally transient, whereas motor neuropathies can take 4 to 6 weeks for recovery. When there is injury to an axon or nerve disruption, and when reversible, recovery can take 2 to 12 months. (334)

65. Electrophysiologic evaluation of an intraoperative nerve injury by a neurologist in the first week may provide information regarding the characteristic and temporal pattern of the injury. Electrophysiologic evaluation after 4 weeks provides more useful information about the site, nature, and severity of the nerve injury. (334)

66. Risk factors for corneal abrasion under general anesthesia include increased age, length of surgery, prone position, Trendelenburg position, and supplemental oxygen delivery in the postanesthesia care unit. (334)

67. Symptoms of a corneal abrasion include the sensation of a foreign body in the eye, photophobia, blurry vision, and erythema. (334)

68. Precautions that can be taken to minimize the risk of corneal abrasion include careful taping of the eyelids soon after the induction of anesthesia, care regarding dangling objects when leaning over patients, ophthalmic ointments, and close observation as patients awaken. Patients may try to rub their eyes with the pulse oximeter on their finger or other equipment before they are fully awake. (334)

69. Central retinal artery occlusion is caused by direct retinal pressure. (334)

70. Ischemic optic neuropathy (ION) accounts for the majority of postoperative visual loss complications. Risk factors for postoperative vision loss due to ischemic optic neuropathy include prolonged hypotension, long duration of surgery, large-volume blood loss, large-volume crystalloid use, anemia or hemodilution, and increased intraocular or venous pressure from the prone position. It is most frequently associated with spine surgery. Patient risk factors for ION include hypertension, diabetes, atherosclerosis, morbid obesity, and tobacco use. (334)

20 ANESTHETIC MONITORING

James Szocik, Magnus Teig, and Kevin K. Tremper

RESPIRATORY SYSTEM

1. What is the purpose of intraoperative patient monitoring?
2. What are four patient parameters that have been mandated to be continually evaluated by the American Society of Anesthesiologists? How frequently is it mandated that intraoperative blood pressure be measured?
3. Do all monitors require calibration?
4. Name two kinds of oxygen sensors that are in use. What are the differences between them?
5. What is the clinical utility of measuring the expired concentration of oxygen?
6. Which law of physics is used in pulse oximetry? Which wavelengths are used?
7. How is a pulse oximeter calibrated?
8. When the absorption ratio of the pulse oximeter is 1.0, that is, equal in both the red and infrared, what percent O_2 saturation will the pulse oximeter read?
9. How do carboxyhemoglobin, methemoglobin, dyes, and motion artifact affect the pulse oximeter readings?
10. How can multiple types of hemoglobin (i.e., carboxyhemoglobin, methemoglobin) be measured?
11. Name several ways ventilation can be assessed without using electronic monitors.
12. What are some possible causes of increased airway pressures?
13. What is the plateau pressure, and how is it measured?
14. When is measuring the plateau pressure clinically useful?
15. What are some possible causes of decreased airway pressures?
16. What is the appropriate tidal volume for adults during positive-pressure ventilation?
17. Does the anesthesia machine "disconnect" alarm ensure detection of esophageal intubation and inadequate tidal volumes?
18. What is the only monitor to ensure adequate ventilation?
19. What are the phases of a normal capnogram?
20. What physiologic patient characteristic can result in upsloping of phase 2 of the capnogram?
21. How would exhausted CO_2 absorbent alter the capnogram?
22. How does the end-tidal CO_2 ($ETco_2$) value compare to the $Paco_2$ value? What is the cause of the difference between the two?
23. What is the approximate difference in mm Hg between the $ETco_2$ and the $Paco_2$ during general anesthesia in healthy patients?
24. What is dead space ventilation?
25. Why does the $ETco_2$ decrease in circulatory collapse?
26. What is the clinical utility of the capnogram during cardiopulmonary resuscitation (CPR) for cardiac arrest?

27. How reliable is the sampled $ETco_2$ from near the mouth in patients whose tracheas are not intubated?

CIRCULATORY SYSTEM

28. Name characteristics of the circulation that can be monitored during anesthesia.
29. Describe proper electrocardiogram (ECG) lead placement.
30. Which ECG leads should be monitored during anesthesia?
31. What information can be gathered from an ECG?
32. What is the clinical utility of the "diagnostic mode" on the ECG?
33. What is the relationship between blood pressure and cardiac output?
34. What is the perfusion pressure?
35. How is the perfusion pressure calculated for each of the following: systemic circulation, pulmonary circulation, brain, and heart?
36. How is mean arterial pressure (MAP) calculated?
37. What is the clinical significance of the MAP?
38. What MAP defines intraoperative hypotension?
39. What is the mechanism by which automatic noninvasive cuffs measure blood pressure?
40. Of the systolic, diastolic, and mean blood pressures, which is most accurately measured by a noninvasive blood pressure cuff?
41. What is the appropriate size of cuff to use for noninvasive blood pressures? How is the blood pressure reading altered by a noninvasive blood pressure cuff that is too large or too small?
42. What is the Riva-Rocci technique for measuring blood pressure?
43. What are some advantages of invasive arterial blood pressure monitoring over noninvasive blood pressure monitoring?
44. Which arteries can be catheterized for invasive blood pressure measurements?
45. How will the blood pressure measurement be altered by invasive arterial measurement increasing distances from the heart?
46. How does increased length of tubing/amount of fluid in the fluid-filled tube transducer setup affect the systolic blood pressure and MAP measurement during invasive arterial blood pressure monitoring?
47. How can arterial blood pressure waveforms be evaluated to assess the patient's intravascular fluid volume status?
48. What is systolic pressure variation (SPV)?
49. What is the clinical use of measuring SPV?
50. What are some situations that limit the clinical use of measuring SPV?
51. What is pulse pressure variation, and what is its clinical use?
52. What is stroke volume variation, and what is its clinical use?
53. What physiologic aspects of the cardiac cycle are reflected by the "waves" and "descents" on the central venous pressure (CVP) waveform?
54. How useful is CVP monitoring in assessing intravascular fluid volume status?
55. What central veins can be catheterized for CVP monitoring? What are some advantages and disadvantages of each?
56. What information does a pulmonary artery (PA) catheter provide? What is the wedge pressure?
57. How is cardiac output measured with a PA catheter?
58. How would hypovolemic, cardiogenic, and septic shock affect the wedge pressure and cardiac output?
59. What are the risks of PA catheterization?
60. What aspects of cardiac physiology can be evaluated by transesophageal echocardiography (TEE)?
61. What are some limitations of TEE?

CENTRAL NERVOUS SYSTEM

62. Why are processed electroencephalograms (EEGs), such as the bispectral index (BIS) monitor, used during anesthesia?

63. What minimal alveolar concentration (MAC) of inhaled anesthetic is recommended to minimize the risk of the intraoperative awareness and postoperative recall during general anesthesia?
64. In large randomized studies, how does monitoring of MAC compare to the BIS monitor in preventing awareness with postoperative recall?
65. When should the intracranial pressure (ICP) be monitored and how?
66. When are cerebral oximeter monitors used?
67. How is a cerebral oximeter different from a pulse oximeter?
68. What is the normal regional oxygen saturation (rSo_2) of the cerebral cortex when using a cerebral oximeter?

PERIPHERAL NERVOUS SYSTEM

69. Describe the various modes of stimulation with a neuromuscular blockade monitor, or "twitch" monitor, and what depth of neuromuscular blockade is appropriately monitored by each mode.
70. What are the potential patient issues with residual postoperative neuromuscular blockade or too little intraoperative neuromuscular blockade?
71. What do somatosensory evoked potentials monitor? How are they affected by anesthetics?
72. What do motor evoked potentials monitor? How are they affected by anesthetics?

TEMPERATURE

73. Which temperature monitoring sites best reflect the core body temperature?
74. Why is patient temperature monitored?
75. What happens to core body temperature during brief anesthesia?

MAGNETIC RESONANCE IMAGING AND ADVERSE CONDITIONS

76. How does the magnetic field decrease with distance from the coil?
77. What are some issues related to monitoring in the magnetic resonance imaging (MRI) suite?

MONITORS AND ALARMS

78. What is the largest problem with monitor alarms?
79. What technological solutions are being proposed to deal with monitor alarm fatigue/false positives?

ANSWERS*

1. The purpose of intraoperative patient monitoring is to continuously assess the patient's physiologic status and the effects of surgery and anesthetic agents. (337)
2. The American Society of Anesthesiologists has mandated that during all anesthetics the patient's oxygenation, ventilation, circulation, and temperature shall be continually evaluated. With general anesthesia, the oxygen (O_2) concentration of the gases administered shall be monitored. With all anesthetics, a quantitative measure of blood oxygenation (pulse oximetry) shall be used. Ventilation during a general anesthetic shall be evaluated qualitatively and, if possible, quantitatively. Breathing device placement must be verified by carbon dioxide (CO_2) identification in the expired gases. Continual, quantitative measurement of CO_2 shall be used until removal of the device. With regional anesthesia, clinical signs of ventilation shall be monitored. For all patients, the arterial blood pressure and heart rate shall be evaluated every 5 minutes. Temperature shall be monitored whenever clinically significant changes are intended, anticipated, or suspected. (337)

*Numbers in parentheses refer to pages, figures, boxes, or tables in Pardo MC, Miller RD, eds. *Basics of Anesthesia.* 7th ed. Philadelphia: Elsevier; 2018.

3. All monitors require calibration. Some monitors need manual calibration, some are autocalibrating, and some are empirically calibrated. (337)

RESPIRATORY SYSTEM

4. Both amperometric and paramagnetic oxygen sensors are in use. Amperometric oxygen sensors require calibration and are slow to respond to changes. Paramagnetic oxygen sensors are autocalibrating and have a rapid response to changes. This rapid response to change allows for the measurement of both inspired and expired oxygen content. (339)

5. Measurement of the expired oxygen concentration (F_{EO_2}) enables the quantification of preoxygenation/denitrogenation prior to the induction of anesthesia and also allows for a rough estimation of oxygen consumption. Denitrogenation is achieved when the F_{EO_2} is greater than 85% or at a plateau for that patient. The 85% value is determined from the alveolar gas equation, $P_{AO_2} = F_{IO_2}$ $(P_{atm} - P_{watervap}) - P_{aCO_2}/RQ$, where P_{AO_2} = alveolar O_2 concentration, F_{IO_2} = F_{IO_2} set by anesthetist, P_{atm} = atmospheric pressure in mm Hg (760 mm Hg at sea level), $P_{watervap}$ = vapor pressure of water (47 mm Hg at 37° C), P_{aCO_2} = 40 mm Hg, and RQ = respiratory quotient (0.8). Solving the equation yields a P_{AO_2} of 663 mm Hg, which is 87% of 760 mm Hg. Comparison of the F_{IO_2} and F_{EO_2} also allows the rough estimation of oxygen consumption if measured simultaneously with minute ventilation (MV): O_2 consumption = $(F_{IO_2} - F_{EO_2}) \times MV$. (339)

6. Beer's law is used as the basic principle of pulse oximetry. Beer's law states that the attenuation of light is related to the properties of the material through which the light is traveling. Two wavelengths are used for conventional pulse oximetry, red at 660 nm and infrared at 940 nm. (339)

7. Pulse oximeters are empirically calibrated using human volunteers and the ratio of absorbances taken from an electronic table to report the percent saturation. (341)

8. When the absorption ratio 660/940 nm of the pulse oximeter is 1.0—that is, equal in both the red and infrared—the pulse oximeter will read an O_2 saturation of 85%. (341)

9. Carboxyhemoglobin, methemoglobin, dyes, and motion artifact all affect the pulse oximeter readings. Because carboxyhemoglobin absorbs light similarly to oxyhemoglobin, the reading will be artificially high (i.e., reading closer to 100% than the true value). Because methemoglobin absorbs at a ratio of 1, it will trend to 85% saturation. This results in a lower observed value if the patient is well oxygenated and a higher observed value in hypoxic patients. Dyes produce an error similar to that seen for methemoglobin (trend to 85%), but because dyes are cleared rapidly from the circulation this error is only transient. Motion artifact will produce noise in the numerator and denominator and force the ratio value to 1.0, also trending the pulse oximeter readings to 85%. (341)

10. Multiple types of hemoglobin can be measured by adding additional wavelengths. A typical two-wavelength oximeter can measure only oxyhemoglobin and deoxyhemoglobin. With the addition of multiple wavelengths, carboxyhemoglobin (especially in burn patients with smoke inhalation) and methemoglobin (from benzocaine or other drug toxicities) can be measured. Newer eight-wavelength pulse oximeters are available that can detect all saturations. (341)

11. Ventilation depth, pattern, and frequency can be assessed by observation, either of the patient's chest or the rebreathing bag on the anesthesia machine. Auscultation with a stethoscope can determine rate and depth as well. A trained clinician can diagnose bronchospasm by hearing wheezing or decreased breath sounds, endobronchial intubation or pneumothorax by unilateral breath sounds, and pulmonary edema by auscultatory rales. (342)

12. An increase in airway pressures can be due to an increase in airflow resistance or a reduction in chest wall compliance. Causes of increased airway pressures can include bronchospasm, endobronchial intubation, pneumothorax, pulmonary edema, a kinked endotracheal tube or circuit, or a malfunctioning valve. (342)

13. The plateau pressure is the pressure in the respiratory circuit when the gases have stopped moving. The plateau pressure is a reflection of lung/chest wall compliance. To measure the plateau pressure during volume-controlled ventilation, an end-inspiratory pause must be set. (342)

14. The plateau pressure is a reflection of lung/chest wall compliance. The difference between the peak inspiratory pressure and the plateau pressure is a reflection of airway resistance only. During incidents of increased airway pressures of unknown cause measurement of changes in the plateau pressure relative to the airway pressure can help determine if the increase in airway pressures is due to lung/chest wall compliance or to airway resistance. (342)

15. Causes of decreased airway pressures include circuit disconnections, leaks in the circuit, extubation of the trachea, failure to deliver fresh gases, ventilator setting error, excess scavenging, or other issues with the anesthesia machine. (342)

16. For adults, a tidal volume of 6 to 8 mL/kg of ideal body weight with the addition of positive end-expiratory pressure is associated with the best pulmonary outcomes in one large study of pulmonary outcomes after major abdominal surgery. Similar tidal volumes have been associated with improved outcomes in patients with acute respiratory distress syndrome. (342)

17. The anesthesia machine "disconnect" alarm does not ensure detection of esophageal intubation or inadequate tidal volumes. The "disconnect" alarm on the anesthesia machine is usually tied to the airway pressure reading. Normal pressures may not provide for adequate ventilation. During pressure support ventilation there can be a significant change in tidal volume without triggering the anesthesia machine alarm. During an esophageal intubation "adequate" airway pressures and volumes may be detected by the anesthesia machine, thereby preventing triggering of the anesthesia machine alarm. (342)

18. Mechanical alarms and tidal volume measurements do not measure the physiologic aspect of ventilation, which is the removal of CO_2 from the body. Pulse oximetry can reflect the oxygenation, but only exhaled CO_2 measurement ensures adequate ventilation. (342)

19. A normal capnogram has three defined phases. Phase 1 reflects the inspired gases and dead space gas (normally both contain no CO_2). Phase 2 is the transition to alveolar gas with rising CO_2. Phase 3 is the alveolar gas reflecting the end-tidal CO_2. The inspiratory segment of the capnogram is referred to as phase 0. (342)

20. Upsloping of phase 2 of the capnogram reflects resistance to expiratory outflow of gas from the alveoli. Physiologic patient characteristic such as chronic obstructive pulmonary disease (COPD) and asthma both result in this upsloping pattern. (342)

21. Exhausted CO_2 absorbent can result in a progressive rise in inspired CO_2, which would be reflected by the capnogram not returning to a baseline of 0 between breaths. (342)

22. The ET_{CO_2} value is lower than the Pa_{CO_2} value because of dead space ventilation. The amount of difference between the two values is related to the proportion of dead space ventilation to alveolar ventilation. (342)

23. The approximate difference between the ET_{CO_2} and the Pa_{CO_2} during general anesthesia in healthy patients is 3 to 5 mm Hg. (343)

24. Dead space ventilation is that portion of the inspired and expired gases that does not participate in gas exchange. There is apparatus dead space (from the equipment), anatomic dead space (from the portion of the airways that do not contain alveoli), and alveolar dead space (the alveoli that are ventilated but not perfused). The exhaled dead space gas is the same as the inhaled dead space gas because no exchange has taken place. Some situations in which there is increased alveolar dead space, and thus an increase in the difference between the ET_{CO_2} and the Pa_{CO_2}, include pulmonary emboli, lateral positioning, and decreased cardiac output. (343)

25. During acute drops in pulmonary blood flow, such as during a pulmonary embolism or cardiac arrest, perfusion of the lung decreases. This causes a decrease in the number of perfused alveoli, and therefore an increase in dead space ventilation. This is reflected as a decrease in the ET_{CO_2}. The Pa_{CO_2} is elevated under these circumstances. (345)

26. The capnogram is the most useful monitor for adequacy of chest compressions during cardiopulmonary resuscitation (CPR) for cardiac arrest. The goal of ET_{CO_2} > 20 should be achieved. A further advantage of following the capnogram during CPR is that it is unaffected by motion artifact, unlike the pulse oximeter and ECG. (345)

27. The sampled ET_{CO_2} from near the mouth in patients whose tracheas are not intubated is diluted by the aspiration of room air and is therefore not a reliable measure. (345)

CIRCULATORY SYSTEM

28. During anesthesia, noninvasive monitors can be used to monitor heart rate and rhythm, systolic blood pressure, diastolic blood pressure, and mean blood pressure. By using invasive monitors, central venous pressure, pulmonary artery pressure, cardiac output, and systolic pressure variation (SPV) can be measured. Circulating blood volume, organ perfusion/blood flow, and venous capacitance are aspects of the circulatory system that cannot be directly measured. (345)

29. When placing ECG leads for a three-lead system, the limb leads should be placed on the shoulders and the third lead on the left abdomen below the rib cage. The five-lead system is preferred, with the single precordial lead (V_5) placed in the fifth intercostal space in the anterior axillary line. (346)

30. Monitoring a combination of ECG leads II and V during anesthesia provides for detection of the majority of dysrhythmias and ischemia. (346)

31. Monitoring the ECG can determine the heart rate (bradycardia, tachycardia, asystole) and rhythm (normal sinus, heart block, atrial fibrillation, ventricular fibrillation). Drugs, electrolytes, temperature, and myocardial ischemia can alter the ECG. (345)

32. The "diagnostic mode" on the ECG removes all filtering and the artifacts that filtering can produce. If the ECG on the monitor looks different from the preoperative ECG, the diagnostic mode may be useful in determining if the changes are real. (345)

33. Blood pressure is directly proportional to cardiac output. This is an Ohm's law system in which blood pressure = flow (cardiac output) × resistance. At any given vascular resistance, an increase in cardiac output will result in an increase in blood pressure. The reciprocal of this also true. (346)

34. The perfusion pressure is the pressure difference across the circulation of any organ. This is calculated as the pressure upstream minus the pressure downstream. (346)

35. The perfusion pressure for the systemic circulation is mean arterial pressure (MAP) minus the central venous pressure (CVP). The perfusion pressure of the pulmonary circulation is mean pulmonary arterial pressure (MPAP) minus the left atrial pressure (usually estimated by pulmonary capillary wedge pressure). The perfusion pressure of the brain is MAP minus the intracranial pressure (ICP). The perfusion pressure of the heart is systemic diastolic pressure minus the right-sided heart (or coronary sinus) pressure. The systemic diastolic pressure is used as the upstream pressure because the heart perfuses itself during diastole. (346)

36. MAP is calculated as two thirds diastolic blood pressure plus one third systolic blood pressure: $MAP = (\frac{2}{3} DBP) + (\frac{1}{3} SBP)$. (346)

37. MAP is the upstream pressure for the perfusion of most vital organs. (346)

38. Intraoperative hypotension may be associated with hypoperfusion, or inadequate delivery of oxygen and nutrients to the tissues. In 2009, an association between MAP less than 50 mm Hg for more than 10 minutes was associated with postoperative cardiac events. In 2013, the cumulative time with a mean MAP less than 55 mm Hg was noted to be associated with increasing incidences of postopera-

tive renal and cardiac injury. In 2015, it was noted that a MAP less than 50 mm Hg for 5 minutes and MAP less than 60 mm Hg for 10 minutes were associated with an increased 30-day postoperative mortality rate. For all these reasons, for adults mean arterial blood pressures below 55 to 60 mm Hg is an accepted definition of intraoperative hypotension. (349)

39. The automatic noninvasive cuff measures blood pressure by the oscillometric method. The cuff first inflates beyond the systolic pressure and then deflates slowly. When the pulse is detected at maximal pulsations, this is the MAP. The cuff then deflates until no pulse is detected. These automated devices use an algorithm to estimate both systolic and diastolic blood pressures. (349)

40. Of the systolic, diastolic, and mean blood pressures, the mean blood pressure is most accurately measured by a noninvasive blood pressure cuff. (352)

41. The appropriate size cuff for noninvasive blood pressures is one for which the width is approximately 40% of the circumference of the arm. If the blood pressure cuff is too large the blood pressure measurement will read artificially low, and if the blood pressure cuff is too small the blood pressure measurement will read artificially high. (352)

42. The Riva-Rocci technique for measuring blood pressure is through insufflation of an occlusive cuff and noting the return of blood flow by palpation (systolic blood pressure) or Doppler. Korotkoff sound auscultation at the antecubital fossa can determine both systolic and diastolic blood pressures. Through the use of a Doppler probe, this technique can measure blood pressure in patients with non-pulsatile flow, such as patients with a left ventricular assist device (LVAD). (352)

43. Invasive arterial blood pressure monitoring allows for continuous measurements of the blood pressure, blood sampling for laboratory analysis, and assessment of the patient's intravascular fluid volume status. (352)

44. Arteries that can be catheterized for invasive blood pressure measurements include the radial, brachial, femoral, and dorsalis pedis arteries. The radial artery is most frequently chosen because of its easy palpation and lower associated risk. (352)

45. Invasive arterial blood pressure measurements will result in higher systolic pressures when measured in arteries at increasing distances from the heart. (352)

46. Increased length of tubing/amount of fluid in the fluid-filled tube transducer setup for invasive arterial blood pressure monitoring will increase amplification artifact in the systolic blood pressure measurement, whereas the MAP measurement remains fairly accurate. (352)

47. Arterial blood pressure waveforms can be evaluated for systolic pressure variation, pulse pressure variation, and stroke volume variation to assess the patient's intravascular fluid volume status. (352)

48. Systolic pressure variation (SPV) is defined as the difference between maximum and minimum systolic blood pressure during a positive-pressure respiratory cycle. The decrease in arterial pressure associated with positive-pressure ventilation is due in part to the positive intrathoracic pressure transiently decreasing venous return to the right side of the heart. SPV is assessed by analyzing the variations in the arterial blood pressure waveform, which can be manually calculated by freezing the arterial waveform on the physiologic monitor and scrolling up and down. Newer generation physiologic monitors automatically calculate SPV. (352)

49. Clinically, measuring SPV can be useful to predict the responsiveness (increase in stroke volume, blood pressure, or cardiac output) of a patient to an intravascular fluid challenge. The SPV is an indirect assessment of venous capacitance. An abnormal number indicates the potential of the blood pressure to improve with fluid administration. (352)

50. Some limitations of SPV include the need for positive-pressure ventilation and a normal sinus heart rhythm. Atrial fibrillation causes irregular variations of the arterial waveform and affects measured SPV values. Increased lung or chest wall compliance, prone positioning, high positive end-expiratory pressure (PEEP), or an open thoracic cavity can also affect the clinical use of SPV measurements. (354)

51. Pulse pressure variation is determined by measuring the relative changes in pulse pressure during positive-pressure ventilation. Pulse pressure variation can be used to predict response to an intravenous fluid bolus similar to SPV. (354)

52. Stroke volume variation is determined by measuring the relative changes in stroke volume during positive-pressure ventilation. The stroke volume is estimated from the arterial pulse wave with a pulse contour algorithm. Stroke volume variation can be used to predict response to an intravenous fluid bolus similar to SPV and pulse pressure variation. (354)

53. Physiologic aspects of the cardiac cycle are reflected by the "waves" and "descents" on the central venous pressure (CVP) waveform. The a wave reflects atrial contraction against the closed tricuspid valve, the c wave reflects tricuspid bulging as the ventricle contracts, the x descent reflects atrial relaxation, the v wave reflects atrial filling, and the y descent reflects atrial emptying. (354)

54. CVP monitoring has not been shown to be useful in assessing intravascular fluid volume status except in the extremes. When the CVP is less than 2 mm Hg the patient may benefit from intravenous fluid administration. Conversely, when the CVP is more than 15 mm Hg the need for additional fluids is not likely. (354-355)

55. Central veins commonly catheterized for CVP monitoring include the internal jugular, subclavian, and femoral veins. The most common site is the internal jugular vein. The advantages of the internal jugular are its accessibility, its compressibility, and the fact that it provides a straight path to the heart for pulmonary artery (PA) catheter placement. Its disadvantage is the potential for carotid artery puncture and injury. The subclavian vein is accessible in patients wearing a cervical collar, and this site is more comfortable for patients. Disadvantages of subclavian vein catheterization include its lack of compressibility, the increased potential for pneumothorax, injury to the brachial plexus, and potential subclavian artery puncture. The femoral vein may be more accessible in some patients and is compressible but carries an increased risk of infection. (356)

56. The PA catheter provides measurements of the right-sided heart filling pressures and the cardiac output. The wedge pressure is measured by wedging the pulmonary catheter in a small arterial branch with an inflated balloon. This provides an indirect measure of the left atrial pressure under normal pulmonary conditions. (356)

57. Cardiac output can be measured with a PA catheter through the thermodilution technique. Cold fluid is injected via the proximal port of the PA catheter, and a thermistor at the distal port measures the temperature. The temperature change over time is recorded as a curve, and the area under the curve is proportional to the cardiac output. (356)

58. Hypovolemic shock would result in a low wedge pressure and low cardiac output. Cardiogenic shock would result in a high wedge pressure and low cardiac output. Septic shock would result in a low wedge pressure and high cardiac output. (356)

59. Risks of PA catheterization include line infection causing sepsis, clot formation, and pulmonary artery rupture. (356)

60. Transesophageal echocardiography (TEE) has become the gold standard for cardiac evaluation. Through TEE one can assess cardiac valves, chamber size, contractile activity and ejection fraction, systolic and diastolic dysfunction, and pericardial pathology such as effusions or tamponade. (357)

61. Limitations of TEE include the need for provider technical expertise, potential for esophageal injuries, and the need for access to the patient's head. (357)

CENTRAL NERVOUS SYSTEM

62. A processed EEG, such as the bispectral index (BIS) monitor, can be used during anesthesia to assess anesthetic depth. The purpose of these monitors is to reduce the risk of intraoperative awareness and recall during general anesthesia. (357)

63. A minimal alveolar concentration (MAC) above 0.5 to 0.7 of inhaled anesthetic is recommended to minimize the risk of the intraoperative awareness and recall during general anesthesia. (357)

64. In large randomized studies, monitoring of MAC with alerts is equivalent to the BIS monitor in preventing awareness with postoperative recall. During total intravenous anesthetics, a BIS monitor may provide an extra layer of protection against recall. (357)

65. Intracranial pressure (ICP) should be measured in the setting of increased cerebrospinal fluid (CSF) pressure, cerebral edema, or intracranial lesions, all of which can markedly increase the ICP and decrease the cerebral perfusion pressure. The ICP can be measured via a ventriculostomy catheter, which provides a method by which to drain CSF and potentially lower the ICP. Another method of measuring ICP uses a catheter with a transducer placed onto the dura, but no fluid can be drained via this method. (357)

66. Cerebral oximeter monitors are used in cardiac or vascular surgical procedures when there is a concern for poor cerebral perfusion reflected by decreased cerebral oxygenation. (357)

67. A cerebral oximeter works by using reflected infrared light through the scalp and skull into a portion of the cerebral cortex beneath it, rather than transmitted light. The cerebral oximeter uses a proprietary algorithm to determine the saturation value, presenting a number between 1% to 100%, similar to the pulse oximeter. (357)

68. The normal regional oxygen saturation (rSo_2) of the cerebral cortex when using a cerebral oximeter is usually around 70%. (358)

PERIPHERAL NERVOUS SYSTEM

69. The neuromuscular blockade monitor has various settings. A post-tetanic count (PTC) is used to assess the deeper levels of block; 5 seconds of tetanic stimulus is given followed by a series of twitches at 1 Hz. Slightly less deep blockade can be followed by a train-of-four (TOF). TOF uses 4 supramaximal stimuli at 2 Hz and the number of responses (twitches) are counted. Deep blockade is 0 to 1 of 4 present. Even with 4 of 4 present, 75% of the receptors can still be blocked. To attempt to show this residual blockade, one can use a double burst stimulation (DBS) of two bursts of 50-Hz tetany separated by 750 ms. Alternatively, a TOF ratio can be measured. This requires a quantitative device to compare the strength of the first and the fourth twitches. The TOF ratio and DBS have overlap in the degree of blockade monitored. Finally, sustained high hertz (100 Hz) tetany can be observed. This is quite painful in an awake patient. (358)

70. Residual postoperative neuromuscular blockade is associated with subclinical aspiration, hypoventilation, and airway obstruction. Too little intraoperative neuromuscular blockade can result in inappropriate patient movement and injury, such as premature extubation, extrusion of ocular contents with a cough or Valsalva maneuver, impalement of the bladder on a rigid cystoscope, and injury of abdominal organs with surgical retractors or instruments. (358)

71. Somatosensory evoked potentials monitor the sensory tracts of the spinal cord. A small current is delivered to a sensory nerve, and the response in the sensory cortex is measured with a scalp electrode. Both halogenated agents and nitrous oxide decrease the amplitude and increase the latency of the measurements, mimicking nerve injury and interfering with monitoring. This is particularly true at higher doses of inhaled anesthetic agents and in patients with preexisting nerve injury. Neuromuscular blockers can improve the signal of somatosensory evoked potentials by decreasing the noise. (358)

72. Motor evoked potentials monitor the motor tracts, or ventral spinal cord. Motor evoked potential are extremely sensitive to the effects of inhaled anesthetic agents such that total intravenous anesthesia is required when using this monitor. In addition, neuromuscular blockers cannot be administered to these patients. (358)

TEMPERATURE

73. True core body temperature is measured by probes in the PA catheter, distal esophagus, nasopharyngeal area, or tympanic membrane area. Sites that can approximate core body temperature include oral, axillary, and bladder. (360)

74. Patient temperature is monitored to manage intraoperative hypothermia, to assess fever, to detect an adverse response to blood products, and to detect malignant hyperthermia. Alterations in body temperature can be deliberate, such as in induced hypothermia for post–cardiac arrest care, cardiopulmonary bypass, or circulatory arrest. Monitoring body temperature intraoperatively is useful to identify and prevent inadvertent hypothermia, which is common if not prevented. (360)

75. Core body temperature drops even with brief anesthesia. The primary mechanism for this is through the redistribution of heat from the core to the periphery. (360)

MAGNETIC RESONANCE IMAGING AND ADVERSE CONDITIONS

76. The magnetic field in a magnetic resonance imaging (MRI) suite is nonlinear and depends upon a multitude of variables. Five feet from the magnet may be safe in one direction but not in another. The safety lines should be clearly marked. (360)

77. MRI-compatible anesthesia monitors must be used for patients undergoing MRI under anesthesia. Normal monitors will not work in an MRI environment. Metal objects (such as an oxygen tank) can be attracted to MRI coil with great force, causing injury. MRI suites can have loud noise levels caused by the rapid changes in magnetic field causing expansion and contraction of the coils (up to 120 dB, similar to a jet aircraft at takeoff). This can affect the ability to hear monitor sounds and alarms. Even a nonmagnetic wire, formed into a loop, can become a hazard from the heating effects. (360-361)

MONTORS AND ALARMS

78. The most common problem with alarms is false positives and negatives. Too many false positive alarms and the caregiver may suffer from the "cry wolf" syndrome and ignore the alarm. A single false negative alarm can result in serious patient harm. (361)

79. Newer generation integrated alarming systems are being developed. Integrating multiple alarms into a single conduit may decrease alarm fatigue. These alarms may delay the notification until a certain time has passed or increase the urgency if multiple conditions are met simultaneously. (361)

21 ACID-BASE BALANCE AND BLOOD GAS ANALYSIS

Emily L. Chanan

DEFINITIONS
1. What is the importance of maintaining a physiologic acid-base status?
2. What are acids and bases?
3. How are acidemia and alkalemia defined?
4. How are acidosis and alkalosis defined?
5. What is the definition of base excess?
6. What is the clinical utility of measuring the base excess?

REGULATION OF THE HYDROGEN ION CONCENTRATION
7. What is the normal plasma H^+ concentration, the normal plasma HCO_3^- concentration, and the normal arterial pH of blood?
8. How does the body regulate acid-base disturbances to maintain normal arterial pH?
9. What is a buffer?
10. What is the pKa?
11. What are the buffering systems in blood? Which buffering system has the greatest contribution to the total buffering capacity of blood?
12. How does the bicarbonate buffering system work? What enzyme facilitates this reaction?
13. How does hemoglobin act as a buffer?
14. How does the respiratory system respond to acid-base disorders?
15. How does the renal system respond to acid-base disorders?
16. How quickly can the buffering system, respiratory system, and renal system respond to physiologic changes in arterial pH?

MEASUREMENT OF ARTERIAL BLOOD GASES
17. What is the relationship between a venous and arterial blood gas drawn from the same patient concurrently?
18. What errors can occur if heparin or air is present in an arterial blood gas sample?
19. What happens if there is a delay in analysis of the blood gas sample?
20. How does temperature affect the arterial blood gas (ABG)?
21. How does an anesthesia provider manage the patient when using alpha stat during cardiopulmonary bypass?
22. How does an anesthesia provider manage the patient when using pH stat during cardiopulmonary bypass?

DIFFERENTIAL DIAGNOSIS OF ACID-BASE DISTURBANCES
23. What is the difference between a primary disturbance and a compensatory disturbance in acid-base status?
24. What defines a primary metabolic acidosis or alkalosis?
25. What defines a primary respiratory acidosis or alkalosis?
26. What adverse responses are associated with severe acidemia?

27. What adverse responses are associated with severe alkalemia?
28. What are the causes of a respiratory acidosis?
29. What is the compensatory response for a respiratory acidosis?
30. What is the treatment for a respiratory acidosis?
31. What are the causes of a respiratory alkalosis?
32. What is the compensatory response for a respiratory alkalosis?
33. What is the treatment for a respiratory alkalosis?
34. What are the causes of a metabolic acidosis?
35. How is the anion gap calculated?
36. How does the Stewart strong ion approach to understanding acid-base status differ from the classic Henderson-Hasselbalch approach?
37. What is the compensatory response for a metabolic acidosis?
38. What is the treatment for a metabolic acidosis?
39. What are some of the concerns regarding the administration of bicarbonate for the treatment of metabolic acidosis?
40. What are the causes of a metabolic alkalosis?
41. What is the compensatory response for a metabolic alkalosis?
42. What is the treatment for a metabolic alkalosis?
43. What are the steps for diagnosing an acid-base disorder?
44. How can an acute respiratory process be distinguished from a chronic process?
45. How is the Δgap determined?
46. What formula is used to determine if there is appropriate respiratory compensation for a metabolic process?

OTHER INFORMATION PROVIDED BY ANALYSIS OF ARTERIAL BLOOD GASES AND pH

47. How does measurement of the Pa_{CO_2} help to determine the adequacy of ventilation?
48. What is the dead space to tidal volume (V_D/V_T) ratio?
49. What are some causes of arterial hypoxemia?
50. What does the alveolar gas equation calculate?
51. How is the alveolar-arterial (A-a) gradient calculated? What is the significance of the gradient?
52. What is the Pa_{O_2}/F_{IO_2} (P/F) ratio?
53. What is the normal mixed venous P_{O_2}?
54. What is the clinical utility of the Fick equation?
55. What is the clinical utility of the arteriovenous difference?

ANSWERS*

DEFINITIONS

1. A physiologic acid-base status optimizes enzyme function, myocardial contractility, and saturation of hemoglobin with oxygen. (363)
2. Brønsted and Lowry defined an acid as a molecule that can act as a proton (H^+) donor and a base as a molecule that can act as a proton acceptor. In biologic molecules, weak acids or bases are molecules that can reversibly donate H^+ or reversibly bind H^+. (363)
3. Acidemia is defined as an arterial pH less than 7.35, and alkalemia is defined as an arterial pH greater than 7.45. (363)
4. An acidosis is the underlying process that lowers the pH, whereas an alkalosis is the process that raises the pH. A patient can have a mixed disorder with both an acidosis and an alkalosis, but it can only be either acidemic or alkalemic. (363)

---

*Numbers in parentheses refer to pages, figures, boxes, or tables in Pardo MC, Miller RD, eds. *Basics of Anesthesia*. 7th ed. Philadelphia: Elsevier; 2018.

5. Base excess is usually defined as the amount of strong acid or strong base required to return 1 L of whole blood exposed in vitro to a P_{CO_2} of 40 mm Hg to a pH of 7.4. (364)

6. The base excess number is supposed to refer to the nonrespiratory, or metabolic, component of an acid-base disorder. A negative base excess (less than zero) suggests the presence of a metabolic acidosis, whereas a positive base excess (greater than zero) suggests the presence of a metabolic alkalosis. It is most often used clinically in the operating room as a surrogate marker for lactic acidosis to help determine the adequacy of volume resuscitation. (364)

REGULATION OF THE HYDROGEN ION CONCENTRATION

7. At 37° C, the normal plasma H^+ concentration is 35 to 45 nmol/L. The normal plasma HCO_3^- concentration is 24 ± 2 mEq/L, and the normal arterial pH of blood is between 7.36 and 7.44. (364)

8. Normal arterial pH is maintained through three systems: buffers, ventilation changes, and renal response. The ventilatory response involves changes in alveolar ventilation and CO_2 concentrations. The renal response involves reabsorption of bicarbonate ions or secretion of hydrogen ions. (364)

9. A buffer is defined as a substance within a solution that can prevent extreme changes in pH. It is composed of a base molecule (which can bind excess hydrogen ions) and its weak conjugate acid (which can protonate excess base molecules). (364)

10. The pKa, or dissociation ionization constant, is the pH at which an acid is 50% protonated and 50% deprotonated. (364)

11. The buffering systems in blood include bicarbonate, hemoglobin, phosphate, plasma proteins, and ammonia. The bicarbonate buffering system is the largest contributor and provides 50% of the total buffering capacity of the body. Hemoglobin is responsible for about 35% of the total buffering capacity, and phosphate, plasma proteins, and ammonia account for the remainder. (364)

12. Carbonic anhydrase facilitates the hydration of carbon dioxide in the plasma and in the erythrocytes into H_2CO_3, which spontaneously dissociates to H^+ and HCO_3^-. The HCO_3^- that is formed then enters the plasma to function as a buffer, and the H^+ that is generated is buffered by hemoglobin. (364)

13. In plasma, hemoglobin exists as a weak acid. It acts as a buffer by binding H^+ generated by the bicarbonate buffering system. Carbon dioxide can also be transported by hemoglobin as carbaminohemoglobin. Deoxyhemoglobin has a greater affinity for carbon dioxide, so venous blood carries more carbon dioxide than arterial blood. (364-365)

14. The respiratory system responds to alterations in blood pH through central and peripheral chemoreceptors. Central chemoreceptors lie on the anterolateral surface of the medulla and respond to changes in cerebrospinal fluid pH. Carbon dioxide diffuses across the blood-brain barrier to change cerebrospinal fluid pH. Minute ventilation increases 1 to 4 L/min for every 1-mm Hg increase in P_{CO_2}. Peripheral chemoreceptors are at the bifurcation of the common carotid arteries and aortic arch. The peripheral chemoreceptors are sensitive to changes in P_{O_2}, P_{CO_2}, pH, and arterial perfusion pressure. They communicate with the central respiratory centers via the glossopharyngeal nerves. The central chemoreceptors are more sensitive to hydrogen ions, whereas the carotid bodies are most sensitive to P_{aO_2}. The stimulus from central and peripheral chemoreceptors to either increase or decrease alveolar ventilation diminishes as the pH approaches 7.4 such that complete correction or overcorrection is not possible. (365)

15. The renal system corrects for pH changes by reabsorbing filtered HCO_3^-, excreting titratable acids, and producing ammonia. (365)

16. The buffering system of the blood responds to physiologic changes in arterial pH almost instantly. Compensatory changes in alveolar ventilation in response to changes in arterial pH occur within minutes. Compensatory changes by the

kidneys in response to changes in arterial pH require 12 to 48 hours and may not be maximal for up to 5 days. (365)

MEASUREMENT OF ARTERIAL BLOOD GASES

17. The correlation between arterial and venous blood gas measurements varies with the hemodynamic stability of the patient. In certain clinically stable situations, peripheral venous blood may serve as an approximation and save an arterial puncture. Venous pH is only 0.03 to 0.04 lower than arterial values. Venous blood cannot be used for estimation of oxygenation because venous Po_2 (Pvo_2) is significantly lower than Pao_2. (366)

18. Excessive amounts of anticoagulant in the sampling syringe could falsely dilute the measured Po_2, Pco_2, and ionized calcium. Air bubbles in the syringe could result in the diffusion of oxygen and carbon dioxide between the air bubble and the blood in the syringe. Typically, this results in a decrease in the carbon dioxide tensions in the blood sample. The change in oxygen tension (either falsely higher or falsely lower) depends on the patient's Po_2. (367)

19. A delay in analysis of the blood gas sample can lead to oxygen consumption and carbon dioxide production by the metabolically active white blood cells. Usually this error is small and can be reduced by placing the sample on ice. In some leukemia patients with markedly elevated white blood cell counts, this error can become significant. This phenomenon is often referred to as leukocyte larceny and has also been reported with extreme thrombocytosis, or platelet larceny. (367)

20. Decreases in temperature decrease the partial pressure of a gas in solution even though the total gas content does not change. A blood gas with a pH of 7.4 and Pco_2 of 40 mm Hg at 37° C will have a pH of 7.58 and Pco_2 of 23 mm Hg at 25° C. The change in Po_2 with respect to temperature depends on the degree that hemoglobin is saturated with oxygen, but as a guideline, the Po_2 is decreased approximately 6% for every 1° C that the patient's body temperature is below 37° C. (367)

21. The term alpha stat developed because as the patient's pH was allowed to drift with temperature, the protonation state of histidine residues remained "static." During cardiopulmonary bypass, an anesthesia provider using alpha stat would manage the patient based on an arterial blood gas (ABG) measured at 37° C and strive to keep that pH at 7.4, although the patient's true pH would be higher. There are no extra adjustments for the patient's hypothermia. (367)

22. pH stat requires keeping a patient's pH static at 7.4 based on the core temperature. During cardiopulmonary bypass, an anesthesia provider using pH stat would manage the patient based on an arterial blood gas that is corrected for the patient's temperature. This usually means adding carbon dioxide so that the patient's temperature-corrected blood gas has a pH of 7.4. (367)

DIFFERENTIAL DIAGNOSIS OF ACID-BASE DISTURBANCES

23. A primary disturbance in acid-base status is the initial deviation in the arterial pH secondary to either respiratory or metabolic causes. A compensatory response occurs in an attempt to reverse the alteration in the arterial pH. Typically the compensatory response is not able to completely reverse the deviation in arterial pH. (368)

24. A primary metabolic acidosis is present when accumulation of any acid other than carbon dioxide results in a pH lower than 7.35. The HCO_3^- concentration is usually less than 22 mEq/L. A primary metabolic alkalosis is present when the pH is higher than 7.45 owing to gain of bicarbonate ions or loss of hydrogen ions. The HCO_3^- concentration is usually greater than 26 mEq/L. (368)

25. A primary respiratory acidosis is accompanied by a Pco_2 above normal, usually greater than 43 mm Hg. A primary respiratory alkalosis is accompanied by a Pco_2 below normal, usually lower than 37 mm Hg. (368)

26. Acidemia usually leads to decreased myocardial contractility and release of catecholamines. When the acidemia is mild, the catecholamine release mitigates the effects of myocardial depression. With severe acidemia, myocardial

depression and hypotension predominate. Respiratory acidosis may produce more rapid and profound myocardial dysfunction than metabolic acidosis because of the rapid entry of carbon dioxide into the cardiac cells. In the brain, this rapid rise in carbon dioxide can lead to confusion, loss of consciousness, or seizures. (369)

27. Severe alkalemia can lead to decreased cerebral and coronary blood flow due to arteriolar vasoconstriction. The consequences are more prominent with respiratory than with metabolic causes because of the rapid movement of carbon dioxide across cell membranes. Acute hyperventilation can produce confusion, myoclonus, depressed consciousness, and seizures. (369)

28. Respiratory acidosis may occur secondary to increased carbon dioxide production, decreased carbon dioxide elimination, or carbon dioxide rebreathing or absorption. Causes of increased carbon dioxide production include malignant hyperthermia, sepsis, hyperthyroidism, and overfeeding. Causes of decreased carbon dioxide elimination include central nervous system (CNS) depressants, decreased skeletal muscle strength, intrinsic pulmonary disease, chest wall restriction, and airway obstruction. Causes of rebreathing or absorption include exhausted soda lime, incompetent one-way valves, and laparoscopic surgery. (369)

29. The kidneys will compensate for a respiratory acidosis by increased hydrogen ion secretion and bicarbonate reabsorption over the course of hours to days. The hallmark of a chronic respiratory acidosis is an elevated P_{CO_2} with a near normal pH. (369)

30. The treatment for a respiratory acidosis is treatment of the underlying disorder. The use of mechanical ventilation to decrease an acutely increased P_{CO_2} may be necessary if the pH is less than 7.2. (369)

31. Respiratory alkalosis may occur with increased minute ventilation relative to carbon dioxide production or decreased carbon dioxide production. Causes of increased minute ventilation relative to carbon dioxide production include CNS disease, sepsis, liver disease, pregnancy, severe anemia, restrictive lung disease, hypoxemia, pain, and anxiety. Causes of decreased carbon dioxide production include hypothermia and skeletal muscle paralysis. (369)

32. Respiratory alkalosis is compensated for by decreased reabsorption of bicarbonate ions from the renal tubules and increased urinary excretion of bicarbonate. (369)

33. Treatment for a respiratory alkalosis should be directed at correcting the underlying cause. Mild alkalemia usually does not require treatment. During general anesthesia, the minute ventilation may be decreased in order to decrease the elimination of carbon dioxide. (369)

34. The causes of metabolic acidosis are divided into anion gap and non–anion gap etiologies. An increase in the anion gap occurs when the anion replacing bicarbonate is not one that is routinely measured. The most common unmeasured anions are lactic acids and ketoacids. Other common anions include methanol, ethylene glycol, uremia, paraldehyde, aspirin, and ethanol. Metabolic acidosis with a normal anion gap occurs when chloride replaces the lost bicarbonate, such as with bicarbonate wasting processes in the kidney (renal tubular acidosis) or gastrointestinal tract (diarrhea). Aggressive fluid resuscitation with normal saline will induce a nongap metabolic acidosis because the chloride administration impairs bicarbonate reabsorption in the kidneys. (369)

35. The anion gap is the difference between the measured cations (sodium) and measured anions (chloride and bicarbonate). A normal gap value is 8 to 12 mEq/L and is mostly composed of albumin. A patient with a low serum albumin will have a lower anion gap. Each 1-g/dL decrease in serum albumin below 4.4 g/dL will lower the actual concentration of unmeasured anions by 2.5 mEq/L. (370)

36. The Stewart strong ion approach to understanding acid-base status distinguished six primary acid-base disturbances (strong ion acidosis and alkalosis, nonvolatile

buffer acidosis and alkalosis, and respiratory acidosis and alkalosis) as opposed to the four differentiated by the Henderson-Hasselbalch equation (metabolic acidosis and alkalosis and respiratory acidosis and alkalosis). The more complex Stewart approach may be similar to the traditional Henderson-Hasselbalch approach if changes in albumin concentration are accounted for in the measurement of the anion gap. (370)

37. Compensatory responses for a metabolic acidosis include increased alveolar ventilation from carotid body stimulation and renal tubule secretion of hydrogen ions into urine. Chronic metabolic acidosis is associated with loss of bone mass because buffers present in bone are used to neutralize the nonvolatile acids. (370)

38. The treatment for metabolic acidosis is based on whether an anion gap is present or not. For a nongap acidosis the intravenous administration of sodium bicarbonate can be instituted because the problem is bicarbonate loss. Management of an anion gap acidosis should be guided by the diagnosis and treatment of the underlying cause in order to remove the nonvolatile acids in the circulation. For example, tissue hypoxia leading to lactic acidosis should be corrected with oxygen, fluid resuscitation, and circulatory support. Diabetic ketoacidosis requires intravenous fluids and insulin therapy. In a mechanically ventilated patient the minute ventilation can be increased until a more definitive treatment takes place. (371)

39. The administration of bicarbonate for the treatment of metabolic acidosis is controversial but may be considered as a temporizing measure in deteriorating patients with severe metabolic acidosis. The concern is that its administration generates carbon dioxide that can worsen any intracellular and extracellular acidosis unless eliminated by ventilation. (371)

40. Metabolic alkalosis can be due to a gain of bicarbonate ions or a loss of hydrogen ions. Causes of a metabolic alkalosis are based on whether the underlying cause is chloride responsive or chloride resistant. Chloride-responsive causes include renal loss from diuretics and gastrointestinal loss from vomiting. Chloride-resistant causes include hyperaldosteronism, refeeding syndrome, hypovolemia, and profound hypokalemia. (371)

41. Compensatory responses for a metabolic alkalosis include increased reabsorption of hydrogen ions, decreased secretion of hydrogen ions by renal tubule cells, and alveolar hypoventilation. The efficiency of the renal compensatory response is dependent on the presence of cations (sodium and potassium) and chloride. (371)

42. Treatment of a metabolic alkalosis should be aimed at reducing the acid loss by stopping gastric drainage or fluid repletion with saline and potassium chloride, which allows the kidneys to excrete excess bicarbonate ions. Occasionally, a trial of acetazolamide may be useful in causing a bicarbonaturia. (371)

43. The steps for diagnosing an acid-base disorder are as follows:
    Step 1: Determine oxygenation by calculating the A-a gradient.
    Step 2: Determine acidemia (pH 7.35) or alkalemia (pH 7.45).
    Step 3: Determine whether the cause is from a respiratory (P_{CO_2} change from 40 mm Hg) or metabolic (HCO_3^- change from 24 mEq/L) process.
    Step 4: If there is a respiratory abnormality, then assess whether the process is acute or chronic. If there is a metabolic acidosis, then skip to step 5. If there is a metabolic alkalosis, then skip to step 7.
    Step 5: If there is a metabolic abnormality, determine the anion gap.
    Step 6: Determine the Δgap.
    Step 7: Determine whether there is adequate respiratory compensation for the metabolic process. (371)

44. An acute respiratory acidosis can be distinguished from a chronic respiratory acidosis by the degree of elevation of HCO_3^-. The renal effects to compensate for a respiratory acidosis take 12 to 48 hours to take effect and are reflected by a more marked increase in the plasma HCO_3^- concentration. During an acute

process, the pH changes 0.08 for every 10-mm Hg change in P_{CO_2} from 40 mm Hg. During a chronic process, the pH changes 0.03 for every 10-mm Hg change in P_{CO_2} from 40 mm Hg. (371)

45. If there is a metabolic acidosis, then it should be determined if there is an anion gap. If so, the Δgap should be determined. The Δgap is the excess anion gap (anion gap minus 12) added back to the serum bicarbonate level. It is used to determine if another concurrent metabolic process is present along with an anion gap metabolic acidosis. If the Δgap is less than 22 mEq/L, then a concurrent nongap metabolic acidosis exists. If the Δgap is greater than 26 mEq/L, then a concurrent metabolic alkalosis exists. (371)

46. There are two formulas (one for metabolic acidosis and another for metabolic alkalosis) to calculate what the P_{CO_2} should be if there is appropriate respiratory compensation. In the presence of metabolic acidosis, the formula is called the Winter formula and is $P_{CO_2} = (1.5 \times HCO_3^-) + 8$. If measured P_{CO_2} is greater than that calculated from the Winter formula, then the compensation is not adequate and respiratory acidosis is also present. If the measured P_{CO_2} is less than the calculated P_{CO_2}, then a respiratory alkalosis is present. In the presence of a metabolic alkalosis, the formula is $P_{CO_2} = (0.7 \times HCO_3^-) + 21$. If the measured P_{CO_2} is greater than the calculated P_{CO_2}, then concurrent respiratory acidosis is present. If the measured P_{CO_2} is less than the calculated P_{CO_2}, then a respiratory alkalosis is present. (371)

OTHER INFORMATION PROVIDED BY ANALYSIS OF ARTERIAL BLOOD GASES AND pH

47. Measurement of the Pa_{CO_2} helps to determine the adequacy of ventilation in removing carbon dioxide from the blood. A Pa_{CO_2} above 45 mm Hg suggests the patient may be hypoventilating relative to carbon dioxide production, whereas a Pa_{CO_2} below 35 mm Hg suggests the patient may be hyperventilating relative to carbon dioxide production. (372)

48. The dead space to tidal volume (V_D/V_T) ratio is the fraction of each tidal volume that is involved in dead space ventilation. Normal V_D/V_T is less than 0.3 and is mostly due to anatomic dead space. This will be reflected by the gradient between Pa_{CO_2} and end-tidal CO_2 when minute ventilation is held constant during anesthesia. An increased dead space will decrease the efficiency of ventilation. Patients with a pulmonary embolus or chronic obstructive pulmonary disease are examples of patients who may have an increased V_D/V_T ratio, which would also be reflected by an increase in the gradient between Pa_{CO_2} and end-tidal CO_2. (372)

49. Arterial hypoxemia is caused by a low P_{O_2} in the inhaled gases, hypoventilation, or venous admixture with or without a decreased mixed venous oxygen content. An increase in the venous admixture involves blood that passes from the pulmonary circulation to the systemic circulation without passing by ventilated alveoli. These right-to-left shunts can be intrapulmonary (atelectasis, pneumonia, one-lung ventilation) or intracardiac (congenital heart disease). (372)

50. The alveolar gas equation estimates the partial pressure of alveolar oxygen (PA_{O_2}) by using barometric pressure, water vapor pressure, the inspired oxygen content, and P_{CO_2}. Changes in the PA_{O_2} can therefore be calculated at different barometric pressure and in the presence of alterations in the P_{CO_2}. (373)

51. The alveolar-arterial (A-a) gradient formula calculates the difference in oxygen partial pressure between alveolar (PA_{O_2}) and arterial (Pa_{O_2}) blood. Calculation of the gradient provides an estimate of venous admixture as the cause of hypoxia. The A-a gradient provides an assessment of the patient's shunt fraction. Larger A-a gradients suggest pathologic shunting, such as atelectasis, pneumonia, or endobronchial intubation. To estimate the amount of shunt present, the shunt fraction is approximately 1% of cardiac output for every 20-mm Hg difference in the A-a gradient when the Pa_{O_2} is higher than 150 mm Hg. (373)

52. The Pa_{O_2}/FI_{O_2} (P/F) ratio is an alternative to the A-a gradient to communicate the degree of hypoxia. Patients with moderate acute respiratory distress syndrome (ARDS) typically have a P/F ratio below 200. A P/F ratio below 200 also corresponds to a shunt fraction greater than 20%. (374)

53. Normal mixed venous P_{O_2} ($P_{\bar{V}O_2}$) is 40 mm Hg. A true mixed venous P_{O_2} should reflect blood from the superior and inferior venae cavae. It is usually obtained from the distal port of an unwedged pulmonary artery catheter. Many physicians use the trend from a venous P_{O_2} obtained from the superior vena cava as a surrogate number. If tissue oxygen consumption is unchanged, then changes in $P_{\bar{V}O_2}$ will reflect direct changes in cardiac output. (374)

54. The Fick equation is used to calculate cardiac output if Pa_{O_2}, Pv_{O_2}, and hemoglobin are known. It basically states that the delivery of oxygen in the veins must equal the delivery of oxygen in the arteries minus the oxygen that is consumed (V_{O_2}). (374)

55. The arteriovenous difference is the difference between the arterial and mixed venous oxygen content. The number is a good estimate of the adequacy of oxygen delivery. The normal arteriovenous difference is 4 to 6 mL of O_2/dL of blood. When tissue oxygen consumption is constant, an increased arteriovenous difference means that there is higher oxygen extraction, which can be seen with decreased cardiac output or congestive heart failure. A lower arteriovenous difference means there is lower extraction or higher cardiac output, which can occur during cyanide poisoning or sepsis, respectively. (375)

22 HEMOSTASIS

Theresa Lo and Lindsey L. Huddleston

PRIMARY HEMOSTASIS

1. What is primary hemostasis?
2. What activates platelets to form the initial platelet plug in primary hemostasis?
3. What is the role of activated platelets in the formation of a platelet plug?
4. What is the role of fibrinogen in the formation of a platelet plug?

SECONDARY HEMOSTASIS

5. What is secondary hemostasis?
6. What is the role of tissue factor in clot formation?
7. Which factors are involved in producing thrombin?'
8. What is the role of thrombin in clot formation?
9. What are the three main regulatory molecules that help terminate the coagulation cascade?
10. What is the role of endogenous heparin in the control of coagulation?
11. What is the role of protein S in the control of coagulation?
12. What is the role of tissue plasminogen activator (tPA) in the termination of coagulation?
13. How is fibrinolysis regulated? What is the potential clinical effect of systemic fibrinolysis?

DISEASES ASSOCIATED WITH BLEEDING

14. What are some historical signs and symptoms that may indicate that a patient has a bleeding disorder?
15. What laboratory value of platelet counts becomes concerning for uncontrolled intraoperative bleeding?
16. What percent of coagulation factors must be present to prevent uncontrolled intraoperative bleeding?
17. Which factors are deficient in each of the inherited diseases hemophilia A and hemophilia B?
18. What percentage of factor activity defines hemophilia A and B as severe disease?
19. What laboratory analysis abnormalities are seen in patients with hemophilia A and B?
20. What laboratory test can be used to distinguish hemophilia A from von Willebrand disease?
21. Which patients are most likely to develop acquired factor deficiencies?
22. Which factors are most commonly affected in acquired factor deficiencies? What are the clinical manifestations of each?
23. What is the most common inherited bleeding disorder? What is its estimated prevalence in the general population?
24. Name two important hemostatic functions of von Willebrand factor.
25. How many types of von Willebrand disease are there? What are they and how are they inherited?

26. Which coagulation factors are dependent on vitamin K for their carboxylation?
27. Which patients are susceptible to vitamin K deficiency?
28. What are some causes of bleeding diastheses in patients with liver disease?
29. What procoagulant and anticoagulant factors are synthesized by the liver?
30. What is the treatment of choice for patients with hemophilia A and hemophilia B? What is the goal of treatment?
31. What is the utility of fresh frozen plasma (FFP) and cryoprecipitate in the treatment of patients with hemophilia A and hemophilia B?
32. What other treatment can be considered to control bleeding in hemophilia B patients if factor IX concentrates are not available?
33. What are some adjuvants that can be used to treat hemophilia A patients in addition to factor VIII concentrates, FFP, and cryoprecipitate?
34. What are the treatments for the different types of inherited von Willebrand disease?
35. What is the treatment for patients who are bleeding with vitamin K deficiency?
36. What is the treatment for patients who are bleeding with liver failure?
37. What is the treatment for patients who are bleeding with acquired factor inhibitors?
38. What are some causes of thrombocytopenia due to decreased platelet production?
39. What are some causes of thrombocytopenia due to increased platelet destruction?
40. What are some causes of thrombocytopenia due to increased platelet sequestration?
41. What diseases in pregnancy can result in thrombocytopenia?
42. What are some causes of qualitative platelet dysfunction?
43. What are some medications that can impair platelet function?
44. What is the mechanism by which uremia can lead to increased clinical bleeding?
45. What are some inherited disorders of platelet function?
46. What is the threshold for transfusing platelets in thrombocytopenic patients?
47. What is the threshold for transfusing platelets in thrombocytopenic patients who are actively bleeding or who require surgical intervention?
48. What is a concern regarding multiple platelet transfusion?

DISEASES ASSOCIATED WITH THROMBOSIS

49. What is the Virchow triad regarding the pathogenesis of venous thromboembolism (VTE)?
50. What are some inherited diseases or acquired conditions that can lead to a venous thromboembolism?
51. What are the two most common inherited thrombophilias?
52. What is the mechanism by which a factor V Leiden mutation can lead to a thrombotic state?
53. What is the mechanism by which a prothrombin gene mutation can lead to a thrombotic state?
54. What are the functions of protein C under normal physiologic conditions?
55. How may a patient with protein C deficiency present clinically?
56. What are the functions of protein S under normal physiologic conditions?
57. What diseases are associated with acquired protein C and S deficiencies?
58. What is antiphospholipid (antibody) syndrome (APS)? What is its clinical manifestation?
59. What are some clinical scenarios in which lupus anticoagulant can be found?
60. What is catastrophic antiphospholipid syndrome?
61. What is disseminated intravascular coagulation (DIC)? What is its clinical manifestation?

62. What laboratory abnormalities are associated with DIC?
63. What is the anticoagulation management in a patient with known thrombophilia?
64. What is the anticoagulation management in patients with APS?
65. What is the treatment for DIC?

LABORATORY EVALUATION OF HEMOSTASIS

66. Name some laboratory tests of coagulation.
67. Low levels of which factors will result in a prolonged prothrombin time?
68. What is the international normalized ratio (INR)? What is it useful for?
69. Low levels of which factors will result in a prolonged activated partial thromboplastin time (aPTT)?
70. What drugs can be monitored by the aPTT?
71. What is evaluated by the thrombin time test?
72. What is tested by the activated clotting time (ACT)? What is its clinical use?
73. Name some laboratory tests of fibrinolysis.
74. What is suggested by elevated D-dimer levels?
75. What is measured by global coagulation assays such as thromboelastography and rotational thromboelastometry?
76. What are some of the limitations of global coagulation assays?
77. Name some laboratory tests of platelet function.
78. What factors may result in an inaccurate platelet count?
79. How is a bleeding time test of platelet function performed?
80. What is a normal bleeding time?
81. What are platelet aggregation studies of platelet function?
82. What is the clinical utility of platelet aggregation studies?
83. What is evaluated by the platelet function analysis test?

ANTITHROMBOTICS AND PROCOAGULANTS

84. What are the three main categories of antithrombotic drugs?
85. What are the three main classes of antiplatelet agents?
86. What are the physiologic effects of the cyclooxygenase isozymes COX-1 and COX-2?
87. What effect does aspirin have on the cyclooxygenase enzymes?
88. What is the duration of the effect of aspirin on platelet function?
89. In what time course is near-normal hemostasis expected after the last dose of aspirin?
90. How can the immediate reversal of the effect of aspirin on platelets be achieved?
91. What effect do nonsteroidal anti-inflammatory drugs (NSAIDs) have on the cyclooxygenase enzymes?
92. What is the duration of the effect of NSAIDs on platelet function?
93. What are the proposed benefit and the potential downside of COX-2 selective antagonists?
94. Is platelet function affected by COX-2 selective antagonists?
95. What are some P2Y12 receptor antagonist drugs and how do they affect platelet function?
96. In what time course does platelet function normalize after discontinuing clopidogrel and ticlopidine?
97. What patient population receiving clopidogrel can have a significantly increased risk of major cardiovascular events leading to the Food and Drug Administration (FDA) black box warning for this drug?
98. How is ticagrelor different from clopidogrel in terms of interindividual variability and dosing regimen?
99. What are some glycoprotein IIb/IIIa receptor antagonist drugs and how do they affect platelet function?
100. What are some clinical uses of intravenous glycoprotein IIb/IIIa (GPIIb/IIIa) receptor antagonists?

101. Of the GPIIb/IIIa receptor antagonist drugs abciximab, eptifibatide, and tirofiban, which bind irreversibly?
102. For each of the GPIIb/IIIa receptor antagonist drugs abciximab, eptifibatide, and tirofiban, how long does it take for platelet aggregation to normalize after discontinuing the drug?
103. What is the mechanism of action of warfarin?
104. What is the duration of the effect of warfarin?
105. What is the INR goal when administering warfarin?
106. What are some concerns with warfarin therapy?
107. What is the mechanism of action of unfractionated heparin?
108. What are some benefits of unfractionated heparin for anticoagulation?
109. Which patient population may be resistant to the effects of unfractionated heparin and how can they be treated?
110. What is the dose of unfractionated heparin prior to the initiation of cardiopulmonary bypass? How is it reversed at the conclusion of cardiopulmonary bypass?
111. What is heparin-induced thrombocytopenia (HIT)?
112. When should HIT be suspected and how do you test for it?
113. What is the treatment for HIT?
114. What is the concern regarding the administration of warfarin for the treatment of patients with HIT?
115. What are some alternatives to anticoagulation in patients with a history of HIT who require cardiac surgery and cardiopulmonary bypass?
116. What is the mechanism of action of low-molecular-weight heparin (LMWH) and fondaparinux?
117. How can the plasma activity levels of LMWH and fondaparinux be assessed? In which patients might this be helpful?
118. How does the duration of action of LMWH and fondaparinux compare to that of heparin?
119. Can protamine be used to reverse LMWH or fondaparinux?
120. What is the recommendation regarding the administration of LMWH and fondaparinux in patients with HIT?
121. What are some direct thrombin inhibitors (DTIs) and what is their mechanism of action?
122. How can the clinical effects of DTIs can be monitored?
123. Of the currently available DTIs, which ones are preferred in patients with renal or hepatic insufficiency?
124. What pharmacologic agents can be used the reverse the effects of DTIs?
125. What is the mechanism of action of the newer oral anticoagulant agents dabigatran (Pradaxa), rivaroxaban (Xarelto), and apixaban (Eliquis)?
126. What are some pharmacologic advantages of the newer oral anticoagulant agents (dabigatran, rivaroxaban, and apixaban) over warfarin?
127. What is the FDA approved indication for dabigatran (Pradaxa)?
128. What is the FDA approved indication for rivaroxaban (Xarelto) and apixaban (Eliquis)?
129. What laboratory tests can be used to monitor the effects of the newer oral anticoagulant agents dabigatran, rivaroxaban, and apixaban?
130. What are some reversal agents for the newer oral anticoagulant agents dabigatran, rivaroxaban, and apixaban?
131. What are some thrombolytic agents and what is their mechanism of action?
132. What are some clinical uses of thrombolytic agents?
133. Why are tissue plasminogen activators both thrombolytics and anticoagulants? What is the clinical implication of this?
134. What negative effects of streptokinase limit its use?
135. What are some potential causes of perioperative bleeding?
136. What is the role of procoagulants in perioperative bleeding?
137. What are some antifibrinolytic agents in use in the United States and what is their mechanism of action?

138. What are some clinical uses of ε-aminocaproic acid (EACA) and tranexamic acid (TXA)?
139. What is the mechanism of action for recombinant factor VIIa (rFVIIa) to enhance hemostasis?
140. What is the duration of action of rFVIIa?
141. What are some clinical uses of rFVIIa?
142. What is a concern with the use of rFVIIa?
143. Which coagulation factors does prothrombin complex concentrate (PCC) contain?
144. What are some clinical uses of PCCs?
145. What is the infectious risk of PCCs?

PERIOPERATIVE MANAGEMENT OF ANTICOAGULATION

146. For patients who are taking vitamin K antagonists (VKAs) and are scheduled to undergo surgery, what is the current recommendation for when to discontinue and restart the administration of the VKAs?
147. How does the perioperative management of patients who are on VKAs differ depending on their risk (high vs. low) of venous thromboembolism?
148. What is the recommendation for the management of perioperative bridging therapy with unfractionated heparin?
149. What is the recommendation for the management of perioperative bridging therapy with LMWH?
150. How should patients on aspirin therapy be managed in the perioperative period?
151. How should patients on dual antiplatelet therapy aspirin and clopidogrel be managed in the perioperative period?
152. What is the recommendation for surgical delay in patients who have undergone recent percutaneous coronary intervention with coronary stent placement?
153. What is the recommendation regarding neuraxial anesthesia procedures in patients who are receiving anticoagulant or antiplatelet therapy?

ANSWERS*

PRIMARY HEMOSTASIS

1. Primary hemostasis refers to the initial platelet deposition, or "platelet plug" formation, at the site of vessel injury. This results from platelet adhesion, activation, and aggregation. (377)
2. Platelets do not adhere to the endothelial surface under normal conditions because thrombogenic substances are separated from platelets by an intact endothelium. When the subendothelial matrix is exposed with vascular injury, platelet adhesion results from activated integrins on the platelet surface binding to multiple ligands, including von Willebrand factor (vWF), collagen, fibrinogen, fibronectin, and vitronectin. These cause the platelets to adhere to the endothelium and become activated. (377)
3. Once activated, platelets recruit and activate additional platelets to the site of vessel injury, where platelet aggregation occurs. This is achieved through the degranulation of activated platelets which in turn induces a change in platelet shape, making them extremely adhesive. (377-378)
4. Fibrinogen has a primary role in platelet aggregation and plug formation. Activated platelets induce a conformational change in glycoprotein IIb/IIIa on its surface, which has a high affinity for fibrinogen. Fibrinogen forms crosslinks with glycoprotein IIb/IIIa on activated platelets to form bridges between

---

*Numbers in parentheses refer to pages, figures, boxes, or tables in Pardo MC, Miller RD, eds. *Basics of Anesthesia*. 7th ed. Philadelphia: Elsevier; 2018.

platelets, thus aggregating and crosslinking platelets to form the platelet plug. This is the final step in primary hemostasis. (378)

SECONDARY HEMOSTASIS

5. Secondary hemostasis refers to the formation of insoluble crosslinked fibrin on the platelet plug to stabilize it and form a clot. This occurs via an interplay of mechanisms including the activation and amplification of clotting factors and the propagation of clot formation. This is commonly referred to as the clotting cascade. (378)

6. Tissue factor is the principal initiator of the coagulation cascade. Tissue factor becomes exposed when the endothelium is disrupted and binds with circulating activated factor VII (factor VIIa) at the site of vessel injury. This complex goes on to activate factors X and IX, further propagating the coagulation cascade. (378)

7. Activated factor X complexes with and activates factor V, forming the pro-thrombinase complex, which converts a small amount of prothrombin to thrombin. The thrombin created further amplifies the cascade by activating factors V, VIII, XI, and platelets. Factor IXa and VIIIa form the tenase complex to activate additional factor X, thus creating increased production of prothrombinase and thrombin. (379)

8. Thrombin cleaves fibrin into fibrinogen once sufficient levels of thrombin are available. Fibrin activates factor XIII to crosslink the fibrin monomers into a fibrin matrix, forming a stable clot. (379)

9. Antithrombin, tissue factor pathway inhibitor (TFPI), and activated protein C (APC) are the three main regulatory molecules that help terminate the coagulation cascade. Antithrombin inhibits thrombin and many of the other activated coagulation factors. TFPI directly inhibits factor Xa and binds with factor Xa to inhibit the TF-VIIa complex. APC inactivates factors Va and VIIIa, thus inactivating the prothrombinase and tenase complexes. (379)

10. Endogenous heparin binds to antithrombin and accelerates its action by over 100-fold. Endogenous heparin is found on normal endothelial cells and prevents spontaneous clot formation on normal endothelial cell surfaces. This helps to limit the coagulation process to only damaged endothelium. (379)

11. Protein S greatly enhances the activity of activated protein C, which acts to terminate the coagulation cascade. (379)

12. Tissue plasminogen activator (tPA), which is secreted by injured endothelium, activates plasminogen to plasmin. Plasmin then degrades fibrin to soluble products such as D-dimers (fibrinolysis). This process is highly regulated and is normally localized to the area of clot. (379)

13. Fibrinolysis is highly regulated to occur only at the site of thrombus. Tissue plasminogen activator binds to fibrin on the clot; thus the generation of plasmin is localized on the fibrin clot surface. Under normal conditions, circulating plasmin that is unbound to the fibrin clot is inhibited by α_2-antiplasmin. However, if plasmin activation goes unchecked, systemic fibrinolysis will occur and massive hemorrhage may develop. (379)

DISEASES ASSOCIATED WITH BLEEDING

14. Some historical signs and symptoms that may indicate that a patient has a bleeding disorder include easy bruising, mucosal bleeding, epistaxis, prolonged bleeding after dental procedures, and menorrhagia. (379)

15. Platelet counts of 50,000 cells/μL or less can be associated with uncontrolled intraoperative bleeding. (379)

16. In general, 20% to 30% of coagulation factors must be present to prevent uncontrolled intraoperative bleeding. (379)

17. Both hemophilia A and hemophilia B are X-linked recessive disorders. Hemophilia A is a deficiency of factor VIII and occurs in approximately 1 in 5000 live male births. Hemophilia B is a deficiency of factor IX and occurs in 1 in 30,000 live male births. (379)

18. Severe disease in hemophilia A and hemophilia B is defined as having less than 1% of factor activity. This occurs in approximately two thirds of patients with hemophilia A and one half of patients with hemophilia B. (379)

19. Laboratory abnormalities seen in patients with hemophilia A and B include a prolonged activated partial thromboplastin time (aPTT) that corrects in mixing studies, with a normal platelet count and prothrombin time (PT). It is important to note that many patients with hemophilia A (up to 25%) and some with hemophilia B (approximately 3-5%) will develop inhibitory antibodies as a response to exogenous factor. In these cases, the aPTT does not correct in mixing studies. (379)

20. To distinguish between hemophilia A (factor VIII deficiency) and von Willebrand disease, plasma von Willebrand factor antigen (VWF:Ag) can be measured. VWF:Ag is normal in hemophilia. (379)

21. Acquired factor deficiencies are caused by autoantibodies. Patients likely to develop acquired factor deficiencies include patients who received infusions of factor concentrates, who are pregnant, who have underlying systemic disease such as rheumatoid arthritis or lupus erythematosus, or as a drug reaction. (380)

22. Factor VIII is the most common acquired factor deficiency and is manifested clinically as bleeding. Other factors associated with acquired deficiency include factors XI (bleeding), XII (clotting), and XIII (delayed bleeding after hemostasis). (380)

23. Von Willebrand disease is the most common inherited bleeding disorder. The estimated prevalence is 1% of the general population; however, the true prevalence is likely higher because of the highly polymorphic von Willebrand gene and variable phenotypes of the disorder. (380)

24. In normal hemostasis, von Willebrand factor (vWF) binds to both platelets and the extracellular matrix at the site of endothelial injury, thus contributing to primary hemostasis by facilitating platelet adhesion. vWF also plays a role in the coagulation cascade and fibrin clot formation by acting as a carrier protein for factor VIII, increasing its concentration and prolonging its half-life. (380)

25. There are three main phenotypes of inherited von Willebrand disease. Types 1 and 2 are autosomal dominant traits. Type 3, the least frequent and most severe form, is transmitted as an autosomal recessive trait. With type 1, there is not enough vWF; with type 2, there are several types of qualitative defects of vWF; and with type 3, vWF is absent. In addition to these inherited types, von Willebrand disease can be acquired through autoantibodies to vWF, increased clearance and proteolysis of vWF, and decreased synthesis of vWF. (380)

26. Vitamin K is an essential fat-soluble vitamin that is required for the carboxylation of factors II, VII, IX, and X and proteins C and S. (380)

27. Vitamin K is in dietary sources such as leafy greens and is synthesized by bacteria in the gastrointestinal tract. Patients who are fasting or have poor dietary intake are susceptible to vitamin K deficiency. Other patients prone to vitamin K deficiency include those with impaired intestinal absorption (obstructive jaundice, intestinal ileus or obstruction, total parenteral nutrition), newborns who have not yet developed normal intestinal flora, and patients undergoing oral antibiotic therapy that alters gut flora. (381)

28. Some causes of bleeding diatheses in patients with liver disease include impairment of hemostasis from thrombocytopenia and platelet dysfunction, deficiencies in coagulation factor synthesis, and increased fibrinolysis. (381)

29. The liver is responsible for the synthesis of all the procoagulant factors except factor VIII. The liver also synthesizes the anticoagulant factors: protein C, protein S, and antithrombin. The result of this is a tenuous hemostatic balance of impaired secondary hemostasis and deficiencies in anticoagulant factors. (381)

30. Factor concentrates are the treatment of choice for patients with hemophilia A (factor VIII concentrate) and hemophilia B (factor IX concentrate). The goal of treatment is to achieve at least 50% of normal factor activity levels for minor surgery and 80% to 100% of normal factor activity levels for major surgery. (381)

31. In resource-limited areas fresh frozen plasma (FFP) and cryoprecipitate may necessarily be used to treat patients with hemophilia A and B, although this treatment is not optimal. FFP can be considered for both hemophilia A and B patients, but it is difficult to achieve sufficient levels of factors with FFP alone because of inadequate levels of factor and the need for large volume administration. Cryoprecipitate contains high quantities of factor VIII, vWF, fibrinogen, and factor XIII, but it does not contain factor IX. It is therefore useful for the treatment of patients with hemophilia A but should not be used for the treatment of patients with hemophilia B. (381)

32. Prothrombin complex concentrates (PCCs) contain factor IX and can be used for bleeding control in patients with hemophilia B when factor IX concentrates are not available. PCCs should be administered with caution as PCCs also induce a thrombotic risk. (381)

33. Adjuvant treatments for hemophilia A patients include desmopressin (DDAVP) and antifibrinolytics (tranexamic acid, ε-aminocaproic acid). DDAVP (0.3 μg/kg) increases plasma levels of factor VIII and vWF and can be used for bleeding management of hemophilia A. Antifibrinolytic treatment with tranexamic acid and ε-aminocaproic acid can help decrease bleeding risk. (381)

34. The different types of inherited von Willebrand disease (vWD) are treated with different agents. Desmopressin (DDAVP) is the treatment of choice in type 1 von Willebrand disease. One dose of DDAVP (0.3 μg/kg) will produce a complete or near-complete response in the majority of patients. In addition, cryoprecipitate and intermediate-purity factor VIII concentrates, which both contain high levels of vWF, can also be used to treat surgical bleeding. DDAVP is contraindicated in type 2b vWD because it causes a transient thrombocytopenia. Patients with severe vWD (type 3) do not respond to DDAVP and should be treated with a combination of factor VIII and vWF concentrates. Antifibrinolytics are also useful adjuvants in the management of perioperative bleeding in this patient population. (381)

35. Vitamin K deficiency can be treated with vitamin K replacement via oral, subcutaneous, intramuscular, or intravenous routes. For isolated vitamin K–deficient patients who are bleeding, the intravenous administration of vitamin K will reverse the prothrombin time within 3 to 4 hours. (381)

36. The treatment of bleeding in patients with liver failure should be guided by the laboratory abnormalities. Platelets are administered for thrombocytopenia, FFP for a prolonged prothrombin time, and cryoprecipitate may be necessary to treat bleeding in the setting of hypofibrinogenemia. The routine administration of blood products solely to correct laboratory values is not recommended because of the complex balance of deficiencies in procoagulant and anticoagulant factors in these patients. (381)

37. Patients with acquired factor inhibitors who are bleeding are difficult to treat because the administration of factors may not lead to an adequate response. Instead, the mainstay of therapy is through the administration of "bypassing agents" that treat bleeding by producing thrombin through pathways independent of factor VIII or factor IX. Currently available bypassing agents include recombinant factor VIIa and prothrombin concentrate complexes (PCCs). Another treatment strategy is "immune tolerance induction" when patients are exposed to prolonged, high concentrations of a factor in an effort to eliminate an inhibitor. Immune tolerance induction can only be used in the nonurgent clinical setting, however. (381)

38. Causes of thrombocytopenia from decreased platelet production include decreased bone marrow production as in myelodysplastic syndromes, infections (especially in the setting of sepsis), nutrient deficiencies, immune thrombocytopenia (ITP), and drug-induced bone marrow suppression. (382)

39. Causes of thrombocytopenia from increased platelet destruction include antiplatelet antibodies (medications or ingested substances) and in the setting of specific autoimmune diseases. Heparin can induce thrombocytopenia in less

than 5% of patients exposed to heparin. Increased platelet consumption within thrombi is seen in disseminated intravascular coagulation (DIC) and thrombotic thrombocytopenic purpura–hemolytic uremic syndromes (TTP-HUS). (382)

40. Causes of thrombocytopenia from increased platelet sequestration are diseases that can result in splenic sequestration of platelets, such as cirrhosis of the liver. (382)

41. Diseases in pregnancy that can result in thrombocytopenia include gestational thrombocytopenia, preeclampsia, and pregnancy-associated hypertensive disorders. The most severe of these disorders is the HELLP syndrome (hemolytic, elevated liver function tests, low platelet counts), which can necessitate emergent delivery before life-threatening maternal complications occur. (382)

42. Some causes of qualitative platelet dysfunction include the ingestion of some drugs, uremia, abnormal circulating proteins (multiple myeloma, dysproteinemia, transfused dextran solutions), and many rare inherited disorders (Glanzmann thrombasthenia, giant platelet disorders, Wiskott-Aldrich syndrome). (382)

43. Some medications that can impair platelet function include aspirin, nonsteroidal anti-inflammatory drugs (NSAIDs), alcohol, dipyridamole, and clopidogrel. (382)

44. Proposed pathophysiologic mechanisms for the mechanism by which uremia can lead to increased clinical bleeding include intrinsic platelet metabolic defects, impaired platelet granule release, and impaired platelet-endothelial cell interactions. (382)

45. Inherited disorders of platelet function are rare. Glanzmann thrombasthenia is an autosomal recessive disorder characterized by defective GPIIb/IIIa receptors on platelets leading to impaired platelet aggregation. Giant platelet disorders include platelet glycoprotein abnormalities, as in Bernard-Soulier syndrome. Wiskott-Aldrich syndrome is an X-linked recessive disorder in which patients have immunodeficiency, severely dysfunctional platelets, and thrombocytopenia. This syndrome is an example of a storage pool disorder, in which granule deficiencies lead to impaired platelet aggregation. (382)

46. Thrombocytopenic patients who are not actively bleeding usually have platelet transfusion withheld until the platelet count is less than 10,000 cells/μL. (382)

47. Thrombocytopenic patients who are actively bleeding or who require surgical intervention are usually transfused platelets to a goal of 50,000 cells/μL. If the location of surgery or active bleeding is in a specific location such as intracranial or intraocular sites, the patient can be transfused platelets to a goal of 100,000 cells/μL. (382)

48. A major concern with the transfusion of multiple platelets is the potential for human leukocyte antigen (HLA) or human platelet antigen antibodies to form. If multiple platelet transfusions are expected, platelets should be HLA-matched whenever possible. (382)

DISEASES ASSOCIATED WITH THROMBOSIS

49. The Virchow triad regarding the pathogenesis of venous thromboembolism (VTE) describes three factors that predispose toward VTE: (1) stasis of blood flow, (2) endothelial injury, and (3) a hypercoagulable state. (382)

50. Inherited diseases that can lead to VTE include deficiencies of protein C, protein S, and antithrombin; factor V Leiden; and prothrombin gene mutations. Numerous other conditions such as malignancy, pregnancy, immobilization, trauma, DIC, antiphospholipid syndrome, infection, drugs (e.g., oral contraceptives), and recent surgery also predispose patients to VTE. (383)

51. The two most common inherited thrombophilias are the factor V Leiden mutation and the prothrombin gene mutation. Together these two diseases account for 50% to 60% of inherited thrombophilias. Patients who are homozygotes for these traits are at the highest risk of forming clots. (383)

52. Individuals with factor V Leiden have an abnormal mutation of factor V that is resistant to the action of activated protein C (APC). APC regulates the coagulation process by inhibiting factor V from forming excessive fibrin in normal

individuals. The lack of inhibition therefore leads to a hypercoagulable or thrombotic state. (383)

53. The prothrombin gene mutation (prothrombin 20210) leads to the overproduction of prothrombin (factor II), leading to a thrombotic state. (383)

54. APC inactivates factors Va and VIIIa (enhanced by protein S). In addition, APC acts directly on cells to protect endothelial barrier function and has anti-inflammatory activities. (383)

55. Clinical manifestations of protein C deficiency include venous thromboembolism, neonatal purpura (in homozygous neonates), fetal loss, and warfarin-induced skin necrosis. Protein C deficiency affects approximately 1 in 500 individuals in the general population and is an autosomal dominant trait. (383)

56. From 40% to 50% of protein S circulates as the free form, the only form with APC cofactor activity. In the presence of protein S, APC inactivates factors Va and VIIIa at an accelerated rate. Protein S also serves as a cofactor for protein C enhancement of fibrinolysis and can directly inhibit prothrombin activation. (383)

57. Acquired protein C deficiency can be seen in liver disease, severe infection (especially meningococcemia), septic shock, and DIC. Acquired protein S deficiency has been associated with pregnancy, use of oral contraceptives, DIC, human immunodeficiency virus (HIV) infection, nephrotic syndromes, and liver disease. (383)

58. The antiphospholipid (antibody) syndrome (APS) is characterized by both venous and arterial thromboses and recurrent pregnancy complications. Patients with this syndrome have persistent circulating antiphospholipid antibodies (aPLs), which include lupus anticoagulant, anticardiolipin antibody, and anti-β_2-glycoprotein I antibodies. It is one of the few prothrombotic states in which arterial and venous thromboses occur. Deep vein thrombosis (DVT) is the most common venous thrombosis, and stroke is the most common arterial thrombosis. (383)

59. Lupus anticoagulant, although often found in patients with systemic lupus erythematosus, can also be associated with medications (phenothiazines, phenytoin, hydralazine, quinine, and antibiotics), inflammatory bowel disease (Crohn disease and ulcerative colitis), infections, and certain kinds of tumors. (383)

60. Catastrophic antiphospholipid syndrome is a rare accelerated form of antiphospholipid syndrome in which patients present with coagulopathy, ischemic necrosis of the extremities, and multiorgan failure in the presence of circulating aPLs. Although the syndrome is rare, the mortality rate in these patients is high, so early recognition and treatment are crucial. (383)

61. DIC is an acquired disorder caused by an underlying condition (most commonly, sepsis) that is characterized by widespread systemic activation of coagulation. This results in uncontrolled intravascular thrombin generation and fibrin deposition in small blood vessels. The formation of microvascular thrombi ultimately leads to end-organ dysfunction and multiorgan failure. Excessive consumption of circulating coagulation factors, platelets, and fibrinogen occurs simultaneously with microvascular thrombi formation, which can result in life-threatening bleeding. Therefore, a patient with DIC may present with both thrombotic and hemorrhagic complications. (383)

62. Although no single laboratory test identifies DIC, a combination of laboratory tests in the setting of a condition known to trigger DIC is sufficient for diagnosis. Laboratory abnormalities that are commonly associated with DIC include thrombocytopenia, elevated fibrin degradation products (D-dimers), prolonged PT and aPTT, and low fibrinogen. (383)

63. In patients with a known thrombophilia but no history of VTE, primary prophylaxis with anticoagulation is not recommended. The exception to this is in the cases of pregnant patients, in whom anticoagulation is often recommended in the antepartum and postpartum settings. Patients who present with VTE and test positive for an inherited thrombophilia are anticoagulated for their acute

presentation. Continuation of anticoagulation after resolution of the acute VTE is determined by severity of presentation, the presence of more than one thrombophilia, and homozygosity or heterozygosity for the thrombophilia. (384)

64. Patients with APS have a high risk of recurrent thrombosis and are most often treated with long-term anticoagulation. The goal for the anticoagulation management in these patients remains controversial. (384)

65. The mainstay of treatment for DIC is to treat the underlying cause. Supportive care for actively bleeding patients is guided by laboratory tests to ensure appropriate transfusion therapy. In patients with active bleeding and suspected fibrinolysis, antifibrinolytics such as tranexamic acid may be used. Transfusions for nonbleeding patients are typically withheld unless platelets, fibrinogen, or coagulation factors are severely low or if patients require an invasive procedure. Treatment with anticoagulation is rare and only initiated in the presence of severe thrombosis. (384)

LABORATORY EVALUATION OF HEMOSTASIS

66. Laboratory tests of coagulation include the prothrombin time, aPTT, thrombin time, fibrinogen levels, activated clotting time (ACT), and global coagulation assays (e.g., thromboelastography). (384)

67. Low levels of tissue factor, factor VII, factor II, factor V, factor X, and fibrinogen (extrinsic pathway) prolong the prothrombin time. (384)

68. The international normalized ratio (INR) is a number that standardizes reagent differences between prothrombin time results across different laboratories. The INR is useful for monitoring oral anticoagulant drug therapy with warfarin. (385)

69. Low levels of factors VIII, IX, XI, and XII (intrinsic pathway) will result in a prolonged aPTT. Adequate levels of factor II, factor X, factor V, and fibrinogen (final common pathway) must also be present for a normal aPTT. (385)

70. Drugs that can be monitored by the aPTT include heparin and parenteral direct thrombin inhibitors such as argatroban. (385)

71. The thrombin time test measures the conversion of fibrinogen to fibrin. Conditions that prolong the thrombin time test include therapy with anticoagulants, hypofibrinogenemia, the presence of abnormal fibrinogen or fibrin degradation products, high concentrations of serum proteins, and circulating bovine thrombus antibodies (after exposure during surgery). (385)

72. The ACT measures the amount of time required for whole blood to clot in a test tube. The ACT test is used clinically to monitor heparin therapy intraoperatively as the aPTT has replaced this test in other clinical situations. (385)

73. Laboratory tests of fibrinolysis include fibrin degradation products such as D-dimer levels and global coagulation assays such as thromboelastography and rotational thromboelastometry. (386)

74. D-dimers are a specific fibrin degradation product and are generated by the fibrinolytic activity of plasmin. Plasmin cleaves crosslinked fibrin. Elevated D-dimer levels are suggestive of some prior formation of crosslinked fibrin (i.e., clot) such as that caused by thrombotic or thromboembolic disorders. (386)

75. Global coagulation assays use viscoelastic measures to analyze time to blood clot formation, maximal clot stability, and resolution of clot due to fibrinolysis. (386)

76. Although viscoelastic measurements obtained by global coagulation assays can assess platelet aggregation, they do not measure platelet dysfunction. In addition, they are unable to detect the effects of vWF. (386)

77. Laboratory tests of platelet function include the platelet count, bleeding time, platelet aggregation studies, and platelet function analysis. (387)

78. Platelet clumping and the presence of giant platelets can lead to artificially decreased platelet counts, whereas the presence of cellular debris (thalassemias, leukemias, TTP) can lead to overestimated platelet counts. (387)

79. The bleeding time test is a standardized test that involves making an incision 9 mm long and 1 mm deep on the volar surface of the forearm. A blood

pressure cuff placed on the upper arm is insufflated to a pressure of 40 mm Hg. Excess blood is blotted away every 30 seconds with filter paper while not touching the edge of the incision. The bleeding time is calculated as the time passed from incision to the end of bleeding. (387)

80. A normal bleeding time is less than 11 minutes. (387)

81. Platelet aggregation studies of platelet function test the response of platelets to aggregating agents such as collagen, adenosine diphosphate (ADP), epinephrine, and ristocetin. (387)

82. A clinical use of platelet aggregation studies is the ability of the test to distinguish between different inherited disorders of platelet aggregation dysfunction. It can also be used to monitor antiplatelet therapy with aspirin or clopidogrel. (387)

83. The platelet function analysis test measures the time to platelet thrombus achieving instrument aperture occlusion. It is useful as a screening test to assess for platelet dysfunction but is not very specific for any disorder. (387)

ANTITHROMBOTICS AND PROCOAGULANTS

84. Antithrombotic drugs can be divided into antiplatelet agents, anticoagulants, and thrombolytics. (387)

85. Antiplatelet agents can be divided into three classes: cyclooxygenase (COX) inhibitors, P2Y12 receptor antagonists, and platelet GPIIb/IIIa antagonists. (387)

86. Cyclooxygenase isozyme COX-1 maintains the integrity of the gastric lining, maintains renal blood flow, and initiates the formation of thromboxane A_2, which is important for platelet aggregation. Cyclooxygenase isozyme COX-2 is responsible for synthesizing prostaglandin mediators in pain and inflammation. (387)

87. Low doses of aspirin irreversibly inhibit COX-1. High doses of aspirin irreversibly inhibit both COX-1 and COX-2, which leads to anti-inflammatory and analgesic effects. (388)

88. Because platelets have no DNA, they are unable to synthesize new COX once aspirin has irreversibly inhibited the enzyme. Despite its short half-life of 15 to 20 minutes, aspirin continues to have an effect on platelet function for its expected lifetime of 7 to 10 days. The recovery of platelet function after aspirin depends on platelet turnover. (388)

89. Megakaryocytes usually generate 10% to 12% of platelets daily, so near-normal hemostasis is expected in 2 to 3 days after the last dose of aspirin, assuming normal platelet turnover. (388)

90. Immediate reversal of the effect of aspirin on platelets can only be achieved with platelet transfusions. (388)

91. Most NSAIDs are nonselective reversible cyclooxygenase enzyme inhibitors. Selective COX-2 antagonists have also been developed. (388)

92. Because NSAIDs inhibit cyclooxygenase enzymes reversibly, platelet function returns to normal 3 days after discontinuing the use of NSAIDs. (388)

93. COX-2 selective antagonists were developed to provide pain relief without the gastrointestinal bleeding complications. A reported downside of COX-2 selective antagonists is their increased risk of cardiovascular complications. (388)

94. Platelet function is not affected by COX-2 selective antagonists because platelets do not express COX-2. The increased cardiovascular risk is likely due to inhibition of prostacyclin without inhibition of thromboxane A_2, thus tipping the balance toward thrombosis. This is why the current recommendation is to use the COX-2 selective inhibitors only when necessary and only the smallest effective dose along with low-dose aspirin. (388)

95. Clopidogrel, ticlopidine, prasugrel, and ticagrelor all belong to the class of P2Y12 receptor antagonists. They interfere with platelet function by inhibiting the P2Y12 receptor, which prevents the expression of GPIIb/IIIa on the surface of activated platelets. This inhibits platelet adhesion and aggregation. (388)

96. Platelet function normalizes 7 days after discontinuing clopidogrel and 14 to 21 days after discontinuing ticlopidine. (388)

97. Patients who are CYP2C19-poor metabolizers, which represents up to 14% of patients, have been shown to have significantly increased risk of major cardiovascular events when taking clopidogrel. This is because clopidogrel is a prodrug that requires CYP2C19 for activation. Genotype testing may be useful prior to initiating treatment with clopidogrel and is the purpose for the FDA black box warning for this drug. (388)

98. Ticagrelor has much lower interindividual variability than clopidogrel because it binds to a different site on the P2Y12 receptor to inhibit G-protein activation and signaling, and ticagrelor is not a prodrug. Because it is much shorter acting than clopidogrel, ticagrelor must be dosed twice daily. (388)

99. Some glycoprotein IIb/IIIa receptor antagonist drugs include abciximab (ReoPro), eptifibatide (Integrilin), and tirofiban (Aggrastat). The glycoprotein IIb/IIIa receptor normally mediates platelet aggregation by binding fibrinogen and von Willebrand factor. (388)

100. Clinical uses of intravenous glycoprotein IIb/IIIa (GPIIb/IIIa) receptor antagonists include stopping ongoing arterial thrombosis and eliminating excessive platelet reactivity in diseased vessels so that occlusive thrombi and restenosis do not occur. (388)

101. Of the GPIIb/IIIa receptor antagonist drugs abciximab, eptifibatide, and tirofiban, only abciximab is a noncompetitive irreversible inhibitor of the receptor. Eptifibatide and tirofiban are competitive, reversible antagonists. (388)

102. Platelet aggregation normalizes in 24 to 48 hours after discontinuing abciximab and 8 hours after discontinuing eptifibatide and tirofiban. (388)

103. Warfarin is an oral vitamin K antagonist. Vitamin K is necessary for the carboxylation of factors II, VII, IX, and X and proteins C and S. Without carboxylation these proteins cannot actively bind to the phospholipid membrane of platelets during hemostasis. (388)

104. Warfarin has a half-life of 40 hours. Complete anticoagulation effects require 48 to 72 hours to develop after its initial administration. This is due to the long half-lives of the coagulation factors it affects. Prothrombin (factor II) has the longest half-life, about 60 hours. (388)

105. The therapeutic range for warfarin is generally an INR of 2.0 to 3.0. Patients with mechanical heart valves require higher values of INR, 2.5 to 3.5. (389)

106. There are multiple concerns with warfarin therapy. Warfarin is difficult to manage because of a very narrow therapeutic window. Frequent laboratory monitoring becomes necessary because drugs, foods, and alcohol can alter the pharmacokinetic profile of warfarin. Factor VII and protein C have the shortest half-lives (3-6 hours) of the proteins affected by warfarin. Protein C is an anticoagulant, so in the early stages of warfarin treatment the balance is tipped to a hypercoagulable state. This can result in thrombosis or warfarin-induced skin necrosis. Patients who are at a high risk for thromboembolism must be bridged with another anticoagulant, usually heparin, until the goal INR is achieved. In addition, there are genetic variations of the metabolism of warfarin, such that pharmacogenetic testing may be considered when there is difficulty achieving the goal INR. Finally, warfarin is contraindicated in pregnancy because fetal exposure can lead to embryopathy. (389)

107. Unfractionated heparin indirectly inhibits thrombin and factor Xa by binding to antithrombin. (389)

108. Some benefits of unfractionated heparin for anticoagulation include its short half-life, that heparin therapy can be monitored with the aPTT or activated clotting time (ACT), and that it can be reversed with protamine, a positively charged protein isolated from salmon. (389)

109. Patients who have a hereditary insufficiency of antithrombin or an acquired deficiency of antithrombin from prolonged heparin administration may be resistant to unfractionated heparin. These patients can be treated with FFP transfusions, which will replenish the antithrombin levels. (389)

110. The full dose of dose of unfractionated heparin for cardiac surgery is 300 to 400 U/kg. An ACT greater than 400 seconds is usually considered safe for initiating cardiopulmonary bypass. At the conclusion of cardiopulmonary bypass heparin is reversed through the administration of protamine at a dose of 1 mg protamine to 100 units of heparin. (389)

111. Heparin-induced thrombocytopenia (HIT) is a hemorrhagic complication with a mortality rate of 20% to 30% caused by unfractionated heparin and, to a lesser degree, low-molecular-weight heparin (LMWH). Unfractionated heparin can stimulate the production of antibodies against the heparin–platelet factor 4 (PF4) complex. These antibodies can activate platelets to induce thrombosis and cause HIT. (389)

112. HIT should be suspected if the platelet count decreases to less than 100,000 cells/μL or less than 50% of baseline 5 to 10 days after the initiation of heparin therapy. If thrombocytopenia or thrombosis develops in a patient on heparin, HIT antibody testing should be undertaken to confirm the diagnosis. The gold standard for testing is the serotonin release assay, which is more specific than the enzyme-linked immunosorbent assay (ELISA), which is sensitive but not as specific. (389)

113. Patients with suspected HIT must be started on an alternate anticoagulant (not heparin or LMWH) immediately, while test results are pending. The most commonly used agents are the parenteral direct thrombin inhibitors such as bivalirudin, argatroban, and lepirudin. Platelet transfusions should be held unless the patient is severely thrombocytopenic (<20,000 cells/μL) with signs of bleeding. (389)

114. Warfarin is contraindicated for HIT treatment because the initial decreased synthesis of proteins C and S enhances the patient's prothrombotic state. (389)

115. Bivalirudin, the shortest acting direct thrombin inhibitor, is an alternative agent for anticoagulation in patients with a history of HIT who require cardiopulmonary bypass. If time allows, antibody titers to the heparin-PF4 complex should be measured. If titers are low, then a single dose of heparin can be considered for cardiopulmonary bypass. Presurgical treatment with plasmapheresis for rapid antibody clearance is an alternative plan, but risks and benefits should be discussed with a hematologist. (389)

116. Low-molecular-weight heparin (LMWH) and fondaparinux both act by specifically inhibiting factor Xa via antithrombin. LMWH is heparin cleaved into shorter fragments, while fondaparinux is a synthetic pentasaccharide. (389)

117. Plasma activity levels of LMWH and fondaparinux can be assessed with factor Xa levels. This may be particularly helpful in patients with renal failure because these drugs are renally excreted. LMWH and fondaparinux do not affect the aPTT assay. (389)

118. LMWH and fondaparinux have longer half-lives than heparin, allowing for their subcutaneous administration to be one to two times daily. (389)

119. Protamine can only partially reverse LMWH and has no effect on fondaparinux. (389)

120. LMWH is contraindicated in patients with HIT. Although the incidence of HIT in patients receiving fondaparinux is rare, case reports exist, so it is not approved for use in patients with HIT. (389)

121. Some direct thrombin inhibitors (DTIs) include hirudin, lepirudin, argatroban, and bivalirudin. All DTIs inhibit thrombin in its free and fibrin-bound states. This is in contrast to heparin, which inhibits only free thrombin. (389)

122. The clinical effects of DTIs can be monitored through the aPTT or ACT. All DTIs will interfere with INR to varying degrees, but argatroban will prolong INR the most, which can complicate the transition to warfarin therapy for long-term anticoagulation. (390)

123. Argatroban, with a half-life of 45 minutes, is the preferred direct thrombin inhibitor in patients with renal insufficiency because it is hepatically eliminated. Bivalirudin is a reversible DTI and is metabolized by plasma proteases

and renally excreted. It has the shortest half-life and is the drug of choice for patients with both renal and hepatic dysfunction. (390)

124. There are no antidotes for any of the DTIs, so reversal depends upon their clearance. (390)

125. Dabigatran (Pradaxa) is an oral direct thrombin inhibitor (DTI). Rivaroxaban (Xarelto) and apixaban (Eliquis) are both factor Xa inhibitors. (390)

126. Some pharmacologic advantages of the newer anticoagulant agents (dabigatran, rivaroxaban, and apixaban) over warfarin include shorter half-life, fewer interactions with food and other drugs, and predictable effects allowing for fixed daily dosing without the need for monitoring. They have also been demonstrated to be as efficient as warfarin in their clinical effects. (390)

127. Dabigatran (Pradaxa) is FDA approved for the prevention of ischemic stroke in patients with nonvalvular atrial fibrillation and for the treatment of venous thromboembolism. (390)

128. Rivaroxaban (Xarelto) and apixaban (Eliquis) are FDA approved for the use of DVT/PE prophylaxis, stroke prophylaxis in patients with atrial fibrillation, and for the treatment of venous thromboembolism. (390)

129. Although laboratory monitoring of the newer oral anticoagulant agents is not routine, it may be useful in some circumstances (life-threatening bleeding, need for emergency surgery, renal insufficiency [dabigatran]). Although not currently available, it would be useful to have tests that measure the ecarin clotting time for the DTI dabigatran or to measure an anti-factor Xa assay for the specific direct factor Xa inhibitors rivaroxaban and apixaban. (390)

130. There are no commercially available reversal agents for the newer oral anticoagulant agents dabigatran, rivaroxaban, and apixaban. There are some agents that may be used in the future, however. Idarucizumab is a specific antidote for dabigatran and acts by binding dabigatran with an affinity 350 times greater than thrombin. Andexanet alfa is a recombinant factor Xa that has been developed to reverse the factor Xa inhibitors. Ciraparatag is a small molecule that binds and neutralizes unfractionated heparin, LMWH, fondaparinux, dabigatran, rivaroxaban, and apixaban. Prothrombin complex concentrates have not yet been tested in randomized, controlled in vivo studies. Fortunately the half-lives of these newer oral anticoagulant agents are short, so supportive care and clinical management of unwanted effects may temporize until the drug effect subsides. (390)

131. Most thrombolytic agents are serine proteases that work by converting plasminogen to plasmin, which then lyses the clot by breaking down fibrinogen and fibrin. Alteplase, reteplase, and tenecteplase are recombinant tissue plasminogen activators and are fibrin-specific drugs. Streptokinase is a non–fibrin-specific drug that catalyzes systemic fibrinolysis. (390)

132. Clinical uses of thrombolytic agents include dissolving blood clots during acute myocardial infarction (within 12 hours), treating strokes (within 3 hours), and treating massive pulmonary emboli. (390)

133. Tissue plasminogen activators can be classified as both thrombolytics and anticoagulants because fibrinolysis generates increased amounts of circulating fibrin degradation products, which inhibit platelet aggregation. Surgery or puncture of noncompressible vessels is contraindicated within a 10-day period after the use of thrombolytic drugs. (390)

134. Streptokinase is highly antigenic and can cause immunologic sensitization and allergic reactions, particularly with repeated use. This limits its use in the United States, but it is still used elsewhere because of its lower cost. (390)

135. Potential causes of perioperative bleeding include surgical bleeding and failure of the hemostatic pathways. Failure of the hemostatic pathways can be due to massive blood transfusion (leading to thrombocytopenia, low fibrinogen, and coagulopathy), fibrinolysis, DIC, transfusion reactions, or an undetected bleeding disorder. (390)

136. Procoagulants may be useful in perioperative bleeding when the patient is bleeding at a rapid rate. (391)

137. Antifibrinolytic agents in use in the United States include ε-aminocaproic acid (EACA) and tranexamic acid (TXA). Both these agents are lysine analogs that competitively inhibit the binding site on plasminogen and prevent its cleavage to plasmin. The antifibrinolytic aprotinin, a serine protease inhibitor, has been removed from the U.S. market and is only available in Canada and Europe. (391)

138. Clinically, both EACA and TXA are used to decrease perioperative blood loss in cardiac surgery, liver transplantation, orthopedic surgery, and trauma. (391)

139. Recombinant factor VIIa enhances hemostasis by acting through both the intrinsic and extrinsic pathways to increase the generation of thrombin (factor II). In the tissue factor–dependent system (extrinsic system), rFVIIa binds to tissue factor at the site of vessel injury, causing activation of factor X. In the tissue factor–independent system (intrinsic system), rFVIIa binds to the surface of the activated platelet, activating factor X. Both mechanisms result in a "burst" of thrombin and fibrin generation, which leads to clot formation. (391)

140. The duration of action of rFVIIa is short, as the half-life of rFVIIa is only 2 to 2.5 hours. The initial dose may need to be repeated until the bleeding is controlled. (391)

141. Recombinant factor VIIa was originally FDA approved for use in hemophiliac patients. This drug has the ability to enhance hemostasis in patients with bleeding who may or may not have a coagulation defect, so there are many variable off-label uses of rFVIIa. These include intracranial hemorrhage, cardiac surgery, trauma, traumatic brain injury, and liver transplantation. (391)

142. A concern with the use of rFVIIa is its potential for arterial and venous thrombosis, making its prophylactic use questionable. This potential risk needs to be weighed against the potential benefit of its administration. In fact, no randomized controlled trial has been able to demonstrate a significant benefit in terms of length of stay in the intensive care unit or hospital or mortality rate with this drug. (391)

143. Prothrombin complex concentrates (PCCs) contain varying amounts of coagulation factors II, VII, IX, and X, as well as one or more types of anticoagulants (protein C or S). Three-factor PCCs differ from four-factor PCCs in that they do not contain significant amounts of factor VII. (391)

144. Clinically, PCCs are now the drug of choice for the reversal of oral anticoagulants in place of rFVIIa or FFP. (391)

145. PCCs are derived from human plasma and carry a risk of infectious and noninfectious transfusion reactions. This risk is reduced, however, through their treatment with at least one viral reduction process. (391)

PERIOPERATIVE MANAGEMENT OF ANTICOAGULATION

146. For patients who are taking vitamin K antagonists and are scheduled to undergo surgery, the current recommendation is to discontinue vitamin K antagonists (VKAs) 5 days prior to surgery and to restart 12 to 24 hours postoperatively. (391)

147. Patients who are at high risk of venous thromboembolism and are on VKAs should be managed with bridging therapy with unfractionated heparin or LMWH after discontinuation of VKAs prior to surgery. There is no clear evidence for patients who are at moderate risk for VTE, so the approach is chosen based on the individual patient and surgical risk factors. (392)

148. For those patients receiving perioperative bridging therapy with unfractionated heparin, the infusion should be stopped 4 to 6 hours prior to surgery and resumed without a bolus dose no sooner than 12 hours postoperatively. In surgeries with high postoperative bleeding risk, the resumption of heparin should be delayed to 48 to 72 hours after surgery. (392)

149. For those patients receiving perioperative bridging therapy with LMWH, the last dose of LMWH should be administered 24 hours prior to surgery, and dosing

should be resumed 24 hours postoperatively. In surgeries with high postoperative bleeding risk, restarting LMWH should be delayed until 48 to 72 hours after surgery. (392)

150. Patients who are undergoing minor surgeries, who are at high or moderate risk for cardiovascular events, or who are undergoing cardiac or vascular surgery should continue their aspirin throughout the perioperative period. Patients who are low risk for cardiovascular events and who are undergoing noncardiac surgery should discontinue aspirin therapy 7 to 10 days prior to surgery. (392)

151. Patients on dual antiplatelet therapy of aspirin and clopidogrel should discontinue clopidogrel 5 days prior to cardiac or noncardiac surgery. (392)

152. Surgery should be delayed for at least 6 weeks after percutaneous coronary placement of a bare-metal stent (BMS) and for at least 6 months after percutaneous coronary placement of a drug-eluting stent (DES). If surgery is required before this time has passed, dual antiplatelet therapy should be continued unless the risk of bleeding outweighs the risk of stent thrombosis. (392)

153. Recommendations regarding neuraxial anesthesia procedures in patients who are receiving anticoagulant or antiplatelet therapy are continually being updated into guidelines as new evidence emerges. Hospital committees may also set local practice guidelines. (393)

BACKGROUND

1. What were the circumstances of the first use of intravenous fluid replacement?
2. Were fluid infusions standard with the onset of intravenous induction agents?

OVERVIEW OF FLUID AND ELECTROLYTE PHYSIOLOGY

3. What are the goals of perioperative fluid management?
4. What percentage of body weight is made up of water?
5. Total body water is divided into which two compartments?
6. What is the average percentage of plasma in blood?
7. What role does plasma play in maintaining intravascular volume?
8. What are the daily water, sodium, glucose, and potassium maintenance requirements for adults?
9. What is the normal electrolyte composition in body compartments?

PERIOPERATIVE FLUID BALANCE

10. What effect does preoperative fasting have on intravascular volume?
11. What are the average fluid requirements on waking after 8 hours of sleep?
12. What are the current preoperative fasting recommendations regarding clear fluids?
13. How does the use of evanescent anesthetic agents alter the amount of intravenous fluids administered?
14. How does antidiuretic hormone release during anesthesia impact the calculations of intravenous fluid administration?
15. How was the concept of the "third space" developed?
16. Are fluid calculations based on the "third space" relevant?

FLUID REPLACEMENT SOLUTIONS

17. How are crystalloids classified?
18. Which crystalloid fluids are balanced salt solutions and hypotonic with respect to sodium?
19. Why are some crystalloid solutions buffered?
20. What are the concerns regarding the administration of normal saline, especially in large volumes?
21. Which fluid(s) should be used to dilute packed red blood cells and why?
22. What are the clinical uses of hypertonic saline? What are some potential drawbacks?
23. What are the indications for dextrose solution?
24. What are colloids?
25. What is the initial volume of distribution of intravenous albumin? How does albumin affect coagulation?
26. What are dextran solutions? What are their clinical uses and side effects?
27. What are hydroxyethyl starch (HES) solutions? What are their clinical uses and side effects?

CRYSTALLOIDS VERSUS COLLOIDS

28. What are the arguments for administering crystalloids versus colloids for fluid replacement?
29. What are the guidelines from the Surviving Sepsis Campaign?
30. What was the Saline versus Albumin Fluid Evaluation (SAFE) study, and what were its conclusions?

PERIOPERATIVE FLUID STRATEGIES

31. Why has it proved difficult to arrive at a simple formula for fluid replacement?
32. How was the 4:2:1 rule devised? Does it have any relevance in current clinical anesthetic practice?
33. What are some general considerations for the management of perioperative fluid replacement in current clinical anesthetic practice?
34. What are some principles for the choice of fluid and volume that should be administered for perioperative fluid replacement?

MONITORING ADEQUACY OF FLUID REPLACEMENT

35. How accurate are arterial blood pressure, heart rate, and central venous pressure measurements in determining intravascular volume status?
36. What is the clinical use of measuring arterial pulse pressure variation or stroke volume variation?
37. What role does transesophageal echocardiography (TEE) play in intravascular volume assessment?
38. Are there any noninvasive means to assess volume status?

ANSWERS*

BACKGROUND

1. Intravenous fluid replacement grew out of the worldwide cholera epidemic in the early to mid 19th century. (395)
2. Induction of anesthesia with intravenous short-acting agents, especially barbiturates, became standard practice during the second half of the 20th century. Fluid infusions were added in difficult cases only; instead, an intravenous site was secured to be used for bolus injections or blood administration, if necessary. (395)

OVERVIEW OF FLUID AND ELECTROLYTE PHYSIOLOGY

3. The goals of perioperative fluid management are to maintain intravascular volume and cardiac preload, oxygen-carrying capacity, optimal coagulation status, acid-base homeostasis, and electrolyte balance. (396)
4. Water approximates 60% of the body's total weight in the average adult. The relative percentage of body water varies, depending on age, gender, and degree of obesity. The average 70-kg individual has about 600 mL/kg, or 40 L, total body water. (396)
5. Body water is found in both intracellular and extracellular compartments. The intracellular fluid volume averages 400 to 450 mL/kg, and the extracellular fluid volume is about 150 to 200 mL/kg. The extracellular compartment comprises blood volume and interstitial volume. (396)
6. Plasma is the noncellular component of blood. The percentage of plasma in blood is a fraction of the blood, according to the hematocrit, and averages about 30 to 35 mL/kg. (396)
7. The higher oncotic pressure of plasma due to the protein component (20 mm Hg greater than interstitial pressure) helps to maintain intravascular volume. (396)

---

*Numbers in parentheses refer to pages, figures, boxes, or tables in Pardo MC, Miller RD, eds. *Basics of Anesthesia.* 7th ed. Philadelphia: Elsevier; 2018.

8. Daily maintenance requirements for adults are about 1.5 to 2.5 L of water, 50 to 100 mEq sodium, 50 to 100 g glucose, and 40 to 80 mEq potassium. (396)

9. Normally, potassium and magnesium are found in greater quantities in intracellular compartments. Sodium and calcium predominate extracellularly. More bicarbonate is also greater in plasma. Chloride is more evenly distributed between the intracellular and extracellular compartments. (396)

PERIOPERATIVE FLUID BALANCE

10. Preoperative fasting has very little effect on intravascular volume. There is a slight decrease in extracellular fluid while intravascular volume is maintained. (396)

11. The average fluid requirements on waking after 8 hours' sleep are about 250 mL in the average patient. (396)

12. Current preoperative fasting recommendations are that patients may have clear fluids for up to 2 hours before anesthesia. (396)

13. The use of evanescent anesthetic agents means that patients have a more rapid return to their preoperative state and are therefore able to drink fluids sooner following anesthesia. (396)

14. Antidiuretic hormone release during anesthesia curtails the ability of the kidneys to remove excess fluid, which makes urine output a poor guide for intravascular fluid replacement. (396)

15. The concept of the "third space" was developed based on a few experiments that do not take into account the surgical and anesthetic techniques used today. (396)

16. Fluid replacement calculations in the perioperative period are based mainly on losses from the surgical site as well as hourly needs. The concept of the "third space" is of questionable validity and relevance. (396)

FLUID REPLACEMENT SOLUTIONS

17. Crystalloids are classified as balanced, isotonic, hypertonic, and hypotonic salt solutions in water depending on the amount of electrolytes they contain. (396)

18. Lactated Ringer solution, Plasma-Lyte, and Normosol are balanced salt solutions, meaning their electrolyte composition is similar to that of extracellular fluid. They are all hypotonic with respect to sodium. (397)

19. Some crystalloid solutions are buffered to generate bicarbonate and reduce the risk of metabolic acidosis and other metabolic derangements. (397)

20. The administration of large volumes of normal saline solution may result in metabolic acidosis, hyperchloremia, and renal dysfunction. This effect may be dose dependent and may be of no clinical significance in otherwise healthy individuals. Avoiding an increased chloride concentration may reduce renal dysfunction, infections, and possibly even fatality. (397)

21. Normal saline or Plasma-Lyte may be used to dilute packed red blood cells. Lactated Ringer solution should not be used because of its calcium content. (397)

22. Hypertonic saline is restricted to use for fast onset volume expansion or control of intracranial hypertension. Potential drawbacks include its short half-life and possible hemolysis at the site of injection. (397)

23. Dextrose solution is seldom used today except for the treatment of hypoglycemia or hypernatremia. (397)

24. Colloids are synthetic starches with large-molecular-weight substances that remain in the intravascular space significantly longer than crystalloids. (398)

25. Albumin comprises 50% of plasma proteins. Administered intravenously as a 5% or 25% solution, albumin has an initial volume of distribution equivalent to the plasma volume. Intravenous albumin has no effect on coagulation. (398)

26. Dextrans are complex branched polysaccharides composed of chains of varying lengths from 3 to 2000 kDa. Clinical uses of intravenous dextran solutions include antithrombotic effects and the reduction of blood viscosity, and as an intravascular volume expander. Potential side effects of dextran solutions include anaphylactic and anaphylactoid reactions, increased bleeding times, and rarely, noncardiogenic pulmonary edema. (398)

27. Hydroxyethyl starch (HES) solutions are nonionic starch derivatives. They are also synthetic starches and modified from polysaccharides, characterized by concentration and molecular weight. Available preparations include Hespan, Hextend, Volvulen, and Volvulyte. Clinically, they are used for volume expansion, although less often than they had been in the past. Side effects of HES include a dose-dependent dilutional coagulopathy, pruritus, and acute kidney injury. (398)

CRYSTALLOIDS VERSUS COLLOIDS

28. Crystalloids, although cheaper than colloids, dilute plasma proteins and plasma oncotic pressure resulting in fluid extravasation into interstitial compartments causing edema. Colloids remain in the intravascular space longer than crystalloids but are expensive and have more complications. In addition, several studies have shown no difference in outcome when either crystalloids or colloids were used for resuscitation in critically ill patients. Resuscitation with HES was associated with increased risk of acute kidney injury and, in some studies, increased risk of mortality. (398)

29. Guidelines from the Surviving Sepsis Campaign were issued for managing patients with severe sepsis and septic shock. Fluid management recommendations include the use of crystalloids as the initial fluid choice, avoidance of HES fluids, and the use of albumin when patients require substantial amounts of crystalloid. (399)

30. The Saline versus Albumin Fluid Evaluation (SAFE) study was a randomized, controlled study that evaluated the use of albumin versus saline in almost 7000 critically ill intensive care unit patients and showed no difference in outcomes. A small subgroup of patients with traumatic brain injury had increased mortality rate when resuscitated with albumin. (399)

PERIOPERATIVE FLUID STRATEGIES

31. It has proved difficult to arrive at a formula for fluid replacement because there is little consensus as to what constitutes liberal or restricted volume amounts, studies have not been standardized, targets are varied, surgical requirements differ, and many health care providers are unwilling to change their current practice. (399)

32. The 4:2:1 rule was based on a rough estimate of a child's fluid requirements over 24 hours. It was suggested over 60 years ago and based on minimal data from the early 20th century. It has no relevance in current clinical anesthetic practice. (399)

33. Considerations for the management of perioperative fluid replacement in current clinical anesthetic practice include that the average, elective patient may not be dehydrated, insensible losses are minimal, the "third space" does not have to be replaced, hypotension after induction is better treated with vasopressors, and urine output is a poor guide. Moreover, the patient will awaken quickly and be able to take fluids orally. (400)

34. Principles for which fluids and in what volume they should be administered for perioperative fluid replacement include preference of balanced salt solutions over normal saline, limiting the volume of crystalloid administered intraoperatively, no fluid replacement of "third space" or urine output, use of colloid on a restricted basis for hypovolemia, and restricting fluid if there is more than a 1-kg weight gain. (400)

MONITORING ADEQUACY OF FLUID REPLACEMENT

35. Although arterial blood pressure and heart rate have been used to assess intravascular volume status and the need for fluid replacement for over 100 years, neither of these monitors is reliable. Arterial blood pressure reacts slowly to changes in intravascular volume status, depending on contractility of the vascular system and the presence of concomitant anesthetic agents. Intravascular fluid challenges may have very little effect on the blood pressure and heart rate, especially in the elderly on cardiovascular drugs. Also, surgical stimulation affects these signs with no change in intravascular volume status.

Central venous pressure records pressure, not volume, from the right atrium and may be maintained, even after arterial blood pressure has fallen. Moreover, it is even more unreliable in the prone or sitting position. (400)

36. Arterial pulse pressure variation and stroke volume variation are dynamic indices that can predict responsiveness to intravascular fluid administration in mechanically ventilated patients. There are several commercially available monitors that measure these indices. (400)

37. Transesophageal echocardiography (TEE) can be used to assess cardiac output and preload, making it useful to guide fluid therapy. (400)

38. Less invasive monitors have been developed and incorporate sensors on endotracheal tubes and on finger probes to measure pulse pressure variation. (400)

1. Describe the terms *lethal triad* and the *50/50 rule*.

BLOOD THERAPY PROCEDURES

2. What is the recipient's blood tested for during the routine typing of blood?
3. What is the risk of transfusing blood to patients without typing the recipient's blood?
4. How is the type and crossmatching of blood accomplished?
5. What are the three steps to the blood type and crossmatch process?
6. What is the time required to type and crossmatch blood?
7. What is type-specific blood?
8. What is the time required to test for type-specific blood?
9. What is the risk of a significant hemolytic reaction with the transfusion of type-specific blood to a patient?
10. Why are O-negative packed red blood cells used in some emergency situations?
11. For which patients is O-positive blood acceptable for emergency transfusion?
12. What is the concern regarding a patient's subsequent transfusions after the administration of O-negative packed red blood cells in an emergency situation?
13. What are the advantages of using fresh whole blood?
14. For emergency clinical events, a massive transfusion protocol may be required. What blood products and quantities can be given?
15. What does it mean to "type and screen" blood?
16. What is the chance of a significant hemolytic reaction with the transfusion of typed and screened blood to a patient?
17. What is contained in preservative solutions for the storage of blood? What is the benefit of adding adenine to the preservative solution?
18. How long can blood be stored?
19. What is the temperature at which blood is stored? Why?

DECISION TO TRANSFUSE

20. What are the considerations when deciding whether to transfuse blood?
21. What is patient blood management (PBM)?
22. What are the indications for the transfusion of blood?
23. Describe the difference between a "restrictive" and a "liberal" blood policy for blood transfusion.

BLOOD COMPONENTS

24. Name the components that can be derived from whole blood.
25. What are some advantages of using components for blood therapy instead of whole blood?
26. What is the hematocrit and total volume in a unit of packed red blood cells?
27. How much will hemoglobin concentration increase with the transfusion of a single unit of packed red blood cells to an adult?

28. Which solutions may be used to reconstitute packed red blood cells for administration?
29. What are some differences in the potential complications associated with the administration of packed red blood cells versus the administration of whole blood?
30. What is the indication for the administration of packed red blood cells?
31. What volume of acute blood loss in an adult may be an indication for transfusion of packed red blood cells?
32. What percentage of blood volume can be lost in a healthy adult before signs of hypovolemia occur?
33. What is the advantage of using whole blood for massive blood loss replacement?
34. What is the recommended ratio of packed red blood cells to fresh frozen plasma (FFP) and platelets when transfusing blood components for massive blood loss replacement?
35. What is an advantage of albumin over crystalloid solutions when administering intravenous fluid to patients with acute blood loss?
36. When is the administration of platelets indicated during surgery?
37. What are some of the risks associated with the administration of platelets?
38. What is FFP? What is contained in FFP?
39. When is the administration of FFP indicated during surgery?
40. What is cryoprecipitate? What is contained in cryoprecipitate?
41. What are some indications for the administration of cryoprecipitate?

COMPLICATIONS OF BLOOD THERAPY

42. Name some potential complications of blood therapy.
43. What is the risk of the transmission of infectious diseases with the transfusion of blood?
44. What is the United Kingdom's National Clinical Guideline Centre (NCGC) published recommendation for hemoglobin concentration as a trigger for blood transfusion in patients who do not have major hemorrhage or acute coronary syndrome?
45. What testing method was the most important factor in reducing the incidence of transfusion-transmitted infectious diseases?
46. Name some noninfectious serious hazards of transfusion (NISHOTs).
47. What is transfusion-related acute lung injury (TRALI)?
48. What are the manifestations of TRALI?
49. What is the treatment of TRALI?
50. What is transfusion-related immunodulation?
51. What is the benefit of leukoreduction?
52. What are some metabolic abnormalities that may accompany the storage of blood?
53. Why do hydrogen ions and potassium concentrations increase during the storage of blood?
54. What is the potential effect of the progressive decrease in concentrations of 2,3-diphosphoglycerate (2,3-DPG) in erythrocytes during the storage of blood?
55. What is the potential effect of citrate in stored blood on the recipient of blood transfusions?
56. What is the potential risk of hypothermia associated with the administration of blood products?
57. What are some ways in which massive blood transfusions can result in coagulation disorders?
58. When should the administration of FFP be considered and at what volume?
59. When should cryoprecipitate be considered in blood therapy?
60. What is the indication for recombinant activated factor VII, and what is its potential risk?
61. What are the various types of transfusion reactions that may occur with blood therapy?

62. What are some signs and symptoms for a transfusion reaction the clinician should monitor for during the administration of a blood transfusion?
63. Why are febrile transfusion reactions thought to occur, and how do they manifest?
64. How are febrile transfusion reactions treated?
65. Why are allergic transfusion reactions thought to occur, and how do they manifest?
66. How are allergic transfusion reactions treated?
67. Why are hemolytic transfusion reactions thought to occur?
68. What are the clinical signs of a hemolytic transfusion reaction? Which of these are masked by anesthesia?
69. What diagnostic tool provides evidence that a hemolytic transfusion reaction has occurred?
70. Why might acute renal failure and disseminated intravascular coagulation result from a hemolytic transfusion reaction?
71. What is the treatment for a hemolytic transfusion reaction?

AUTOLOGOUS BLOOD TRANSFUSIONS

72. Name the types of autologous blood transfusions.
73. Why is autologous blood used?
74. What is an acceptable schedule for the collection of predeposited blood for autologous blood transfusion?
75. How can anemia secondary to the donation of autologous blood be minimized?
76. How is the intraoperative salvage of blood for autologous blood transfusions accomplished?
77. What are some relative contraindications to the intraoperative salvage of blood?
78. What are some complications that may accompany the intraoperative salvage of blood for autologous blood transfusions?
79. What is the normovolemic hemodilution technique for blood transfusions? What are some advantages of this technique?

FUTURE DIRECTIONS

80. Describe some of the trends for transfusion of blood products.

ANSWERS*

1. A few terms have evolved to emphasize that severe complications can occur when multiple transfusions are given to a patient. The *lethal triad* is a combination of hypothermia, acidosis, and coagulopathy and indicates poor outcome in a patient. Another indicator of severity is the *50/50 rule*, which this is based on the observation that there is a 10% increase in mortality rate with every 10 units of blood given. Although an individual clinician rarely gives 50 units of blood to a patient, the 50/50 rule simply confirms the logical conclusion that patients who require increasing numbers of transfusions have very serious medical or surgical conditions with increasing mortality rates. (402)

BLOOD THERAPY PROCEDURES

2. Determination of the blood types of the recipient and donor is the first step in selecting blood for transfusion therapy. Routine typing of blood is performed to identify the antigens (A, B, Rh) on the membranes of erythrocytes. Naturally occurring antibodies (anti-B, anti-A) are formed whenever erythrocyte membranes lack A or B antigens (or both). The antibodies can cause the rapid intravascular destruction of erythrocytes that contain the corresponding antigens. (402)

---

*Numbers in parentheses refer to pages, figures, boxes, or tables in Pardo MC, Miller RD, eds. *Basics of Anesthesia*. 7th ed. Philadelphia: Elsevier; 2018.

3. The risk of transfusing blood to patients without typing the recipient's blood is a dramatic and life-threatening transfusion reaction. In this case, the transfusion would result in disastrous, rapid intravascular hemolysis and possibly death. (402)

4. Typing and crossmatching of blood are performed to test for a potential serious transfusion reaction before the administration of the blood to the recipient. The major crossmatch occurs when the donor's erythrocytes are incubated with the recipient's plasma. Incubation of the donor's plasma with the recipient's erythrocytes constitutes a minor crossmatch. Agglutination occurs if either the major or minor crossmatch is incompatible. (403)

5. There are three steps to the blood type and crossmatch process. The first phase is the *immediate* phase, in which the blood is tested for ABO compatibility at room temperature. It also tests for incompatibilities in the M, N, P, and Lewis groups. The second phase is the *incubation* phase, which tests for the presence of antibodies at 37° C. Albumin or a low ionic strength saline solution is added to the products of the first phase to cause the agglutination of weak or incomplete antibodies that are present. The last phase is the *antiglobulin* phase, in which antiglobulin is added to the products of the second phase. Incomplete antibodies in the Rh, Kell, and Kidd systems will be detected by this step. In each phase, incompatible blood will result in agglutination during the crossmatch test. (403)

6. The three steps to the blood type and crossmatch process (immediate, incubation, and antiglobulin phases) take about 45 minutes to perform. (403)

7. Type-specific blood refers to blood that has been tested and is compatible with the recipient's ABO-Rh types. The donor erythrocytes are mixed with recipient plasma, centrifuged, and observed for macroscopic agglutination. (403)

8. The time required to test for type-specific blood is typically less than 10 minutes. (403)

9. The risk of a significant hemolytic reaction related to the transfusion of type-specific blood is 1 in 1000 units transfused. (404)

10. O-negative packed red blood cells are used for transfusion in some emergency situations in which acute large-volume blood loss requires the rapid administration of blood and there is not sufficient time to perform compatibility testing for either type-specific or typed and crossmatched blood. (404)

11. O-positive blood is acceptable for emergency transfusion in all patients of adult age other than female patients of childbearing age. (404)

12. O-negative packed red blood cells can be administered in emergency situations. Because they lack the A, B, and Rh antigens, O-negative red blood cells cannot be hemolyzed by anti-A or anti-B antibodies that may be present in the patient's blood. After the administration of 2 units of O-negative packed red blood cells there is a concern that the transfusion of blood that is the patient's type may result in major intravascular hemolysis of donor red blood cells by increasing titers of transfused anti-A and anti-B antibodies. However, it is not clear if the classic practice of continuing transfusions with O-negative blood is necessary. The generally recommended approach is to switch to type-specific blood when it is available. Of note, the risk of continued use of O-negative packed red blood cells under these conditions is minor hemolysis of donor red blood cells and perhaps hyperbilirubinemia. (404)

13. "Fresh whole blood" is extremely effective in restoring normal coagulation after severe injury, and its use is associated with improved survival compared to component therapy without platelets. The effectiveness of "fresh whole blood" depends on how long it has been stored and its temperature. (404)

14. Most acute care hospitals have a massive transfusion and emergency release protocol. At the University of California, San Francisco (UCSF), the policy is to release 4 units of uncrossmatched red blood cells (type O-negative), 4 units of fresh frozen plasma (FFP), and 1 unit of platelets. The red blood cells are released in 5 minutes, and the other products are available in 10 minutes. (404)

15. Typed and screened blood refers to blood that has only been typed for the A, B, and Rh antigens and screened for common antibodies. This approach is

used when the scheduled procedure is unlikely to require transfusion of blood (hysterectomy, cholecystectomy) but is one in which blood should be available. (404)

16. The chance of a significant hemolytic reaction related to the use of typed and screened blood is approximately 1 in 10,000 units transfused. (404)

17. Solutions used to preserve blood include phosphate, dextrose, and possibly adenine. Phosphate acts as a buffer, and dextrose provides energy to the red blood cells. Adenine increases erythrocyte survival by allowing the cells to resynthesize the adenosine triphosphate needed to fuel metabolic reactions. (404)

18. Blood can be stored for 21 to 35 days depending on the storage medium. The duration of the storage of blood is determined by the requirement that there be at least 70% viability of transfused erythrocytes 24 hours after transfusion. The clinician must consider duration of storage as a criterion for selection of a blood product for transfusion. (404)

19. Blood is stored at a temperature of 1° to 6° C. This slows down the rate of glycolysis in red blood cells and increases their survival time in storage. (404)

DECISION TO TRANSFUSE

20. The decision to transfuse should be based on a combination of factors: (1) patient blood management (PBM) and preoperative anemia; (2) monitoring of blood loss; (3) assessment of how much additional blood loss may occur; (4) monitoring for inadequate perfusion and oxygenation of vital organs; (5) quantitation of intravenous fluids given overall; and (6) monitoring for transfusion indicators, especially the hemoglobin concentration. (404)

21. PBM is a multidisciplinary evidence-based approach to optimizing the care of patients who may need a blood transfusion. PBM includes all aspects of patient evaluation and clinical (medical and surgical) management surrounding the transfusion decision-making process, including the application of appropriate indications, as well as minimization of blood loss and hemoglobin concentrations. For example, patients with preoperative anemia can be treated with recombinant human erythropoietin and iron. This action can decrease the need for blood transfusions. PBM can improve patient outcomes, implement better blood utilization, and optimize cost efficiency for a hospital's laboratory. (404)

22. The fundamental indication for the transfusion of blood is to increase the oxygen-carrying capacity of the blood. Because there are no direct measures of the oxygen-carrying capacity, the hemoglobin concentration is usually the basis on which the decision to transfuse is made. A general standard of care has evolved that healthy patients with hemoglobin values greater than 10 g/dL rarely require transfusion. Those with hemoglobin values less than 6 g/dL almost always require transfusion. Blood transfusion is almost always justified when the hemoglobin value is less than 6 g/dL and is rarely justified when the hemoglobin value is greater than 10 g/dL. Oxygen transport is maximized when the hemoglobin level is 10 g/dL, such that the transfusion of blood at hemoglobin levels above 10 g/dL may provide no further benefit to the patient. The threshold for the transfusion of blood between hemoglobin values of 6 g/dL and 10 g/dL is further modified by several factors, including the patient's age and medical status, the surgical procedure, the potential for ongoing losses, and the extent to which the patient's current anemia is chronic or is due to blood loss that is acute. For example, patients with coronary artery disease who are at risk for myocardial ischemia may benefit from keeping the hemoglobin level to no less than 10 g/dL, whereas a young healthy patient may not be transfused until the hemoglobin level is 6 to 7 g/dL. The decision to transfuse blood must therefore be made on an individual basis. (405)

23. PBM has focused on the terms "*restrictive*" and "*liberal*" policies for blood transfusions that are dominated by hemoglobin value as the indicator. A liberal policy would allow giving blood when hemoglobin levels are more than 9 g/dL. A restrictive policy would allow giving of blood only when the hemoglobin value levels were 8 g/dL or lower. However, the decision to administer blood

requires a careful thought process that is based on objective clinical indications and a knowledge of transfusion medicine overall. (405)

BLOOD COMPONENTS

24. Components that can be derived from whole blood include packed red blood cells, platelet concentrates, FFP, cryoprecipitate, albumin, plasma protein fraction, leukocyte-poor blood, factor VIII, and antibody concentrates. (405)

25. The primary advantage of using components for blood therapy instead of whole blood is that a patient's specific deficiency can be directly corrected. It also allows for prolonged storage, the retention of unnecessary components for other patients who may need them, and the avoidance of transfusing unnecessary components that could potentially contain antigens or antibodies. (405)

26. In each unit of packed red blood cells, the total volume is about 250 to 300 mL, and the hematocrit is about 70% to 80%. (405)

27. A single unit of packed red blood cells will increase adult hemoglobin levels by 1 to 1.5 g/dL. (405)

28. Packed red blood cells can be administered either alone or reconstituted in crystalloid or colloid. Reconstitution with 50 to 100 mL of saline facilitates the administration of packed red blood cells. Crystalloid solutions that are hypotonic can result in red blood cell swelling and lysis and should not be used to reconstitute packed red blood cells. Examples of hypotonic solutions include glucose-containing solutions and Plasmanate. The reconstitution of packed red blood cells in solutions containing calcium (e.g., lactated Ringer solution) may result in clotting. (405)

29. Complications associated with the administration of packed red blood cells and whole blood are similar. There are some differences, however. The potential for citrate toxicity that can result from the administration of whole blood is less likely to occur with the administration of packed red blood cells simply because there is less volume of citrate infused with each unit of packed red blood cells. The removal of plasma from packed red blood cells decreases the concentration of factors I (fibrinogen), V, and VIII as compared with whole blood. (406)

30. The administration of packed red blood cells is indicated for the treatment of anemia (i.e., hemoglobin <10 g/dL). The purpose of transfusing packed red blood cells is based on measured blood loss and is used to augment the oxygen-carrying capacity of the blood by increasing the hemoglobin concentration. (406)

31. Acute blood loss in the range of 1500 to 2000 mL (approximately 30% of the patient's blood volume) may be an indication for the transfusion of packed red blood cells. The administration of crystalloids alone in this situation may jeopardize the oxygen-carrying capacity of the blood. (406)

32. In a healthy adult, up to 20% of the blood volume can be lost before signs of hypovolemia may occur in part because of compensatory vasoconstriction. (406)

33. Whole blood transfusion may be advantageous over packed red blood cell transfusion when blood losses are more than 30% of the blood volume or when massive, as in the case of trauma. Whole blood transfusion under these circumstances is associated with a decreased incidence of hypofibrinogenemia and possibly coagulopathies as compared to the administration of packed red blood cells alone. (406)

34. When transfusing blood components to replace massive blood loss as in trauma, a proposed recommended ratio is 1.5 units packed red blood cells to 1.0 unit of FFP, and 1.0 unit of platelets for every 6.0 units of packed red blood cells. (406)

35. An advantage of albumin over crystalloid solutions when administering intravenous fluid to patients with acute blood loss is that the expansion of intravascular volume can be achieved more rapidly, as well as for a longer duration (about 12 hours). In large volumes (>20 mL/kg) the administration of colloids such as albumin may result in coagulation defects. (406)

36. The administration of platelets during surgery is usually indicated for platelet counts less than 50,000 cells/mm³. Both laboratory analysis and the clinical situation must be taken into consideration. For instance, in cases of surgical

trauma or in cases of bleeding in the brain, eye, or airway, the transfusion of platelets at a larger number may be warranted. (406)

37. Risks associated with the administration of platelets include the transmission of viral diseases and sensitization to the human leukocyte antigens present on the platelet cell membranes. Bacterial contamination is more likely with platelet transfusion than with any other blood product because they are stored at room temperature. Although the risk is small (<1/5000), platelet-related sepsis should be considered in a patient who develops a fever a few hours after receiving platelet therapy. The proper diagnosis can be confused with transfusion-related acute lung injury (TRALI). (406)

38. FFP is the plasma portion of 1 unit of donated blood. The plasma is frozen within 6 hours of collection. All plasma proteins are contained in FFP, including all the coagulation factors except platelets. This includes factors V and VIII, which decrease in concentration during the storage of packed red blood cells. (407)

39. The administration of FFP is indicated during surgery when the prothrombin time (PT) and partial thromboplastin time are longer than 1.5 times normal and there is a clinical indication of the need to transfuse. Other indications include the need to reverse warfarin therapy, for the management of heparin resistance, or for the correction of known factor deficiencies. (407)

40. Cryoprecipitate is the plasma fraction that precipitates when FFP is thawed. Cryoprecipitate contains high concentrations of factor VIII, von Willebrand factor, factor XIII, fibrinogen, and fibronectin. (407)

41. Cryoprecipitate is useful for the treatment of factor VIII deficiency as in hemophilia A, von Willebrand factor deficiency, and fibrinogen deficiency (e.g., from FFP). The transfusion of cryoprecipitate should be considered when fibrinogen levels are less than 100 mg/dL. (407)

COMPLICATIONS OF BLOOD THERAPY

42. The leading causes of fatal outcomes associated with blood therapy are TRALI, transfusion-associated circulatory overload (TACO), and hemolytic transfusion reactions. Fatal complications are rare. Additional complications include the transmission of infectious diseases, noninfectious hazards of transfusion (NISHOTs), metabolic abnormalities, hypothermia, coagulation, and transfusion reactions. (407)

43. Historically, the transmission of infectious diseases, hepatitis, and human immunodeficiency virus (HIV) and hemolytic transfusion reactions have probably been the most feared complications of transfusion therapy. The risk of transmission of hepatitis C and HIV have dramatically decreased to less than 1 in 1 million transfusions. In 2002, transfusion-transmitted West Nile virus occurred, but by 2003 universal screening reduced the risk to that of HIV. As of November 2016, there were no confirmed Zika virus transmissions via blood transfusion, yet the Zika virus has been transmitted via platelet transfusion in Brazil. Other less commonly transmitted infections include Chagas disease, hepatitis B, human T-cell lymphotropic virus, cytomegalovirus, malaria, and possibly variant Creutzfeldt-Jakob disease. Health care–associated infections also exist, the concept being that transfusions make a patient increasingly susceptible to infections. Patients who are older or sicker may require more transfusions and are therefore at an increased risk for infectivity. (407)

44. The United Kingdom's National Clinical Guideline Centre (NCGC) has published major recommendations in JAMA (*Journal of the American Medical Association*). Among these guidelines is to use restrictive red blood cell transfusion hemoglobin thresholds (7 to 9 g/dL) for patients who do not have major hemorrhage or acute coronary syndrome. (407)

45. The most important factor accounting for the decrease in the transmission of infectious disease from blood transfusions is improved testing of donor blood by nucleic acid technology. Currently hepatitis C, HIV, and West Nile virus are all tested by nucleic acid technology. (407)

46. There are numerous NISHOTs, with the list dominated by TRALI and transfusion-related immunodulation (TRIM). (408)

47. TRALI is acute lung injury that occurs within 6 hours after transfusion of a blood product, especially packed red blood cells or FFP. The risk of TRALI may be decreased by excluding female blood donors and using fresher blood (i.e., storage <14 days). TRALI is the leading cause of transfusion-related deaths. (408)

48. TRALI is characterized by dyspnea and arterial hypoxemia secondary to noncardiogenic pulmonary edema. The diagnosis of TRALI is confirmed when pulmonary edema occurs in the absence of left atrial hypertension and the pulmonary edema fluid has a high protein content. (408)

49. When TRALI is suspected immediate actions to take include (1) stopping the transfusion, (2) supporting the patient's vital signs, (3) determining the protein concentration of the pulmonary edema fluid via the endotracheal tube, (4) obtaining a complete blood count and chest radiograph, and (5) notifying the blood bank of possible TRALI so that other associated units can be quarantined. (408)

50. TRIM refers to the blood transfusion suppression of cell-mediated immunity, which when combined with similar effects produced by surgical trauma, may place the patient at risk for postoperative infection. There is a suggestion of a correlation between cancer tumor recurrence and blood transfusion. However, patients who receive blood transfusions may have more extensive disease and a poorer prognosis independent of the administration of blood. Packed red blood cells may produce less immunosuppression than whole blood, suggesting that plasma contains an unidentified immunosuppressive factor. Still, it is difficult to ascertain the role of blood transfusions in postoperative infections and cancer. (408)

51. The practice of leukoreduction, the removal of white blood cells and platelets from blood, is becoming increasingly common. This reduces the incidence of nonhemolytic febrile transfusion reactions and the transmission of leukocyte-associated viruses. Speculative benefits include reductions in cancer recurrence and postoperative infections. (408)

52. Metabolic abnormalities that accompany the storage of whole blood include (1) the accumulation of hydrogen ions, (2) the accumulation of potassium, (3) decreased 2,3-diphosphoglycerate (2,3-DPG) concentrations, and (4) citrate present in the blood preservative producing changes in the recipient. (408)

53. The addition of most preservatives promptly increases the hydrogen ion content of stored whole blood. Hydrogen ions are also produced as a byproduct of continued metabolic function of erythrocytes. The net effect is a lowered pH of stored blood to as low as 7.0. The potassium content of stored blood increases progressively with the duration of storage because of a slow but constant leakage of potassium from the cells into the surrounding plasma along a concentration gradient. Despite this, the amount of potassium present in 1 unit of whole blood is usually small. (408)

54. In stored blood, there is a progressive decrease in concentrations of 2,3-DPG in erythrocytes, which results in increased affinity of hemoglobin for oxygen (decreased P_{50} values). Conceivably, this increased affinity could make less oxygen available for tissues and jeopardize tissue oxygen delivery. The clinical significance of the 2,3-DPG oxygen affinity changes remains unconfirmed. (408)

55. Citrate contained in transfused blood can be metabolized to bicarbonate and may contribute to metabolic alkalosis in the recipient, whereas binding of calcium by citrate could result in hypocalcemia. Protective mechanisms against hypocalcemia include mobilization of calcium from stores in the bone and the rapid metabolism of citrate to bicarbonate by the liver. Prior to the administration of calcium, the clinician should evaluate for objective evidence of hypocalcemia (prolonged QT intervals on the electrocardiogram and decreased plasma ionized calcium concentration measurements). Supplemental calcium may

be needed when (1) the rate of blood infusion is more rapid than 50 mL/min, (2) hypothermia or liver disease interferes with the metabolism of citrate, or (3) the patient is a neonate. Citrate intoxication is likely to occur in patients undergoing liver transplantation, and these patients may require calcium administration during a massive transfusion. (409)

56. Because blood is stored at a temperature below 6° C, the administration of stored blood to a patient can result in decreases in body temperature. Intraoperative hypothermia can lead to intraoperative cardiac irritability, especially in the presence of arterial pH abnormalities. Postoperative hypothermia can lead to shivering and increased myocardial oxygen demand. This risk can be minimized by administering the blood through warmers. It is prudent to confirm that the blood is being warmed to an appropriate temperature of 37° C to 38° C because red blood cells will hemolyze if overheated. Blood warmers are designed to make this unlikely. (409)

57. Massive blood transfusions can result in two different coagulation disorders: a dilutional thrombocytopenia and a dilution of some of the coagulation factors necessary to clot blood. Either case may manifest clinically as continued frank bleeding without clotting in the surgical site. It may also manifest as hematuria, gingival bleeding, and spontaneous oozing from various puncture areas in both surgical and nonsurgical sites, such as sites of intravenous access. If this clinical situation is noted, disseminated intravascular coagulation and a hemolytic transfusion reaction should also be considered as a potential source for the bleeding abnormalities. (409)

58. The administration of FFP should be considered when the PT is longer than 1.5 times normal, or the international normalized ratio is more than 2.0. If laboratory tests are unavailable, FFP administration should be considered after the transfusion of one blood volume (about 70 mL/kg) in the presence of microvascular bleeding. The dose of FFP should achieve at least 30% of most plasma factor concentrations. This amounts to about 10 to 15 mL/kg volume of FFP. (409)

59. Low blood fibrinogen levels are associated with coagulopathies and massive blood transfusions. Cryoprecipitate should be considered if fibrinogen levels are less than 100 mg/dL. Also, a highly purified lyophilized virus-inactivated fibrinogen concentrate from human plasma can be used to treat hypofibrinogenemia and is effective in some broader coagulopathies. (409)

60. Recombinant activated factor VII may be considered as a "rescue" drug when standard therapy has failed to treat coagulopathy manifested as microvascular bleeding. Recombinant activated factor VII seems to enhance thrombin formation on already activated platelets but also carries the potential risk of inducing thromboembolic complications. (409)

61. The types of transfusion reactions that may occur with blood therapy include febrile, allergic, and hemolytic transfusion reactions. (409)

62. During the administration of a blood transfusion, the clinician should monitor for signs and symptoms of bacterial contamination and TRALI, as well as for other transfusion reactions including urticaria, hypotension, tachycardia, increased peak airway pressure, hyperthermia, an acute change in urine output, hemoglobinuria, and microvascular bleeding. However, anesthesia, particularly general anesthesia, can mask the signs and symptoms for all types of transfusion reactions. (409)

63. Febrile transfusion reactions are thought to occur from antibodies in the recipient's serum interacting with antigens from the donor's cells. Febrile transfusion reactions are the most frequently occurring transfusion reaction, accompanying 0.5% to 1% of transfusions. A febrile transfusion reaction may manifest as fever (rarely above 38° C), chills, headache, myalgia, nausea, and a nonproductive cough occurring after the initiation of the transfusion of blood. (410)

64. Febrile transfusion reactions are treated by slowing the infusion of blood and administering antipyretics. Severe cases accompanied by chills and shivering may require discontinuation of the blood transfusion. (410)

65. Allergic transfusion reactions are thought to occur because of the presence of incompatible plasma proteins in the donor blood. Allergic transfusion reactions manifest as increases in body temperature, urticaria, pruritus, and occasionally facial swelling. (410)

66. The treatment of an allergic transfusion reaction is through the intravenous administration of antihistamines. There are more severe cases of allergic transfusion reactions that are anaphylactic without red blood cell destruction. Those cases are believed to be due to the transfusion of IgA to patients who are IgA deficient. In such situations, the blood transfusion should be discontinued. (410)

67. Hemolytic transfusion reactions occur when the wrong type of blood is administered to a patient. Transfused donor cells are attacked by the recipient's antibody, resulting in intravascular hemolysis and the development of spontaneous hemorrhage by activation of the complement system. As little as 10 mL of donor blood can result in a hemolytic transfusion reaction, which can be fatal. The severity of a transfusion reaction can be proportional to the volume of transfused blood. (410)

68. The immediate clinical signs of a hemolytic transfusion reaction include hypotension, lumbar and substernal pain, fever, chills, dyspnea, and skin flushing. These signs, except possibly hypotension, can be masked by anesthesia. (410)

69. The appearance of hemoglobin in plasma or urine (sometimes a brown color) is presumptive evidence of a hemolytic reaction. Hemoglobinuria is often the first clear sign of a hemolytic transfusion reaction. When a fever occurs after a transfusion has been started, a febrile transfusion reaction can be distinguished from a hemolytic transfusion reaction by evaluating the serum and the urine for hemolysis. (410)

70. Following a hemolytic transfusion reaction acute renal failure reflects precipitation of stromal and lipid contents (not free hemoglobin) of hemolyzed erythrocytes in distal renal tubules. Disseminated intravascular coagulation causing a coagulopathy can be initiated by material released from hemolyzed erythrocytes. (410)

71. Treatment of a hemolytic transfusion reaction is immediate discontinuation of the incompatible blood transfusion and maintenance of urine output by infusion of crystalloid solutions and mannitol or furosemide. The use of sodium bicarbonate to alkalinize the urine and improve solubility of hemoglobin degradation products in the renal tubules is of unproven value. The administration of corticosteroids for treatment is also unproved. (410)

AUTOLOGOUS BLOOD TRANSFUSIONS

72. The types of autologous blood transfusion are (1) predeposited (preoperative) autologous donation (PAD), (2) intraoperative and postoperative blood salvage, and (3) normovolemic hemodilution. (410)

73. There are two primary reasons to use autologous blood. One is to decrease or eliminate complications from allogeneic blood transfusions such as transfusion reactions and transmission of blood-borne diseases. The second reason is to conserve blood resources. Autologous blood donations reserve blood bank stores for other patients, thus decreasing the strain on blood bank resources. Of note, PAD is more expensive and not very effective in reducing allogeneic blood transfusions. (410)

74. For patients to donate autologous blood for transfusion, they must have a hemoglobin concentration of at least 11 g/dL. Most patients can donate 10.5 mL/kg of blood approximately every 5 to 7 days (maximum 2 to 3 units), with the last unit collected 72 hours or more prior to surgery to permit restoration of plasma volume. (410)

75. Anemia secondary to the donation of autologous blood can be minimized with oral iron supplementation, which is recommended when blood is withdrawn within a few days preceding surgery. Treatment with recombinant erythropoietin is very expensive, but it increases the amount of blood that patients can predeposit by as much as 25%. (410)

76. Typically, the intraoperative salvage of blood for autologous blood transfusions is accomplished using semiautomated systems, in which the red blood cells are collected and washed. The washed red blood cells are then delivered to a reservoir for future administration intraoperatively or postoperatively. (410)

77. The presence of infection or malignant disease at the operative site is considered a contraindication to the intraoperative salvage of blood. (410)

78. Complications that may accompany the intraoperative salvage of blood for autologous blood transfusions include dilutional coagulopathy, reinfusion of excessive anticoagulant (heparin), hemolysis, air embolism, and disseminated intravascular coagulation. A documented quality assurance program, as recommended by the American Association of Blood Banks, is required for those using intraoperative blood salvage techniques. (410)

79. Normovolemic hemodilution consists of withdrawing a portion of the patient's blood volume early in the intraoperative period with the concurrent infusion of crystalloids or colloids to maintain intravascular volume. The end point is a hematocrit value of 27% to 33%, depending on the patient's cardiovascular and respiratory status. At the conclusion of surgery, the patient's blood is reinfused. The patient's blood has enhanced oxygen-carrying capacity because of a higher hematocrit and greater clotting ability owing to platelets and other coagulation factors. Besides the enhanced oxygen-carrying capacity and greater clotting ability, another advantage of the normovolemic hemodilution technique is that fewer red blood cells are lost per millimeter of blood loss during surgery. (410)

FUTURE DIRECTIONS

80. Transfusion of blood products is safer, especially as a result of the dramatic decrease of incidence of infectious disease transmission. Emphasis is being placed on defining ratios of blood products that should be given (e.g., 1:1 packed red blood cells with FFP or platelets). Whole blood may be given more often. Other possibilities include hemoglobin-based oxygen carriers (HBOCs) (synthetic blood). However, in the near feature, HBOC products may not be available. It is not clear what the impact of the length of time blood is stored will have on transfusion practice. Consistent with the practice of medicine overall, well-designed protocols will increasingly be the basis upon which transfusion practice is based. (411)

25 CARDIOVASCULAR DISEASE

Arthur W. Wallace

CORONARY ARTERY DISEASE

1. What percent of adult patients undergoing surgery are estimated to have, or be at risk for, coronary artery disease?
2. What are some components of a routine preoperative cardiac evaluation? What are some more specialized methods of cardiac evaluation?
3. What is the ultimate purpose of a preoperative cardiac evaluation?
4. What are some important aspects of the preoperative history taken from patients with coronary artery disease with respect to their cardiac status?
5. What are some coexisting noncardiac diseases that are frequently present in patients with coronary artery disease?
6. By what percent can a major coronary artery be stenosed in an asymptomatic patient?
7. What is the best indicator for a patient's cardiac reserve?
8. When is angina pectoris considered "stable"?
9. When is angina pectoris considered "unstable"? What is the clinical implication of unstable angina?
10. What is it likely an indication of when dyspnea follows the onset of angina pectoris?
11. How does angina pectoris due to spasm of the coronary arteries differ from classic angina pectoris?
12. What is silent myocardial ischemia?
13. What is the most common symptom of angina in men and women?
14. Approximately what percent of myocardial ischemic episodes are not associated with angina pectoris? Approximately what percent of myocardial infarctions are not associated with angina pectoris?
15. Is hypertension or tachycardia more likely to result in myocardial ischemia in the patient with coronary artery disease? What is the physiologic explanation for this?
16. What is the basis for the common recommendation that elective surgery be delayed until 6 months or more after a prior myocardial infarction?
17. What is the approximate incidence of perioperative myocardial infarction 6 months after a myocardial infarction? What is the approximate incidence of perioperative myocardial infarction in patients who have not had a prior myocardial infarction?
18. Within what time period after surgery do most perioperative myocardial infarctions occur?
19. What cardiac medications are patients with coronary artery disease likely to be taking? What is the recommendation regarding the patient's preoperative medicine regimen with regard to their regular cardiac medicines?
20. Which patients may benefit from receiving preoperative β-adrenergic blockers? When should they be started, and how long should they be given to the patient?

21. What information can be gained from a preoperative electrocardiogram?
22. How might myocardial ischemia appear on the electrocardiogram?
23. Complete the following table:

Electrocardiogram Lead	Coronary Artery Responsible for Myocardial Ischemia	Area of Myocardium That May Be Involved
II, III, aVF		
V_3-V_5		
I, aVL		

24. Which patients should be referred for cardiology consultation prior to surgery?
25. Name some determinants of myocardial oxygen requirements and delivery.
26. What is the difference between risk stratification and risk reduction?
27. What are the risks of recent percutaneous coronary angioplasty in surgical patients, and how do they differ with bare metal versus drug-eluting intracoronary stents?
28. What are two potential benefits of administering premedication preoperatively to patients with coronary artery disease?
29. How should anesthesia be induced in patients at risk for myocardial ischemia?
30. Why is there an increased risk of myocardial ischemia during direct laryngoscopy? What are some things the anesthesiologist may do during this time to minimize this risk?
31. What are some methods of maintenance of anesthesia that may be employed by the anesthesiologist for the patient with coronary artery disease?
32. What are some intraoperative goals for the anesthesiologist in an attempt to decrease the risk of myocardial ischemia in patients at risk?
33. What is coronary artery steal syndrome? What is its clinical significance?
34. What is a concern regarding the administration of a regional (spinal or epidural) anesthetic to patients with coronary artery disease?
35. What are some considerations an anesthesiologist should take when selecting a neuromuscular blocking drug for patients with coronary artery disease? What is unique about pancuronium in this situation?
36. How should neuromuscular blockade be reversed in patients with coronary artery disease?
37. What are some factors that influence the intensity of intraoperative monitoring by the anesthesiologist?
38. When might an intraoperative pulmonary artery catheter be useful? What information does it provide?
39. What is some information that may be provided by an intraoperative transesophageal echocardiogram?
40. What are some treatment options when myocardial ischemia is detected intraoperatively?
41. What is the problem with decreases in body temperature that may occur intraoperatively in patients with coronary artery disease?
42. Why is it important to monitor heart rate postoperatively in the patient with coronary artery disease?

VALVULAR HEART DISEASE

43. What information can be gained from Doppler echocardiography in patients with valvular heart disease?
44. How should anesthetic drugs and neuromuscular blocking drugs be selected for the patient with valvular heart disease?
45. When is it important to administer antibiotics to patients with known valvular heart disease?
46. What is mitral stenosis? How does it affect left atrial and pulmonary venous pressures? At what chronic left atrial pressure is an increase in pulmonary vascular resistance likely to be seen?

47. What is the most common cause of mitral stenosis? How does it present?
48. Why are patients with mitral stenosis at an increased risk of atrial fibrillation?
49. Why are patients with mitral stenosis at an increased risk of thrombus formation in the left atrium?
50. How should medication therapy for mitral stenosis be managed in the perioperative period?
51. What are some anesthetic considerations for patients with mitral stenosis?
52. How can the maintenance of anesthesia be achieved in patients with mitral stenosis?
53. How might the adequacy of intravascular fluid replacement be monitored in patients with mitral stenosis? Why is this important?
54. Why might the mechanical support of ventilation be required postoperatively in patients with mitral stenosis?
55. What is mitral regurgitation? How is mitral regurgitation reflected on the recording of pulmonary artery occlusion pressure tracings?
56. What are the most common causes of mitral regurgitation?
57. What are some anesthetic considerations for patients with mitral regurgitation?
58. How can the maintenance of anesthesia be achieved in patients with mitral regurgitation?
59. What is aortic stenosis? How is the severity of aortic stenosis estimated? What is considered to be hemodynamically significant aortic stenosis?
60. Name at least two causes of aortic stenosis. What is the natural course of aortic stenosis?
61. Why might patients with aortic stenosis have angina pectoris despite the absence of coronary artery disease?
62. How is aortic stenosis diagnosed on cardiac auscultation? Why is it important for the anesthesiologist to rule out aortic stenosis by auscultation preoperatively?
63. What are some anesthetic considerations for the patient with aortic stenosis?
64. What would result from tachycardia, bradycardia, or decreases in systemic vascular resistance in the patient with aortic stenosis?
65. How can the maintenance of anesthesia be achieved in patients with aortic stenosis?
66. How should the intravascular fluid status be managed intraoperatively in patients with aortic stenosis?
67. In patients with chronic aortic stenosis, why might the pulmonary artery occlusion pressure not be reflective of the left ventricular end-diastolic volume?
68. How effective are external cardiac compressions in patients with aortic stenosis during cardiopulmonary arrest?
69. What is aortic regurgitation? What is the effect of chronic aortic regurgitation on the left ventricle?
70. What is acute aortic regurgitation most likely due to? What is chronic aortic regurgitation most likely due to?
71. Why might a patient with aortic regurgitation have angina pectoris despite the absence of coronary artery disease?
72. What are the goals for the anesthetic management of aortic regurgitation? The anesthetic management of aortic regurgitation resembles the anesthetic management for which other valvular disease?
73. What is mitral valve prolapse? What percent of the adult population is estimated to have mitral valve prolapse?
74. What are some other conditions associated with mitral valve prolapse?
75. What symptoms do most patients with mitral valve prolapse have?
76. What are some potential complications of mitral valve prolapse?
77. What is the goal of the maintenance of anesthesia in patients with mitral valve prolapse? How should the intravascular fluid volume status be managed in patients with mitral valve prolapse?

78. What is the potential problem with regional anesthesia in patients with mitral valve prolapse?

DISTURBANCES OF CARDIAC CONDUCTION AND RHYTHM

79. What are some tools available to the clinician for the diagnosis of disturbances in cardiac conduction and rhythm?

80. What are some types of conduction defects? Are conduction defects above or below the atrioventricular node usually permanent?

81. Is the placement of a prophylactic artificial cardiac pacemaker before surgery indicated in a patient with a bifascicular block? Why or why not? What is the theoretical concern?

82. How is third-degree atrioventricular heart block treated? What are the various methods by which this can be accomplished? How can third-degree heart block be treated pharmacologically?

83. What is sick sinus syndrome? How does it present? How is it treated?

84. What are ventricular premature beats? What are the hallmark features of a ventricular premature beat on an electrocardiogram?

85. When do premature ventricular beats warrant treatment? How are they treated under these circumstances?

86. What may be some causes of ventricular premature beats?

87. When is ventricular tachycardia diagnosed? How can it be treated?

88. What are preexcitation syndromes?

89. What is Wolff-Parkinson-White (WPW) syndrome? What is the incidence of WPW syndrome in the general population? How is it characterized on the electrocardiogram?

90. What is the most common cardiac dysrhythmia associated with WPW syndrome? How can it be treated?

91. What is the goal of the anesthetic management of a patient with WPW syndrome?

92. What are the various methods by which paroxysmal atrial tachycardia or fibrillation may be treated in the perioperative period in patients with WPW syndrome?

93. What is prolonged QT interval syndrome? What adverse events are associated with a prolonged QT interval? How can they be treated pharmacologically?

94. What is a congenital cause of prolonged QT interval syndrome? How is a stellate ganglion block thought to work for this?

95. What is the goal of the anesthetic management of a patient with a chronically prolonged QT interval?

ARTIFICIAL CARDIAC PACEMAKERS

96. What should be included in the preoperative evaluation of the patient with an artificial cardiac pacemaker?

97. How should the pacemaker be evaluated by the anesthesiologist preoperatively?

98. Why might an automatic defibrillator device need to be inactivated for surgery requiring electrocautery?

99. What intraoperative monitoring is important in a patient with an artificial cardiac pacemaker?

100. What can occur if the ground plate for electrocautery is placed too near the pulse generator of the artificial cardiac pacemaker?

101. How is the selection of drugs or anesthetic techniques altered by the presence of an artificial cardiac pacemaker in a patient?

102. Why should a magnet be kept in the operating room intraoperatively for a patient with an artificial cardiac pacemaker undergoing anesthesia?

103. What are some causes of temporary pacemaker malfunction? When is placement of a pulmonary artery catheter in a patient with an artificial cardiac pacemaker a risk?

104. How should intraoperative artificial cardiac pacemaker failure be managed?

ESSENTIAL HYPERTENSION

105. What is the definition of essential hypertension? What is the benefit of the long-term treatment of patients with essential hypertension?
106. What should be included in the preoperative evaluation of a patient with essential hypertension?
107. How should blood pressure medications be managed in the perioperative period in the patient with essential hypertension?
108. What other medical problems are frequently seen in patients with essential hypertension? Approximately what percent of patients with peripheral vascular disease can be assumed to have 50% or greater stenosis of one or more coronary arteries even in the absence of symptoms?
109. How is the curve for the autoregulation of cerebral blood flow altered in patients with essential hypertension?
110. What is the value of treating essential hypertension in patients before an elective procedure?
111. How do patients with essential hypertension frequently respond physiologically to the induction of anesthesia with intravenous medications? Why is this thought to occur?
112. How do patients with essential hypertension frequently respond physiologically to direct laryngoscopy? What are these patients at risk for during this time? How can this response be attenuated?
113. What is the goal of the anesthetic management of patients with essential hypertension?
114. How can the maintenance of anesthesia in patients with essential hypertension be achieved?
115. How might intraoperative hypotension be managed by the anesthesiologist in patients with essential hypertension?
116. What is the potential problem with regional anesthesia in patients with essential hypertension?
117. How frequently does hypertension occur in the early postoperative period in patients with essential hypertension? How can it be managed?

CONGESTIVE HEART FAILURE

118. What is the correlation between congestive heart failure and postoperative morbidity? What does this suggest for the patient scheduled for elective surgery in the presence of congestive heart failure?
119. What is the goal of the anesthetic management of patients with congestive heart failure who are undergoing urgent or emergent surgery? What medicines may be useful to achieve this?
120. How does positive-pressure ventilation of the lungs affect patients in congestive heart failure?
121. For major surgery in patients with congestive heart failure, what monitoring may be necessary?
122. For peripheral surgery in patients with congestive heart failure, can regional anesthesia be selected as an anesthetic option?

HYPERTROPHIC CARDIOMYOPATHY

123. What is another name for hypertrophic cardiomyopathy? What pathophysiology defines hypertrophic cardiomyopathy? What is the stroke volume in patients with hypertrophic cardiomyopathy?
124. What is the goal of the anesthetic management of patients with hypertrophic cardiomyopathy?
125. How can intraoperative hypotension be treated in patients with hypertrophic cardiomyopathy?
126. How can intraoperative hypertension be treated in patients with hypertrophic cardiomyopathy?
127. What is the problem with using β-adrenergic agonists for the treatment of hypotension or using nitrates for the treatment of hypertension in patients with hypertrophic cardiomyopathy?

PULMONARY HYPERTENSION AND COR PULMONALE

128. What is cor pulmonale? What are some causes of cor pulmonale?
129. What are some signs and symptoms associated with cor pulmonale?
130. What are some treatment methods for cor pulmonale?
131. What is the recommendation for the patient with cor pulmonale who is scheduled for an elective surgical procedure?
132. What is the goal of the anesthetic management of patients with cor pulmonale? How can this be achieved?
133. What is the advantage of monitoring pulmonary artery pressure during surgery in patients with cor pulmonale?

CARDIAC TAMPONADE

134. What is cardiac tamponade?
135. Name some manifestations of cardiac tamponade.
136. What is the treatment for cardiac tamponade? What are some temporizing measures for patients with cardiac tamponade awaiting definitive treatment?
137. What is the goal of the anesthetic management of cardiac tamponade?
138. What effect can the induction of anesthesia and positive-pressure ventilation of the lungs have on patients with cardiac tamponade?
139. What is the recommendation for anesthesia in patients with cardiac tamponade?
140. What pharmacologic agents may be useful in patients with cardiac tamponade?

ANEURYSMS OF THE AORTA

141. What is the most frequent cause of aortic aneurysms? Do most aortic aneurysms involve the thoracic or abdominal aorta?
142. What is a dissecting aneurysm?
143. When is elective resection of an abdominal aortic aneurysm recommended?
144. What are some medical problems frequently associated with aortic aneurysms?
145. What is the goal of the anesthetic management of patients undergoing resection of an abdominal aortic aneurysm? What monitoring is warranted in these procedures?
146. When are patients with coronary artery disease especially at risk of myocardial ischemia during surgery for resection of an aortic aneurysm?
147. How should intraoperative fluids be managed during surgery for resection of an aortic aneurysm?
148. Why does hypotension frequently accompany unclamping of the abdominal aorta during surgery for the resection of an aortic aneurysm? What are some methods for minimizing the hypotension?
149. What are some concerns regarding renal function in patients undergoing aortic aneurysm repair?
150. What are some concerns regarding spinal cord function in patients undergoing aortic aneurysm repair?

CARDIOPULMONARY BYPASS

151. How is blood drained from the venae cavae during cardiopulmonary bypass?
152. What are two different types of pumps that are used to return blood to the arterial system during cardiopulmonary bypass? Which results in less trauma to blood?
153. How is blood kept from entering the heart from the superior and inferior venae cavae during cardiopulmonary bypass for mitral valve or intracardiac surgery?
154. Why does the aorta need to be cross-clamped distal to the aortic valve and proximal to the systemic arterial inflow cannula during cardiopulmonary bypass?
155. Why might the left ventricle need a vent during cardiopulmonary bypass? How might this be achieved?
156. How can venous drainage from the inferior and superior venae cavae during cardiopulmonary bypass be facilitated?

157. What is the required cardiac index delivered by the systemic pump on the cardiopulmonary bypass machine dependent upon? What approximate cardiac index is usually sufficient?
158. What is the advantage of low flows during cardiopulmonary bypass?
159. What are two different types of oxygenators that are used to oxygenate blood that is returning to the arterial system during cardiopulmonary bypass?
160. What is the advantage of a bubble oxygenator? What is the disadvantage of a bubble oxygenator?
161. What is the advantage of a membrane oxygenator? What is the disadvantage of a membrane oxygenator?
162. How are the patient's Pa_{O_2} and carbon dioxide levels controlled during cardiopulmonary bypass?
163. How can the patient's body be heated or cooled by the cardiopulmonary bypass machine?
164. What is the optimal patient temperature for cardiopulmonary bypass?
165. How is blood loss from the field recirculated to the patient during cardiopulmonary bypass?
166. What is a problem with the cardiotomy suction used during cardiopulmonary bypass?
167. How are systemic emboli from cellular debris prevented from occurring during cardiopulmonary bypass?
168. What does priming of the cardiopulmonary bypass system refer to? What is the cardiopulmonary bypass system primed with?
169. What hematocrit percent is maintained during cardiopulmonary bypass? Why is it important to hemodilute the patient's blood during cardiopulmonary bypass?
170. Why is it important to remove all air from the cardiopulmonary bypass system during cardiopulmonary bypass?
171. Why is heparin-induced anticoagulation of the patient's blood necessary during cardiopulmonary bypass? What dose of heparin is usually administered? How is the adequacy of anticoagulation confirmed?
172. What are some explanations for the low mean arterial pressure often seen after the institution of cardiopulmonary bypass?
173. What mean arterial blood pressure is typically considered acceptable during cardiopulmonary bypass?
174. Why does blood pressure slowly rise spontaneously after some time on cardiopulmonary bypass?
175. What are the dangers of hypertension while on cardiopulmonary bypass? How can hypertension under these circumstances be treated?
176. What are some methods for evaluating the adequacy of tissue perfusion during cardiopulmonary bypass?
177. Why is diuresis induced during cardiopulmonary bypass?
178. What may be the cause of an increasing central venous pressure with or without facial edema while on cardiopulmonary bypass? How can this be confirmed?
179. What may be the cause of increasing abdominal distention while on cardiopulmonary bypass?
180. What are some complications of extracorporeal circulatory support or cardiopulmonary bypass?
181. How should ventilation of the lungs be managed during cardiopulmonary bypass?
182. What is the goal of myocardial preservation during cardiopulmonary bypass?
183. What are some methods by which myocardial preservation during cardiopulmonary bypass can be achieved?

184. What is the oxygen consumption of a normally contracting heart at 30° C? What is the oxygen consumption of a fibrillating heart at 22° C? What is the oxygen consumption of an electromechanically quiet heart at 22° C?

185. How does the infusion of cardioplegia solution exert its effect of myocardial protection?

186. How is correct placement of the cardioplegia catheter confirmed?

187. How is the effectiveness of cold cardioplegia of the heart measured?

188. What are two potential negative effects of intramyocardial hyperkalemia due to cold cardioplegia after cardiopulmonary bypass? How can they be treated?

189. What are two potential sources for systemic hyperkalemia during cardiopulmonary bypass? How can the hyperkalemia be treated if it were to persist at the conclusion of cardiopulmonary bypass?

190. Why might supplemental intravenous anesthetics be administered during cardiopulmonary bypass?

191. Why is it important to monitor glucose levels in patients undergoing cardiopulmonary bypass? What is the target glucose level, and how can this be achieved?

192. Why might supplemental neuromuscular blocking drugs be administered during cardiopulmonary bypass?

193. Is supplemental anesthesia routinely required during rewarming after the conclusion of cardiopulmonary bypass?

194. What conditions in the patient must be present for cardiopulmonary bypass to be discontinued?

195. When are the aortic and vena cava cannulae removed after cardiopulmonary bypass?

196. What are some potential problems associated with persistent hypothermia after cardiopulmonary bypass?

197. What special precautions must be taken before discontinuing cardiopulmonary bypass in patients who have had the left side of the heart opened, as during valve replacement surgery?

198. What is the potential risk of air remaining in the heart at the conclusion of cardiopulmonary bypass?

199. For each of the following situations, please complete the diagnosis and appropriate therapy:

Blood Pressure	Atrial Pressure	Cardiac Output	Diagnosis	Therapy
Decreased	Increased	Decreased	–	–
Decreased	Decreased	Decreased	–	–
Decreased	Decreased	Increased	–	–
Increased	Increased	Decreased	–	–
Increased	Decreased	Increased	–	–

200. Why might a patient have posterior papillary muscle dysfunction after cardiopulmonary bypass? How would this be manifest on the pulmonary artery occlusion pressure tracing?

201. What is a mechanical addition to the pharmacologic support of cardiac output in patients with a poor cardiac output after cardiopulmonary bypass? How does it work? What physiologic alterations may interfere with its efficacy?

202. When is protamine administered after cardiopulmonary bypass? Why?

203. What are some possible side effects of protamine administration?

204. What are some pharmacologic measures than can be taken to decrease bleeding after cardiopulmonary bypass?

205. What does the perfusionist do with blood and fluid that remain in the cardiopulmonary bypass circuit after cardiopulmonary bypass?

206. Why might there be a gradient between central aortic and radial artery blood pressures in the early period after cardiopulmonary bypass? How long can this effect persist?
207. What are some intravenous anesthetics that can be used to provide sedation after cardiac surgery and in the intensive care unit prior to extubation? Which of these may reduce the risk of postoperative delirium in these patients?
208. What is off-pump coronary artery bypass graft (CABG) surgery?
209. What are some problems with off-pump CABG surgery?
210. What is the role of ischemic preconditioning during off-pump CABG surgery?
211. What are some similarities between anesthesia management for CABG surgery using cardiopulmonary bypass versus off-pump CABG surgery?
212. What are some differences between anesthesia management for CABG surgery using cardiopulmonary bypass versus off-pump CABG surgery?

ANSWERS*

CORONARY ARTERY DISEASE

1. It is estimated that 40% of adult patients undergoing surgery have, or are at risk for, coronary artery disease (CAD). (415)
2. Components of a routine preoperative cardiac evaluation include the history and physical examination, evaluation of the patient's electrocardiogram, and reviewing or ordering more specialized procedures. Specialized methods of cardiac evaluation include a Holter monitor, exercise electrocardiogram, echocardiogram, radioisotope imaging, cardiac catheterization, and angiography. (416)
3. The ultimate purpose of a preoperative cardiac evaluation is to assess the patient's risk of an adverse perioperative cardiac event, to determine whether the patient is in optimal medical condition for surgery, and to reduce operative risk. There is little to no evidence that specialized invasive cardiac testing reduces cardiac risk. Optimization of medical therapy reduces cardiac risk. (416)
4. Important aspects of the preoperative history taken from patients with CAD with respect to their cardiac status include their exercise tolerance, characteristics of their angina, and the presence of a previous myocardial infarction. It is also important to learn what cardiac medicines, including antiplatelet and anticoagulants, the patient may be taking and what the potential interactions of these are with anesthetics that may be administered for surgery. (416)
5. Noncardiac diseases that are frequently present in patients with CAD include peripheral vascular disease (PVD), chronic obstructive pulmonary disease, renal dysfunction, chronic hypertension, and diabetes mellitus. (416)
6. A major coronary artery can be stenosed by as much as 50% to 70% in an asymptomatic patient. (416)
7. The best indicator for a patient's cardiac reserve is by evaluation of the exercise tolerance. A limited exercise tolerance in the absence of significant pulmonary disease gives evidence of a decrease in a patient's cardiac reserve. Alternatively, the cardiac reserve of a patient who is able to climb two to three flights of stairs without stopping is probably adequate. Walking on level ground is a poor indicator of cardiac reserve. Shortness of breath with climbing one to two flights of stairs may indicate significant cardiac disease. (416)

*Numbers in parentheses refer to pages, figures, boxes, or tables in Pardo MC, Miller RD, eds. *Basics of Anesthesia.* 7th ed. Philadelphia: Elsevier; 2018.

8. Angina pectoris is considered "stable" when there has been no change in the patient's anginal symptoms for at least 60 days. Factors related to the angina that should be evaluated include the precipitating factors, frequency, and duration. (416)

9. Angina pectoris is considered "unstable" when there has been a recent change in the patient's anginal symptoms. Changes that should be evaluated include the degree of activity a patient can do before the onset of angina and the duration of each anginal episode. Another symptom of unstable angina is chest pain occurring at rest. The clinical implication of unstable angina is that the patient may be at risk of an impending myocardial infarction. (416)

10. Dyspnea after the onset of angina pectoris is likely an indication of acute left ventricular dysfunction due to myocardial ischemia and acute transient cardiac failure. Shortness of breath with ischemia may be secondary to acute mitral regurgitation secondary to lateral wall ischemia and papillary muscle dysfunction. (416)

11. Angina pectoris due to spasm of the coronary arteries differs from classic angina pectoris in that the pain may occur at rest but may not occur during periods of exertion. Angina of this type is associated with ST-segment changes on the electrocardiogram. This type of angina is referred to as Prinzmetal or variant angina. (416)

12. Silent myocardial ischemia is myocardial ischemia that occurs in the absence of angina. This type of angina is more common in patients with diabetes mellitus and carries the same prognosis as myocardial ischemia associated with angina. (416)

13. The most common symptom of angina in men is dyspnea on exertion. Shortness of breath with climbing stairs is very common. Walking on a flat surface does not seem to be sufficient to elicit shortness of breath until the symptoms are severe. Waking from sleep with angina is also a symptom of severe angina. Women most commonly complain of nonspecific fatigue, making identification of angina more difficult. (416)

14. Approximately 70% of myocardial ischemic episodes are not associated with angina pectoris, and myocardial infarctions are not associated with angina pectoris approximately 15% of the time. (416)

15. Tachycardia is more likely than hypertension to result in myocardial ischemia in the patient with CAD secondary to an increased oxygen consumption with a decreased duration for coronary blood flow to the left ventricle. Tachycardia results in an increased myocardial oxygen requirement as oxygen consumption is per beat combined with a decreased myocardial perfusion time. Myocardial perfusion to the left ventricle, and thus myocardial oxygen supply, occurs during diastole. Hypertension, on the other hand, leads to an increased myocardial oxygen requirement but also simultaneously increases myocardial perfusion. (417)

16. The basis for the common recommendation that elective surgery be delayed until 6 months after a prior myocardial infarction is based on numerous epidemiologic studies. These studies have shown that there is a 5% to 86% reinfarction rate in the perioperative period if previous myocardial infarction preceded the surgical procedure by less than 6 months. This rate of myocardial infarction is 1.5 to 10 times higher than if more than 6 months separated the previous myocardial infarction and the surgical procedure. (417)

17. The approximate incidence of perioperative myocardial infarction 6 months or more after a myocardial infarction is 5% to 6%, whereas the approximate incidence of perioperative myocardial infarction in patients who have not had a prior myocardial infarction is 0.13%. (417)

18. Most perioperative myocardial infarctions occur in the first 48 to 72 hours after surgery. (417)

19. Cardiac medications that patients with CAD are likely to be taking include β-adrenergic antagonists, nitrates, calcium channel blockers, antihypertensives, antiplatelet agents, anticoagulants, and diuretics. Recent work suggests a

reduction in risk if angiotensin-converting enzyme (ACE) inhibitors are held on the day of surgery and restarted soon after surgery. The overall recommendation is that patients continue taking their regular cardiac medicines throughout the perioperative period. (417)

20. Patients who have either CAD or PVD, or who have two risk factors for CAD (age ≥60 years, cigarette smoking, diabetes, hypertension, cholesterol ≥240 mg/dL), may benefit from receiving preoperative β-adrenergic blockers. Care should be taken for patients with congestive heart failure (CHF) or aortic stenosis; these patients may need slow titration of β-adrenergic blockade under the supervision of a cardiologist. Patients with a history of atrioventricular block without a pacemaker, reactive asthma, or an intolerance to β-adrenergic blockers should be excluded. The optimal time to start therapy is at the time of identification of the risk, usually by the surgeon. If not instituted sooner, atenolol or metoprolol can be started on the day of surgery (for heart rate more rapid than 55 beats/min, and systolic blood pressure higher than 100 mm Hg); however, large-dose β-adrenergic blocker therapy should not be started on the day of surgery. β-Adrenergic blockade should be continued for at least 30 days, if not longer, for patients with CAD or PVD. For patients with risk factors only, 7 days of β-adrenergic blockade may be sufficient. (417)

21. Preoperative electrocardiograms may provide evidence of myocardial ischemia, prior myocardial infarction, cardiac hypertrophy, abnormal cardiac rhythm or conduction disturbances, and electrolyte abnormalities. (418)

22. Myocardial ischemia may appear as ST-segment changes or T-wave changes on an electrocardiogram. (418)

23.

Electrocardiogram Lead	Coronary Artery Responsible for Myocardial Ischemia	Area of Myocardium That May Be Involved
II, III, aVF	Right coronary artery	Right atrium, atrioventricular node, right ventricle
V_3-V_5	Left anterior descending coronary artery	Anterolateral portion of left ventricle
I, aVL	Circumflex coronary artery	Lateral aspects of the left ventricle

(418)

24. Patients with new-onset angina, a change in angina pattern, unstable angina, angina without medical therapy, aortic stenosis, CHF, or an intracoronary stent receiving a platelet inhibitor should be referred for cardiology consultation prior to surgery. (418)

25. Determinants of myocardial oxygen requirements and delivery are related to factors that affect myocardial oxygen supply or myocardial oxygen demand. Myocardial oxygen supply is decreased by tachycardia, hypotension, increased preload, hypocapnia, coronary artery spasm, anemia, and hypoxemia. Myocardial oxygen demand is increased by tachycardia, increased wall tension, and increased myocardial contractility. A goal of the anesthetic management of patients with CAD is maintenance of the balance between myocardial oxygen supply and demand to minimize the risk of myocardial ischemia. (418)

26. Risk stratification is the identification of risk factors in patients that lead to the determination of preoperative risk. Risk stratification does not actually decrease risk, it simply identifies it. Risk reduction requires changing the care provided to the patient either through medications such as the administration of perioperative β-adrenergic blockade or through an alteration in the anesthetic or surgical plan. (418)

27. Patients with recent intracoronary stents have an increased risk of myocardial infarction and death if platelet inhibitors are withdrawn for surgery. Patients

with bare metal intracoronary stents require 1 to 3 or more months of antiplatelet therapy, and those with drug-eluting intracoronary stents may require a year or more before risk is acceptable to discontinue platelet inhibitors for surgery. Many patients who have had percutaneous intervention should be operated on while on dual antiplatelet therapy (aspirin and clopidogrel) if surgical conditions allow. (420)

28. Two benefits of administering premedication preoperatively to patients with CAD are the decrease in the secretion of potentially harmful catecholamines and the potential to prevent the increase in myocardial oxygen requirements that may occur with tachycardia and hypertension related to anxiety. (420)

29. The induction of anesthesia in patients at risk for myocardial ischemia is typically achieved with great care. The patient's standard daily medications should be reviewed and administered if there are no specific contraindications. Patients on β-adrenergic blockers should receive them. A preinduction intra-arterial line may help recognize hemodynamic perturbations reducing risk. Prophylactic initiation of infusions of phenylephrine are helpful to reduce hypotension on induction. Careful administration of intravenous induction agents, narcotics, and inhaled agents, combined with monitoring and careful vasoconstrictor use, is essential. It is important to avoid tachycardia with associated increases in myocardial oxygen requirements. (420)

30. Direct laryngoscopy is associated with an increased risk of myocardial ischemia because it often produces intense sympathetic nervous system stimulation leading to tachycardia and hypertension. To minimize this risk, there must be adequate levels of anesthesia to suppress sympathetic nervous system stimulation. Volatile anesthetics, intravenous anesthetics other than ketamine, opioids, and lidocaine may all be used to blunt the response to direct laryngoscopy. β-Adrenergic antagonists may be administered before induction to attenuate the increase in heart rate and blood pressure that can occur. (420)

31. The maintenance of anesthesia for the patient with CAD may be achieved through the administration of volatile anesthetics, propofol, dexmedetomidine, and opioids, with or without nitrous oxide. The key goal is to avoid tachycardia and hypotension. (421)

32. In an attempt to decrease the risk of a perioperative myocardial infarction in patients at risk, the anesthesiologist should attempt to maintain stable patient hemodynamics. In general, the desired hemodynamics to minimize the risk of intraoperative ischemia include slower heart rates, lower filling pressures, and normal systolic blood pressures. A common recommendation for patients at risk of myocardial ischemia is that heart rate and blood pressure be maintained within 20% of awake values intraoperatively. Even so, approximately 50% of all new perioperative myocardial ischemic episodes are not preceded by or associated with changes in heart rate or blood pressure. Heart rates above 100 beats/min may increase risk of cardiac morbidity. Heart rates above 120 beats/ min, in patients at risk, increase perioperative cardiac risk. Systolic blood pressure below 60 mm Hg or mean blood pressure below 65 mm Hg increases risk. Diastolic blood pressure below 30 mm Hg increases risk. The duration of tachycardia and hypotension increases risk in a dose-response–related fashion. The anesthesiologist may choose to closely monitor the patient's more limited hemodynamic status using invasive monitors to achieve these goals. He or she should also be prepared to intervene quickly with pharmacologic interventions should they become necessary. (422)

33. Coronary artery steal syndrome is a theoretical risk in which administration of a coronary artery vasodilator to a patient with CAD could result in diversion of blood flow from the ischemic areas, in which stenotic coronary arteries are maximally dilated, to areas in which the coronary arteries are patent and able to vasodilate. Isoflurane is a potent coronary vasodilator, and it was once thought that isoflurane might lead to coronary steal. Clinical testing of the administration of isoflurane to patients with CAD has not been shown

to increase the risk of myocardial ischemia through the coronary artery steal syndrome. (422)

34. The administration of a regional (spinal or epidural) anesthetic to patients with CAD can result in hypotension, which may in turn lead to decreased blood flow through pressure-dependent stenosed coronary arteries. For this reason, it is important for the anesthesiologist to be prepared to treat decreases in blood pressure that may accompany the induction of any anesthetic. An advantage of regional anesthesia for patients with CAD is that the anesthesiologist may continue to monitor the patient for symptoms of angina and treat them accordingly. (422-424)

35. Considerations in the selection of a neuromuscular blocking drug for patients with CAD should take into account the effects of the neuromuscular blocking drug on the cardiovascular system. For example, a neuromuscular blocking drug that may lower blood pressure through the release of histamine should be administered slowly to minimize those effects. Pancuronium causes mild increases in heart rate and blood pressure that may or may not be beneficial, depending on the status of the patient. (422-424)

36. Neuromuscular blockade may be reversed in patients with CAD in the usual manner with an anticholinesterase-anticholinergic drug combination. Care should be taken to avoid tachycardia and subsequent myocardial ischemia with reversal. Glycopyrrolate has less of a chronotropic effect on the heart than atropine, but either glycopyrrolate or atropine is acceptable for the reversal of neuromuscular blockade. Alternatively, avoiding reversal by appropriate timing and choice of nondepolarizing muscle relaxants can reduce the risk of tachycardia and other side effects of nondepolarizing muscle relaxant reversal. Sugammadex may allow reversal of nondepolarizing muscle relaxants without the risk of tachycardia or other side effects from the combination of cholinesterase inhibitor and anticholinergic. (422-424)

37. The intensity of intraoperative monitoring the anesthesiologist chooses to implement for a surgical procedure in a patient with CAD is influenced by the type of procedure the patient is undergoing, the severity of the patient's disease, the choice of anesthetic technique, and a risk-benefit analysis of each type of potential monitoring. One must remember that the induction of general anesthesia for even a "simple" case may result in hemodynamic collapse. The risk from the induction of general anesthesia is independent of the scheduled case, case type, case complexity, case duration, or surgical service caring for the patient. (422-424)

38. There is no proven clinical benefit to the use of a pulmonary artery (PA) catheter. PA catheters may be useful in patients with poor left ventricular function, valvular heart disease, a recent myocardial infarction, pulmonary vascular disease, in situations of massive trauma, or in major vascular surgery. Information provided by a PA catheter includes more accurate assessment of cardiac filling pressures than a central venous monitor in the presence of pulmonary vascular disease, left-sided heart dysfunction, or potential left-sided heart dysfunction due to myocardial ischemia. The PA catheter can be used to measure cardiac output and calculate systemic vascular resistance (SVR). If a patient has cardiac risk that supports the use of a PA catheter, he or she likely should have simultaneous continuous transesophageal echocardiography (TEE) to provide context to the PA catheter measurements. (422-424)

39. Information provided by an intraoperative transesophageal echocardiogram includes both functional and anatomic information including early detection of myocardial ischemia through the presence of new-onset regional wall motion abnormalities, an assessment of the intravascular fluid volume status of the patient, an estimation of the cardiac output, an estimation of left ventricular afterload, and an evaluation of the cardiac valves. (422-424)

40. The detection of intraoperative myocardial ischemia should promptly lead to the treatment of any hemodynamic alterations in an attempt to increase

myocardial oxygen supply while decreasing myocardial oxygen demand. Stabilizing hemodynamics with control of heart rate and blood pressure is critical. Tachycardia may be treated with a β-adrenergic antagonist. These drugs decrease the demand of the myocardium for oxygen through its effects of decreases in heart rate and myocardial contractility. Administration of any medication should be judicious in patients with left ventricular dysfunction. Hypertension may be treated with a nitrate. Nitroglycerin may also be used in a situation in which there are ischemic changes on the electrocardiogram but blood pressure remains normal to high. Intravenous nitroglycerin administration may lead to reflex tachycardia. Hypotension may be treated with a sympathomimetic drug and intravascular fluids. Anticoagulation with a heparin bolus and infusion, combined with the administration of aspirin, may be appropriate. (424-425)

41. Decreases in body temperature that may occur intraoperatively in patients with CAD can result in shivering on awakening. Shivering can significantly increase myocardial and systemic oxygen requirements and can be especially detrimental to patients with CAD because it is often accompanied by tachycardia. (425)

42. It is important to control heart rate postoperatively to avoid myocardial ischemia. Control of pain, stress, volume status, and administration of anti-ischemic agents is essential in the patient with CAD. Intensive monitoring may need to be continued in the postoperative period in selected patients. Tachycardia from any cause (including pain, hypovolemia, atrial fibrillation, and stress) increases myocardial oxygen requirements and is detrimental to the patient with CAD. (425)

VALVULAR HEART DISEASE

43. Information that can be gained from Doppler echocardiography in patients with valvular heart disease includes the significance of cardiac murmurs, hemodynamic abnormalities, transvalvular pressure gradients, the orifice area of the cardiac valve, and the evaluation of prosthetic valve function. (425)

44. Anesthetic drugs and neuromuscular blocking drugs should be selected for the patient with valvular heart disease based on the effects they may have on cardiac rhythm, heart rate, blood pressure, SVR, and pulmonary vascular resistance. The objective is to choose anesthetic drugs and neuromuscular blocking drugs that will not compromise cardiac output with their administration. (425)

45. Antibiotics are administered to patients with known valvular heart disease prophylactically to protect the patient from infective endocarditis. Administration of prophylactic antibiotics is now recommended for patients with congenital heart disease, prosthetic heart valves, patients with a history of infective endocarditis, or heart transplant patients with a developing cardiac valvulopathy. Prophylaxis is recommended to minimize the risk of infection from a bacteremic event, such as surgical or dental procedures. Bacteremia does not seem to occur with orotracheal intubation, but it may occur with nasotracheal intubation independent of any surgical event. The specific recommended prophylaxis regimens vary depending on the site of surgery, mechanism of administration, and any history of allergies to antibiotics the patient may have. (425)

46. Mitral stenosis is a mechanical obstruction to left ventricular diastolic filling secondary to a decrease in the orifice of the mitral valve. Measurement of the mitral valve area provides for the best indication of the severity of the disease. Mitral stenosis is classified as severe when the mitral valve area is less than 1 cm^2. Left atrial and pulmonary venous pressures are increased in patients with mitral stenosis. An increase in pulmonary vascular resistance is likely to be seen when the left atrial pressure is higher than 25 mm Hg on a chronic basis. (425)

47. The most common cause for mitral stenosis is rheumatic heart disease. The mitral valve leaflets often fuse, scar, and fibrose during the healing process of acute rheumatic carditis. Mitral stenosis presents after a prolonged course of development, usually about 20 years after the initial episode of rheumatic fever. Often the disease presents with atrial fibrillation or when there is an increased demand for cardiac output, as may occur during pregnancy or exercise. Patients with mitral stenosis may have recurrent episodes of pulmonary edema, dyspnea, paroxysmal nocturnal dyspnea, chest pains, palpitations, and fatigue. (426)

48. Patients with mitral stenosis are at an increased risk of atrial fibrillation secondary to the distention and stretch of the left atrium. (426)

49. Patients with mitral stenosis are at an increased risk of thrombus formation in the left atrium because of the stasis of blood in the atrium. Thrombi in the left atrium may be ejected from the heart as systemic emboli. (426)

50. Patients with mitral stenosis are commonly on medication for heart rate control (e.g., digitalis), diuretics, and anticoagulants. Medications for rate control should be continued throughout the perioperative period, with a goal for ventricular rate less than 80 beats/min. Diuretic medications may be held preoperatively on a case-dependent basis. Anticoagulants should be discussed with the surgeon, and depending on the surgical case, patients may be switched to heparin therapy prior to surgery. (426)

51. Considerations for the anesthetic management of patients with mitral stenosis include maintenance of a normal sinus rhythm and heart rate, maintenance of a normal intravascular fluid volume, and the avoidance of increases in pulmonary vascular resistance. A preinduction intra-arterial line may facilitate identification and treatment of hemodynamic changes in patients with significant disease. Patients with mitral stenosis have a greater reliance on atrial contraction for left ventricular filling. Alterations from sinus rhythm should be promptly treated chemically or with cardioversion. Tachycardia and bradycardia may both result in decreases in left ventricular filling. The intravascular fluid volume should be maintained at near-normal or maximally tolerated levels, while avoiding pulmonary edema. Increases in pulmonary vascular resistance and pulmonary hypertension may place the patient at an increased risk for pulmonary artery rupture with placement of a pulmonary artery catheter and repeated wedge pressure measurements. Care should be taken to avoid overtransfusion and the head-down position in these patients. Arterial hypoxemia or hypercarbia may exacerbate pulmonary hypertension and precipitate right ventricular failure and should be avoided. Central venous pressure monitoring may be useful to detect changes in the right ventricular pressure. (426)

52. The maintenance of anesthesia can be achieved in patients with mitral stenosis through the administration of volatile anesthetics, nitrous oxide, and opioids. Of greater importance is the management of the cardiovascular effects of these drugs to achieve the goal of the anesthetic management of patients with mitral stenosis and treatment of the unfavorable effects of these drugs, accordingly. For example, pancuronium may not be an appropriate choice for neuromuscular blockade in patients with mitral stenosis secondary to the increased speed of transmission of cardiac impulses through the atrioventricular node that results from this drug. This increased speed of transmission may be detrimental to patients prone to atrial fibrillation. Likewise, the administration of ketamine to these patients should be avoided. The increase in pulmonary vascular resistance that is associated with nitrous oxide is not usually sufficient to detract from its utility in patients with mitral stenosis. Nitrous oxide use lowers F_{IO_2} and may not be optimal in patients with mitral stenosis. Drugs that are being administered for heart rate control should be continued throughout the perioperative period. (426)

53. Intraoperative monitoring of the right atrial pressure may be useful in assessing the adequacy of intravascular fluid replacement in patients with mitral stenosis. In patients in normal sinus rhythm, monitoring of pulse pressure variation (PPV) or stroke volume variation (SVV) may provide information regarding fluid status and responsiveness of cardiac output to fluid boluses. The monitoring of intraoperative fluid therapy in these patients is important because they are prone to intravascular fluid overload, leading to right-sided heart failure and pulmonary edema. (426)

54. The mechanical support of ventilation may be required postoperatively in patients with mitral stenosis because they are susceptible to developing pulmonary edema and right-sided heart failure, particularly when shifting from positive-pressure ventilation to spontaneous ventilation. This may be especially true in patients with mitral stenosis after major thoracic or abdominal surgery. (426)

55. Mitral regurgitation occurs as a result of an incompetent mitral valve. Physiologically, there is left atrial overload and a decreased effective left ventricular stroke volume in these patients. When mitral regurgitation develops over time, left ventricular dilation and left ventricular hypertrophy develop to maintain the left ventricular stroke volume. With progression of the disease, however, CHF can occur. Patients with chronic mitral regurgitation are frequently in atrial fibrillation. Acute mitral regurgitation results in acute increases in left atrial pressure and pulmonary artery pressures and can present as pulmonary congestion, pulmonary hypertension, and right-sided heart failure. Measurement of the regurgitant fraction provides for an estimate of the severity of the disease. For instance, a regurgitant fraction of 0.6 or greater is typically associated with CHF. A recording of pulmonary artery occlusion pressure tracings in a patient with mitral regurgitation would show prominent v waves that are characteristic of mitral regurgitation. (427)

56. The most common causes of mitral regurgitation include mitral valve prolapse, rheumatic heart disease, infective endocarditis, annular calcification, cardiomyopathy, and ischemic heart disease. When mitral regurgitation is secondary to rheumatic heart disease it is often chronic, is accompanied by mitral stenosis, and progresses over years. The most common cause of isolated mitral regurgitation is papillary muscle dysfunction, which is usually acute in onset with a corresponding acute onset of symptoms. Papillary muscle dysfunction usually occurs after a myocardial infarction or after rupture of the chordae tendineae secondary to infective endocarditis. (427)

57. Considerations for the anesthetic management of patients with mitral regurgitation include the avoidance of sudden decreases in heart rate, the avoidance of sudden increases in SVR, and minimizing drug-induced myocardial depression, because each of these will increase regurgitant flow. The size of the v wave on the pulmonary artery catheter tracing may be monitored as a reflection of mitral regurgitant flow. (427)

58. The maintenance of anesthesia in patients with mitral regurgitation can be achieved through the administration of a volatile anesthetic, nitrous oxide, and an opioid. Of greater importance is the management of the cardiovascular effects of these drugs to achieve the goal of the anesthetic management of patients with mitral regurgitation and treatment of the unfavorable effects of these drugs accordingly. The goals include maintenance of normal to increased heart rate, normal to reduced SVR, and maintenance of myocardial contractility. Nondepolarizing neuromuscular blocking drugs, including pancuronium, may be safely used in patients with mitral regurgitation. The increase in heart rate that can result from the administration of pancuronium can be beneficial to patients with mitral regurgitation. (427)

59. Aortic stenosis is the mechanical obstruction to the ejection of blood from the left ventricle secondary to a decrease in the orifice of the aortic valve. Increased left ventricular systolic pressure necessarily results from the chronic attempt of

this chamber to maintain an adequate stroke volume through a narrowed aortic valve in aortic stenosis. The increased thickness of the left ventricular wall that is often seen in patients with aortic stenosis occurs in response to chronically increased intraventricular pressures. The severity of aortic stenosis is estimated by the degree of stenosis of the valve. A mean pressure gradient across the aortic valve that is in excess of 40 mm Hg or valve area less than 1 cm^2 is considered severe aortic stenosis. Aortic valve area of less than 0.75 cm^2 or a mean gradient greater than 50 mm Hg is considered critical. (427)

60. Two causes of aortic stenosis are rheumatic heart disease and the progressive calcification and stenosis of a congenitally abnormal valve. The congenital valve abnormality most often associated with aortic stenosis is a bicuspid valve. The natural course of aortic stenosis is one of an insidious, long progression of asymptomatic disease before the onset of symptoms. Symptoms may include angina, syncope, dyspnea on exertion, CHF, stroke, and death. (427)

61. Patients with aortic stenosis may have angina pectoris, which typically occurs with exertion, despite the absence of CAD. Myocardial ischemia and angina occur because of an increased demand for, and decreased supply of, myocardial oxygen. The increase in myocardial oxygen demand is due to left ventricular hypertrophy combined with increased left ventricular pressures and increased myocardial work. The decrease in myocardial oxygen delivery results from the increased gradient in pressure from the left ventricle to the coronary ostia caused by the stenotic valve. (427)

62. A systolic murmur heard best in the second right intercostal space that may radiate to the right carotid artery characterizes the murmur of aortic stenosis heard on cardiac auscultation. It is important for the anesthesiologist to rule out aortic stenosis by auscultation preoperatively to best manage the patient. For instance, a precipitous drop in SVR, as may occur with a regional anesthetic or induction of general anesthesia, could be lethal to the patient with aortic stenosis. (427)

63. A consideration for the anesthetic management of a patient with aortic stenosis includes the maintenance of a stable blood pressure. Avoiding hypotension and tachycardia is critical. The goal of the anesthetic management of patients with aortic stenosis is the maintenance of normal sinus rhythm, normal heart rates, and normal myocardial contractility, while avoiding sudden decreases in SVR or hypovolemia. All patients with aortic stenosis should have invasive arterial pressure monitoring prior to the induction of general anesthesia. (427)

64. Tachycardia in the patient with aortic stenosis increases oxygen consumption and decreases coronary filling time by shortening diastole. Tachycardia also decreases the amount of time for left ventricular filling, leading to a decrease in the stroke volume. Bradycardia can lead to an acute overdistention of the left ventricle in these patients. Sinus rhythm is desired because the contribution of the atrial contraction to left ventricular filling is greater in these patients. Decreases in SVR with diastolic hypotension in patients with aortic stenosis can lead to decreases in coronary blood flow with myocardial ischemia, with rapid ventricular decompensation and death. (427)

65. The maintenance of anesthesia in patients with aortic stenosis can be achieved through the administration of narcotics, volatile agents, or intravenous anesthetics. Volatile anesthetic administered carefully to avoid excessive decreases in SVR and tachycardia is common. The most important point in patients with aortic stenosis is to carefully manage hemodynamics to avoid hypotension, tachycardia, myocardial ischemia, and ventricular dysfunction. Intra-arterial pressure monitoring prior to the induction of anesthesia is mandatory, as is the availability of vasoconstrictors (e.g., phenylephrine) both as a bolus and as an infusion. (428)

66. Management of the intravascular fluid status of patients with aortic stenosis should be geared toward the maintenance of an adequate intravascular volume through the prompt, liberal correction of blood and fluid losses. (428)

67. The pulmonary artery occlusion pressure may not be reflective of the left ventricular end-diastolic volume in patients with chronic aortic stenosis secondary to the decrease in left ventricular compliance seen in these patients. (428)

68. External cardiac compressions administered during cardiopulmonary arrest are not effective in patients with aortic stenosis because of the greater pressures that are necessary to create forward flow through the stenosed aortic valve. (428)

69. Aortic regurgitation results from an incompetent aortic valve. Patients with aortic regurgitation have a decrease in effective left ventricular stroke volume due to regurgitation of part of the ejected stroke volume from the aorta back into the left ventricle. The regurgitated volume places an increased volume load on the left ventricle. Chronic aortic regurgitation results in eccentric hypertrophy of the left ventricle in an attempt to compensate for the regurgitation by increasing the stroke volume. Symptoms may include dyspnea, fatigue, and palpitations. (428)

70. Acute aortic regurgitation is most likely due to infective endocarditis, trauma, connective tissue disease, or a dissecting thoracic aortic aneurysm. Chronic aortic regurgitation is most likely due to prior rheumatic fever, but it may also be due to hypertension, syphilis, and other causes. (428)

71. Angina pectoris despite the absence of CAD in a patient with aortic regurgitation may occur as a result of increased myocardial oxygen requirements in the presence of a decreased supply. The increase in myocardial oxygen requirements is due to left ventricular hypertrophy. The decrease in myocardial oxygen supply is due to a decrease in aortic diastolic pressure, which decreases coronary blood flow to the left ventricle. Coronary blood flow to the left ventricle occurs during diastole, so lower diastolic pressures compromise it. Angina resulting from aortic regurgitation is typically a late and dismal sign. (428-429)

72. The anesthetic management of aortic regurgitation resembles the anesthetic management for mitral regurgitation. Considerations for the anesthetic management of patients with aortic regurgitation include the avoidance of sudden decreases in heart rate, the avoidance of sudden increases in SVR, and minimizing drug-induced myocardial depression. (429)

73. Mitral valve prolapse is a valvular disease in which the valve prolapses into the left atrium during contraction of the left ventricle. Valve prolapse is caused by an abnormality of the valve support structure. Mitral valve prolapse on cardiac auscultation is characterized by a systolic murmur with a clicking sound. It has been estimated that 5% to 15% of the adult population has mitral valve prolapse, also called click-murmur syndrome. Currently, this estimate is believed to be higher than the true prevalence. The diagnosis of mitral valve prolapse can be confirmed through echocardiography. (429)

74. Mitral valve prolapse is associated with atrial secundum defects, von Willebrand syndrome, and polycystic kidney disease, as well as with musculoskeletal abnormalities such as Marfan syndrome, pectus excavatum, and kyphoscoliosis. Females are more likely than males to have mitral valve prolapse. (429)

75. Patients with mitral valve prolapse typically are asymptomatic. Symptoms that can be associated with mitral valve prolapse include palpitations, dyspnea, atypical chest pain, dizziness, and syncope. (429)

76. Potential complications of mitral valve prolapse include mitral regurgitation, infective endocarditis, transient cerebral ischemic events, cardiac dysrhythmias, and sudden death. Sudden death is extremely rare, however. Cardiac dysrhythmias associated with atrioventricular bypass tracts and preexcitation syndromes are fairly common in these patients. Transient cerebral ischemic events may lead to the prescription of aspirin or anticoagulants for patients with mitral valve prolapse. (429)

77. The maintenance of anesthesia in patients with mitral valve prolapse should be geared toward the avoidance of cardiac emptying. Cardiac emptying results in increased prolapse of the mitral valve into the left atrium. Avoidance of sympathetic nervous system stimulation, decreases in SVR, and the performance of surgery with patients in the head-up or sitting position will all minimize cardiac emptying. The intravascular fluid volume of the patient should be maintained at normal or high normal for the same reason. Hypotension in patients with mitral valve prolapse can be treated with phenylephrine. Cardiac dysrhythmias that occur intraoperatively should be promptly treated. Ketamine is not recommended in patients with mitral valve prolapse because of its propensity to increase myocardial contractility and heart rate. (429)

78. The potential problem with regional anesthesia in patients with mitral valve prolapse is the decrease in SVR that can be detrimental to these patients. Appropriate monitoring can make regional anesthesia the preferred anesthetic approach for some surgical patients with valvular heart disease. (429)

DISTURBANCES OF CARDIAC CONDUCTION AND RHYTHM

79. Tools available to the clinician for the diagnosis of disturbances in cardiac conduction and rhythm include an electrocardiogram, Holter monitoring, continuous adhesive-patch electrocardiogram monitoring (Zio Patch), or an electrophysiology (EP) study. A Holter monitor is an ambulatory electrocardiogram that can be worn for days to document the occurrence of cardiac dysrhythmias and to assess the efficacy of treatment interventions. (429)

80. The conduction system of the heart includes the sinoatrial node, atrioventricular node, the bundle of His, and Purkinje fibers of the right and left bundle branches. Types of conduction defects include sinus node block, atrioventricular conduction defects, and intraventricular conduction defects. Atrioventricular conduction defects are classified as first-, second-, or third-degree heart blocks. Intraventricular conduction defects include right bundle branch block, left bundle branch block, and left fascicular hemiblock. Heart block below the atrioventricular node is usually progressive and permanent, whereas heart block above the atrioventricular node is usually transient and benign. (430)

81. The placement of a prophylactic artificial cardiac pacemaker before surgery is not indicated in a patient with a bifascicular block. The theoretical concern in preoperative patients with a bifascicular block is that the single remaining intact fascicle will become compromised by perioperative events, such as changes in hemodynamics, oxygenation, or electrolytes. This would lead to acute third-degree atrioventricular heart block. Third-degree atrioventricular block is also referred to as complete heart block because all the electrical activity from the atria fails to be conducted to the ventricles. Ventricular contractions in patients with third-degree atrioventricular block occur at a rate of about 40 beats/min, typically too slow to maintain an adequate cardiac output. Fortunately, there is no evidence that bifascicular blocks proceed to third-degree atrioventricular block with enough consistency to warrant the prophylactic placement of a pacemaker. (430)

82. Third-degree atrioventricular heart block is treated by the placement of an artificial cardiac pacemaker. There are various methods by which this can be accomplished. An endocardial pacemaker lead may be inserted intravenously, an epicardial or myocardial lead may be placed by the subcostal approach, or noninvasive transcutaneous cardiac pacing can be started. The pharmacologic treatment of third-degree heart block involves a continuous infusion of isoproterenol, which can act as a medical pacemaker until artificial electrical cardiac pacing is implemented. (430)

83. Sick sinus syndrome occurs as a result of degenerative changes in the sinoatrial node and is associated with an inappropriate sinus bradycardia. In sick sinus syndrome, rapid heart rates inhibit the normal pacemaker activity of the sinoatrial node and lead to periods of asystole. Sick sinus syndrome therefore usually presents as bradycardia with episodes of supraventricular tachycardia.

Treatment is by administering medicines to control tachycardia. When these medicines result in bradycardia, medical management is said to have failed, and artificial cardiac pacemakers become the next line of treatment. Patients with sick sinus syndrome may be at a high risk for pulmonary embolism and may therefore be started on anticoagulants. (430)

84. Ventricular premature beats occur as a result of ectopic pacemaker activity at a level below the atrioventricular node. The premature ventricular contraction then spreads through the ventricular conducting system. The premature ventricular contraction often blocks the sinoatrial node's subsequent depolarization, leading to a characteristic pause until the next normal sinus beat is generated. The hallmark features of a ventricular premature beat on an electrocardiogram are representative of the aberrant conduction associated with the ventricular contraction. They include a premature occurrence, the absence of a P wave preceding the QRS complex, a wide and bizarre appearing QRS complex, an inverted T wave, and a compensatory pause after the premature beat. (430)

85. Premature ventricular beats warrant treatment when they occur more frequently than six times a minute, are multifocal, occur in a train of three or more, or take place during the ascending limb of the T wave, that is, during the refractory period of the ventricle. Treatment is typically with lidocaine at a dose of 1 to 2 mg/kg. Recurrent premature ventricular beats can be treated with a lidocaine infusion. Additional therapy, if necessary, may include amiodarone, β-adrenergic antagonists, bretylium, procainamide, quinidine, verapamil, or overdrive pacing. A search for an underlying cause of the premature beats, such as myocardial ischemia or electrolyte abnormalities, should be the primary goal. (430)

86. Causes of ventricular premature beats include myocardial ischemia, arterial hypoxemia, hypercarbia, hypertension, hypokalemia, and mechanical irritation of the ventricles. (430)

87. Ventricular tachycardia may be diagnosed with the appearance of three or more consecutive, wide QRS complexes on the electrocardiogram occurring at an effective heart rate higher than 120 beats/min. The QRS complexes must be greater than 0.12 second. The P waves have no fixed relationship to the QRS complex because the beat originates in the ventricle. The onset of ventricular tachycardia can be life threatening. Ventricular tachycardia should be treated with intravenous amiodarone as a bolus followed by an infusion if the patient is hemodynamically stable. Hemodynamic instability, loss of consciousness, or myocardial ischemia should prompt immediate electrical cardioversion. (430)

88. Preexcitation syndromes are defined as an activation of a portion of the ventricles by cardiac impulses that have originated in the atria but were conducted to the ventricles by an accessory conduction pathway. Activation of the ventricles during this syndrome occurs sooner than it otherwise would have because of the accessory pathway, making the QRS complex appear sooner than it would have if sinus rhythm were maintained. (431)

89. Wolff-Parkinson-White (WPW) syndrome is the most commonly occurring preexcitation syndrome. The incidence of this syndrome is 0.3% in the general population. These patients may have sporadic supraventricular tachycardia or atrial fibrillation. In extreme cases, the rapid heart rate may be associated with syncope or CHF. On the electrocardiogram, WPW syndrome is characterized by a short PR interval and a wide QRS complex. There is also a characteristic delta wave that appears on the electrocardiogram. The delta wave, together with the QRS complex, represents the composite of cardiac impulses conducted by both the normal and accessory pathways. (431)

90. The most common cardiac dysrhythmia associated with WPW syndrome is paroxysmal atrial tachycardia. WPW syndrome is most frequently treated by catheter ablation of the accessory pathway. Identification of the accessory pathway is accomplished by electrophysiologic mapping. (431)

91. The goal of the anesthetic management of a patient with WPW syndrome is the avoidance of any events, such as anxiety or drugs, that can result in sympathetic nervous system stimulation. Any cardiac antidysrhythmic drugs should be continued throughout the perioperative period. An adequate depth of anesthesia should be achieved before direct laryngoscopy to ensure that the patient does not respond to the noxious stimulus with sympathetic nervous system activity, placing the patient at an increased risk of tachyarrhythmias. Reduction in the stimulation of laryngoscopy can be achieved with adequate doses of an intravenous induction agent, such as propofol, thiopental, benzodiazepines, opioids, or β-adrenergic blockers, or with a bolus of lidocaine just before direct laryngoscopy. Ketamine is not recommended as it stimulates the sympathetic nervous system. The duration of laryngoscopy should also be as short as possible. (431)

92. Methods for the treatment of paroxysmal atrial tachycardia or fibrillation that can occur in the perioperative period in patients with WPW syndrome include the administration of adenosine or procainamide. Adenosine acts by prolonging the refractory period of the atrioventricular node, whereas procainamide acts by increasing the refractory period of the accessory pathways. β-Adrenergic antagonists can be used to control the heart rate. When the tachydysrhythmias become life threatening, emergent electrical cardioversion is indicated. Of note, drugs such as verapamil and digitalis may actually result in an increase in ventricular response during the dysrhythmia by accelerating the conduction in the accessory atrioventricular pathway. (431)

93. Prolonged QT interval syndrome can be congenital or acquired. Acquired prolonged QT interval syndrome can be due to quinidine, tricyclic anti-depressants, subarachnoid hemorrhage, hypokalemia, hypocalcemia, or hypomagnesemia. It may also present in the postoperative period after right radical neck dissection. The diagnosis of prolonged QT interval syndrome is made when the QT interval is chronically greater than 0.44 second. Adverse events that are associated with a prolonged QT interval include ventricular dysrhythmias, syncope, and sudden death. The pharmacologic treatment of a chronically prolonged QT interval can include β-adrenergic antagonists or a left stellate ganglion block. These treatments are empirical. The most important treatment is to search for and discontinue medications that prolong the QT interval. (431)

94. A congenital cause of a prolonged QT interval is thought to be due to an imbalance of autonomic innervation to the heart caused by decreases in right cardiac sympathetic nerve activity. A left stellate ganglion block is thought to work by decreasing left cardiac sympathetic nerve activity, thereby balancing the autonomic innervation to the heart. (431)

95. The goal of the anesthetic management of a patient with a chronically prolonged QT interval includes the avoidance of any events or drugs that are likely to cause sympathetic nervous system stimulation. General anesthesia has triggered life-threatening ventricular dysrhythmia and cardiac arrest in patients with this syndrome. β-Adrenergic blockade may be instituted preoperatively to minimize this risk. Although thiopental prolongs the QT interval in normal patients, it has been used for the induction of anesthesia in patients with the syndrome without any problems. Direct laryngoscopy should be performed with the patient deeply anesthetized. Should acute ventricular dysrhythmias occur, they can be treated with a β-adrenergic antagonist. Procainamide and quinidine are both known to prolong the QT interval in normal patients and should probably be avoided. Lidocaine, which also prolongs the QT interval in normal patients, has been used to successfully treat ventricular dysrhythmias in these patients. Electrical cardioversion may be necessary in the event of dysrhythmias that become life threatening. (431)

96. The preoperative evaluation of a patient with an artificial cardiac pacemaker should include an understanding of the underlying cardiac condition that required placement of the pacemaker and an assessment of the current function of the pacemaker, brand, model, make, and magnet mode. (431)

97. A pacemaker should be evaluated by the anesthesiologist preoperatively so that the anesthesiologist has a good understanding of the pacemaker and its programming. For instance, the anesthesiologist should be aware of what the default rhythm is (should the pacemaker not capture), the type of pacemaker, the chamber paced, the chamber sensed, how to detect deterioration in battery function, who can reprogram the pacemaker, and the current rate and sensitivity settings of the pacemaker and magnet mode. A discussion with the electrophysiology service or the pacemaker company representative can quickly resolve any issues. (431)

98. An automatic defibrillator device may need to be inactivated for surgery requiring electrocautery because the electrocautery may be misinterpreted as a ventricular dysrhythmia, triggering unnecessary shocks and decreasing battery life. (432)

99. Intraoperative monitoring that is important in a patient with an artificial cardiac pacemaker includes the electrocardiogram, pulse oximeter, and possibly an intra-arterial catheter. Intra-arterial catheters or a pulse oximeter that are not affected by electrocautery may allow for diagnosis of interference of the pacemaker by electrocautery. In a patient with third-degree heart block and no escape rhythm, intra-arterial catheters can be quite helpful. Inhibition of the pacemaker by electrocautery may lead to pacemaker inhibition and asystole in patients with third-degree heart block. The intra-arterial catheter or pulse oximeter provides a measure of blood flow and cardiac output during that period allowing rapid diagnosis of the interference between the electrocautery and the pacemaker. (432)

100. If the ground plate for the electrocautery is placed too near the pulse generator of the artificial cardiac pacemaker, there could be electromagnetic interference that is interpreted as spontaneous cardiac activity by the pacemaker. This interference may result in asystole due to an inhibition of pulse generator activity by the pacemaker. The ground plate should be placed as far away as possible from the pulse generator, at least 15 cm away. Bipolar electrocautery may also be useful to reduce interference between the electrocautery and the pacemaker. Other potential sources of mechanical interference include electroconvulsive shock therapy, succinylcholine-induced fasciculations, and myoclonic movements. (432)

101. The selection of drugs or anesthetic techniques for a patient should not be altered by the presence of an artificial cardiac pacemaker. However, patients with pacemakers or implantable cardiac defibrillators (ICDs) have an increased risk of CAD and ventricular dysfunction and should be monitored and anesthetized with added caution. (432)

102. A pacemaker magnet should be kept in the operating room intraoperatively for patients with artificial cardiac pacemakers to convert the pacemaker modes to an asynchronous mode, or fixed rate, should it become necessary. For instance, if the patient's pacemaker stops functioning intraoperatively, placement of an external converter magnet over the pulse generator may convert the pacemaker to an asynchronous mode. The magnet does not "magically" solve all pacemaker problems; the magnet throws a switch in the pacemaker that changes its function. In a pacemaker, magnet mode is commonly DOO (dual pace [atrium and ventricle], no sensing, no inhibitions) at a rate of 99 beats/min. In an ICD magnet mode is commonly DDD (dual pace, dual sense, dual inhibit) at a rate of 80 beats/min. However, these modes should not be assumed because some devices allow magnet mode to be programmed or shut off. The specific magnet mode for the device the patient has should be reviewed by the anesthesiologist prior to surgery. (432)

103. The most common cause of temporary pacemaker malfunction is the disruption of contact between the pacemaker electrode wires and the endocardium. Some causes of this disruption include muscular exertion, blunt trauma, cardioversion, and positive-pressure ventilation. When this occurs, pacemaker spikes will continue to be seen on the electrocardiogram, although there is no myocardial activity or pulse. Placement of a pulmonary artery catheter in a patient with an artificial cardiac pacemaker may disrupt the placement of transvenous endocardial electrodes if they have been placed in the 2 weeks preceding the procedure. (432)

104. Artificial cardiac pacemaker failure intraoperatively can be treated with atropine, isoproterenol, or an external pacemaker, which should all be available. (432)

ESSENTIAL HYPERTENSION

105. Essential hypertension has been defined as a sustained elevated blood pressure on two or more measurements without any known cause. Systolic blood pressure greater than 160 mm Hg or diastolic blood pressure greater than 90 mm Hg have been arbitrarily defined as the limits at which hypertension begins. The benefits of the long-term treatment of patients with essential hypertension include decreases in the incidence of cerebrovascular accidents, CHF, and renal disease. (432)

106. The preoperative evaluation of a patient with essential hypertension should include a determination of the adequacy of blood pressure control, a review of the pharmacology of the antihypertensive drugs, and an evaluation of effects of the hypertension on other organs. (432)

107. Antihypertensives include ACE inhibitors, calcium channel blockers, β-adrenergic antagonists, diuretics, and vasodilators. It is generally recommended that blood pressure medications be administered on their routine schedule in the perioperative period in the patient with essential hypertension. This includes medicines on the morning of the surgical procedure. Withdrawal of medications in the perioperative period can lead to an increase in complications and should be avoided. Recent studies have suggested that ACE inhibitors be withheld on the day of surgery but should be restarted after surgery. (432)

108. Medical problems that are frequently seen in patients with essential hypertension include CHF, CAD, cerebral ischemia, renal dysfunction, and PVD. Approximately 50% of patients with PVD can be assumed to have 50% or greater stenosis of one or more coronary arteries, even in the absence of symptoms. (432)

109. The curve for the autoregulation of cerebral blood flow in patients with essential hypertension is shifted to the right, such that autoregulation occurs at a higher pressure than it would for a normotensive patient. This implies that the same degree of absolute hypotension in patients with a history of hypertension may be more harmful than the same blood pressure would be for a normotensive patient. Thus maintenance of blood pressure in the perioperative period should be relative to what the preoperative resting blood pressure is specific to that patient. Recent work has demonstrated that there are absolute thresholds for blood pressure: diastolic pressure below 30 mm Hg, systolic blood pressure below 60 mm Hg, and mean blood pressure below 65 mm Hg all increase morbidity and mortality rates. These thresholds are not varied by preoperative blood pressure ranges. (433)

110. Treating essential hypertension in patients before an elective procedure has been shown to be beneficial in decreasing the risk of intraoperative hypotension and myocardial ischemia. There have been multiple studies conducted regarding this topic. Studies have also shown that there is no increased incidence of cardiac complications in hypertensive patients in the perioperative period as long as the diastolic blood pressure was not higher than 110 mm Hg preoperatively. (433)

111. Patients with essential hypertension frequently respond to the induction of anesthesia with an exaggerated decrease in blood pressure. This hypotension is thought to occur as a result of an unmasking of a decreased intravascular fluid volume status. (433)

112. Patients with essential hypertension are especially likely to respond to direct laryngoscopy with exaggerated increases in blood pressure, placing them at risk for myocardial ischemia. This response can be attenuated with adequate levels of anesthesia. It must be done with caution in hypertensive patients, because an excessive depth of anesthesia may produce hypotension in these patients as well. Other methods may be used to attenuate the sympathetic nervous system response to direct laryngoscopy and the associated exaggerated hypertension. For instance, esmolol or lidocaine may be administered just before direct laryngoscopy. In addition, the duration of direct laryngoscopy should be minimized. (433)

113. The goal of the anesthetic management of patients with essential hypertension is to minimize the fluctuations in blood pressure that is characteristic of these patients. This can be accomplished with anesthetics and antihypertensive medications as appropriate. The patient should also be continually monitored for evidence of myocardial ischemia via a continuous electrocardiogram. (433)

114. The maintenance of anesthesia in patients with essential hypertension can be achieved through the administration of a volatile anesthetic in conjunction with an opioid, intravenous agents, or nitrous oxide. An anesthetic dose sufficient to attenuate hypertensive responses to surgical stimulation should be administered. The maintenance of normotension intraoperatively may also require the administration of other medicines, such as β-adrenergic antagonists, vasoconstrictors, or nitrates. (433)

115. Intraoperative hypotension in patients with essential hypertension can be managed by the administration of intravenous fluids, by decreasing the concentration of volatile anesthetics, and by the administration of vasopressors as necessary. (434)

116. Regional anesthesia is frequently an excellent choice in appropriate surgical cases for patients with cardiovascular disease. The administration of regional anesthesia in patients with essential hypertension has the theoretical problem of causing excessive decreases in systemic blood pressure. Hypotension can occur secondary to vasodilation associated with the sympathetic nervous system blockade in combination with the decreased intravascular fluid volume status often seen in patients with chronic hypertension. The anesthesiologist must be prepared to support the blood pressure as necessary when a regional anesthetic is administered to these patients. (434)

117. Hypertension occurs frequently in the early postoperative period in patients with a diagnosis of essential hypertension. Hypertension secondary to inadequate pain control should be considered. If hypertension persists despite adequate analgesia, the administration of additional doses of antihypertensives is likely necessary. (435)

CONGESTIVE HEART FAILURE

118. CHF is highly correlated with postoperative morbidity. In fact, preoperative CHF is the single greatest preoperative risk factor for predicting postoperative morbidity. This suggests that the preoperative patient with CHF scheduled for elective surgery should not have his or her surgery until treatment of the CHF can be instituted and the patient's medical status optimized. (435)

119. The goal of the anesthetic management of patients with CHF who are undergoing urgent or emergent surgery is the optimization of cardiac output without increasing stress or workload or tachycardia. Optimal cardiac output in patients with CHF undergoing anesthesia may be best achieved with careful hemodynamic management. The patient's chronic medications should be given preoperatively if there are no specific contraindications. Volatile anesthetics may produce a dose-dependent depression of cardiac muscle

function that is greater in patients with CHF than in patients without CHF. In addition, the maintenance of myocardial contractility may necessitate the continuous administration of β-adrenergic agonists and vasoactive agents in the perioperative period. Avoidance of the administration of β-adrenergic agonists may reduce overall risk and should only be used if necessary. (435)

120. Positive-pressure ventilation of the lungs of patients in CHF may be beneficial because of its effect of decreasing pulmonary vascular congestion, reducing volume overload through decreased venous return, and improvement in arterial oxygenation. Alternatively, positive-pressure ventilation may reduce volume loading and reduce cardiac output. Careful monitoring and control of hemodynamics during institution and discontinuation of positive-pressure ventilation are essential. (435)

121. Monitors in the patient with CHF undergoing major surgery include an intra-arterial catheter. Although there is no evidence to support the use of pulmonary artery catheters to monitor central filling pressures and cardiac output, they can be used to monitor the effects of inotropic, vasoactive agents, and volume status. TEE may be more useful than pulmonary artery catheterization but is not required. Monitors chosen should be influenced by the patient's medical status, risk-benefit ratios, and surgical procedure. (435)

122. Regional anesthesia for peripheral surgery in patients with CHF can be administered safely, but it has not been proved to have reliably better outcomes than general anesthesia for these patients. Mild decreases in the SVR produced by an epidural or spinal anesthetic may provide for improvement in cardiac output in the patient with CHF. Greater decreases in the SVR should be avoided if possible. (435)

HYPERTROPHIC CARDIOMYOPATHY

123. Hypertrophic cardiomyopathy is a genetically transmitted disease also known as idiopathic hypertrophic subaortic stenosis. The pathology that defines hypertrophic cardiomyopathy is the obstruction to left ventricular outflow produced by asymmetric hypertrophy of the intraventricular septal muscle. As a result of the obstruction to ventricular outflow, left ventricular hypertrophy develops to the degree that the volume of the left chamber is decreased. As the disease advances, the increased muscle mass in the subaortic region can lead to complete obstruction of left ventricular outflow. The stroke volume in patients with hypertrophic cardiomyopathy remains normal despite the physiologic changes. The normal stroke volume is reflective of the hypercontractile state of the myocardium. (435)

124. The goal of the anesthetic management of patients with hypertrophic cardio-myopathy is geared toward decreasing the pressure gradient across the obstructed left ventricular outflow tract. There are several methods of decreasing the left ventricular outflow obstruction in patients with hyper-trophic cardiomyopathy. These include decreasing myocardial contractility, as with the administration of β-adrenergic antagonists; increasing the dose of volatile agents; increasing preload with increased intravascular fluid volume; and increasing afterload with α-adrenergic stimulation as is pro-duced by phenylephrine. (436)

125. Intraoperative hypotension in patients with hypertrophic cardiomyopathy can be treated with the administration of intravascular fluids as well as phenylephrine. (436)

126. Intraoperative hypertension in patients with hypertrophic cardiomyopathy can be treated with the administration of increased concentrations of volatile anesthetics. (436)

127. The administration of β-adrenergic agonists for the treatment of hypotension in patients with hypertrophic cardiomyopathy can result in an increase in myocardial contractility and a corresponding increase in left ventricular outflow obstruction. Likewise, the administration of nitrates such as nitroprusside or nitroglycerin to these patients can increase left ventricular

outflow obstruction by decreasing SVR, making them an unlikely choice for the treatment of hypertension. (436)

PULMONARY HYPERTENSION AND COR PULMONALE

128. Cor pulmonale is right ventricular hypertrophy and cardiac dysfunction that occurs as a result of pulmonary hypertension. The most likely cause of cor pulmonale is chronic obstructive pulmonary disease with associated chronic arterial hypoxemia leading to chronic pulmonary vascular vasoconstriction. Vascular smooth muscle hypertrophy and permanently increased pulmonary vascular resistance result from sustained pulmonary vascular vasoconstriction. When systemic acidosis is also present, there is a synergistic effect between arterial hypoxemia and acidosis on the pulmonary vasculature. In general, when the increased pulmonary vasculature resistance is due to arterial hypoxemia from chronic obstructive pulmonary disease, the prognosis is somewhat favorable if the arterial hypoxemia can be reversed with the administration of oxygen. Other causes of increased pulmonary vascular resistance leading to cor pulmonale, such as primary pulmonary hypertension or pulmonary fibrosis, have less favorable outcomes. (436)

129. Symptoms of cor pulmonale are often masked by the symptoms associated with coexisting chronic obstructive pulmonary disease. As the right ventricle becomes increasingly impaired, patients may experience syncope with exertion. Patients may also have chronic dependent edema, an enlarged liver, ascites, and dilated neck veins. On the lateral chest radiograph, right ventricular hypertrophy may present as a decrease in the retrosternal space. There may also be a decrease in pulmonary vascular markings. Right ventricular hypertrophy on the electrocardiogram would show peaked P waves in leads II, III, and aVF. Often there will also be right-axis deviation. On right-sided heart catheterization, the mean pulmonary artery pressure will be elevated, whereas the pulmonary artery occlusion pressure is normal. Pulmonary hypertension is considered mild with mean pulmonary artery pressure between 20 and 35 mm Hg and is considered moderate when the pressure is greater than 35 mm Hg. (436)

130. The treatment of cor pulmonale is directed toward decreasing right ventricular work by decreasing the pulmonary vascular resistance. This reduction in pulmonary vascular resistance may be achieved through the correction of the patient's pH and through the administration of oxygen to reverse arterial hypoxemia if possible. Diuretics may also be administered for patients with CHF. Nitroglycerin administration may result in lowering of the pulmonary artery pressure and a decrease in pulmonary vascular resistance. Pulmonary vasodilation with prostaglandins, endothelial receptor antagonists, inhaled nitric oxide, type 5 phosphodiesterase inhibitors, or soluble guanylate cyclase inhibitors have been tried with variable success. (436)

131. Just as in any other patient, the patient with cor pulmonale who is scheduled for an elective surgical procedure should be medically optimized before the procedure. Any pulmonary infections should be treated. Patients should have any bronchospasm reversed, be well hydrated, and have electrolytes evaluated and corrected if necessary. (436)

132. The goal of the anesthetic management of patients with cor pulmonale is the avoidance of events or drugs that could result in an increase in pulmonary vascular resistance, thereby worsening right ventricular failure. Events that may result in an increase in pulmonary vascular resistance include arterial hypoxemia, hypercapnia, acidosis, and decreases in body temperature. An abrupt or significant decrease in the SVR should be avoided. Nitrous oxide should be avoided because of its potential for increasing pulmonary vascular resistance. Although positive-pressure ventilation may increase pulmonary vascular resistance, its potential benefit for improving arterial oxygenation likely outweighs its risk. An intra-arterial catheter allows for arterial blood

gas analysis to assess the effects of any interventions on the patient's arterial oxygenation and pH and should be considered essential. (436)

133. The advantage of monitoring pulmonary artery and central venous pressure during surgery in patients with cor pulmonale is the ability of the anesthesiologist to assess the hemodynamic effects of the surgical procedure and optimize pharmacologic and hemodynamic management. (436)

CARDIAC TAMPONADE

134. Cardiac tamponade occurs as a result of increased intrapericardial pressure from the accumulation of fluid in the pericardial space. The increase in pericardial pressures causes a decrease in compliance of the right ventricle, reducing right ventricular filling, stroke volume, and cardiac output, thus causing hypotension. The decrease in stroke volume results in sympathetic nervous system activation in an attempt to maintain cardiac output. Cardiac output and systemic blood pressure in these patients become dependent on heart rate and on a central venous pressure that exceeds the right ventricular end-diastolic pressure. (436)

135. Manifestations of cardiac tamponade include hypotension, tachycardia, vasoconstriction, equalization of diastolic filling pressures, increased central venous pressure, and a fixed, decreased stroke volume with low cardiac output. These patients also have pulsus paradoxus. Pulsus paradoxus is a decrease in the arterial blood pressure by greater than 10 mm Hg during inspiration. This change in pressure is the opposite of what would be expected in normal patients and reflects the decrease in ventricular stroke volume that occurs with inspiration. On the chest radiograph, there may be a change in the cardiac silhouette when 250 mL or greater of fluid has accumulated in the pericardial space. Decreased voltages through all leads may be seen in patients with cardiac tamponade. Cardiac tamponade is best diagnosed through echocardiography. (437)

136. The definitive treatment of cardiac tamponade is the drainage of the pericardial fluid. Drainage can be achieved either percutaneously or by a pericardiotomy in the operating room under general or local anesthesia. Temporizing measures until definitive treatment include the expansion of the intravascular fluid volume; the administration of agents that will increase myocardial contractility, such as epinephrine, norepinephrine, or dopamine; and the correction of metabolic acidosis, which may depress myocardial contractility. Definitive care requires drainage of the pericardial fluid and may be lifesaving. (437)

137. Prior to the induction of general anesthesia, the patient should be prepped and draped and the surgeons scrubbed and ready to make an incision. Immediate hemodynamic collapse may occur with induction of general anesthesia that can only be resolved with surgical relief of the pericardial tamponade. The goal of the anesthetic management of patients with cardiac tamponade is the avoidance of events or drugs that could result in a decrease in cardiac output. Myocardial contractility, arterial blood pressure, increased heart rate, and venous return must all be maintained. Rapid surgical drainage of the tamponade is critical to avoid hemodynamic collapse and death. (437)

138. The induction of anesthesia and positive-pressure ventilation of the lungs of patients with cardiac tamponade can result in profound, irreversible hypotension. Hypotension that occurs in response to positive-pressure ventilation of the lungs of these patients results from anesthetic-induced peripheral vasodilation, direct myocardial depression, and decreases in venous return from positive intrathoracic pressure. The recommendation for patients with cardiac tamponade is that, if at all possible, percutaneous pericardiocentesis be performed under local anesthesia to relieve some of the tamponade before the induction of anesthesia. This drainage should be done in the operating room with the patient spontaneously breathing and continually monitored. If time permits, monitors may include an intra-arterial catheter for continuous arterial blood pressure monitoring and a central venous catheter to monitor central venous pressures. The ability to

immediately surgically drain the pericardium should be established prior to the induction of general anesthesia. (437)

139. The recommendation for anesthesia in patients with cardiac tamponade is that percutaneous pericardiocentesis be performed if possible under local anesthesia before the induction of anesthesia. One must be careful with percutaneous drainage of cardiac tamponade because it is common for there to be secondary injury to the ventricle or even a coronary artery with needle placement. It is difficult to establish if the blood drained from percutaneous drainage is from the ventricle or the pericardial space without echocardiography. Percutaneous drainage of major hemorrhage into the pericardium is temporizing. Percutaneous catheters are commonly small diameter, and suction is required for adequate drainage. Administration of procoagulants such as fresh frozen plasma, platelets, and factor VII may cause clotting of the blood in the pericardial space, making drainage impossible, worsening tamponade, and causing cardiac arrest. If there is more than minimal continuous drainage, the patient should be taken for definitive, open surgical repair in an operating room. Induction of general anesthesia is extremely dangerous in patients with tamponade secondary to vasodilation combined with increased pleural pressures from positive-pressure ventilation, reducing venous return, and resulting in hemodynamic collapse. The patient should be prepped, draped, and the surgeons ready for incision prior to induction. If the patient suffers cardiac arrest prior to induction, then intubation can proceed as part of the code, but intubation should be delayed until the patient is ready for incision and definitive drainage if possible. An awake orotracheal intubation can be considered with spontaneous ventilation if possible. The patient should have the urgency of the need to perform the procedure explained and the airway anesthetized topically. After confirmed orotracheal intubation, the patient can then be gently sedated while maintaining spontaneous ventilation. Small doses of ketamine may be administered to the patient to provide analgesia and sedation during pericardiocentesis. Alternatively, once the patient is prepped and draped for surgery, a rapid sequence induction with small anesthetic doses and succinylcholine with rapid intubation and immediate pericardiocentesis can be considered. Positive-pressure ventilation in this situation may cause profound hemodynamic collapse that will only be resolved by rapid, definitive, pericardial drainage. The induction of anesthesia and positive-pressure ventilation, if required for further surgical exploration, should not be instituted until immediate drainage of the pericardial space can be achieved. (437)

140. Sympathetic nervous system stimulants, such as epinephrine, norepinephrine, dopamine, dobutamine, or isoproterenol administered as continuous infusions may be useful in patients with cardiac tamponade, although they will not preclude or prevent hemodynamic collapse and cardiac arrest with loss of ventricular filling. The pericardium must be drained as soon as possible to allow venous filling and cardiac output. (437)

ANEURYSMS OF THE AORTA

141. Most aortic aneurysms involve the abdominal aorta. About 95% of abdominal aortic aneurysms are due to atherosclerosis, in contrast to about 50% of thoracic aortic aneurysms. Other causes of aortic aneurysms include trauma, mycotic infection, connective tissue disorders such as Marfan syndrome, and syphilis. Only about 0.5% of abdominal aortic aneurysms extend into the renal arteries. (437)

142. A dissecting aneurysm occurs when a tear in the intima of the aorta separates the layers of the wall of the aorta. Blood is then allowed to enter and penetrate between the intima on one side and the media and adventitia layers on the other, creating a false lumen. The dissection can then reenter the true lumen through another tear in the intima, or it may rupture through the adventitia. Acute dissection may present as excruciating chest pain, and patients may appear to be in shock. Peripheral pulses may be difficult to palpate. The treatment

for aortic dissection is either surgical excision, usually followed by placement of a graft, or endovascular graft placement. Short-term management until a definitive treatment can take place may include decreasing blood pressure to the lowest acceptable level and the relief of pain. (437)

143. The risk of rupture of an abdominal aortic aneurysm is best predicted by the diameter of the aneurysm, as well as its rate of expansion. Elective resection of an abdominal aortic aneurysm is recommended when the diameter of the aneurysm is estimated to be 5 cm or greater. This recommendation is made based on the dramatic increase in the likelihood of spontaneous rupture of the aneurysm when the size of the aneurysm exceeds 5 cm. Abdominal aortic aneurysms with a diameter less than 5 cm are typically followed with serial measurements to evaluate their rate of expansion. If the aneurysm expands by more than 0.5 cm in a 6-month period, or if the patient becomes symptomatic, surgical repair is recommended. (437)

144. Medical problems frequently associated with aortic aneurysms include hypertension, diabetes mellitus, ischemic heart disease, and atherosclerosis. (437)

145. The goal of the anesthetic management of patients undergoing resection of an abdominal aortic aneurysm is aimed toward the maintenance of cardiovascular and hemodynamic parameters at or near normal. Aggressive intraoperative monitoring is necessary to achieve this goal. Patients should have their intra-arterial blood pressure closely monitored throughout the case. Perioperative administration of β-adrenergic antagonists, statins, and aspirin may reduce cardiac risk. (437)

146. Patients with CAD are especially at risk of myocardial ischemia during surgery for resection of an aortic aneurysm during cross-clamping of the aorta. Cross-clamping of the aorta at the suprarenal or supraceliac level creates the greatest increase in SVR and central venous pressure and a decrease in cardiac output. On the pulmonary artery catheter, cross-clamping of the aorta would result in an increase in the pulmonary artery occlusion pressure. In contrast, cross-clamping the aorta below the level of the renal arteries creates minimal hemodynamic changes. The hemodynamic response to aortic cross-clamping is influenced by the patient's cardiac status, intravascular fluid volume, and anesthetic drugs and technique. Management of the patient during aortic cross-clamping should be aimed toward decreasing the systolic blood pressure and cardiac filling pressures. Pharmacologic agents that could be administered might include inhaled anesthetic agents, nitroprusside, or nitroglycerin. (438)

147. Intraoperative fluid management during surgery for resection of an aortic aneurysm is best guided by the data obtained from hemodynamic monitors, either from arterial PPV, SVV, central venous and pulmonary arterial pressures, or TEE. Optimal fluid management can be administered with appropriate hemodynamic monitoring. (438)

148. Hypotension frequently accompanies unclamping of the abdominal aorta during the resection of an aortic aneurysm. The hypotension is believed to occur as a result of the sudden increase in venous capacitance that accompanies unclamping. Even when the aortic cross-clamp is infrarenal, unclamping can result in a decrease in the systolic blood pressure by about 40 mm Hg. Methods for minimizing the hypotension include adequate volume replacement before unclamping and the gradual removal of the aortic cross-clamp to allow time for the pooled venous blood to circulate. It is prudent to use only short-acting vasodilators, such as inhaled agents, nitroprusside, or nitroglycerin, to treat increases in the SVR during aortic cross-clamping so that their effects can be reversed with titration or by discontinuation before unclamping of the aorta. The SVR may be increased after unclamping with the administration of phenylephrine if necessary. (438)

149. Renal function may become impaired postoperatively to the extent that hemodialysis is required after aortic aneurysm repair, particularly if the aortic

cross-clamp was suprarenal. Coexisting renal disease appears to place the patient at the greatest risk of postoperative renal dysfunction, but other risk factors include the duration of aortic cross-clamp time, thrombotic or embolic interruption of renal blood flow, hypovolemia, and hypotension. Hypothermia may protect the kidneys during periods of ischemia. In an effort to decrease the risk of postoperative renal dysfunction, the intravascular fluid volume should be maintained and the urine output should be closely monitored during aortic aneurysm repair. Mannitol is frequently given just before aortic cross-clamping to facilitate diuresis and maintain glomerular function. A loop diuretic may also be administered in selected cases if the urine output is unsatisfactory. Alternatively, a continuous dopamine infusion at low doses may be started to dilate renal blood vessels to maintain renal blood flow and urine output. Unfortunately, none of these therapies have been definitively demonstrated to have efficacy for the prevention of renal dysfunction. (438)

150. Spinal cord ischemia and paraplegia can occur after supraceliac aortic cross-clamping for thoracic aortic aneurysm repair. The mechanism for the ischemia is most likely due to an interruption of a portion of the blood supply to the spinal cord. The spinal cord blood supply is from two posterior arteries and one anterior spinal artery. The greatest contributor to the blood supply of the anterior spinal artery is the artery of Adamkiewicz, whose origin is between T9 and T12 in 75% of patients. The anterior spinal artery supplies the motor tracts in the spinal cord. Mechanisms employed to reduce the risk of spinal cord ischemia include cerebrospinal fluid drainage, intrathecal papaverine injection, naloxone administration, barbiturate administration, hypothermia, and partial bypass. Hypothermia is believed to be the most effective method of neuroprotection through its effects of decreasing oxygen requirements. Cerebrospinal fluid drainage is thought to improve spinal cord perfusion because the spinal cord perfusion pressure is the distal mean aortic pressure minus the cerebrospinal fluid pressure. Cerebrospinal fluid drainage to improve spinal cord perfusion during aortic aneurysm repair remains controversial. (438)

CARDIOPULMONARY BYPASS

151. Blood is drained from the venae cavae during cardiopulmonary bypass by siphon action caused by gravity. The blood then passes from the cardiotomy reservoir, through a pump, a heat exchanger, an oxygenator, and a filter before it is returned to the arterial system. (438)

152. The two different types of pumps that are used to return blood to the arterial system during cardiopulmonary bypass are the roller pump and the centrifugal pump. The roller pump works by compressing the tubing that contains the fluid between a roller and curved metal back plate, producing flow. In contrast, the centrifugal pump produces flow and less trauma to blood. The flow rate generated by the centrifugal pump is affected by the resistance of the tubing and the patient's SVR. (438)

153. Blood is kept from entering the heart from the superior and inferior venae cavae during cardiopulmonary bypass for open heart or intracardiac surgery by placing both a superior and inferior vena caval cannula, as well as ligatures placed around the superior and inferior vena cava proximal to the cannulae, thereby occluding the cava and preventing flow into the heart. All returning blood from the patient's venous system enters the cardiopulmonary bypass machine via the two large cannulae, which are placed in the superior and inferior venae cavae. (438)

154. The aorta is cross-clamped distal to the aortic valve and proximal to the systemic arterial inflow cannula during cardiopulmonary bypass to allow cardioplegic arrest. Cardioplegic solution is administered through a catheter placed in the ascending aorta proximal to the aortic cross-clamp. Cardioplegia may also be administered retrograde through a coronary sinus catheter. An incompetent aortic valve in an arrested heart without this cross-clamp would allow blood to flow retrograde from the aorta into the heart, stretching the

myocardium and causing permanent muscle injury and ventricular dysfunction. (438)

155. Venting of the left ventricle may be necessary to prevent harmful left ventricular distention during cardiac surgery in which the heart is not opened. Persistent left ventricular distention may lead to permanent damage to the myocardial contractile elements. There are at least three reasons why the left ventricle might need a vent during cardiopulmonary bypass. First, incompetence of the aortic valve can lead to the retrograde flow of blood from the aorta to the heart. Second, there may be a large degree of blood flow from the coronary sinus and bronchial circulation back to the heart. Third, surgical positioning may result in backward flow from the aorta into the heart, or from the heart into the pulmonary veins. Finally, venting of the ventricle or pulmonary artery can help reduce risks of elevated pulmonary artery pressures during cardiopulmonary bypass. Venting of the left ventricle can be achieved through the placement of a catheter into the left ventricle, usually through a pulmonary vein or via the left atrium. Alternatively, incising the pulmonary artery can vent the circuit. The most common venting of the left ventricle is suction on the antegrade cardioplegia line placed in the ascending aorta proximal to the systemic inflow cannula. (438)

156. Venous drainage from the inferior and superior venae cavae during cardiopulmonary bypass, which is achieved by gravity, can be facilitated by raising the operating table to a higher level (creating a larger vertical distance between the operating room table and the cardiopulmonary bypass machine), or by adding negative pressure or suction to the cardiotomy reservoir. (438)

157. The required cardiac index that is delivered to the patient by the roller pump on the cardiopulmonary bypass machine depends on the patient's body temperature and oxygen consumption. A cardiac index of 2 to 2.4 L/min/m^2 is usually sufficient in the normothermic or slightly hypothermic patient. Flows of about half these levels have also been used without adverse effects. (438)

158. The advantage of low flows during cardiopulmonary bypass is that less trauma is sustained to the blood. Less noncoronary collateral blood flow returns to the heart as well, which may lead to better myocardial protection because less warm blood is entering the heart and counteracting the cold myocardial preservation solutions. (438)

159. Two different types of oxygenators that are used to oxygenate blood that is returning to the arterial system during cardiopulmonary bypass are a bubble oxygenator and a membrane oxygenator, although bubble oxygenators are rarely used at the present time. (439)

160. Advantages of a bubble oxygenator over a membrane oxygenator include its relative simplicity and lower cost. Disadvantages of a bubble oxygenator include an increase in the amount of turbulence and foaming it produces and denaturing of blood proteins by direct contact with gas, resulting in trauma to blood that increases with the duration of the bypass time. Bubble oxygenators are rarely used in the current era. (439)

161. An advantage of a membrane oxygenator includes the relatively less trauma produced to the blood than that produced by a bubble oxygenator by avoiding direct exposure of blood to gas. Disadvantages of a membrane oxygenator include its increased complexity and cost. (439)

162. During cardiopulmonary bypass the patient's Pao$_2$ is maintained by adjusting the concentration of oxygen into the oxygenator, and the carbon dioxide levels are maintained between 35 and 45 mm Hg by controlling the sweep (the total free gas flow through the oxygenator). (439)

163. In addition to the usual methods of heating a patient's body intraoperatively, the body can also be heated or cooled during cardiopulmonary bypass through the use of heat exchangers that are incorporated into the extracorporeal circuit. These heat exchangers are able to heat or cool blood as it circulates through the extracorporeal circuit via a countercurrent flow system. (440)

164. The optimal patient temperature for cardiopulmonary bypass is not clear. Metabolic requirements decrease by about 8% for every degree Celsius decrease in body temperature. Normothermic cardiopulmonary bypass is associated with an increased risk of cerebrovascular accidents. Prior to circulatory arrest 18° C is commonly used, during aortic cross-clamping 28° C is commonly used, and prior to weaning from bypass the patient is warmed to 37° C. Body temperature is maintained between 31° C and 33° C with newer protocols. (440)

165. Blood loss from the field can be recirculated to the patient during cardiopulmonary bypass by having the blood that is suctioned return to a cardiotomy reservoir. In the cardiotomy reservoir the blood is filtered, defoamed, and returned to the oxygenator. The blood is then recirculated to the patient after oxygenation. (440)

166. A problem with the cardiotomy suction used during cardiopulmonary bypass is that it is a significant contributor to the hemolysis and particulate emboli that occur during cardiopulmonary bypass. (440)

167. Systemic emboli from cellular debris are prevented from occurring during cardiopulmonary bypass through the use of filters that are incorporated into the extracorporeal circuit in the cardiotomy reservoir and downstream after the oxygenator. (440)

168. Priming of the cardiopulmonary bypass system refers to the filling of the tubing of the cardiopulmonary bypass system with fluid and sometimes blood. The bypass system is flushed with carbon dioxide prior to priming to remove low-solubility gas (the nitrogen in air). The system is then filled with crystalloid fluid and additives. The fluid consists of an osmotically active substance, an osmotic diuretic, an antibiotic, and electrolyte supplements. The additives are prescribed by protocol by the surgeon. Review of prime and bypass additives on a regular basis (at least yearly) is important to understand their osmotic, diuretic, hemodynamic, and coagulation effects. Blood is added if the patient's hematocrit necessitates it. (440)

169. Hemodilution of the patient's blood to a hematocrit of 20% to 30% during cardiopulmonary bypass lessens the viscosity of the blood. This decrease is important to facilitate circulation through the small vessels during hypothermia. (440)

170. It is essential to remove all air from the cardiopulmonary bypass system during cardiopulmonary bypass to prevent the pumping of air into the arterial system of the patient. (440)

171. Heparin-induced anticoagulation of the patient is mandatory before the institution of cardiopulmonary bypass to prevent patient death through clotting of the blood both in the patient and in the cardiopulmonary bypass machine. The dose of heparin that is usually administered is 300 to 400 U/kg. The adequacy of anticoagulation must be confirmed before the placement of the venous and aortic cannulae used for cardiopulmonary bypass. The adequacy of anticoagulation is usually confirmed by evaluating the activated clotting time, which should remain longer than 450 seconds throughout the course of cardiopulmonary bypass. The activated clotting time should be evaluated periodically during the course of cardiopulmonary bypass and additional heparin administered as necessary. After the cannulae are removed from the patient and cardiopulmonary bypass terminated, the effects of heparin may be reversed with the administration of protamine. The activated clotting time should return to baseline, typically between 90 to 120 seconds, after the administration of protamine. (440)

172. The low mean arterial pressure often seen after the institution of cardiopulmonary bypass is believed to be due to the peripheral vasodilation caused by the decreased viscosity, decreased temperature, and low oxygen content of infused priming solution. (440)

173. What mean arterial blood pressures during cardiopulmonary bypass are sufficient to allow for coronary and cerebral perfusion is a subject of great

debate. Most institutions prefer the mean arterial pressures to be about 60 mm Hg and to administer phenylephrine if blood pressure support is needed. There are many standard ranges of mean pressure on bypass: some use 40 to 60 mm Hg while cold and 60 to 80 mm Hg while warm. Other institutions allow the mean arterial blood pressure greater ranges without adverse effect. The perfusion pressures for extracorporeal circulatory support are even lower in infants and children. (441)

174. Blood pressure slowly rises spontaneously after some time on cardiopulmonary bypass as a result of vasoconstriction. The vasoconstriction may be in response to stimulation of the sympathetic nervous system or the renin-angiotensin system. It may also be an indication of inadequate perfusion to some tissues. (441)

175. The potential dangers of hypertension while on cardiopulmonary bypass include aortic dissection, intracerebral hemorrhage, and an increase in coronary and bronchial artery circulation, leading to increased return of warm blood to the heart during a time of cold cardioplegia. Hypertension under these circumstances can be treated by decreasing the SVR with a nitrate or a volatile anesthetic. Vaporizers have been incorporated into the cardiopulmonary bypass circuit for the administration of a volatile anesthetic to patients while on cardiopulmonary bypass. (441)

176. The patient can be monitored for adequate tissue perfusion during cardiopulmonary bypass using renal output as a guide to renal perfusion. A renal output of 1 mL/kg/h is considered sufficient. Second, the patient's acid-base status can be monitored for any evidence of a progressive metabolic acidosis. Third, the patient's mixed venous oxygen tension can be monitored for evidence of excessive oxygen extraction. A mixed venous Po_2 lower than 40 mm Hg is generally regarded as evidence of inadequate tissue perfusion. Finally, the nasopharyngeal temperature can be compared with a core temperature such as the bladder, rectum, skeletal muscle, or skin temperature. Whereas bladder temperature represents core temperature, the nasopharyngeal temperature is an indicator of perfusion to the brain. The greater the discrepancy between these two, the greater the indication of poor cerebral perfusion. Cerebral oximetry using infrared light can monitor adequacy of cerebral perfusion and may reduce risk of central nervous system injury. (441)

177. Diuresis is induced during cardiopulmonary bypass by the inclusion of mannitol in the priming solution, hypothermia which interferes with renal tubular absorption, and well-perfused renal glomeruli with blood low in oncotic pressure due to hemodilution. For this reason during cardiopulmonary bypass the minimally acceptable urine output is 1 mL/kg/h. Adequate urine output is important for the excretion of potassium administered in the cardioplegia solution. When the urine output is less than desired, a mechanical obstruction to urine flow in the catheter should be considered before instituting methods to increase the urine output. (441)

178. Causes of an increasing central venous pressure with or without facial edema while on cardiopulmonary bypass include aortic cannula flow into the carotid artery, obstruction of the superior vena cava cannula, and obstruction of jugular venous drainage by either a cannula, head position, or neck compression. Inadequate venous return from the patient to the cardiopulmonary bypass machine is an indication that one of these may have occurred. (441)

179. Causes of increasing abdominal distention while on cardiopulmonary bypass include obstruction of the inferior vena cava cannula, intra-abdominal hemorrhage or ascites, or gastrointestinal distention by gas or fluid. (441)

180. The most serious complications of cardiopulmonary bypass include aortic dissection, carotid artery dissection, air in the aortic inflow tubing, clotting of the bypass circuit, and systemic gas, atherosclerotic, or blood clot emboli. (441)

181. Ventilation of the lungs of a patient is not necessary during cardiopulmonary bypass. The lungs can be ventilated with oxygen during partial

cardiopulmonary bypass or when there is significant pulmonary blood flow. Evidence of pulmonary blood flow is seen as pulsatile pulmonary artery flow on the pulmonary artery catheter tracing. (441)

182. The goal of myocardial preservation during cardiopulmonary bypass is the minimization of the effects of ischemia on the heart. (441)

183. Myocardial protection is achieved in a variety of ways, all of which are aimed toward reducing the myocardial oxygen requirement of the heart during that period. Myocardial cooling can be achieved by hypothermic cardiopulmonary bypass, by the direct placement of ice on the epicardium, through pericardial irrigation with iced fluid, and by the intracoronary infusion of a cold cardioplegia solution at 200 mL/min. Myocardial arrest is achieved by the infusion of cold cardioplegia solution containing potassium both anterograde through a cannula at the aortic root and by retrograde flow through the coronary sinuses. The prevention of myocardial rewarming during cardiopulmonary bypass can be achieved by redosing of cardioplegia, ice packs next to the heart, pericardial slush, placing a vent in the left ventricle, and placing a cross-clamp in the aorta distal to the aortic valve. (441)

184. The oxygen consumption of a normally contracting heart at 30° C is 8 to 10 mL/100 g of heart muscle in a minute. The oxygen consumption of a fibrillating heart at 22° C is 2 mL/100 g/min, and the oxygen consumption of an electromechanically quiet heart at 22° C is approximately 0.3 mL/100 g/min. (441)

185. The potassium in cardioplegia solution causes cessation of electrical and mechanical cardiac activity by blocking the initial phase of myocardial depolarization, resulting in cessation of electrical and mechanical activity. The cold solution produces selective hypothermia of cardiac muscle. Cardioplegia solution may contain many additives (e.g., blood, insulin, glucose, aspartate, glutamate, calcium, magnesium, nitroglycerin) at the surgeon's discretion, but none of these additives has provided any proven benefit over cold cardioplegia with a short cross-clamp time. (441)

186. The correct placement of the cardioplegia catheter during retrograde cardioplegia administration can be confirmed through monitoring of coronary sinus pressures at the distal tip of the coronary sinus catheter. The goal is a distal pressure of 40 to 60 mm Hg. If the distal pressure is equal to central venous pressure, the catheter tip is likely in the right atrium. If the distal pressure is too high, the catheter tip is likely up against a vascular wall. Alternative methods of confirming positioning of the coronary sinus catheter are through TEE and manual feel by the surgeon. (442)

187. The effectiveness of cold cardioplegia of the heart can be measured by placing a temperature probe in the left ventricle and directly measuring the temperature of the heart. The absence of any electrical activity on the heart is also a good indication that the heart muscle is effectively quiescent. (442)

188. Two potential negative effects of the intramyocardial hyperkalemia of the cold cardioplegia solutions after cardiopulmonary bypass are decreased myocardial contractility and an increased incidence of atrioventricular heart block while coming off cardiopulmonary bypass. These can both be treated with the administration of calcium and, if necessary, insulin with or without glucose. In addition, the atrioventricular block can be treated through the use of an artificial cardiac pacemaker. The pacemaker is usually only needed temporarily because the atrioventricular block typically only lasts for 1 to 2 hours after discontinuing cardiopulmonary bypass. (442)

189. Two potential sources for systemic hyperkalemia during cardiopulmonary bypass are the recirculation of cardioplegia solution that has drained into the blood and decreased renal function. Hyperkalemia that persists at the conclusion of cardiopulmonary bypass can be treated with the administration of insulin and glucose in addition to calcium, by ultrafiltration on the

extracorporeal bypass circuit, or by administration of diuretics such as furosemide. (442)

190. Although there is a decreased minimum alveolar concentration (MAC) under hypothermic conditions, the decrease in MAC may not be sufficient to offset the sudden dilution of anesthetics that occurs when the patient is placed on cardiopulmonary bypass. For this reason, supplemental intravenous anesthetics may be needed during cardiopulmonary bypass in some cases to ensure an adequate depth of anesthesia. Dexmedetomidine infusions during this time are associated with a reduced risk of delirium. (442)

191. It is important to monitor glucose levels in patients undergoing cardiopulmonary bypass because abnormalities can have detrimental effects. Hypoglycemia has been associated with an increased risk of neurologic injury, and hyperglycemia may lead to an increased risk of infections and neurologic sequelae. The target goal of glucose level during cardiopulmonary bypass is between 120 and 180 mg/dL. This can be achieved through insulin infusions if necessary. (442)

192. There is a sudden dilution of the neuromuscular blocking drug level that occurs when the patient is placed on cardiopulmonary bypass. Supplemental neuromuscular blocking drug should be administered just prior to the initiation of extracorporeal circulatory support or cardiopulmonary bypass to ensure there is a neuromuscular blocking drug level sufficient to prevent patient movement during this important portion of the procedure. (442)

193. Although supplemental anesthesia is not routinely required during rewarming after the conclusion of cardiopulmonary bypass, it is important that the anesthesiologist be aware that the rewarming patient could be returning to consciousness in a paralyzed state. Low-dose inhaled agents reduce the risk of intraoperative awareness. There are a number of choices for post-bypass anesthesia, including dexmedetomidine, propofol, opiates, benzodiazepines, volatile agents, or a combination of agents. Intravenous infusions allowing continued sedation into the intensive care unit (ICU) are commonly chosen. (442)

194. Conditions in the patient that must be present for the discontinuation of cardiopulmonary bypass include SVR normalization; hemodynamic stability; normothermia; the venting of all arterial air; an adequate cardiac rate, rhythm, and output; normal acid-base status and electrolyte levels; ventilation of the lungs; and an adequate intravascular status and hematocrit. (442)

195. The aortic and vena cava cannulae are removed after an adequate blood pressure and cardiac output have been maintained by the heart for several minutes. For optimal safety, the ability to rapidly reestablish cardiopulmonary bypass should be maintained for some time after the discontinuation of cardiopulmonary bypass. Administration of protamine can cause profound hypotension from systemic vasodilation. In severe reactions there can be profound pulmonary hypertension and right ventricular failure. For these reasons the arterial inflow cannula is commonly removed after protamine has been successfully administered without major problems. (442)

196. Potential problems associated with persistent hypothermia after cardiopulmonary bypass include coagulopathy, hypertension, tachycardia and sympathetic nervous system stimulation, shivering, metabolic acidosis, and difficulty in defibrillating the heart and maintaining a normal cardiac rhythm. The effects of persistent hypothermia on the heart are particularly evident at temperatures less than 34° C. Rewarming a patient's body can be achieved more rapidly after systemic vasodilation through the administration of a vasodilator, such as nitroprusside, or a volatile anesthetic. It is common to try to avoid rapid reheating, high temperature gradients between in-flow blood temperatures and body temperatures, to avoid gas emboli. Overheating the patient, above 37° C, may be associated with neurologic complications. (442)

197. A special precaution that must be taken before discontinuing cardiopulmonary bypass in patients who have had the heart opened, as during valve replacement surgery, is the venting of all air from the heart. This can be accomplished by surgical massage of the left atrium and ventricle. In addition, rotating the table from side to side simultaneous with the maintenance of positive-pressure ventilation of the lungs and placement of the patient's head at a lower level than the heart may assist in venting any air from the heart. Positive pressure of the lungs should be maintained during the removal of the left ventricle vent cannula. The avoidance of nitrous oxide administration after cardiopulmonary bypass might minimize the potential increase in the size of microemboli that may have occurred. (442)

198. The potential risk of air remaining in the heart at the conclusion of cardiopulmonary bypass is the embolization of air to the arterial circulation, especially the coronary and cerebral circulations. Air is most likely to embolize from the heart after cardiopulmonary bypass during manipulation of the heart and alterations in the anatomy, closure of the sternum, and movement of the patient. Air embolism to the coronary arteries can cause rapid and profound heart failure requiring a return to cardiopulmonary bypass with extracorporeal support. Air embolism to the brain may be manifest by failure to awaken and status epilepticus. Treatment with hyperbaric oxygen can eliminate central nervous system gas emboli and improve outcomes. Treatment with hyperbaric oxygen should not be delayed but has been efficacious even 24 to 48 hours after the embolic event and may be lifesaving. (443)

199.

Blood Pressure	Atrial Pressure	Cardiac Output	Diagnosis	Therapy
Decreased	Increased	Decreased	Left ventricular dysfunction	Inotrope Vasodilator Mechanical assistance
Decreased	Decreased	Decreased	Hypovolemia	Intravascular fluid administration
Decreased	Decreased	Increased	Vasodilation, low blood viscosity	Erythrocyte administration
Increased	Increased	Decreased	Vasoconstriction, left ventricular dysfunction	Vasodilator Inotrope
Increased	Decreased	Increased	Hyperdynamic	Volatile anesthetic β-Adrenergic antagonist

(443)

200. Posterior papillary muscle dysfunction after cardiopulmonary bypass can occur as a result of inadequate cooling of the posterior myocardium during cardiopulmonary bypass. The posterior myocardium is the portion of the heart muscle that is most vulnerable to inadvertent warming of the heart from the return of blood from the coronary and bronchial circulations, as well as any potential blood that flows retrograde via an incompetent aortic valve. Posterior papillary muscle function impairment would manifest as mitral regurgitation. In addition, prominent v waves would be evident on the pulmonary artery occlusion pressure tracing. Acute mitral regurgitation

can be managed by reverse Trendelenburg positioning to reduce venous return to the heart. (433)

201. In some situations the cardiac output of the patient on discontinuation of cardiopulmonary bypass is inadequate because of either poor myocardial function or refractory myocardial ischemia. Under these circumstances the intra-aortic balloon pump is a mechanical addition to the pharmacologic support of cardiac output. An intra-aortic balloon pump is a balloon that is 25 cm long and mounted on a long plastic catheter. The pump is advanced from the left femoral artery to the aorta. The pump inflates and deflates timed to the electrocardiogram. Inflation of the balloon, which occurs during diastole, increases the diastolic blood pressure and increases the coronary perfusion pressure gradient. Deflation of the balloon occurs just before systole. This allows for a reduction of afterload and the pressure against which the heart has to pump. Overall the intra-aortic balloon pump increases coronary blood flow by increasing diastolic pressure while decreasing the work of the myocardium and thus the myocardial oxygen requirement. The efficacy of the balloon pump is altered by rapid heart rates, cardiac dysrhythmias, and aortic insufficiency. (444)

202. Protamine administration to reverse heparin anticoagulation after termination of cardiopulmonary bypass should take place after systemic arterial blood pressure and cardiac output have been maintained for several minutes and the vena cava cannula has been removed. Protamine administration is prior to the removal of the aortic cannulae to allow rapid return to extracorporeal circulatory support in the case of a severe protamine reaction. If a protamine reaction occurs and return to extracorporeal circulatory support is required, additional heparin in doses of 300 to 400 U/kg may be required depending on the dose of protamine administered. Treatment of protamine reactions may include the combination of diphenhydramine (H_1 blocker), ranitidine (H_2 blocker), and hydrocortisone or other steroid. Protamine is administered to reverse the anticoagulant effects produced by heparin. (444)

203. Side effects associated with the administration of protamine include hypotension due to vasodilation, myocardial depression, pulmonary hypertension, histamine release, and, rarely, anaphylactic or anaphylactoid reactions. Anaphylactic and anaphylactoid reactions can be associated with bronchospasm and pulmonary edema. Diabetics who use NPH insulin (which is made with protamine) may be at an increased risk for protamine reactions. These potential effects of protamine call for the careful, slow titration of protamine administration after an initial test dose. (444)

204. Pharmacologic measures than can be taken to decrease bleeding after cardio-pulmonary bypass include the administration of antifibrinolytics (aminocaproic acid, tranexamic acid) and desmopressin. Blood loss throughout the procedure can be salvaged, washed, and retransfused using "cell-saver" devices. (444)

205. Blood and fluid that remain in the cardiopulmonary bypass circuit after cardiopulmonary bypass are washed, collected, and placed in plastic bags by the perfusionist. The blood and fluid can then be administered to the patient. (444)

206. A gradient between central aortic and radial artery blood pressures can exist in the early period after cardiopulmonary bypass. Although the exact mechanism for this is not known, it is believed to be due to vasoconstriction in the extremity. The discrepancy can be determined by the surgical placement of a needle in the aorta and transduction of the pressure. Although the duration of this effect is typically only about 60 minutes, a femoral artery catheter can be placed for the transduction of arterial pressure if the discrepancy is large. (444)

207. Propofol infusions, dexmedetomidine infusions, opioids, or benzodiazepines can all be continued after bypass to provide sedation in the ICU prior to extubation. Of these, dexmedetomidine may reduce postoperative delirium in these patients. (444)

208. Off-pump coronary artery bypass graft (CABG) surgery is CABG surgery done without cardiopulmonary bypass in the presence of a spontaneously beating heart and normothermia. It was developed to reduce the sequelae of extracorporeal circulatory support, which may include stroke, global encephalopathy, renal failure, pulmonary injury, and death. (445)

209. There are several problems with off-pump CABG surgery. First, motion of the coronary artery can make suture placement difficult. Appropriate ACT (activated clotting time) levels are under debate, with some surgeons using doses much smaller than those used for cardiopulmonary bypass. Blood flow to the target coronary artery is usually stopped, and this may cause myocardial ischemia, hemodynamic collapse, and cardiac arrest. Prophylactic antiarrhythmic therapy (lidocaine and magnesium or amiodarone) is necessary to avoid arrhythmias that can occur with surgical manual manipulation of the heart, ischemia during distal coronary artery anastomosis, and upon reperfusion after completion of the anastomosis. To stabilize the heart for surgery ventricular filling can be compromised by the retractors. To displace the heart for the difficult to reach lateral and inferior coronary arteries, steep Trendelenburg positioning may be necessary. Because of these issues, the ability to immediately go on extracorporeal circulatory support must be available during off-pump CABG surgery. Indeed, the use of off-pump CABG surgery is becoming less frequent as a result of the ROOBY (*r*andomized *on/off by*pass) trial, which showed a reduction in graft patency and poorer outcomes in the off-pump group. (445)

210. Ischemic preconditioning may reduce ischemic injury caused by the 10- to 15-minute time necessary for anastomosis of the coronary artery. The 5-minute preconditioning is used to optimize hemodynamics and test to see if the patient will tolerate the anastomosis. A 5-minute recovery period follows the anastomosis. (445)

211. Some similarities between anesthesia management for CABG surgery using cardiopulmonary bypass versus off-pump CABG surgery include the continuance of preoperative medications, sedation and induction medications, neuromuscular blocking drugs, and airway management. (446)

212. There are several differences between the anesthesia management for CABG surgery using cardiopulmonary bypass versus off-pump CABG surgery. In off-pump surgery there is a greater intolerance of tachycardia, hypotension, and hypertension. Myocardial ischemia, ventricular arrhythmias, and hemodynamic collapse are all possible rapidly developing complications. Anesthetic agents that can cause cardiac depression should be minimized or avoided. Hemodynamic stability during the distal anastomosis may require surgical manipulation and retraction of the heart, table positioning, vasoconstrictor infusion, and volume. β-Adrenergic agonists can raise the heart rate and should be avoided. Prophylactic antiarrhythmic therapy is administered to avoid arrhythmias. Finally, the duration and requirements for postoperative ventilation and sedation may be reduced in off-pump CABG surgery. (446)

Chapter

26 CONGENITAL HEART DISEASE

Stephen D. Weston, Jin J. Huang, and
Scott R. Schulman

FUNDAMENTAL PATHOPHYSIOLOGY IN CONGENITAL HEART DISEASE

1. How does shunting in congenital heart disease differ from the normal circulatory pattern?
2. What factors determine the direction and volume of shunt flow?
3. What is a left-to-right shunt, and what are some examples?
4. Explain the concepts of recirculated pulmonary blood flow and effective pulmonary blood flow in a left-to-right shunt.
5. Describe the short-term and long-term effects of increased pulmonary blood flow from a left-to-right shunt.
6. What is a right-to-left shunt? What are the physiologic effects of such a shunt?
7. What are mixing lesions in congenital heart disease, and what are some examples?
8. What determines the systemic arterial oxygen saturation in patients with mixing lesions?
9. What factors can decrease the pulmonary venous oxygen content? The systemic venous oxygen content?
10. What is the ideal Qp:Qs ratio in mixing lesions? Why?
11. What are some factors that can increase systemic vascular resistance?
12. What are some factors that can decrease systemic vascular resistance?
13. What are five factors that increase pulmonary vascular resistance?
14. What are five factors that decrease pulmonary vascular resistance?
15. Why might a patient with a mixing lesion be dependent on a patent ductus arteriosus?
16. Describe the significance of diastolic flow through a patent ductus arteriosus in mixing lesions.
17. What is Eisenmenger syndrome?
18. What are the two most common types of obstructive lesions in congenital heart disease?
19. Describe the spectrum of presentations that might be encountered in aortic stenosis.
20. In coarctation of the aorta, where is the lesion usually found? How should infants with critical coarctation be managed?
21. What are some possible long-term sequelae of repaired coarctation of the aorta?

PERIOPERATIVE MANAGEMENT

22. How can an anesthesiologist participate in the preoperative planning for a patient requiring surgery for congenital heart disease?
23. What preexisting conditions might be important to the care of patients with congenital heart disease?
24. What information might be gained from preoperative echocardiograms or magnetic resonance imaging (MRI)?

25. What are some aspects of the preoperative physical examination that are important to assess in patients with congenital heart disease?
26. Previous sternotomy is a risk factor for what intraoperative complications?
27. What are the fasting recommendations for infants and children scheduled for congenital heart surgery?
28. What is the most important feature of intravenous fluid line preparation for the patient scheduled for congenital heart surgery?
29. What are some common benefits and pitfalls of an inhaled induction of anesthesia in patients with congenital heart disease?
30. Describe the advantages and disadvantages of nitrous oxide for induction of anesthesia in congenital heart disease.
31. Why might an opioid induction of anesthesia be selected for a patient with congenital heart disease? What are some deleterious side effects of an intravenous induction using opioids such as fentanyl?
32. Why might a ketamine induction of anesthesia be selected for a patient with congenital heart disease? What are some deleterious side effects of an intravenous induction using ketamine?
33. What are some general principles for the induction of anesthesia that might apply to all patients with congenital heart disease?
34. What are some congenital cardiac lesions that result in increased pulmonary blood flow and increased pulmonary artery pressure? Describe the overall goals of anesthetic management in such patients.
35. What are some congenital cardiac lesions that result in inadequate pulmonary blood flow? Describe the overall goals of anesthetic management in such patients.
36. What are some considerations for the ventilatory management in patients with congenital heart disease?
37. Describe the overall goals of anesthetic management for patients with obstructive congenital cardiac lesions, such as aortic stenosis or coarctation.
38. For critically ill patients such as those with truncus arteriosus, what is an important feature of ventilator management prior to cardiopulmonary bypass?
39. Describe the stage I procedure for hypoplastic left heart syndrome (Norwood procedure). Describe the important goals of anesthetic management prior to cardiopulmonary bypass.
40. Describe the stage II procedure for hypoplastic left heart syndrome (Glenn procedure). What are some important aspects of anesthetic management?
41. Describe the stage III procedure for hypoplastic left heart syndrome (Fontan procedure). What are poor prognostic factors of a successful Fontan procedure?
42. What are some common abnormalities seen in patients with Williams syndrome?
43. What are some monitors that might be required for children undergoing surgery for congenital heart disease?
44. What are some general requirements for the selection of blood products for infants requiring cardiac surgery?
45. What are some antifibrinolytic drugs used in congenital heart surgery?
46. How is anesthesia maintained prior to cardiopulmonary bypass?
47. What patients may be able to have early extubation of the trachea following congenital heart surgery?
48. Describe the role of arterial blood gas sampling in the operating room during surgery for congenital heart disease.
49. How is anticoagulation for cardiopulmonary bypass achieved?
50. What is the target activated clotting time (ACT) value?
51. Describe the cardiopulmonary bypass circuit.
52. How are flow rates adjusted during cardiopulmonary bypass for infants and children?
53. How does the perfusionist control oxygenation and ventilation during cardiopulmonary bypass?
54. How is body temperature adjusted during cardiopulmonary bypass?

55. How are mechanical quiescence and myocardial protection provided during cardiopulmonary bypass?
56. What is the lowest acceptable level of anemia during cardiopulmonary bypass?
57. What measures are used to provide cerebral and myocardial protection during cardiopulmonary bypass?
58. In what kinds of surgical repairs would deep hypothermic circulatory arrest be employed? Describe an alternative approach.
59. What are some potential negative effects of persistent hypothermia after cardiopulmonary bypass?
60. How can ventricular fibrillation, relative bradycardia, or atrioventricular node conduction failure during separation from cardiopulmonary bypass be treated?
61. How are patients with long-standing excessive pulmonary blood flow treated on separation from bypass?
62. What is the best approach to the management of a patient who has had a palliative procedure and is left with a mixing lesion? What is an effective monitoring tool in these patients?
63. What are some common vasoactive drugs used during separation from cardiopulmonary bypass?
64. What are some causes of difficulty in separation from cardiopulmonary bypass in congenital heart surgery?
65. What rescue measures can be employed if a patient cannot be weaned from cardiopulmonary bypass?
66. What are important complications of protamine administration?
67. What are contributors to coagulopathy after cardiopulmonary bypass in congenital heart surgery?
68. How should blood component therapy be approached in infants? What are common considerations to blood component therapy?
69. What agents can be used for refractory bleeding after cardiopulmonary bypass?
70. What are common parameters to be actively managed after congenital heart surgery in the intensive care unit?

ANSWERS*

FUNDAMENTAL PATHOPHYSIOLOGY IN CONGENITAL HEART DISEASE

1. Pulmonary blood flow and systemic blood flow are normally in series and do not mix. Shunting occurs when there is an abnormal communication between two structures that do not normally communicate, creating abnormal flow between the systemic and pulmonary circulations. A portion of the venous return of one circulation is redirected back to the arterial outflow of that same circulation. (450)
2. The direction and volume of shunt flow depend upon the size of the abnormal communication and the pressure gradient across that communication. Small defects tend to be *restrictive*, with limited flow, whereas large defects tend to be *nonrestrictive*, with unimpeded flow. (450)
3. A left-to-right shunt occurs when a portion of the pulmonary venous return is recirculated to the pulmonary arterial system. Examples include anomalous pulmonary venous return, atrial septal defect, ventricular septal defect, and patent ductus arteriosus. (450)
4. In a left-to-right shunt, the portion of pulmonary venous return (oxygenated blood) that returns to the pulmonary artery is *recirculated* pulmonary blood flow. The portion that is appropriately directed into the systemic circulation is *effective* pulmonary blood flow. The total pulmonary blood flow (Qp) is the sum of the recirculated and effective pulmonary blood flows. (451)

*Numbers in parentheses refer to pages, figures, boxes, or tables in Pardo MC, Miller RD, eds. *Basics of Anesthesia*. 7th ed. Philadelphia: Elsevier; 2018.

5. Patients with left-to-right shunts are typically acyanotic. Pulmonary overflow can lead to pulmonary edema, and systemic underflow can manifest as hypotension, lactic acidosis, and shock. Over time, a left-to-right shunt can cause an increase in pulmonary vascular resistance and ventricular dilation. If the pulmonary vascular resistance becomes sufficiently high, the shunt flow may reverse direction and convert to a cyanotic lesion. This is known as Eisenmenger physiology. (451)

6. A right-to-left shunt occurs when a portion of the systemic venous return is redirected to the systemic arterial outflow without first circulating through the lungs. This results in arterial oxygen desaturation due to an oxygen-poor admixture of systemic venous blood to the oxygen-rich pulmonary venous blood. The degree of desaturation depends on the magnitude of the shunt and the degree of desaturation of the systemic venous return. (451)

7. Mixing lesions are conditions in which oxygen saturation is identical, or nearly identical, at both the pulmonary and systemic arterial level. In mixing lesions, therefore, the systemic arterial oxygen saturation is decreased. Examples include unpalliated single-ventricle anatomy such as hypoplastic left heart syndrome and truncus arteriosus. (452)

8. In mixing lesions, the systemic arterial oxygen saturation is determined by the ratio of the blood flow through the pulmonary and systemic circulatory systems (Qp:Qs) and by the pulmonary venous and systemic venous oxygen saturations. The ratio of resistance to flow (pulmonary vascular resistance/systemic vascular resistance) determines the ratio of flow through each circuit. If pulmonary vascular resistance (PVR) exceeds systemic vascular resistance (SVR), systemic blood flow will exceed pulmonary blood flow (Qs > Qp). The opposite is also true; that is, if SVR exceeds PVR, Qp will exceed Qs. (452)

9. Factors that cause a decrease in pulmonary venous oxygen content (pulmonary veins) include apnea, atelectasis, and pneumonia. Factors that cause a decrease in systemic venous oxygen content (venae cavae) include increased oxygen consumption (e.g., fever, exercise), increased oxygen extraction (low cardiac output), and decreased oxygen delivery (anemia, low systemic arterial oxygen saturation). (452)

10. The ideal Qp:Qs ratio in mixing lesions is close to 1. This minimizes wasteful recirculation to either circuit. When Qp:Qs is >1, the higher pulmonary blood flow results in a higher systemic oxygen saturation, but at the expense of a lower systemic cardiac output, with lower oxygen delivery. When Qp:Qs is <1, the higher blood flow directed out the aorta results in improved systemic perfusion pressure, but at the expense of a lower oxygen saturation, with lower oxygen delivery. (452)

11. Factors that can increase systemic vascular resistance are light anesthesia, sympathetic nervous system activation, administration of α-agonists, and physical manipulations such as flexing the hips of infants and small children. (452)

12. Factors that can decrease systemic vascular resistance are deep anesthesia and the administration of vasodilating drugs, such as nitrates and inhaled anesthetics. (452)

13. Five readily manipulated factors that increase pulmonary vascular resistance are alveolar hypoxemia, hypercapnia, acidosis, sympathetic nervous system stimulation (e.g., light anesthesia), and hypothermia. Other factors include high lung volumes and pressures, or low lung volumes with atelectasis. (452)

14. Five readily manipulated factors that decrease pulmonary vascular resistance are oxygenation, hyperventilation/hypocarbia, alkalosis, warmth, and pulmonary vasodilators such as inhaled nitric oxide. Bronchodilators such as albuterol or inhaled anesthetics reduce pulmonary vascular resistance as well. (452)

15. The ductus arteriosus connects the pulmonary artery to the descending aorta. In patients with mixing lesions and one functional ventricle, a patent ductus arteriosus (PDA) is often required to supply blood flow to the underdeveloped

side. Shunting through the PDA in systole is either left to right (e.g., pulmonary atresia with intact ventricular septum) or right to left (e.g., hypoplastic left heart syndrome) depending on which side of the heart is hypoplastic. In these patients, systemic blood flow is dependent on the patent duct. The duct patency can be maintained with a continuous infusion of prostaglandin E_1. (452)

16. During diastole, shunting through a PDA is usually left to right, because the aorta typically has a higher resting tone than the pulmonary artery. This can cause poor coronary blood flow during diastole, with risk of ischemic or infarcted myocardium. Any maneuvers that decrease pulmonary vascular resistance will cause more diastolic runoff, exacerbating coronary ischemia. (452)

17. When the pulmonary vasculature is exposed to abnormally high flow or pressure, a process of vascular remodeling may occur, with resultant increase in pulmonary vascular resistance. When pulmonary hypertension becomes irreversible, and pulmonary pressures become supersystemic, left-to-right shunts may be converted to right-to-left shunts. This is known as Eisenmenger syndrome and often represents a contraindication to surgical repair of the lesion. (452)

18. The two most common obstructive lesions in congenital heart disease are left ventricular outflow tract obstruction and coarctation of the aorta. Left ventricular outflow tract obstruction is most commonly due to valvar aortic stenosis. (453)

19. Critical aortic stenosis (AS) in utero can lead to hypoplastic left heart syndrome. Severe AS may present with heart failure and failure to thrive. Many patients with AS are asymptomatic but will develop left ventricular hypertrophy, premature coronary atherosclerosis, and congestive heart failure later in life. Bicuspid aortic stenosis is the most prevalent abnormality in this disease, with clinical manifestations in early adulthood. (453)

20. Coarctation of the aorta is a discrete narrowing of the thoracic aorta just distal to the takeoff of the left subclavian artery, where the ductus arteriosus attaches to the aorta. Coarctation of the aorta can occur in isolation or in conjunction with other lesions such as aortic stenosis and ventricular septal defects. Many infants with critical coarctation need a continuous intravenous prostaglandin E_1 infusion to maintain patency of the ductus arteriosus, as they are at risk of developing heart failure and death when the duct closes. (453)

21. Long-term sequelae of repaired coarctation of the aorta include recoarctation, hypertension, aortic aneurysm, coronary artery disease, and stroke. Preeclampsia is more common in parturients with history of coarctation, even if repaired. Long-term follow-up of patients with history of coarctation is imperative. (453)

PERIOPERATIVE MANAGEMENT

22. Most important, the anesthesiologist should understand the physiology of the congenital heart lesion and the subsequent effects of the planned surgery. Aspects of the patient's condition that can be improved prior to surgery should be identified. Cardiac medicines are generally continued, with some variation by anesthesia provider for diuretics, angiotensin-converting enzyme inhibitors, and angiotensin receptor blocking drugs. Anticoagulants and antiplatelet medications are typically held for several days before surgery. (453)

23. Preexisting conditions that might be important to the care of patients with congenital heart disease include a history of prematurity, syndromes such as trisomy 21 or DiGeorge syndrome, and chronic illness such as renal dysfunction, pulmonary edema, and electrolyte abnormalities. For outpatient elective procedures, a day-of-surgery evaluation should investigate for new problems, such as upper respiratory tract infections. (454)

24. Review of the preoperative imaging allows the anesthesiologist to understand the anatomy of the patient's lesion(s) as well as the severity of physiologic derangements such as degree of pulmonary arterial hypertension or ventricular hypertrophy. (454)

25. The preoperative physical examination in patients with congenital heart disease should include an airway evaluation (especially in patients with genetic syndromes), signs of congestive heart failure (tachypnea, wheezing, dilated heart veins), cyanosis, nutritional status, and other coexisting conditions. (454)

26. Previous sternotomy is a risk factor for increased intraoperative blood loss and cardiac trauma during opening of the sternum and dissection of the intrathoracic structures because of adhesions and poor operating conditions caused by scar tissue. (454)

27. The standard American Society of Anesthesiologists guidelines regarding preoperative fasting should be followed for patients preparing for congenital heart surgery. (454)

28. Intravenous administration sets must be meticulously flushed and de-aired prior to use in congenital heart surgery. Systemic air embolus is of particular concern in patients with mixing lesions or right-to-left shunts. However, even left-to-right shunts can be intermittently reversed by such actions as coughing or surgical manipulation of the heart. (455)

29. Advantages of an inhaled induction include no need for venous access prior to induction and ability to slowly titrate the induction. Disadvantages include myocardial depression, decreased heart rate, and decreased systemic vascular resistance. Dose-dependent decrease in myocardial contractility is common to all of the volatile anesthetics; thus, an inhaled induction may not be tolerated in patients with limited cardiac reserve. (455)

30. Nitrous oxide may be used to speed up the inhaled induction and to lower the concentration of volatile anesthetic (e.g., sevoflurane) needed for induction. Disadvantages of nitrous oxide include a lower inspired oxygen concentration during induction, and the concern that intravascular air bubbles will expand. For these reasons its administration is often discontinued shortly after the induction of anesthesia. (455)

31. An opioid induction tends to be hemodynamically stable, because opioids cause little or no myocardial depression or systemic vasodilation. This may make it a preferable induction choice in patients with poorly controlled congestive heart failure, moderately impaired ventricular function, significant right-to-left shunting, or complete mixing lesions. These patients are often critically ill and have intravenous access already in place. Bradycardia is a common side effect of an opioid induction. In patients who are reliant on sympathetic tone to maintain their hemodynamics, opioids can cause hypotension. (455)

32. Ketamine preserves or augments sympathetic nervous system tone and therefore maintains a high degree of cardiovascular stability. In addition, it may be administered intramuscularly, allowing a stable induction of anesthesia in patients without intravascular access. Ketamine's direct negative inotropic effects are typically counteracted by its sympathetic stimulation; in patients with depleted catecholamine stores, ketamine may cause hemodynamic instability. Ketamine causes increased salivary and tracheobronchial secretion, an effect that may be treated with an anticholinergic such as atropine or glycopyrrolate. (455)

33. General principles for the induction of anesthesia in patients with congenital heart disease include avoidance of dehydration, maintenance of sinus rhythm, avoidance of myocardial depression, careful attention to the avoidance of air bubbles in intravenous lines, and appropriate sedation with close monitoring in the preoperative setting after sedation. Increased anxiety, crying, coughing, or breath-holding should be avoided as these states can aggravate unfavorable physiologic effects in susceptible patients. (455-456)

34. Congenital cardiac lesions that result in increased pulmonary blood flow include atrial septal defect and anomalous venous return. Congenital cardiac lesions that result in increased pulmonary artery pressure include ventricular septal defect, atrioventricular canal defect, truncus arteriosus, transposition of the great arteries, and patent ductus arteriosus. The most important additional goal of anesthetic management in such patients is to avoid increasing the degree of

pulmonary overflow. Thus, avoid decreased pulmonary vascular resistance (high inspired oxygen content, hyperventilation), and avoid excessively increased systemic vascular resistance. (457)

35. Congenital cardiac lesions that result in inadequate pulmonary blood flow include tetralogy of Fallot, tricuspid atresia, and pulmonary atresia with intact ventricular septum. Important goals of anesthetic care include maintaining systemic vascular resistance, avoiding increased pulmonary vascular resistance (e.g., avoiding pain, cold, hypoventilation), and treating with high fraction of inspired oxygen when needed. (457)

36. Ventilatory management of the patient with congenital heart disease depends on how the circulatory system will be affected by changes in the pulmonary vascular resistance relative to the systemic vascular resistance. The goal is to minimize the impact on blood flow across shunts, and the cardiac lesion must be understood to best manage the patient. Pulse oximetry is a valuable tool to guide ventilator management. Pulse oximetry provides a continuous monitor of the balance between pulmonary and systemic blood flow and changes in this balance that reflect changes in shunt direction or magnitude. Adjustments in the fractional inspired oxygen concentration, minute ventilation, peak inspiratory pressure, and the possible use of the positive end-expiratory pressure are all considerations. (457)

37. For left-sided obstructive lesions such as coarctation of the aorta and aortic stenosis, goals are to decrease myocardial oxygen demand and support coronary perfusion, accomplished by avoiding tachycardia, dysrhythmias, and hypotension. In coarctation of the aorta, a right-sided arterial line is preferred, and careful attention to ventilation and the avoidance or correction of acidosis is needed in the thoracotomy position. (457)

38. For critically ill patients such as those with truncus arteriosus, an important feature of ventilator management prior to cardiopulmonary bypass is to closely manage the ratio of systemic to pulmonary vascular resistance. (457)

39. The stage I procedure for palliation of hypoplastic left heart syndrome (Norwood procedure) involves reconstruction of the ascending aorta and aortic arch, ligation of the ductus arteriosus, and establishment of pulmonary blood flow, either by a subclavian-to-pulmonary artery shunt (Blalock-Taussig shunt) or a right ventricle–to–pulmonary artery shunt (Sano shunt). Important prebypass anesthetic considerations include maintaining prostaglandin infusion; balancing systemic and pulmonary blood flow with goal Qp:Qs of 1 (Spo_2 80% to 85%); avoidance of myocardial depression; and protection against air embolism. (457)

40. The stage II procedure for palliation of hypoplastic left heart syndrome (Glenn procedure) involves the creation of a direct connection between the superior vena cava and the pulmonary artery. The Blalock-Taussig or Sano shunt is typically ligated during the Glenn procedure. Thus, in Glenn physiology, all pulmonary blood flow comes from the superior vena cava. Important goals of anesthetic management include maintaining a high hematocrit and avoidance of central lines in the superior vena cava distribution. A mild respiratory *acidosis* is sometimes targeted because it increases cerebral blood flow and thus pulmonary blood flow. A metabolic alkalosis is targeted, in compensation, in order to keep pulmonary vascular resistance low. Because positive-pressure ventilation can reduce pulmonary blood flow, early extubation is desirable. (457)

41. The stage III procedure for hypoplastic left heart syndrome (Fontan procedure) involves the creation of a direct connection between the inferior vena cava and the pulmonary artery. This may be accomplished by an extracardiac conduit or (now less commonly) an intracardiac baffle. In Fontan physiology, all systemic venous return drains passively to the lungs and then returns by the pulmonary veins to the common atrium. This physiology is poorly tolerated when there is high pulmonary vascular resistance, atrioventricular valve regurgitation, or poor ventricular function. (457)

42. Common cardiac abnormalities seen in patients with Williams syndrome include supravalvar aortic stenosis, pulmonary arterial stenosis, and abnormalities of the coronary arteries. (457)

43. Monitors for surgery for congenital heart disease, in addition to standard American Society of Anesthesiologists monitors, often include arterial and central venous pressure monitoring and transesophageal echocardiography. The cardiac lesion may dictate the site for arterial line placement. A central line might be placed by the anesthesiologist prior to incision, or the surgeon might place a transthoracic line prior to separation from bypass. Transesophageal echocardiography helps with evaluating anatomy, checking for additional defects, and to assess the quality of the repair. (457)

44. Factors that increase the likelihood of the need for packed red blood cells for infants undergoing cardiac surgery include smaller infants, lower preoperative hematocrit levels, repeat sternotomy incisions, and long cardiopulmonary bypass times. In general, packed red blood cells should be the freshest possible (less than 5 days of storage) or washed. Potassium levels are higher in older packed cells, and older product also exhibits a leftward shift in the oxygen-hemoglobin dissociation curve. Blood products must be administered with proper filters and should be warmed if possible. Other blood products (e.g., fresh frozen plasma, platelets, cryoprecipitate) are often administered after weaning from cardiopulmonary bypass. (457)

45. Aminocaproic acid and tranexamic acid are two antifibrinolytic drugs that may be used to reduce blood loss and transfusion requirements in congenital heart surgery. (457)

46. Maintenance of anesthesia prior to cardiopulmonary bypass is typically achieved with a combination of intravenous opioids and benzodiazepines, volatile anesthetics, and neuromuscular blocking drugs. Nitrous oxide is generally not used for maintenance of anesthesia because of its propensity to expand unintentional intravascular air emboli. Because volatile anesthetics are myocardial depressants, the balance of opioid and volatile agent depends on the patient's myocardial reserve. In more robust patients, opioid dose may be reduced in the expectation of early extubation. In contrast, high-dose opioid techniques may be beneficial in patients who are critically ill or with complex cardiac anomalies so as to minimize the hypotensive and myocardial depressant effects of volatile anesthetics. (458)

47. Good candidates for early extubation of the trachea include patients with good cardiac reserve and simple defects (e.g., atrial septal defect, ventricular septal defect, patent ductus arteriosus, coarctation of the aorta). Another group of patients who may benefit from early extubation are those who have Glenn or Fontan physiology, for whom spontaneous ventilation is likely to improve pulmonary blood flow and cardiac output. (458)

48. The potential for significant hemodynamic, respiratory, and metabolic derangements warrants early, and often repeated, arterial blood gas analysis. (458)

49. Anticoagulation for cardiopulmonary bypass is achieved with unfractionated heparin, with the typical dose of 3 to 4 mg/kg. (458)

50. The target activated clotting time (ACT) may vary with institutional preference but is typically 480 seconds. (458)

51. During cardiopulmonary bypass systemic venous blood returns to the cardiopulmonary bypass machine, and oxygenated blood is returned from the cardiopulmonary bypass machine to the arterial system. The patient's systemic venous return is diverted away from the heart; this is typically achieved by placing two cannulas, one in each vena cava. The systemic venous blood is drained by gravity (passively) to a venous reservoir. The venous reservoir serves as a volume buffer against fluctuations or interruptions in venous drainage; it also allows for rapid administration of blood products, crystalloid or colloid solutions, blood suctioned from the field by the surgeon, and medications. Blood

from the reservoir is conducted to a pump mechanism, generally a centrifugal pump. The blood is pumped at an adjustable, specified flow rate through a membrane oxygenator to equilibrate with supplied fresh gas, adding oxygen and removing carbon dioxide. The blood is also pumped through a heat exchanger. An arterial filter is usually placed downstream from the oxygenator to prevent microembolization to the systemic arterial system. Finally, blood is conducted back to the patient via the arterial cannula, typically in the aorta, to create systemic arterial flow. (458)

52. The target flow rate is based on the patient's weight and adjusted to maintain an age-appropriate mean arterial blood pressure. (458)

53. The perfusionist controls oxygenation during cardiopulmonary bypass by adjusting the oxygen concentration (F_{IO_2}) of the flow to the oxygenator and controls the ventilation by adjusting the flow rate of the gas (sweep) to the oxygenator. (458)

54. Rapid adjustment of blood temperature, and thus body temperature, during cardiopulmonary bypass is achieved by running cooled or warmed water through a coil in contact with the blood path of the systemic arterial flow. (458)

55. When a still heart or bloodless field is required, the heart may be arrested immediately after aortic cross-clamping. Mechanical quiescence and myocardial protection are dually provided during cross-clamp by the administration of cardioplegia. Cardioplegia is cold (4° C) hyperkalemic crystalloid solution. Both the hypothermia and electromechanical arrest contribute to decreasing myocardial oxygen requirements and prolonging tolerable time of myocardial ischemia. (458)

56. The lowest acceptable level of anemia during cardiopulmonary bypass varies from institution to institution but is commonly in the range of 20% to 30%. Because the cardiopulmonary bypass circuit requires an obligatory "priming volume," the hematocrit will be reduced when the patient's blood is diluted upon commencing bypass. In infants and small children, the bypass pump will often require priming with blood products to avoid an unacceptably low hematocrit. Factors that influence the amount of blood product required include the patient's starting hematocrit, estimated blood volume, circuit prime volume, and lowest level of acceptable hematocrit. (458)

57. Because systemic hypothermia reduces cellular metabolism, mild (30° C to 35.5° C) to moderate (25° C to 30° C) systemic hypothermia is used to achieve cerebral and myocardial protection. Metabolic oxygen requirements decrease 7% per degree Celsius. Active rewarming is usually initiated toward the end of cardiopulmonary bypass. (458)

58. For surgical repairs of the ascending aorta and aortic arch, placement of an aortic cannula for cardiopulmonary bypass may obstruct the surgical field. These repairs were traditionally performed under deep hypothermic circulatory arrest, consisting of active cooling on bypass to 18° C to 20° C, then cessation of bypass flow and removal of the aortic cannula for the duration of the repair. Because of adverse outcomes, many centers now provide regional low-flow antegrade cerebral perfusion via cannulation of the innominate (brachiocephalic) artery instead of circulatory arrest. After surgical repair, cardiopulmonary bypass is reinstituted, and the patient is rewarmed and reperfused. (459)

59. Potential negative effects of persistent hypothermia after cardiopulmonary bypass include myocardial ischemia, cardiac dysrhythmias, elevated pulmonary vascular resistance, coagulopathies, and renal dysfunction. (459)

60. Ventricular fibrillation can occur after the aortic cross-clamp is removed and coronary arteries are initially reperfused. Electrical defibrillation is often required to convert to sinus rhythm. Cardiac pacing via temporary epicardial pacing wires is a common intervention to treat relative bradycardia or atrioventricular node dysfunction after cardiopulmonary bypass. Hypothermia, acid-base, and electrolyte disturbances can contribute to cardiac dysrhythmias and should be treated. (459)

61. Long-standing excessive pulmonary blood flow is a risk factor for the development of pulmonary arterial hypertension, and these patients are at risk for a pulmonary hypertensive crisis upon separation from cardiopulmonary bypass. These patients may benefit from maneuvers that reduce pulmonary vascular resistance, including the implementation of inhaled nitric oxide. (459)

62. In the setting of a palliative procedure (such as the Norwood operation), in which a patient is left with a mixing lesion, pulmonary vascular resistance and systemic vascular resistance must continue to be adjusted to optimize both systemic and pulmonary blood flows (balanced Qp:Qs). An effective monitoring tool in these patients is the pulse oximeter. A balanced circulatory system in these patients will result in a systemic oxygen saturation near 80%. When systemic oxygen saturation is greater than 85%, excessive pulmonary blood flow exists, with possible concomitant systemic hypoperfusion. Systemic oxygen saturation less than 75% suggests inadequate pulmonary blood flow. (459)

63. Some common vasoactive drugs used to achieve adequate cardiac output and systemic blood pressure during separation from cardiopulmonary bypass in congenital heart surgery are dopamine, epinephrine, milrinone, and calcium. (460)

64. Difficulty in separation from cardiopulmonary bypass in congenital heart surgery may be caused by inadequate pulmonary blood flow (arterial hypoxemia); inadequate systemic blood flow (hypotension and metabolic acidosis); valvar dysfunction; decreased cardiac output; decreased systemic vascular resistance; abnormal cardiac rhythm; and hypovolemia. (460)

65. If a patient cannot be weaned from cardiopulmonary bypass, surgical revision of the repair must be considered. Otherwise, a return to bypass for a short period of "rest" may allow for improvement in myocardial function induced by the cardiopulmonary bypass run. If the patient still cannot separate from cardiopulmonary bypass despite surgical revision, maximal inotropic support, and ventilation management, implementation of extracorporeal life support may be established. (460)

66. Protamine administration is associated with anaphylactic/anaphylactoid reactions, hypotension, and pulmonary hypertensive crises. However, the incidence of such reactions seems to be lower in children than in adults. (460)

67. Coagulopathy after cardiopulmonary bypass is commonly caused by coagulation factor deficiencies, hypothermia, hypocalcemia, and platelet dysfunction caused by the cardiopulmonary bypass circuit. (460)

68. Empiric blood component therapy is often necessary before laboratory data are available. Such therapy in infants must take account of the patient's small intravascular volume: hypervolemia and ventricular dysfunction may result from aggressive transfusion. Administration of products in 5-mL/kg aliquots or by continuous infusion may avoid this. In addition, hypocalcemia may result from the transfusion of citrated blood products, dilutional anemia from platelet or plasma transfusions, and hypothermia from large volumes of cold blood products. Calcium replacement may be necessary, and fluid-warming devices should be used. (460)

69. Refractory bleeding after cardiopulmonary bypass can be treated with recombinant activated factor VII when conventional hemostatic therapy has failed to stop the bleeding. Recombinant activated factor VII is associated with an increased risk of thromboembolic complications and is of particular concern for risk to the coronary arteries in patients who have undergone the arterial switch operation. (460)

70. Postoperative intensive care for congenital heart surgery includes monitoring and correction of ventilatory, metabolic (electrolytes, glucose), and hematologic parameters. Hemodynamic drug infusions and electrical pacing of the cardiac rhythm may need to be continued. Appropriate sedation both while intubated and after tracheal extubation is required for patient comfort and safety. The repair, and the patient's adaptation to the repair, are monitored with invasive and noninvasive monitoring, including readily available echocardiography. (461)

27 CHRONIC PULMONARY DISEASE AND THORACIC ANESTHESIA

Andrew J. Deacon and Peter D. Slinger

CHRONIC PULMONARY DISEASE

INTRODUCTION

1. What are the major common types of chronic pulmonary diseases encountered in clinical practice?
2. What is the optimal method of anesthesia for patients with moderate or severe chronic lung disease?
3. What history, physical, and laboratory examinations and tests should be considered in patients with moderate or severe chronic lung disease?

ASTHMA

4. What characterizes asthma?
5. What percent of the population has asthma?
6. Which medications are commonly used to treat asthma?
7. What contributes to exacerbations of asthma?
8. What is a concern for the patient with asthma coming for surgery after a recent respiratory infection?
9. How can the severity of asthma be assessed?
10. What are some concerns for the perioperative management of patients on chronic steroids for severe asthma?
11. What doses of corticosteroids for asthma may result in suppression of the hypothalamic-pituitary-adrenal (HPA) axis?
12. Do inhaled steroids suppress the HPA axis?
13. What are some basic principles of the perioperative management of anesthesia for the patient with asthma?

CHRONIC OBSTRUCTIVE PULMONARY DISEASE

14. How is the severity of chronic obstructive pulmonary disease (COPD) classified?
15. What baseline Pa_{CO_2} defines carbon dioxide retention?
16. How can carbon dioxide retention be diagnosed on history and physical examination?
17. When "CO_2 retainers" are given supplemental oxygen, their Pa_{CO_2} levels rise. Why does this occur?
18. What is the risk of an exacerbation of baseline hypercapnia in patients who retain CO_2?
19. How can supplemental oxygen be delivered safely to patients who retain CO_2?
20. What is the cause of the right ventricular dysfunction seen in some severe COPD patients?
21. What Pa_{O_2} should be maintained in COPD patients who have right ventricular dysfunction?

22. What is the pathogenesis of bullae in patients with COPD?
23. What are the symptoms of COPD patients with bullae?
24. What is the concern for positive-pressure ventilation in a patient with bullae?
25. Which inhaled anesthetic agent is contraindicated in patients with bullae?
26. What is the pathogenesis of "flow-limited" breathing seen in COPD patients?
27. What is the concern for positive-pressure ventilation in COPD patients with "flow-limited" breathing?
28. List four treatable complications of COPD that must be evaluated preoperatively.
29. What preoperative management can reduce the risk of postoperative pulmonary complications in patients with severe COPD?

INTERSTITIAL LUNG DISEASE

30. What confirms the diagnosis of a restrictive lung disease on pulmonary function testing?
31. What are the major causes of interstitial lung disease (ILD)?
32. What is the cause of the chronic hypoxemia in patients with severe ILD?
33. What is the optimal strategy for intraoperative ventilation for a patient with ILD?

CYSTIC FIBROSIS

34. What is the cause of cystic fibrosis (CF)?
35. What factors contribute to early fatality in patients with cystic fibrosis?
36. How should patients with cystic fibrosis be managed preoperatively?

OBSTRUCTIVE SLEEP APNEA

37. What are some risk factors for obstructive sleep apnea (OSA)?
38. What are some signs and symptoms associated with OSA?
39. What is the pathophysiology of OSA?
40. How can the diagnosis of OSA be made?
41. What is the treatment for OSA?
42. What are some preoperative considerations for patients with OSA?
43. Which anesthetic medications should be avoided or used in reduced doses in patients with OSA?
44. What are some intraoperative anesthetic concerns for patients with OSA?
45. What airway management difficulties should be anticipated in patients with OSA?
46. Which anesthetic agents are useful in patients with OSA?
47. What are some airway management strategies that should be used at the end of surgery in patients with OSA?
48. How should postoperative analgesia be managed for the patient with OSA?
49. What factors should be considered when planning postoperative disposition of a patient with OSA?
50. What is the obesity hypoventilation syndrome?
51. What are some perioperative concerns for patients with obesity hypoventilation syndrome?

PULMONARY HYPERTENSION

52. What are the criteria for diagnosis of pulmonary hypertension?
53. What are the main types of pulmonary hypertension?
54. What are the main hemodynamic goals on induction in patients with pulmonary hypertension secondary to lung disease?
55. What anesthetic induction agents are useful in patients with pulmonary hypertension?
56. What vasopressors, inotropes, and vasodilators are useful in patients with pulmonary hypertension?
57. Is neuraxial anesthesia/analgesia useful in patients with pulmonary hypertension?

THORACIC ANESTHESIA

ANESTHESIA FOR LUNG RESECTION

58. Describe objective assessments of lung function that may aid assessment of suitability for pneumonectomy and timing of postoperative tracheal extubation.
59. How are respiratory mechanics evaluated prior to anesthesia for lung resection?
60. How is lung parenchymal function evaluated prior to anesthesia for lung resection?
61. How is cardiopulmonary interaction evaluated prior to anesthesia for lung resection?
62. How can ventilation-perfusion scintigraphy help predict postresection pulmonary function?
63. A patient is scheduled to undergo a left upper lobectomy. His forced expiratory volume in 1 second (FEV_1) is 62%. What is his predicted postoperative FEV_1 ($ppoFEV_1$)?
64. In what circumstances are formal lung function tests required for a patient scheduled for lung resection?
65. What preoperative interventions decrease the risk of postoperative pulmonary complications for a patient scheduled for lobectomy?
66. What preoperative interventions decrease the risk of cardiac complications for a patient scheduled for lobectomy?
67. Describe some preoperative considerations specific to patients with lung cancer scheduled to undergo a lobectomy.
68. Describe the physiologic and pharmacologic effects of cigarette smoking.
69. Describe the indications for lung isolation.
70. A double-lumen endobronchial tube (DLT), bronchial blocker (BB), and single-lumen tube (SLT) advanced into a bronchus may all be used for lung isolation. What are the advantages and disadvantages of each?
71. How do you estimate the correct size of DLT for a patient?
72. What are the indications for a right-sided DLT?
73. What are some potential problems associated with use of a right-sided DLT for lung isolation?
74. Describe the design features of the endobronchial portion of a right-sided DLT that differentiate it from a left-sided DLT.
75. Describe the insertion technique for a left-sided DLT using direct laryngoscopy. Describe an alternate insertion technique for a left-sided DLT using direct laryngoscopy and aided by a bronchoscope.
76. Describe the features on bronchoscopy of a correctly placed left-sided DLT.
77. Describe the insertion of a bronchial blocker through a single-lumen endotracheal tube. What features on bronchoscopy confirm correct positioning?
78. Describe the changes in $\dot{V}/\dot{Q}$ matching that occur in an anesthetized patient in the lateral decubitus position upon initiation of one-lung ventilation (OLV) with an open chest.
79. List some potentially serious complications that can occur during thoracotomy and OLV for intrathoracic surgery. What are their causes?
80. What are some surgical considerations for patient monitoring during OLV in addition to standard monitoring?
81. Does the risk of impairment of hypoxic pulmonary vasoconstriction by volatile anesthetics preclude their use during general anesthesia for OLV?
82. Describe the management approach to each of the following during OLV: mode of ventilation, FiO_2, tidal volume, respiratory rate, PCO_2, positive end-expiratory pressure (PEEP), and recruitment maneuvers.
83. How should intravenous fluids be managed for patients undergoing thoracic surgery?
84. Describe an approach to analgesia for a patient undergoing thoracotomy for lung resection.

85. What factors predict patients at increased risk of hypoxemia during OLV?
86. Describe the management of severe and rapid-onset hypoxemia during OLV.
87. Describe the management of slow-onset hypoxemia during OLV.
88. What factors would guide your decision making as to timing of extubation at the conclusion of surgery for a patient undergoing pneumonectomy?

MEDIASTINOSCOPY

89. What structures may be compressed or injured during mediastinoscopy?
90. How does the positioning of patient monitors allow detection of intraoperative innominate artery compression during mediastinoscopy?
91. Describe the management of major hemorrhage during mediastinoscopy.

MEDIASTINAL MASSES

92. What factors on history, examination, and investigations are useful in assessing the risk of anesthesia for resection of a mediastinal mass?
93. Describe the principles of management of a patient with a lower airway obstruction due to a large mediastinal mass.
94. Describe the principles of management of a patient with a large mediastinal mass close to the right atrium or ventricle.

ANSWERS*

CHRONIC PULMONARY DISEASE

INTRODUCTION

1. Chronic pulmonary diseases include obstructive and restrictive lung diseases, obstructive sleep apnea, and pulmonary hypertension. Obstructive lung diseases are commonly divided into reactive airway disorders (asthma) and chronic obstructive pulmonary disease (COPD). However, many patients have more than one type of lung disease. (462)
2. Avoiding general anesthesia with regional or local anesthesia is usually preferable for patients with chronic respiratory diseases. (462)
3. Common symptoms to be elicited in patients with lung disease include cough, wheezing, shortness of breath, chest tightness, sputum production, and reduced exercise tolerance. Also important are recent exacerbations, current and previous therapies including hospital admissions and emergency room visits, and tobacco use. Signs of chronic respiratory disease include tachypnea, cyanosis, use of accessory muscles of respiration, and finger clubbing. On auscultation, signs to be elicited include unequal breath sounds, wheezing, and rales.

   A recent preoperative chest radiograph is not required for all patients but should be considered in any patient with a chronic respiratory disease or a patient with a recent change in respiratory symptoms or signs.

   Simple spirometry (expired volume or flow vs. time), forced vital capacity (FVC), and forced expiratory volume in 1 second (FEV_1) are not required in all stable patients but should be ordered if there is any doubt about the severity of disease (e.g., a recent change in symptoms, if the patient is unable to give a clear history, or if any patient with chronic lung disease is having lung surgery). Full pulmonary function tests (plethysmography) including measurement of residual volume (RV), functional residual capacity (FRC), and measurement of the lung diffusing capacity for carbon monoxide (D_{LCO}) are only indicated if the diagnosis or severity of the lung disease is unclear from simple spirometry.

*Numbers in parentheses refer to pages, figures, boxes, or tables in Pardo MC, Miller RD, eds. *Basics of Anesthesia*. 7th ed. Philadelphia: Elsevier; 2018.

Oxygen saturation (pulse oximetry, $Spo_2\%$) should be documented preoperatively in every patient with a chronic respiratory disease. Arterial blood gases are required preoperatively in patients with moderate or severe chronic respiratory disease who are at risk of requiring postoperative mechanical ventilation (major abdominal, thoracic, cardiac, spine, or neurosurgery), or if there has been a recent worsening of symptoms. (463)

ASTHMA

4. Inflammation of the airways is a hallmark of asthma. (463)
5. Asthma is a common form of episodic recurrent lower airway obstruction that affects 3% to 5% of the population; 65% of people with asthma become symptomatic before age 5. Patients with childhood asthma often become quiescent with time but can have recurrences. (463)
6. Steroids (inhaled and oral) are the most effective medications in controlling airway inflammation associated with asthma. β-Adrenergic bronchodilators are useful for symptomatic relief. (463)
7. Exacerbations of asthma are caused by inflamed airways becoming hyperresponsive to irritant stimuli, with subsequent bronchospasm and mucous secretions. Bronchospastic stimuli can include allergens, dust, cold air, instrumentation of the airways, and medications (aspirin or histamine-releasing drugs). (463)
8. Asthmatics are at risk for life-threatening bronchospasm during anesthesia if improperly managed, particularly during or recently after a respiratory tract infection. Elective surgery should therefore be delayed at least 6 weeks after a respiratory infection in these patients. (463)
9. The severity of asthma is defined by the amount of treatment required to control symptoms. Most patients will be on steps 1 or 2 of this treatment protocol, which include patients using short-acting β_2-agonists with or without inhaled steroids at up to 400 µg/day. Caution is required when anesthetizing patients on steps 4 or 5, such as those using high-dose inhaled or oral steroids daily. Peak expiratory flow (PEF) rate is another very simple and useful measurement of the severity of asthma, and many patients measure their own PEFs to guide their therapy. PEF rates less than 50% predicted (corrected for age/gender/height) indicate severe asthma. A PEF increase greater than 15% after bronchodilator use suggests inadequate treatment of asthma. Eliciting a previous history of severe or life-threatening exacerbations (e.g., requiring intensive care or intubation) is indicative of patients at increased risk. (464)
10. Patients on chronic steroids for severe asthma may have suppression of the hypothalamic-pituitary-adrenal (HPA) axis. The stress of surgery may precipitate an adrenal crisis in these patients. (464)
11. Short courses of oral prednisone used to treat asthma exacerbations can affect HPA function for up to 10 days. In patients who are taking larger doses, prolonged therapy of more than 3 weeks, evening dosing, and continuous daily dosing may have HPA suppression for up to a year. (464)
12. Inhaled steroids are unlikely to suppress the HPA axis. (464)
13. There are some basic principles of the perioperative management of patients with asthma. During the preoperative evaluation the adequacy of asthma control needs to be assessed. On the day of surgery patients should use their inhalers on their normal schedule. Inhaled β_2-agonists can be administered prior to anesthesia. Endotracheal intubation should be avoided if possible through the use of an LMA (laryngeal mask airway) and/or regional anesthesia if possible. If endotracheal intubation is necessary, instrumentation of the airway should be done after an adequate level of anesthesia is achieved to decrease airway reflexes. Anesthetic drugs that promote bronchodilation, such as sevoflurane and propofol, should be chosen. Drugs that cause histamine release, such as morphine, should be avoided. (464)

CHRONIC OBSTRUCTIVE PULMONARY DISEASE

14. Chronic obstructive pulmonary disease (COPD) incorporates three disorders: emphysema, peripheral airway disease, and chronic bronchitis. The FEV_1/FVC ratio will be less than 70%, and RV will be increased. The severity of COPD is assessed by the FEV1%: stage I, more than 50% predicted (this category includes both "mild" and "moderate" COPD); stage II, 35% to 50% predicted; stage III, less than 35% predicted. Stage I patients should not have significant dyspnea, hypoxemia, or hypercarbia. (464)

15. Carbon dioxide retention is defined as a baseline $Paco_2$ greater than 45 mm Hg on an arterial blood gas measurement. (465)

16. Many stage II or III COPD patients have an elevated $Paco_2$ at rest. It is not possible to differentiate these "CO_2 retainers" from nonretainers on the basis of history, physical examination, or spirometry. A preoperative arterial blood gas measurement is necessary for diagnosis. (465)

17. Patients who retain CO_2 will have an exacerbation of their hypercapnia when given supplemental oxygen for two reasons. Mainly, the administration of oxygen leads to a decrease in regional hypoxic pulmonary vasoconstriction, which in turn leads to an increase in alveolar dead space. In smaller part, the rise in $Paco_2$ is also due to the Haldane effect. The Haldane effect is that increased oxygenation of hemoglobin promotes dissociation of carbon dioxide or decreases the ability of CO_2 to bind to hemoglobin for transport. (465)

18. Increased $Paco_2$ levels above baseline lead to respiratory acidosis, which causes cardiovascular changes (tachycardia, hypotension, and pulmonary vasoconstriction) and $Paco_2$ levels higher than 80 mm Hg, which cause a decreased level of consciousness. (465)

19. When supplemental oxygen is administered to patients who retain CO_2, a rise in CO_2 levels above baseline should be anticipated. Oxygen administration should be slowly titrated and monitored with serial examinations of $Paco_2$ and level of consciousness. (465)

20. Chronic recurrent hypoxemia is the cause of RV dysfunction that occurs in up to 50% of patients with severe COPD. These patients can progress to cor pulmonale or right-sided heart failure. Cor pulmonale occurs in 70% of adult COPD patients with an FEV_1 less than 0.6. (465)

21. Mortality risk in COPD patients with right ventricular dysfunction is primarily related to chronic hypoxemia. The only therapy that has been shown to improve long-term survival and decrease right-sided heart strain in COPD is oxygen. COPD patients who have resting Pao_2 lower than 55 mm Hg should receive supplemental home oxygen to maintain a Pao_2 60 to 65 mm Hg. (465)

22. Patients with moderate or severe COPD develop cystic air spaces in the lung parenchyma known as *bullae*. A bulla is a localized loss of structural support tissue in the lung with elastic recoil of surrounding parenchyma. (465)

23. COPD patients with bullae are often asymptomatic in the early stages. When bullae occupy more than 50% of the hemithorax the patient may present with findings of restrictive pulmonary disease in addition to their obstructive disease. (465)

24. COPD patients with bullae are at risk for bulla rupture, tension pneumothorax, and bronchopleural fistula with positive-pressure ventilation. The pressure in a bulla is the mean pressure in the surrounding alveoli averaged over the respiratory cycle. Whenever positive-pressure ventilation is used, the pressure in a bulla will become positive in relation to the adjacent lung tissue and the bulla will expand, leading to these potential complications. Positive-pressure ventilation can be used safely in patients with bullae, provided the airway pressures are kept low and there is adequate expertise and equipment immediately available to insert a chest drain and obtain lung isolation if necessary. (465)

25. Nitrous oxide will diffuse into a bulla more quickly than the less soluble nitrogen can diffuse out and may lead to rupture of the bulla. Nitrous oxide is thus contraindicated in patients with bullae. (465)

26. Severe COPD patients are often "flow limited" even during normal breathing. Flow limitation occurs when any increase in expiratory effort will not produce an increase in flow at that given lung volume. Flow limitation is present in normal patients only during a forced expiratory maneuver. In patients with COPD, because of the loss of lung elastic recoil and collapse of distal airways, flow limitation may be present at all times. (465)

27. During positive-pressure ventilation COPD patients with flow-limited breathing can develop an intrinsic positive end-expiratory pressure (auto-PEEP). Severely flow-limited patients are at risk of hemodynamic collapse during positive-pressure ventilation as a result of "breath stacking," dynamic hyperinflation of the lungs leading to obstruction of pulmonary blood flow and decreased central venous return. (466)

28. Four treatable complications of COPD that must be actively sought and managed at the time of preoperative assessment are atelectasis, bronchospasm, respiratory tract infections, and congestive heart failure. Atelectasis impairs local lung lymphocyte and macrophage function, predisposing to infection. Wheezing may be a symptom both of airway obstruction and congestive heart failure. All COPD patients should receive bronchodilator therapy as guided by their symptoms. A patient who is poorly controlled on sympathomimetic and anticholinergic bronchodilators should receive a trial of corticosteroids. (466)

29. Patients with severe COPD have fewer postoperative pulmonary complications when intensive chest physiotherapy is initiated preoperatively. Even in patients with severe COPD, it is possible to improve exercise tolerance with physiotherapy, though little improvement is seen before 1 month. Among patients with COPD, those with excessive sputum benefit the most from chest physiotherapy. A comprehensive program of pulmonary rehabilitation involving physiotherapy, exercise, nutrition, and education has been shown consistently to improve functional capacity for these patients. Programs are typically of several months' duration and are generally not an option in resections for malignancy. (466)

INTERSTITIAL LUNG DISEASE

30. Restrictive pulmonary disease will have findings of an FEV_1 less than 70% predicted, FEV_1/FVC ratio normal or increased, and RV decreased on pulmonary function testing. Interstitial lung disease (ILD) is a chronic restrictive pulmonary disease. (466)

31. About 35% of ILD is attributable to an identifiable cause—for example, exposure to inorganic dust, organic antigen, drugs, or radiation. The inciting agent in the remaining 65% of patients is unknown. In many of these patients the lung is affected as part of an autoimmune disorder. (466)

32. In ILD, elastic recoil of the lungs increases as a consequence of inflammation and fibrosis of the alveolar walls, which results in contraction of lung volumes. Early in the disease, patients adapt to lower tidal volumes by increasing their respiratory rate. As the disease progresses, increased respiratory effort and energy are required to maintain sufficient tidal volumes to prevent alveolar hypoventilation. Uneven disease distribution throughout the lung can cause significant ventilation-perfusion mismatch and is the primary cause of hypoxemia in patients with ILD. (466)

33. Controlled ventilation through an endotracheal tube is often the most reliable and safest approach to optimize oxygenation and ventilation in patients with ILD when a general anesthetic is required. The goal of mechanical ventilation in patients with ILD is to maintain adequate ventilation and oxygenation while minimizing the risks of barotrauma and acute lung injury. Potential strategies to minimize airway pressures include the use of long duration of inspiration compared to the duration of expiration ratios (e.g., ratios of 1:1 to 1:1.5), small tidal volumes, and rapid respiratory rates. In contrast to obstructive lung disease, positive end-expiratory pressure (PEEP) can be used safely in ILD. (466)

CYSTIC FIBROSIS

34. Cystic fibrosis (CF) is an autosomal recessive disorder that results in impaired transport of sodium, chloride, and water across epithelial tissue. This leads to exocrine gland malfunction with abnormally viscous secretions, which can cause obstruction of the respiratory tracts, pancreas, biliary system, intestines, and sweat glands. It presents as a mixed obstructive and restrictive lung disease. Inability to clear the thick purulent secretions enhances bacterial growth and, as the disease advances, leads to bronchiectasis. (466)

35. The early fatality of CF is primarily the result of pulmonary complications: air trapping, pneumothorax, massive hemoptysis, and respiratory failure. (466)

36. Effective sputum elimination is a key goal in the management of CF. To optimize CF patients for anesthesia, chest physiotherapy should be performed immediately prior to surgery. Intubation with a large endotracheal tube is preferred because it facilitates endobronchial toileting with a suction catheter or bronchoscopy. (466)

OBSTRUCTIVE SLEEP APNEA

37. Risk factors for obstructive sleep apnea (OSA) include obesity, male gender, middle age, BMI more than 28 kg/m^2, alcohol use, and sedative use. Patients with these risk factors presenting for surgery should be screened for signs and symptoms of OSA. (466)

38. Clinical characteristics associated with OSA include BMI greater than 35 kg/m^2, neck circumference larger than 17 inches, airway craniofacial abnormalities, anatomic nasal obstruction, and tonsils touching or nearly touching at midline. Clinical history suggestive of OSA includes frequent snoring, observed pauses in breathing, awakening from sleep with choking sensation, frequent arousals from sleep, and daytime somnolence or fatigue. (466)

39. The pathophysiology of the airflow obstruction of OSA is related primarily to upper airway pharyngeal collapse. Upper airway patency depends on the action of dilator muscles (i.e., tensor palatine, genioglossus muscle, and hyoid muscles). During sleep, laryngeal muscle tone is decreased, and apnea occurs when the upper airway collapses. Nonobese patients may develop OSA as a result of adenotonsillar hypertrophy or craniofacial abnormalities (retrognathia). Recurrent episodes of apnea or hypopnea lead to hypoxia, hypercapnia, increased sympathetic stimulation, and arousal from sleep. Patients may develop cardiopulmonary dysfunction manifesting as systemic or pulmonary hypertension and cor pulmonale. Nonrestoration of sleep can lead to cognitive dysfunction manifesting as intellectual impairment and hypersomnolence. (466)

40. The diagnosis of OSA can be based on clinical impression or a formal sleep study. OSA should be suspected when a patient with predisposing clinical risk factors reports heavy snoring and excessive daytime sleepiness, which are the cardinal features of OSA. OSA is characterized by frequent episodes of apnea or hypopnea during sleep. Apnea is defined as complete cessation of breathing for 10 seconds or more and hypopnea is defined as greater than 50% decrease in ventilation or oxygen desaturation of 3% to 4% for 10 seconds or more. OSA is definitively diagnosed by polysomnography in a sleep laboratory. The severity of OSA is measured by using the apnea-hypopnea index (AHI), which is the number of apneic or hypopneic episodes occurring per hour of sleep. (467)

41. Treatment for OSA should include correction of reversible exacerbating factors by means of weight reduction, avoidance of alcohol and sedatives, and nasal decongestants, if needed. Patients with mild OSA can achieve clinical improvement through lifestyle modification. For severe OSA, the three main therapeutic options are continuous positive airway pressure (CPAP), dental appliances, and upper airway surgery. (467)

42. Preoperative considerations for patients with OSA include the following:
    a. Airway: Anticipated difficulties with airway management include difficult face mask ventilation and tracheal intubation.
    b. Respiratory system: Patients with obesity will have evidence of restrictive lung disease on pulmonary function testing secondary to decreased chest wall compliance.

    c. Cardiovascular system: Preoperative evaluation should be directed toward the detection of end-organ dysfunction resulting from chronic hypoxemia, hypercarbia, and polycythemia. Systemic hypertension, pulmonary hypertension, and signs of biventricular dysfunction (cor pulmonale and congestive heart failure) should be sought.

    d. Endocrine and gastrointestinal systems: Fasting blood glucose levels should be sought to screen for type II diabetes. Symptoms of esophageal reflux should lead to aspiration prophylaxis prior to induction of anesthesia. Liver function tests may indicate fatty liver infiltration causing hepatic dysfunction in severe cases. (467)

43. Patients with OSA are exquisitely sensitive to the respiratory depressant and sedative effects of benzodiazepines and opioids, which can cause upper airway obstruction or apnea. These medications should be withheld preoperatively or used with caution in a monitored environment. (468)

44. Intraoperative anesthetic concerns for patients with OSA include airway management, anesthetic technique, patient positioning, monitoring, and vascular access. (468)

45. Difficulties with airway management should be anticipated in patients with OSA. Upper airway abnormalities or increased airway adiposity in patients with OSA predisposes them to difficult hand ventilation by bag and mask following induction of anesthesia. Oral and nasopharyngeal airways and video laryngoscopy should be readily available. Excessive pharyngeal adipose tissue can make exposure of the glottic opening difficult during direct laryngoscopy and intubation. (468)

46. The use of short-acting inhaled (sevoflurane and desflurane) and injected (propofol, remifentanil) drugs is recommended for intraoperative use to minimize postoperative respiratory depression in patients with OSA. Nitrous oxide is best avoided in patients with coexisting pulmonary hypertension. Short- to intermediate-acting neuromuscular blocking drugs can be used for muscle relaxation if required. (468)

47. At the end of surgery in patients with OSA, the anesthesiologist should consider tracheal extubation with the patient in a semiupright position with an oral or nasopharyngeal airway in place to facilitate spontaneous ventilation. It is likely that two-person bag and mask ventilation and possible reintubation will be required should acute airway obstruction develop. Supplemental oxygen by face mask should be provided during patient transfer to the postanesthesia recovery unit (PACU). CPAP must be available for postoperative use in patients on CPAP or BiPAP (bilevel positive airway pressure) preoperatively. (468)

48. For patients with OSA, multimodal analgesia with NSAIDs, acetaminophen, and regional analgesia to minimize opiate analgesia and resultant respiratory depression should be used postoperatively. CPAP should be reinstituted postoperatively. Surveillance in a high-dependency unit such as the PACU, step-down unit, or intensive care unit (ICU) is prudent for patients with severe OSA. (468)

49. Postoperative disposition of OSA is influenced by three things:
    a. Severity of the OSA (either by historical information or objective findings of a sleep study)
    b. Invasiveness of the surgical procedure and anesthesia
    c. Predicted postoperative opioid use
    A patient with increased perioperative risk of airway obstruction and resultant hypoxemia (perioperative OSA risk score greater than 4) should receive continuous oxygen saturation monitoring in either the ICU, a step-down unit, or telemetry unit. (468)

50. Obesity hypoventilation syndrome (OHS) is defined by chronic daytime hypoxemia ($Pa_{O_2} < 65$ mm Hg) and hypoventilation ($Pa_{CO_2} > 45$ mm Hg) in an obese patient without coexisting COPD. It is a long-term consequence of OSA. Patients exhibit signs of central sleep apnea (apnea without respiratory efforts).

This may culminate in the pickwickian syndrome characterized by obesity, daytime hypersomnolence, hypoxemia, and hypercarbia. (469)

51. Preoperatively, obese patients should be screened for OHS with pulse oximetry. Patients with an oxygen saturation less than 96% warrant arterial blood gas analysis to assess carbon dioxide retention. Preoperative interventions may include treatment of coexisting conditions (systemic hypertension, cardiac dysrhythmias, congestive heart failure) and initiation of CPAP. A 2-week period of CPAP therapy is usually effective in correcting the abnormal ventilatory drive of patients with OHS. Postoperative care should also be planned, such as postoperative monitoring or hospital bed (i.e., step-down bed or ICU) arrangements. (469)

PULMONARY HYPERTENSION

52. Pulmonary hypertension is defined as mean pulmonary artery pressure greater than 25 mm Hg by catheterization or a peak systolic pulmonary artery pressure more than 35 mm Hg. A right ventricular systolic pressure on echocardiography higher than 50 mm Hg is not diagnostic but is consistent with the diagnosis of pulmonary hypertension. (469)

53. Although five different types of pulmonary hypertension are included in the cardiology literature, for the anesthesiologist there are essentially two main types of pulmonary hypertension: pulmonary hypertension due to left-sided heart disease and pulmonary hypertension due to lung disease. Patients who present for noncardiac surgery are more likely to have pulmonary hypertension due to lung disease. (469)

54. Avoiding hypotension is the key to managing patients with pulmonary hypertension secondary to lung disease. The increased right ventricular transmural and intracavitary pressures associated with pulmonary hypertension may restrict perfusion of the right coronary artery during systole, especially as pulmonary artery pressures approach systemic levels. The impact of pulmonary hypertension on right ventricular dysfunction has several anesthetic implications. The hemodynamic goals are similar to other conditions in which cardiac output is relatively fixed. Care should be taken to avoid physiologic states that will worsen pulmonary hypertension such as hypoxemia, hypercarbia, acidosis, and hypothermia. Conditions that impair right ventricular filling such as tachycardia and arrhythmias are not well tolerated. Ideally, under anesthesia, right ventricular contractility and systemic vascular resistance are maintained or increased, whereas pulmonary vascular resistance is decreased. (469)

55. Although basically any common anesthetic induction agent can be used for the induction of anesthesia in patients with pulmonary hypertension, hypotension must be avoided. Ketamine can be a useful anesthetic agent in these patients. (469)

56. Inotropes and inodilators such as dobutamine and milrinone may improve hemodynamics in patients with pulmonary hypertension due to left-sided heart disease; however, they decrease systemic vascular tone and tachycardia and can lead to a deterioration in the hemodynamics of patients with pulmonary hypertension due to lung disease. For pulmonary hypertension secondary to lung disease, vasopressors such as phenylephrine, norepinephrine, and vasopressin are commonly used to maintain a systemic blood pressure greater than pulmonary pressures. Vasopressin may be preferable as it appears to increase systemic blood pressure significantly without affecting pulmonary artery pressure in patients with pulmonary hypertension. In patients with severe pulmonary hypertension, selective inhaled pulmonary vasodilators including nitric oxide (10-40 ppm) or nebulized prostaglandins (prostacyclin 50 ng/kg/min) should be considered. (469)

57. There have been multiple case reports of the successful use of lumbar epidural analgesia and anesthesia in obstetric patients with pulmonary hypertension. There are very few reports of the use of thoracic epidural analgesia in pulmonary hypertension. Patients with pulmonary hypertension from lung disease seem to be extremely dependent on tonic cardiac sympathetic innervation for normal hemodynamic stability. These patients will often require a low-dose infusion of inotropes or vasopressors during thoracic epidural local analgesia. (469)

THORACIC ANESTHESIA

ANESTHESIA FOR LUNG RESECTION

58. No test of respiratory function has proved to be adequate as a sole preoperative assessment for patient suitability for pneumonectomy and timing for postoperative tracheal extubation. Before surgery, respiratory function should be assessed in three related but independent areas: respiratory mechanics, lung parenchymal function, and cardiopulmonary interaction. (470)

59. The most useful test of respiratory mechanics is forced expiratory volume in 1 second (FEV_1) calculated from spirometry. This can be used to calculate a predicted postoperative FEV_1 ($ppoFEV_1$). Patients with a $ppoFEV_1$ greater than 40% are at low risk of postoperative pulmonary complications, whereas those with a $ppoFEV_1$ less than 30% are at high risk. (470)

60. Lung parenchymal function refers to the ability of the lung to exchange oxygen and carbon dioxide. Lung parenchymal function can be assessed by diffusion capacity of the lungs for carbon monoxide (D_{LCO}) and arterial blood gas analysis. A $ppoD_{LCO}$ of greater than 40%, Pao_2 more than 60 mm Hg, and $Paco_2$ less than 45 mm Hg are associated with a low risk of postoperative pulmonary complications. (470)

61. Cardiopulmonary interaction is most accurately assessed with exercise testing to calculate a $\dot{V}o_{2max}$, though several surrogates may be used. Patients with a $\dot{V}o_{2max}$ of less than 15 mL/kg/min are at an increased risk of postoperative pulmonary complications. (471)

62. Ventilation-perfusion scintigraphy may further modify the $ppoFEV_1$ by providing an assessment of the functional contribution of the lung or lobe to be resected. (471)

63. The predicted postoperative FEV_1 ($ppoFEV_1$) is calculated using the following equation:

$$ppoFEV_1\% = \text{preoperative } FEV_1\% \times (100 - \% \text{ of function tissue removed}/100)$$

The proportion of functional lung removed will be 10/42 = 24% (10 lung subsegments in the left upper lobe and 42 in total). A patient with an FEV_1 of 62% undergoing a left upper lobectomy will therefore have a $ppoFEV_1$ of 47% ($ppoFEV_1$ = 62% × (100 − 24/100) = 62% × 0.76 = 47%). (471)

64. All patients scheduled for lung resection should undergo simple spirometry allowing assessment of FVC and FEV_1 preoperatively. Formal lung function testing additionally allows for an assessment of lung volumes, airway resistance, and diffusion capacity (D_{LCO}). This assists in confirmation of the clinical diagnosis and assessment of disease severity. The decision to refer for formal lung function testing should be based on the likelihood of the patient having a $ppoFEV_1$ less than 40% (i.e., patients at increased risk of postoperative pulmonary complications). Patients with underlying lung disease or those undergoing more extensive resections (e.g., lobectomy and pneumonectomy) should therefore be referred. (471)

65. A number of preoperative interventions can decrease postoperative pulmonary complications for patients scheduled for lobectomy.

Smoking cessation reduces pulmonary complications regardless of the timing of cessation prior to surgery. The anesthesiologist should encourage the patient to stop smoking at the preoperative assessment, when patients may be more receptive to the message.

Symptoms and signs of a current respiratory tract infection should be sought, and if present, the patient should be treated and the surgery rescheduled if feasible.

All patients with COPD should receive bronchodilator therapy as guided by their symptoms. A patient who is poorly controlled on sympathomimetic and anticholinergic bronchodilators should receive a trial of corticosteroids. Further, patients with COPD have fewer postoperative pulmonary complications when intensive chest physiotherapy is initiated preoperatively. Even in patients with severe COPD, it is possible to improve exercise tolerance with physiotherapy, though little improvement is seen before 1 month. Among patients with COPD, those with excessive sputum benefit the most from chest physiotherapy. A comprehensive program of pulmonary rehabilitation involves physiotherapy, exercise, nutrition, and education and has been shown to improve functional capacity in patients with severe COPD. These programs are usually of several months' duration and are generally not an option in resections for malignancy. (471)

66. Assessment of cardiac risk should follow the American College of Cardiology/American Heart Association (ACC/AHA) Guideline on Perioperative Cardiovascular Evaluation and Management of Patients Undergoing Noncardiac Surgery. Thoracic surgery is identified as a risk factor for major adverse cardiac events. Further, postoperative arrhythmia is common following thoracic or esophageal surgery, occurring in 12% to 44% of patients. The most common dysrhythmia seen is atrial fibrillation, typically occurring on postoperative day 2 or 3. Risk factors for postoperative atrial fibrillation include male sex, older age, magnitude of lung or esophagus resected, history of congestive cardiac failure, concomitant lung disease, and length of procedure. It may be reasonable to give high-risk patients (e.g., older patients undergoing pneumonectomy) prophylactic diltiazem to decrease the incidence of postoperative atrial fibrillation. (471)

67. Patients undergoing lung resection for malignancy should be assessed for the "four Ms": *m*ass effects, *m*etabolic abnormalities, *m*etastases, and *m*edications. Mass effects include obstructive pneumonia, lung abscess, superior vena cava syndrome, tracheobronchial distortion, Pancoast syndrome, recurrent laryngeal nerve or phrenic nerve paresis, chest wall or mediastinal extension. Metabolic effects include Lambert-Eaton syndrome, hypercalcemia, hyponatremia, and Cushing syndrome. Metastases are particularly likely to brain, bone, liver, and adrenal glands. Medications (i.e., chemotherapy) may cause pulmonary toxicity (bleomycin, mitomycin), cardiac toxicity (doxorubicin), and renal toxicity (cisplatin). (471)

68. Nicotine and carbon monoxide are the principal substances of harm when cigarettes are smoked. Nicotine increases sympathetic outflow and catecholamine release, resulting in increased heart rate, cardiac inotropy, peripheral vascular resistance, blood pressure, and therefore myocardial oxygen consumption. Carbon monoxide decreases oxygen transport and utilization. Other components of cigarette smoke increase mucous secretion and viscosity and damage the respiratory epithelium. Long-term smoking alters lung elasticity, resulting in emphysema.
The half-life of nicotine is 30 to 60 minutes. The half-life of carbon monoxide is 4 to 6 hours and depends chiefly on pulmonary ventilation. Carbon monoxide binds hemoglobin, myoglobin, and cytochrome oxidase, resulting in decreased oxygen-carrying capacity in the blood and muscle and decreased mitochondrial oxygen utilization. (471)

69. Lung isolation is indicated to (1) allow one-lung ventilation and surgical access to the thorax and adjacent structures (lung resection, mediastinal, cardiac, vascular, esophageal, and spinal surgery); (2) control ventilation (bronchopleural fistula); (3) prevent contralateral lung soiling (pulmonary hemorrhage, bronchopleural fistula, and whole lung lavage); and (4) allow for differential patterns of ventilation in patients with unilateral lung injury. (471)

70. Advantages of a double-lumen tube (DLT) compared to a bronchial blocker (BB) or single-lumen, standard endotracheal tube (SLT) include the following: successful placement is easy, repositioning is rarely required, bronchoscopy can be performed to the isolated lung, suction to the isolated lung is possible, CPAP is easily applied, one-lung ventilation can be performed easily to either lung, and placement is possible if a bronchoscope is not available. Disadvantages of a DLT include the following: size selection is more difficult than for a BB or SLT, it is challenging to place

in patients with difficult airways or abnormal tracheas, it is not optimal for postoperative ventilation, and it has the potential for laryngeal and bronchial trauma.

Advantages of a BB compared to a DLT include that size selection is rarely an issue, it can be easily added to a regular ETT, it allows ventilation during placement, and it is easier to place in patients with difficult airways and in children. Additionally, postoperative two-lung ventilation is easy by withdrawing the BB, selective lobar isolation is possible, and CPAP is possible to the isolated lung. Disadvantages of a BB include that more time is required to position, repositioning is required more often, a bronchoscope is essential for positioning, right lung isolation is limited owing to the relatively short right main bronchus in many people, bronchoscopy to the isolated lung is not possible, minimal suction can be applied to the isolated lung, and it is difficult to alternate one-lung ventilation to either lung.

An advantage of an SLT advanced into a bronchus compared to a DLT is the ease of placement in patients with difficult airways. Disadvantages of an SLT include that bronchoscopy is necessary for placement; it does not allow for bronchoscopy, suctioning, or CPAP to the isolated lung; the cuff is not designed for lung isolation; and one-lung ventilation to the right lung is extremely difficult owing to the short right main bronchus. (473)

71. There is no consensus as to the optimal method to size a DLT. An ideally sized DLT should have a bronchial external diameter 1 to 2 mm smaller than the bronchial diameter in order to fit the deflated bronchial cuff. A chest radiograph may be used to assist DLT selection. The authors' preference is a simplified method based on patient sex and height. For females taller than 160 cm use a 37 Fr, and for those shorter than 160 cm use a 35 Fr. For females shorter than 152 cm consider a 32 Fr. For males taller than 170 cm use a 41 Fr, and for those shorter than 170 cm use a 39 Fr. For males shorter than 160 cm consider a 37 Fr. A further important step prior to placement is to check a chest radiograph, or ideally a computed tomography (CT) chest coronal slice, to exclude aberrant anatomy (e.g., endoluminal obstruction, significant tracheal deviation, or aberrant right upper lobe takeoff). It is important to appreciate that compared to an SLT, a DLT has a large external diameter and should not be advanced against resistance. (473)

72. There are two main indications for a right-sided DLT. Distorted anatomy of the entrance of the left main bronchus may preclude using a left-sided DLT (e.g., external or intraluminal tumor compression or descending thoracic aortic aneurysm). Further, the site of surgery may involve the left main bronchus (e.g., left lung transplantation, left-sided tracheobronchial disruption, left-sided pneumonectomy, or left-sided sleeve resection). It is possible to manage a left pneumonectomy with a left-sided DLT or BB, but the DLT or BB will have to be withdrawn before stapling the left main bronchus. (475)

73. A right-sided DLT must be positioned with the slot in the endobronchial lumen at the orifice of the right upper lobe. A small movement of the DLT distally may occlude the right upper lobe, resulting in hypoxemia, whereas migration proximally may result in loss of lung isolation. Further, there is anatomic variation in the distance of the right upper lobe orifice from the carina (1 in 250 patients have a right upper lobe originating at or proximal to the carina). Tracheobronchial anatomy must be checked prior to insertion of the right-sided DLT (coronal slice of a CT scan or bronchoscopy) to confirm normal positioning of the right upper lobe orifice. If the right upper lobe orifice originates more than 1.5 cm from the carina, successful use of a right-sided DLT is likely. (475)

74. A right-sided DLT incorporates a modified cuff and slot in the endobronchial lumen that allows ventilation of the right upper lobe. (475)

75. Two techniques are commonly used when inserting a left-sided DLT. One is a blind technique, in which the endobronchial lumen of the DLT is passed through the glottis by laryngoscopy and the DLT is then turned 90 degrees

counterclockwise and advanced until resistance is felt. Blind insertion alone results in malposition in approximately 35% of cases, and therefore, confirmation of position with a flexible bronchoscope is important. An alternate technique for DLT insertion is performed under direct vision using a bronchoscope. The tip of the endobronchial lumen is passed through the glottis, the DLT is rotated 90 degrees counterclockwise, and the DLT is then advanced so the tracheal cuff is just past the glottis. A flexible bronchoscope is then inserted into the endobronchial lumen to its opening, and the DLT and bronchoscope are advanced simultaneously into the correct bronchus. Alternatively the bronchoscope may be advanced through the endobronchial lumen and into the left main bronchus, with the DLT advanced over it. (473)

76. Bronchoscopy using a pediatric bronchoscope (≤3.5 mm diameter) is first performed through the tracheal lumen to ensure the endobronchial portion of the left-sided DLT is in the left bronchus and the blue endobronchial cuff is approximately 5 mm below the tracheal carina. It is important to identify the right upper lobe takeoff at this time to confirm anatomic landmarks. The bronchoscope is removed and reinserted into the bronchial lumen, ensuring the division of the left upper and lower lobes can be seen. Both lobes must be identified to ensure that distal migration of the endobronchial lumen has not led to insertion into the left lower lobe and occlusion of the left upper lobe. (474)

77. The method of insertion of a BB depends on the blocker's design. The unifying principle of a BB is that it is inserted within a SLT and advanced into the left or right main bronchus or, less commonly, into a lobe. The cuff of the BB is inflated to obstruct the lumen, allowing lung isolation, and ideally sits 5 mm distal to the carina. A small channel within the blocker may be used to apply suction to the lung, intermittently insufflate oxygen, and apply PEEP. An adaptor attaches to the SLT, allowing insertion of the BB, flexible bronchoscope, and attachment to the anesthetic circuit. (475)

78. Initiation of one-lung ventilation (OLV) with an open chest in the lateral position sees physiologic changes that improve ventilation and perfusion matching compared to two-lung ventilation with a closed chest. Perfusion to the nonventilated, nondependent lung is decreased owing to hypoxic pulmonary vasoconstriction and gravity, thereby favoring perfusion of the dependent, ventilated lung and decreasing shunt. Changes in cardiac output can have varying effects, but typically shunt is lowest (and arterial Po_2 is greatest) at a "normal" cardiac output during OLV. Ventilation of the nondependent lung is stopped by virtue of lung isolation. The compliance of the dependent lung decreases because of the cephalad shift of the diaphragm after induction of anesthesia and muscle relaxation, mediastinal shift following opening of the chest, and surgical pushing and manipulation of the mediastinum. This decrease in compliance and functional residual capacity can be improved with the application of PEEP. PEEP (5 to 10 cm H_2O) to the dependent lung also helps to reduce blood flow to the nondependent lung as pulmonary vascular resistance is lowest at FRC. Excessive PEEP may increase pulmonary vascular resistance, thereby increasing blood flow to the nondependent lung and worsening shunt. (475)

79. There are several intraoperative complications that occur with increased frequency during thoracotomy, including hypoxemia, sudden hypotension, sudden changes in ventilating pressure or volume, arrhythmia, bronchospasm, hemorrhage, and hypothermia. Hypoxemia can be due to intrapulmonary shunt during OLV. Sudden hypotension can be due to surgical compression of the heart or great vessels. Sudden changes in ventilating pressure or volume can be due to movement of the endobronchial tube/blocker or a new air leak from the lung parenchyma. Arrhythmia can be due to mechanical irritation of the heart. Bronchospasm can be due to direct airway stimulation and increased frequency of reactive airway disease. Hemorrhage can be due to surgical blood loss from

great vessels or inflamed pleura. Hypothermia can be due to heat loss from an open hemithorax. (475)

80. Choice of monitoring should be guided by a knowledge of which complications are likely to occur, the duration of the procedure (typically 2 to 4 hours), lateral position that makes intraoperative access to the patient challenging, and the surgeon operating in close proximity to the heart and major vessels. In addition to standard monitoring (pulse oximeter, electrocardiogram, noninvasive blood pressure), an intra-arterial catheter allows hemodynamic monitoring and analysis of arterial blood gases. It is the authors' practice to place intra-arterial catheters in all but the simplest thoracic cases (e.g., wedge resection) being performed on patients without comorbid disease. Central venous catheters allow vasoactive agents to be infused, assisting hemodynamic stability in patients who are at risk of intraoperative hemorrhage or postoperative hypervolemia, such as for pneumonectomy, complex procedures, and redo-thoracotomy. The open hemithorax provides a large surface area for evaporative cooling, and therefore, devices to measure and maintain patient normothermia are required.
Another useful monitor during OLV is continuous spirometry. Available on most modern ventilators, this allows for continuous monitoring of inspiratory and expiratory volumes, pressures, and flows. The difference between the inspired and expired volumes during OLV may indicate an air leak and loss of lung isolation (>30 mL/breath). During two-lung ventilation after lung resection, this difference correlates to an air leak through the lung parenchyma. The development of gas trapping in patients with obstructive lung disease is indicated by persistent end-expiratory flow. (476)

81. Volatile anesthetics impair hypoxic vasoconstriction at MAC levels greater than those of routine use, making their use during general anesthesia for OLV safe. There is no clear advantage of a propofol total intravenous anesthetic compared to volatile anesthetic in terms of shunt fraction or hypoxemia. (477)

82. During OLV the mode of ventilation can be volume controlled or pressure controlled. Pressure controlled may be preferred for patients at risk of lung injury, such as those with bullae, preexisting lung disease, pneumonectomy, or lung transplantation. The FIO_2 should ideally be decreased during OLV if tolerated to minimize absorption atelectasis in the nondependent lung. The tidal volume should be between 4 and 6 mL/kg during OLV guided by keeping peak airway pressure less than 35 cm H_2O and plateau airway pressure less than 25 cm H_2O. The respiratory rate should be 12 to 16 breaths per minute but may be higher if necessary. Permissive hypercapnia is usually employed during OLV, but PCO_2 should be adjusted to keep the pH higher than 7.20. PEEP of 4 to 10 cm H_2O is usually applied to the dependent lung except in cases of obstructive lung disease. Recruitment maneuvers employed prior to lung isolation and during OLV as needed may reverse atelectasis in the ventilated lung, improving PO_2 during OLV. (477–478)

83. Intravenous fluids during thoracic surgery should be aimed at maintaining euvolemia—that is, replacement of intravascular fluid volume deficits and maintenance only. A positive fluid balance in excess of 3 to 4 L in the first 24 hours has been associated with postpneumonectomy acute lung injury. (477)

84. Posterolateral thoracotomy is one of the most painful surgical incisions. It is likely that improvements in analgesic techniques over the past 30 years have contributed to a decrease in the postoperative mortality rate for these procedures. No single analgesic technique can block the multiple sensory afferents that transmit nociceptive stimuli after thoracotomy (thoracic and cervical, vagus, and phrenic nerves), and therefore, analgesia should be multimodal. The optimal choice for a patient will be based on patient factors (contraindications, preferences), surgical factors (type of incision), and system factors (available equipment, monitoring, nursing support, institutional familiarity with techniques). The ideal post-thoracotomy analgesic technique will include opioids, anti-inflammatory agents, and regional anesthesia. (478)

85. There are a number of patient and surgical predictors of intraoperative hypoxemia during OLV. Patient predictors include a higher percentage of ventilation or perfusion to the operative lung on preoperative $\dot{V}/\dot{Q}$ scan, poor Pao_2 during two-lung ventilation, and normal preoperative spirometry (FEV_1 or FVC) or restrictive lung disease. Surgical predictors include right-sided thoracotomy and supine position during OLV. (478)

86. Sudden and severe hypoxemia should be managed by informing the surgeon of the problem, reinflation of the isolated lung provided it is safe to do so, and two-lung ventilation while attempting to identify and manage the cause. (478)

87. The management of slow-onset hypoxemia is described from least intrusive to most intrusive to surgical access. It should be reinforced that the most common cause of hypoxemia during OLV is distal migration of the DLT causing obstruction of an upper lobe, and therefore, bronchoscopy should be performed to confirm correct positioning.
The Fio_2 should be increased to 1.0 until the situation is controlled and the DLT position checked via a bronchoscope. Cardiac output should be optimized as high or low cardiac output and volatile anesthesia greater than 1 MAC may contribute to hypoxemia. A recruitment maneuver may be applied to the dependent (ventilated) lung + application of PEEP 5 to 10 cm H_2O if not already done so. Passive O_2 insufflation can be provided to the operative lung via a suction catheter inserted in to the DLT and connected to O_2 1 to 2 L/min. This is more effective if the operative lung is partially reinflated prior to oxygenation. A partial recruitment maneuver to the operative lung followed by CPAP 1 to 5 cm H_2O is more effective still, though it potentially obscures surgical access during video-assisted thoracic surgery (VATS). Lobar O_2 insufflation using a bronchoscope can be performed with O_2 connected to the working port of bronchoscope and intermittently insufflated during the period of OLV. Lobar rather than lung collapse is possible using a BB. If hypoxia persists then the lung can be intermittently reinflated, and finally the pulmonary artery may be temporarily occluded. (478)

88. Prior to extubation after thoracotomy, the patient should be awake, warm, and comfortable (AWaC). For a patient undergoing pneumonectomy, the $ppoFEV_1$ is useful to guide extubation. Patients with a $ppoFEV_1$ greater than 40% can be extubated in the operating room. Patients with a $ppoFEV_1$ less than 30% will likely require staged weaning from mechanical ventilation. For patients with a $ppoFEV_1$ of 30% to 40%, consider extubation based on $ppoD_{LCO}$, exercise tolerance, $\dot{V}/\dot{Q}$ scan, and the patient's comorbid conditions. (478)

MEDIASTINOSCOPY

89. During mediastinoscopy there are many structures that may be compressed or transected. These include the trachea and bronchi, pleura, great vessels (particularly the innominate artery and vein), lymphatic vessels, phrenic and recurrent laryngeal nerves, and esophagus. It is important that the patient be still during the procedure, as movement or coughing may result in surgical complications. (479)

90. It is useful to monitor the pulse in the right hand (pulse oximeter, arterial line, anesthesiologist's finger) as compression of the innominate artery supplying blood to the carotid artery and right upper limb may occur by the mediastinoscope. A noninvasive blood pressure cuff is placed on the left arm to confirm innominate compression. (480)

91. Massive mediastinal hemorrhage is perhaps the most feared complication of mediastinoscopy and requires a median sternotomy or thoracotomy to control. There is a serious risk of hemodynamic collapse if the surgery-anesthesia team does not realize soon enough that there is a problem. Surgery should stop and the wound should be packed. Resuscitation should begin and both anesthetic and surgical help should be called. Large-bore intravenous access should be obtained in the lower limbs. An arterial line should be inserted if not placed at induction. Cross-matched blood should be made available in the operating

room. If the surgeon thinks thoracotomy is a possibility then insertion of a DLT or BB is required. Once the patient is stabilized and all preparations are made, the surgeon can reexplore the surgical incision with conversion to sternotomy or thoracotomy if indicated. (480)

MEDIASTINAL MASSES

92. Risk factors for anesthesia complications during resection of mediastinal mass include a history of positional dyspnea, stridor, wheeze, cough, or supine presyncope. Examination findings of relevance include superior vena cava syndrome, syncope during a Valsalva maneuver, and cardiac murmur. The size of the mass, its location, and relations to vital structures can be assessed by imaging such as CT scan, magnetic resonance imaging (MRI), and transthoracic echocardiography. Patients who are symptomatic or have significant compression on CT of major airways, main pulmonary arteries, atria, and superior vena cava are likely to be at high risk of life-threatening respiratory or cardiovascular collapse. Flow-volume loops for assessment of severity of intrathoracic airway obstruction are unreliable and not recommended for decision making. (480)

93. A patient with lower airway compression from a large mediastinal mass is at risk of airway collapse on induction of anesthesia. Awake fiberoptic intubation with an SLT or endobronchial tube may be used to ensure the tip of the endotracheal tube is placed distal to the obstruction. Induction and maintenance of anesthesia should aim for maintenance of spontaneous ventilation and avoidance of muscle relaxants. If airway obstruction does occur, the patient should be repositioned based on the symptoms. Rigid bronchoscopy may be necessary to negotiate and lift the obstruction, allowing ventilation distal to the obstruction. An experienced bronchoscopist and necessary equipment should be in the room at induction. (480)

94. A patient with a large mediastinal mass close to the right atrium or ventricle is at risk of cardiovascular collapse on induction of anesthesia. Lower limb intravenous access (large-bore intravenous ± central line) should be inserted to ensure vascular access if the superior vena cava is obstructed. If hemodynamic instability occurs, then the patient should be repositioned based on the symptoms. In extreme cases, elective cardiopulmonary bypass prior to induction can be used. (480)

28 RENAL, LIVER, AND BILIARY TRACT DISEASE

Anup Pamnani and Vinod Malhotra

RENAL DISEASE

1. What are some essential physiologic functions of the kidneys?
2. Name some factors that place patients at an increased risk of acute renal failure in the perioperative period.
3. What percent of the cardiac output normally goes to the kidneys? What fraction of this goes to the renal cortex?
4. Over what range of mean arterial blood pressures do renal blood flow and the glomerular filtration rate (GFR) remain constant? How is this accomplished by the kidneys? Why is it important?
5. Even during normal kidney autoregulatory function, what two factors can alter renal blood flow?
6. What is renin? What is the secretion of renin usually in response to? What effect does renin have on renal blood flow?
7. What is the physiologic effect of the secretion of renin?
8. What triggers the release of prostaglandins that are produced by the renal medulla? What is the effect of prostaglandins released by the renal medulla?
9. What is the renal effect of arginine vasopressin released by the hypothalamus?
10. What is the effect of atrial natriuretic peptide? What is the secretion of atrial natriuretic peptide usually in response to?
11. What is glomerular filtration? What is glomerular filtration dependent on? What is a normal glomerular filtration rate (GFR)?
12. About what percent of the fluid shift from glomerular filtration is reabsorbed from renal tubules and ultimately returned to the circulation?
13. How is the GFR influenced by the renal blood flow?
14. What are the three mechanisms upon which the renal clearance of drugs depends?
15. Name some conventional tests used for the evaluation of renal function. How sensitive are these conventional tests of renal function?
16. What degree of renal disease can exist before renal function tests begin to indicate possible decreases in renal function?
17. What factors may influence the blood urea nitrogen (BUN) level?
18. Why does the BUN concentration increase in dehydrated states? What is the serum creatinine level under these circumstances?
19. What do BUN concentrations higher than 50 mg/dL almost always indicate?
20. What is the source of serum creatinine? How is the serum creatinine level related to the GFR?
21. Why might a normal creatinine level be seen in elderly patients despite a decreased GFR?

22. Why might normal serum creatinine levels not accurately reflect the GFR in patients with chronic renal failure?
23. What is the creatinine clearance a measurement of?
24. Why is the creatinine clearance a more reliable measurement of the GFR than serum creatinine levels? What is a disadvantage of creatinine clearance measurements?
25. What are some nonrenal causes of proteinuria?
26. Name some newly identified markers of renal function. How are they advantageous over conventional tests of renal function?
27. What are the differences in site of action of thiazide, spironolactone, and loop and osmotic diuretics?
28. What are the differences in pharmacologic action between dopamine and fenoldopam?
29. What are the systemic changes that frequently accompany end-stage renal disease (ESRD)?
30. What are some anesthetic considerations for the anesthetic management of patients with ESRD?
31. Should succinylcholine be avoided in patients with ESRD?
32. Is lactated Ringer solution contraindicated for fluid resuscitation in patients with ESRD?
33. Is sevoflurane contraindicated in patients with ESRD?
34. What are some causes of prerenal oliguria?
35. What is the treatment for prerenal causes of oliguria?
36. What are some causes of oliguria due to intrinsic renal disease?
37. For oliguria that is secondary to renal causes such as acute tubular necrosis, is the urine typically concentrated or dilute? Does the urine typically contain excessive or minimal stores of sodium?
38. What are some causes of postrenal oliguria?

LIVER AND BILIARY TRACT DISEASE

39. What are some physiologic functions of the liver?
40. What is the blood supply to the liver? What percent of the cardiac output goes to the liver?
41. What are some determinants of hepatic blood flow?
42. What is the hepatic arterial buffer response? How is this hepatic response affected by anesthesia?
43. What results from sympathetic nervous stimulation of the liver?
44. How does positive-pressure ventilation of the lungs affect hepatic blood flow?
45. How does congestive heart failure affect hepatic blood flow?
46. How do changes in cardiac output or myocardial contractility affect hepatic blood flow?
47. How do changes in arterial blood pressure affect hepatic blood flow?
48. How does the liver store glucose?
49. How does the liver maintain glucose homeostasis in times of starvation?
50. Why might patients with cirrhosis be more likely to develop hypoglycemia in the perioperative period?
51. What role does the liver play in blood coagulation? What is the clinical implication of this for the patient with liver disease?
52. How significant must liver dysfunction be before abnormal blood coagulation is noted? How can this be evaluated preoperatively?
53. What is the role of vitamin K in coagulation?
54. What are some mechanisms of drug metabolism by the liver?
55. How does chronic drug therapy affect the metabolism of anesthetic drugs by the liver?
56. How does chronic liver disease impact drug metabolism?
57. Why may hepatic drug metabolism be accelerated after the administration of certain medications?

58. What role does the liver play in heme synthesis and elimination? What is the clinical implication of this for the patient with liver disease?
59. What proteins are synthesized in the hepatocytes?
60. What is the role of the urea cycle in the hepatocytes?
61. What pathophysiologic changes are associated with end-stage liver disease (ESLD)?
62. What are the hemodynamic changes associated with ESLD?
63. What are some consequences of the portal hypertension seen in ESLD?
64. What are some of the symptoms of portal hypertension?
65. What are some complications that can occur as a result of the portal hypertension seen in ELSD?
66. What are some pulmonary complications that can be seen in ESLD?
67. What are some reasons why a patient with hepatic cirrhosis may have arterial hypoxemia? Does the administration of supplemental oxygen increase the oxygen saturation in these patients?
68. What are some causes of hepatic encephalopathy seen in patients with ESLD?
69. What is the therapy for hepatic encephalopathy? Is it effective?
70. What role does the liver play in drug binding to serum proteins? What is the clinical implication of this for the patient with liver disease?
71. Why is ascites thought to accumulate in patients with hepatic cirrhosis?
72. What are some complications associated with ascites?
73. What is the treatment for ascites?
74. How might renal function be affected in patients with hepatic cirrhosis?
75. What categories of hepatorenal syndrome have been described? Are there any therapies?
76. In the absence of surgical stimulation, how do regional and inhaled anesthetics affect hepatic blood flow?
77. Is there any evidence to suggest that one inhaled anesthetic preserves hepatic autoregulation more than others?
78. What is halothane hepatitis? Are pediatric patients or adult patients more likely to develop halothane hepatitis?
79. What is the cause of halothane hepatitis?
80. Can volatile anesthetics, other than halothane, cause hepatotoxicity?
81. What are some commonly ordered liver function tests? What is the utility of liver function tests in the perioperative period?
82. What are some preoperative findings in patients with liver disease that are associated with increased postoperative morbidity?
83. What monitoring may be useful intraoperatively for patients with hepatic cirrhosis undergoing surgical procedures?
84. Why is the intraoperative maintenance of the arterial blood pressure particularly important in patients with hepatic cirrhosis?
85. When liver function tests become abnormal postoperatively, what is the most likely mechanism for the postoperative liver dysfunction? In what patients and types of surgeries are liver function tests most likely to become elevated postoperatively?
86. What is the advantage of point-of-care coagulation testing relative to standard laboratory testing in the perioperative setting?
87. What are the most likely causes of postoperative liver dysfunction?
88. What laboratory values indicate an intrahepatic cause of liver dysfunction?
89. What are some causes of postoperative jaundice?
90. What is delirium tremens? How does it usually present?
91. What is the treatment of delirium tremens?
92. What is the mortality rate associated with delirium tremens? What is the usual cause of death in these patients?
93. What approximate percentage of females and males aged 55 to 65 years are believed to have gallstones?
94. What is the potential problem with the use of opioids intraoperatively during a cholecystectomy or common bile duct exploration?

95. How can intraoperative spasm of the sphincter of Oddi be treated?
96. What are some anesthetic considerations for patients undergoing laparoscopic procedures?

ANSWERS*

RENAL DISEASE

1. Essential physiologic functions of the kidneys include the excretion of metabolic wastes; the retention of nutrients; the regulation of water, tonicity, and electrolyte and hydrogen ion concentrations in the blood; and the production of hormones that contribute to water regulation and bone metabolism. (483)
2. Factors that place patients at an increased risk of acute renal failure in the perioperative period include advanced age, emergent surgery, liver disease, high-risk surgery, high body mass index (≥32), peripheral vascular occlusive disease, and chronic obstructive pulmonary disease (COPD). (483)
3. Although the kidneys typically constitute only 0.5% of body weight, about 20% of the cardiac output normally goes to the kidneys. Of the 20%, more than two thirds goes to the renal cortex and the remaining blood flow supplies the renal medulla. (483)
4. Renal blood flow and the glomerular filtration rate (GFR) remain constant when mean arterial blood pressures range between 80 and 180 mm Hg. This autoregulatory function of the kidneys is accomplished by the afferent arteriolar vascular bed. The afferent arterioles are able to adjust their tone in response to changes in blood pressure, such that during times of higher mean arterial blood pressure the afferent arterioles vasoconstrict, whereas the opposite occurs during times of lower mean arterial blood pressure. This is important for two reasons. The ability of the kidneys to maintain constant renal blood flow despite fluctuations in blood pressure ensures continued renal tubular function in the face of changes, especially decreases, in blood pressure. In addition, autoregulatory responses of the afferent arterioles protect the glomerular capillaries from large increases in blood pressure during times of hypertension, as may occur with direct laryngoscopy. When mean arterial blood pressures are less than 80 mm Hg or greater than 180 mm Hg renal blood flow is blood pressure dependent. (484)
5. Even during normal kidney autoregulatory function, renal blood flow can be altered by sympathetic nervous system activity and by circulating renin. (484)
6. Renin is a proteolytic enzyme secreted by the juxtaglomerular apparatus of the kidney. At least three things stimulate the release of renin from the endothelial cells of the afferent arteriole: (1) sympathetic nervous stimulation; (2) decreased renal perfusion; and (3) decreased delivery of sodium to distal convoluted renal tubules. Renin increases efferent renal arterial arteriolar tone at low levels and causes afferent arteriolar constriction at higher levels. (484)
7. Renin is the rate-limiting enzyme in the production of angiotensin II. After its secretion from the juxtaglomerular apparatus of the kidneys, renin acts on angiotensinogen. Angiotensinogen is a large glycoprotein released by the liver to the circulation. After being cleaved by renin, angiotensin I is formed from angiotensinogen. Angiotensin I is in turn cleaved by angiotensin-converting enzyme in the lungs to form angiotensin II. Angiotensin II stimulates the release of aldosterone from the adrenal cortex and is a potent vasoconstrictor. It also inhibits renin secretion as part of a negative feedback loop. Aldosterone stimulates reabsorption of sodium and water in the distal tubule and collecting ducts. (484)

---

*Numbers in parentheses refer to pages, figures, boxes, or tables in Pardo MC, Miller RD, eds. *Basics of Anesthesia.* 7th ed. Philadelphia: Elsevier; 2018.

8. Prostaglandins are released from the renal medulla in response to angiotensin II, hypotension, and sympathetic nervous system stimulation. Prostaglandins attenuate the actions of the sympathetic nervous system, arginine vasopressin, norepinephrine, and the renin-angiotensin system on the kidney by maintaining cortical blood flow. Drugs that inhibit prostaglandins, such as nonsteroidal anti-inflammatory agents and aspirin, may impair this protective effect of prostaglandins. (484)

9. Arginine vasopressin (previously known as antidiuretic hormone) release by the hypothalamus results in the renal tubular conservation of water, an increased urine osmolality, and a decrease in plasma osmolality. It is typically secreted in response to small increases in serum osmolality. (484)

10. Atrial natriuretic peptide relaxes vascular smooth muscle to cause vasodilation, inhibits the renin-angiotensin system, and stimulates diuresis and natriuresis. It is secreted when stretch receptors in the atria of the heart, and other organs, are stimulated by increased intravascular volume. The net effect of atrial natriuretic peptide is to decrease systemic blood pressure and intravascular volume. (485)

11. Glomerular filtration is the filtration of water and low-molecular-weight substances from the blood in the renal afferent arterioles into the Bowman space through the glomerulus. Glomerular filtration is dependent on two things: the permeability of the filtration barrier (the glomerular membrane) and the net difference between the hydrostatic forces pushing fluid into the Bowman space and the osmotic forces keeping fluid in the plasma. Normal GFR is approximately 125 mL/min. (485)

12. About 90% of the fluids that have been filtered by the glomerulus into Bowman capsule are reabsorbed from renal tubules and ultimately returned to the circulation. (485)

13. The GFR is decreased during times of decreased renal blood flow or decreased mean arterial blood pressure. (485)

14. The renal clearance of drugs or their metabolites depends on three things: glomerular filtration (GFR and protein binding), active secretion by the renal tubules, and passive reabsorption (favors nonionized compounds) by the tubules. (485)

15. Tests that are commonly used for the preoperative evaluation of renal function include a serum creatinine level, a blood urea nitrogen (BUN) level, creatinine clearance, and urine protein levels. Tests that are commonly used for the preoperative evaluation of renal tubular function include the urine specific gravity, urine osmolarity, and urine sodium excretion. Most tests of renal function are not very sensitive. (486)

16. A significant degree of renal disease can exist before it is reflected in renal function tests. It is estimated that more than a 50% decrease in renal function may exist before these tests become abnormal. (486)

17. Factors that may influence the BUN level include dietary protein intake, gastrointestinal bleeding, decreased urinary flow, hepatic function, and increased catabolism as during trauma, sepsis, or febrile illness. (486)

18. The BUN concentration increases in dehydrated states as a result of the corresponding decrease in urinary flow through renal tubules. During low urinary flow rates, a greater fraction of the urea is reabsorbed by the kidney. During low urinary flow rates the serum creatinine level remains normal, such that the ratio of serum BUN to creatinine is increased during times of low urinary flow associated with hypovolemia. (486)

19. BUN concentrations higher than 50 mg/dL are almost always a reflection of decreased GFR. (486)

20. Serum creatinine is a product of skeletal muscle protein catabolism, and creatinine levels reflect the balance between creatinine production by muscle and its renal excretion. Serum creatinine levels are dependent on a patient's total body water, creatinine generation rate, and creatinine excretion rate. The generation of creatinine is relatively constant within an individual, making its release into the

circulation relatively constant as well. Serum creatinine levels are believed to be reliable indicators of the GFR, because its rate of clearance from the circulation is directly dependent on the GFR. (486)

21. Elderly patients may have a normal creatinine level despite a decreased GFR secondary to the decrease in muscle mass that commonly accompanies aging. For this reason, even mild increases in the serum creatinine level of elderly patients may be an indication of significant renal dysfunction. (486)

22. Normal serum creatinine levels may not accurately reflect the GFR in patients with chronic renal failure for two reasons. First, patients with chronic renal failure may have decreased skeletal muscle mass, resulting in a decrease in creatinine production. Second, the excretion of creatinine occurs via nonrenal means in these patients. (486)

23. The creatinine clearance is a measurement of the excretion of creatinine into the urine after being filtered by the glomerulus. (486)

24. The creatinine clearance is a more reliable measurement of GFR than serum creatinine levels because the clearance does not depend on corrections for age or the presence of a steady state. A disadvantage of creatinine clearance measurements is the requirement of accurate, timed urine collections. (486)

25. Intermittent proteinuria occurs in healthy individuals after standing for long periods of time and after strenuous exercise. Proteinuria may also occur during febrile states and congestive heart failure. (486)

26. Serum cystatin C, N-acetyl-β-D-glucosaminidase, kidney injury molecule-1, and interleukin-18 are newly identified markers of renal function. They are advantageous over conventional renal function tests because they allow earlier detection of kidney injury and are less influenced by variations in muscle mass and nutrition. (487)

27. Thiazide diuretics cause diuresis by inhibition of reabsorption of sodium and chloride ions from the early distal renal tubules. Spironolactone, an aldosterone antagonist, blocks the renal tubular effects of aldosterone. Spironolactone is a potassium-sparing diuretic. Loop diuretics inhibit the reabsorption of sodium and chloride and augment the secretion of potassium primarily in the loop of Henle. Osmotic diuretics, such as mannitol, produce diuresis by being filtered at the glomeruli but not reabsorbed by the renal tubules. The excess osmolarity of the renal tubular fluid leads to excretion of water. (487)

28. Dopamine dilates renal arterioles by its agonist action at the D_1 receptor and causes adrenergic stimulation, leading to an increase in renal blood flow and GFR. Dopamine therapy when used to augment urine output has not been shown to alter the course of renal failure. Dopamine also potentially leads to tachydysrhythmias, pulmonary shunting, and tissue ischemia. Fenoldopam is a dopamine analog that also possesses D_1 agonist activity but lacks the adrenergic activity of dopamine. (487)

29. Several systemic changes accompany end-stage renal disease (ESRD). Cardiovascular disease is the predominant cause of death in patients with ESRD. Acute myocardial infarction (MI), cardiac arrest/dysfunction, and cardiomyopathy account for more than 50% of deaths in patients maintained on dialysis. Systemic hypertension is very common and can be severe and refractory to therapy. Diabetes mellitus frequently presents concomitantly with ESRD. Electrolyte abnormalities also occur commonly as patients develop difficulty excreting their dietary fluid and electrolyte loads. A normochromic normocytic anemia is frequently present because of decreased erythropoiesis. Uremia-induced platelet dysfunction can lead to clinical coagulopathy. (487–488)

30. There are several considerations for the anesthetic management of patients with ESRD. These patients may benefit from extensive monitoring, such as direct arterial blood pressure monitoring and perhaps central venous pressure monitoring, depending on the surgical case, comorbid conditions, and other factors. Patients with symptomatic coronary artery disease or a history of congestive heart failure may benefit from monitoring with a pulmonary artery catheter or transesophageal echocardiography. Hypotension can commonly occur in patients with ESRD, particularly after hemodialysis. Patients with arteriovenous fistulas should have

the presence of the thrill monitored during positioning and intraoperatively. Patients with gastroparesis should be considered at increased risk for the aspiration of gastric contents. Electrolytes, especially potassium, should be evaluated preoperatively and intraoperatively if necessary. Finally, drugs or their metabolites that are renally excreted should be administered judiciously or avoided if possible. (488)

31. Succinylcholine is not necessarily contraindicated in patients with ESRD unless the baseline serum potassium level is severely elevated. The increase in serum potassium after a large dose of succinylcholine is approximately 0.6 mEq/L for patients both with and without ESRD. This increase can be tolerated without imposing a significant cardiac risk, even in the presence of an initial serum potassium concentration as high as 5 mEq/L. (488)

32. Normal saline (NS) had previously been recommended over lactated Ringer (LR) solution for fluid resuscitation in patients with ESRD. This choice was due to the hypothesized risk of hyperkalemia from the potassium contained in LR solution. The concern appears unfounded, however, as prospective randomized clinical testing comparing the two fluid therapies has shown greater hyperkalemia and acidosis with intraoperative therapy utilizing NS. (488)

33. The metabolism of sevoflurane to inorganic fluoride has been thought to cause renal toxicity in experimental studies, but no controlled human studies are available and it is an acceptable choice of inhaled anesthetic for patients with ESRD. (489)

34. Prerenal oliguria is indicative of a decrease in renal blood flow, the most common causes of which include a decrease in the intravascular fluid volume and a decrease in the cardiac output. Another intraoperative cause may be surgical compression of the renal arteries leading to obstructed blood flow to the kidneys, either directly through clamping or inadvertently through retraction or manual traction. Other causes of decreased renal blood flow are sepsis, liver failure, and congestive heart failure. Whatever the cause, the duration of oliguria should be minimized to decrease the risk of acute renal failure. (489)

35. The treatment of prerenal causes of oliguria is dependent on whether the cause is secondary to a decrease in intravascular fluid volume or in cardiac output. A crystalloid fluid bolus would result in a brisk diuresis if in fact the cause was hypovolemia. A lack of response to the fluid bolus would indicate that perhaps the cause of the oliguria is a decrease in cardiac output or is a result of the secretion of antidiuretic hormone in response to surgical stress. A small dose of furosemide, 0.1 mg/kg intravenously, will lead to diuresis if the cause of the oliguria is antidiuretic hormone secretion. If there is no response to the intravenous administration of furosemide, a determination should be made as to whether the patient remains hypovolemic or there is a decrease in cardiac output. If the patient is at risk for a decrease in cardiac output, it may be worthwhile to monitor cardiac filling pressures to guide intravascular fluid replacement. If the cardiac filling pressure is high, a cause for the decrease in cardiac output should be sought. (489)

36. Acute tubular necrosis, glomerulonephritis, and acute interstitial nephritis are intrinsic renal causes of oliguria. (490)

37. Oliguria owing to acute tubular necrosis is characterized by urine that is typically dilute and contains excessive sodium. (490)

38. Causes of postrenal oliguria include ureteral obstruction, bladder outlet obstruction, and obstruction or kinking of the Foley catheter. Surgical ligation, renal calculi, and edema are other causes. Postrenal causes of oliguria are frequently reversible once the source of the obstruction is removed. (490)

LIVER AND BILIARY TRACT DISEASE

39. Physiologic functions of the liver include protein synthesis, drug metabolism, fat metabolism, hormone metabolism, bilirubin formation and excretion, and glucose homeostasis. (490)

40. The liver receives its blood supply via the portal vein (70%) and hepatic artery (30%). Approximately 25% of the cardiac output goes to the liver. Although the portal vein supplies 70% of hepatic blood supply, it only contributes 50% of the liver's oxygen supply. The remaining 50% of the liver's oxygen supply comes from the hepatic artery. (490)

41. Total hepatic blood flow is directly proportional to the perfusion pressure across the liver and is inversely proportional to splanchnic vascular resistance. There are many determinants of hepatic blood flow. Determinants intrinsic to the liver include hepatic autoregulation, metabolic control, and the hepatic arterial buffer response. Determinants extrinsic to the liver include sympathetic nervous system activity, surgical stimulation, and humoral factors. (490)

42. Portal blood flow is a major intrinsic regulator of hepatic arterial tone. The hepatic arterial buffer response refers to the capacity of the liver to increase or decrease hepatic artery blood flow in response to decreases or increases in portal venous flow. For example, when portal venous flow decreases, the resistance of the hepatic artery decreases and hepatic artery blood flow increases. This reciprocal relationship allows for the hepatic oxygen supply and total hepatic blood flow to be maintained despite alterations in portal venous flow. This compensatory mechanism does not completely compensate for changes in portal venous flow, however. In addition, the hepatic arterial buffer response can be disrupted by several factors, including neural, humoral, and metabolic changes. This hepatic response is also disrupted by hepatic cirrhosis and volatile anesthetics. Of note, there does not appear to be autoregulation of the portal venous system. Instead portal venous blood flow parallels cardiac output. (490)

43. Innervation of the liver is by both the parasympathetic nervous system and the sympathetic nervous system. Generalized sympathetic nervous system stimulation, as can occur with arterial hypoxemia or hypercarbia, pain, or surgical stress, results in an increase in the splanchnic vascular resistance. The increase in splanchnic vascular resistance yields a decrease in liver blood flow and blood volume. (490)

44. Positive-pressure ventilation of the lungs decreases hepatic blood flow through its increase in hepatic venous pressure. Hepatic blood flow is decreased further by the application of positive end-expiratory pressure through the same mechanism. (491)

45. Congestive heart failure, particularly right-sided heart failure, decreases hepatic blood flow through its increase in hepatic venous pressure. (491)

46. Decreases in cardiac output or myocardial contractility result in decreases in hepatic blood flow. (491)

47. Decreases in arterial blood pressure result in decreases in hepatic blood flow. (491)

48. The liver stores glucose as glycogen in the hepatocytes. The liver is the main organ for the storage and release of glucose. (491)

49. Glucose homeostasis is maintained during times of starvation by the breakdown of the glycogen to glucose in the hepatocytes. Glucose is then released into the circulation. The glycogen stores of the liver correspond to 24 to 48 hours of glucose supply during times of starvation. Prolonged starvation that results in the depletion of the glycogen stores requires that the liver convert lactate, glycerol, and amino acids to glucose. This is termed *gluconeogenesis*. (491)

50. Patients with cirrhosis may be more likely to develop hypoglycemia in the perioperative period as gluconeogenesis may be impaired. (491)

51. A normal liver synthesizes most of the proteins responsible for the coagulation of blood. A diseased liver may therefore manifest as coagulopathy in the patient. (491)

52. Bleeding can be prevented with only 20% to 30% of normal levels of clotting factors, so that abnormal blood coagulation manifests only after significant liver disease. The coagulation status of a patient can be evaluated preoperatively by checking the patient's prothrombin time, partial thromboplastin time, and

bleeding time. Indeed, the prothrombin time is frequently used as an evaluation of the synthetic function of the liver. (491)

53. Vitamin K plays an important role in the catalysis of some of the procoagulant proteins to produce factors II, VII, IX, and X. (491)

54. Mechanisms of drug metabolism by the liver include facilitation of the renal excretion of lipid-soluble drugs to more water-soluble forms via conjugation, the transformation to pharmacologically less active drugs, and the excretion of drugs in the bile. (491)

55. Chronic drug therapy can inhibit anesthetic drug metabolism by inhibiting hepatic enzymes. Conversely, it can also enhance drug metabolism by inducing hepatic enzymes (particularly cytochrome P isoforms). (491)

56. Chronic liver disease may interfere with the metabolism of drugs because of the decreased number of enzyme-containing hepatocytes or the decreased hepatic blood flow that typically accompanies cirrhosis of the liver. (491)

57. Accelerated drug metabolism may be noted after the administration of certain drugs such as phenytoin. It is believed that exposure of the microsomal enzymes to these drugs causes an upregulation, or induction, of their own synthesis. (491)

58. The liver is responsible for almost all erythrocyte production in the fetus and about 20% of adult heme synthesis, with the remainder produced in the bone marrow. Heme degradation results in bilirubin as an end product. The conjugation of bilirubin with glucuronic acid takes place in the liver through the action of glucuronyl transferase. The conjugation of bilirubin allows it to become water soluble for renal excretion. Impairment of this function of the liver, as with liver disease, can lead to increased serum levels of unconjugated bilirubin. The liver is also responsible for the excretion of conjugated bilirubin into bile. This explains the elevated serum levels of conjugated bilirubin in the presence of liver disease. (491)

59. All proteins are synthesized in hepatocytes except for gamma globulins and factor VIII. (491)

60. The urea cycle is used by hepatocytes to convert the end products of amino acid degradation, such as ammonia and other nitrogenous waste products, to urea, which is readily excreted by the kidneys. (491)

61. End-stage liver disease (ESLD) is associated with portopulmonary hypertension, hepatopulmonary syndrome (shunting due to impairment of hypoxic pulmonary vasoconstriction), atelectasis, pleural effusions, hepatic encephalopathy, impaired drug binding, coagulopathy, ascites, and renal dysfunction (due to various factors including the hepatorenal syndrome). (492)

62. Severe liver disease that has advanced to cirrhosis is associated with a hyperdynamic circulation. Patients typically have normal to low systemic blood pressure, increased cardiac output, and decreased systemic vascular resistance due to vasodilation and shunting. (492)

63. Portal hypertension, as seen in ESLD, is the high resistance of blood flow through the liver. This results in an accumulation of blood in the vascular beds that normally drain to the liver, and these vessels become dilated and hypertrophic. Vessels draining the esophagus, stomach, spleen, and intestines are affected, resulting in splenomegaly and esophageal, gastric, and intra-abdominal varices. (492)

64. Some of the symptoms of portal hypertension include anorexia, nausea, ascites, esophageal varices, spider nevi, and hepatic encephalopathy. (492)

65. Complications that can occur as a result of the portal hypertension seen in ELSD include increased susceptibility to infection, renal failure, mental status changes, and massive hemorrhage through the rupture of the engorged dilated submucosal veins. Gastroesophageal varices are at the greatest risk of rupture. (492)

66. Pulmonary complications that can be seen in ESLD include pulmonary arteriovenous communications that are not ventilated (hepatopulmonary syndrome), the impairment of hypoxic pulmonary vasoconstriction, atelectasis, and restrictive pulmonary disease due to ascites and pleural effusions. In less than 5% of

patients with ESLD portopulmonary hypertension develops, but its cause is not well established. Portopulmonary hypertension is an increase in intrapulmonary vascular pressure in patients with portal hypertension. (492)

67. Patients with hepatic cirrhosis may have arterial hypoxemia for several reasons. Often, patients with hepatic cirrhosis have right-to-left pulmonary shunting in response to the portal vein hypertension. Patients with ascites and hepatomegaly may also have impairment of diaphragmatic excursion from the weight of the abdominal contents, particularly in the supine position. In patients with significant ascites, pleural effusions may impair lung expansion. In the early stages of ESLD, supplemental oxygen may improve arterial hypoxemia, but as the disease progresses oxygen therapy may not be effective. (492)

68. The cause of hepatic encephalopathy seen in patients with ESLD is multifactorial. Hepatic encephalopathy is in part due to increased serum concentrations of chemicals normally cleared by the liver, especially ammonia. Other factors include disruption of the blood-brain barrier, increased central nervous system inhibitory neurotransmission, and altered cerebral energy metabolism. (492)

69. Therapy for hepatic encephalopathy revolves around reducing the production and absorption of ammonia. Neomycin is used to reduce ammonia production by urease-producing bacteria, and lactulose is administered to reduce ammonia absorption. Some symptoms of hepatic encephalopathy are reversible with flumazenil therapy. These therapies are not completely effective because multiple other etiologic factors are associated with hepatic encephalopathy. It is also important to rule out other causes of altered mental status in the patient with ESLD. Other causes may include intracranial bleeding, hypoglycemia, or a postictal state (492).

70. The liver synthesizes albumin, which binds drugs in the plasma. The binding of drugs to albumin decreases the free, or pharmacologically active, portion of the drug. When the liver is diseased the synthesis of albumin becomes impaired, decreasing the albumin available in the plasma for binding. As a result there is an increased concentration of free, unbound drug in the plasma. Patients with liver disease may manifest a more pronounced drug effect than patients with normal liver function after an intravenous injection of a specific drug dose. Increased drug effect secondary to a decrease in protein binding is more likely to be seen when the serum albumin concentration is less than 2.5 g/dL. (492)

71. Ascites affects up to 50% of patients with hepatic cirrhosis. Ascites is thought to accumulate secondary to a decrease in plasma oncotic pressure, a corresponding increase in the hydrostatic pressure in the hepatic sinusoids, and an increase in sodium retention by the kidneys owing to increased circulating levels of antidiuretic hormone. (492)

72. Complications associated with ascites include marked abdominal distention that can lead to atelectasis and restrictive pulmonary disease, spontaneous bacterial peritonitis, and circulatory instability as a result of compression of the inferior vena cava and right atrium. (492)

73. The treatment for ascites is initially fluid restriction, reduced sodium intake, and diuretic therapy. In severe cases abdominal paracentesis temporarily effectively reduces abdominal distention and restores hemodynamic stability. Some patients with refractory ascites are candidates for the interventional radiologic procedure transjugular intrahepatic portosystemic shunt (TIPS), in which a stent is placed between a branch of the hepatic vein and the portal vein. (493)

74. Patients with hepatic cirrhosis tend to have a decrease in arterial blood volume and consequently a decrease in renal blood flow and GFR. Because of this patients with hepatic cirrhosis are at risk of developing hepatorenal syndrome, a serious complication that is often fatal. The syndrome is characterized by intravascular fluid depletion, intrarenal vasoconstriction, worsening hyponatremia, hypotension, and oliguria. (493)

75. Two types of hepatorenal syndromes have been described. Type 1 hepatorenal syndrome presents as rapidly progressing prerenal failure. It is associated with a poor prognosis in the absence of therapeutic intervention. Type 2 hepatorenal

syndrome presents with a milder degree of renal dysfunction. Treatment with octreotide, glucagon, and midodrine has shown promise at reversing type 1 hepatorenal syndrome. (493)

76. In the absence of surgical stimulation, regional and inhaled anesthetics decrease hepatic blood flow by 20% to 30%. Changes in hepatic blood flow in response to regional and inhaled anesthetics are believed to result from decreases in cardiac output, mean arterial pressure, or both. Volatile anesthetics may also decrease hepatic blood flow by impairing intrinsic hepatic mechanisms to maintain hepatic blood flow to varying degrees. (493)

77. There is some evidence to suggest that isoflurane inhibits hepatic autoregulation less than other inhaled anesthetics. (493)

78. Two different forms of hepatotoxicity can result from the administration of halothane. Type I is benign and self limiting and more common. Type II is a severe, immune-mediated form that can lead to fulminant liver failure. Halothane hepatitis typically refers to the second more severe hepatotoxicity that can result in hepatic necrosis and death. Halothane hepatitis is extremely rare. Adult patients are more likely to develop halothane hepatitis than pediatric patients. Patients most likely to be affected are middle-aged, obese women who have had repeated administration of halothane anesthesia. (493)

79. Although the exact cause of halothane hepatitis is unclear, it is believed to be due to an immunologic response to a toxic metabolite of halothane. (493)

80. The administration of all volatile anesthetics can result in a mild, self-limited form of hepatotoxicity. It can be seen in up to 20% of patients but is associated with minimal sequelae. (493)

81. Commonly ordered liver function tests include serum bilirubin, aminotransferase enzymes, alkaline phosphatase, albumin, and the prothrombin time. Liver tests are very nonspecific, and significant liver dysfunction must occur before it is reflected in the majority of tests. Despite this, liver function tests have some utility in the perioperative period. Liver function tests may be useful preoperatively in detecting the presence of liver disease. Perioperatively, liver dysfunction may be classified as prehepatic, intrahepatic, or posthepatic through the evaluation of the results of the various liver function tests. (493)

82. Preoperative findings in patients with liver disease that are associated with increased postoperative morbidity include marked ascites, markedly elevated prothrombin time and serum bilirubin level, markedly decreased serum albumin level, and encephalopathy. (493)

83. Intraoperative monitoring for patients with hepatic cirrhosis should be guided by the surgical procedure. In general, monitoring of the arterial blood pressure with an intra-arterial catheter may be useful. This allows for monitoring of the arterial blood gases, pH, coagulation status, and glucose as well as the blood pressure. In addition, the urine output should be closely monitored owing to the risk of postoperative renal dysfunction that can occur in patients with severe liver disease. Central venous pressure or pulmonary artery catheter monitoring might be useful in the fluid management of patients with cardiomyopathy and congestive heart failure. The intravascular fluid balance of patients with liver disease and especially ascites can be difficult to manage. Finally, the use of an intraoperative transesophageal echocardiogram may be useful to monitor myocardial function and intravascular fluid status, but in patients with esophageal varices there exists a risk of bleeding with its insertion. (494)

84. The intraoperative maintenance of the arterial blood pressure is particularly important in patients with hepatic cirrhosis because these patients are dependent on hepatic arterial blood flow to provide oxygen to the hepatocytes. In the presence of portal hypertension, hepatic arterial blood flow is typically reduced from normal levels. The addition of anesthetics and the surgical procedure can exacerbate this reduction in hepatic blood flow and may contribute to postoperative liver dysfunction. (494)

85. Liver function tests are most likely to become abnormal secondary to an inadequate supply of oxygen to the hepatocytes intraoperatively. This is the most likely mechanism for mild, self-limited postoperative liver dysfunction. Abnormal postoperative liver function tests are most likely to occur in patients with preexisting liver disease whose hepatic oxygenation was marginal preoperatively or after surgery in which the operative site was in close proximity to the liver. (494)

86. Recent advances in point of care coagulation technology allow the clinician to rapidly diagnose and manage coagulopathy associated with ESLD in the perioperative setting. Additional information, unavailable through conventional laboratory tests, such as clot strength, platelet function, and hyperfibrinolysis, can be assessed rapidly at the bedside with these newer techniques. (495)

87. The most likely causes of postoperative liver dysfunction include drugs, arterial hypoxemia, sepsis, congestive heart failure, cirrhosis, and a history of preexisting hepatic viruses. (495)

88. Elevated aminotransferase enzymes, decreased albumin, and a prolonged prothrombin time are all indicative of an intrahepatic cause of liver dysfunction. These alterations are reflective of direct hepatocellular damage. (495)

89. Operations on the liver or biliary tract, multiple blood transfusions, resorption of surgical hematoma, antibiotics and other perioperative drugs, and metabolic and infectious causes can all lead to postoperative jaundice. Rarely, inhaled anesthetic agents may be implicated. (495)

90. Delirium tremens is a severe withdrawal syndrome in patients with a history of chronic alcohol abuse. The onset of delirium tremens is typically 48 to 72 hours after cessation of the ingestion of alcohol. Delirium tremens presents clinically as tremulousness, hallucinations, agitation, confusion, disorientation, and increased activity of the sympathetic nervous system. Increased activity of the sympathetic nervous system in these patients is manifest as diaphoresis, fever, tachycardia, and hypertension. In severe cases the syndrome may progress to seizures and death. (495)

91. The treatment of delirium tremens is primarily with the administration of central nervous system depressants, usually a benzodiazepine. If necessary, a β-adrenergic antagonist may be administered to offset sympathetic nervous system hyperactivity. The trachea may be intubated if indicated for airway protection. Other treatment is supportive as necessary, including hydration and the correction of electrolyte disorders. (495)

92. The mortality rate associated with delirium tremens can be as high as 10%. The usual cause of death in these patients is cardiac dysrhythmias or seizures. (495)

93. Approximately 20% of women and 10% of men aged 55 to 65 years are believed to have gallstones. Elevated serum bilirubin and alkaline phosphatase levels in these patients imply the presence of a stone in the common bile duct causing obstruction to the flow of bile. (495)

94. Opioids such as morphine, meperidine, and fentanyl may produce spasm in the sphincter of Oddi. This increases the pressure in the common bile duct in a dose-dependent manner and may be painful to an awake patient. The administration of these medicines intraoperatively could hinder the passage of contrast medium for exploration of the common bile duct. In clinical practice, however, the administration of opioids to these patients rarely results in difficulty with intraoperative cholangiograms. (495)

95. Intraoperative spasm of the sphincter of Oddi can be treated with naloxone, glucagon, or nitroglycerin. (495)

96. Anesthetic considerations for patients undergoing laparoscopic procedures are multiple. Included are the insufflation of the abdomen with carbon dioxide and the possible impairment of ventilation of the lungs in the presence of increased ventilatory requirements, the probable placement of the patient in the Trendelenburg position, the risk of puncture of bowel or vessels, and the potential for nitrous oxide to expand bowel gas. (495)

Chapter

29 NUTRITIONAL, GASTROINTESTINAL, AND ENDOCRINE DISEASE

Amy C. Robertson and William R. Furman

NUTRITIONAL DISORDERS

1. What is a desired body mass index (BMI)? What BMI defines morbid obesity, superobese and super-superobese?
2. What organ systems can be affected by obesity?
3. What is the metabolic syndrome, and what is its significance?
4. How is the diagnosis of metabolic syndrome made?
5. What are the contributory factors to morbid obesity?
6. What are some considerations in the anesthetic management of a morbidly obese patient?
7. What are the characteristics of gastric contents in fasted obese patients?
8. What are potential challenges with venous access and blood pressure monitoring in an obese patient?
9. What are potential challenges associated with positioning an obese patient?
10. How does obesity affect laryngeal intubation?
11. How does obesity influence induction, maintenance, and emergence of anesthesia?
12. What were some of the complications with the early weight loss operations such as jejunoileal bypass?
13. What surgical procedures are commonly performed for weight reduction? Why are laparoscopic bariatric procedures favored over open procedures?
14. What are three significant and beneficial effects of modern gastric bypass?
15. What is the definition of malnutrition? Why might malnutrition be present in surgical patients?
16. Is enteral or intravenous nutrition preferable for most patients who require supplemental feedings? Why?
17. When is intravenous feeding (total parenteral nutrition [TPN]) preferred? What are the risks of long-term TPN?
18. What is refeeding syndrome? What are the clinical signs of refeeding syndrome?
19. What are some perioperative considerations for the malnourished patient? What are the considerations for the enterally fed critically ill patient?

GASTROINTESTINAL DISEASE

20. What is the presumed pathophysiology of inflammatory bowel disease (IBD)? What are some of the factors that are associated with IBD?
21. What are the major differences between ulcerative colitis and Crohn disease?
22. What is the preferred anesthetic technique for a patient with IBD?
23. How do drugs used in the treatment of IBD interact with anesthetic drugs?
24. What is the definition of gastroesophageal reflux disease (GERD)?
25. What is the pathophysiology of GERD?
26. How is GERD diagnosed? What are the signs and symptoms of GERD?
27. What are some other conditions associated with GERD?

28. What are the incidence and cause of GERD among pregnant women?
29. What is the risk of pulmonary aspiration of gastric contents in patients with GERD on induction of anesthesia?
30. Does the rapid-sequence induction (RSI) with cricoid pressure (CP) prevent pulmonary aspiration of gastric contents? Why or why not?
31. What are potential intraoperative and postoperative complications associated with Nissen fundoplication?

ENDOCRINE DISORDERS

32. What is the definition of diabetes?
33. What types of complications are associated with long-standing diabetes?
34. Why are the historical classifications of insulin-dependent and non–insulin-dependent diabetes inferior to type 1 diabetes mellitis (T1DM) and type 2 diabetes mellitis?
35. What is the major treatment goal in T1DM and T2DM?
36. What is the preferred initial pharmacologic agent for the treatment of T2DM?
37. What is hemoglobin A_{1C} (glycated hemoglobin)? What is its significance in the management of diabetes?
38. What is the recommended preoperative management of diabetes medicines?
39. What blood glucose levels should be maintained in the perioperative period?
40. What are some potential causes and complications of perioperative hyperglycemia?
41. What laboratory values define hyperthyroidism?
42. What are some common causes of hyperthyroidism?
43. What is Graves disease?
44. What are the signs and symptoms of hyperthyroidism?
45. What is the difference between hyperthyroidism and thyroid storm?
46. What are the signs and symptoms of thyroid storm?
47. What conditions may cause a thyrotoxic patient to develop thyroid storm?
48. What medications are used in the management of thyroid storm?
49. What is the Wolff-Chaikoff effect?
50. What are the anesthetic considerations for a patient with hyperthyroidism?
51. How should perioperative thyroid storm be managed?
52. What laboratory values define hypothyroidism?
53. What are the causes of hypothyroidism?
54. What are the signs and symptoms of hypothyroidism?
55. What is the difference between primary and secondary hypothyroidism?
56. What is the treatment for hypothyroidism?
57. Is it necessary to delay surgery in hypothyroid patients and achieve a euthyroid state before operating?
58. What are the preoperative airway considerations in a patient undergoing thyroid surgery?
59. What are the postoperative airway considerations in a patient undergoing thyroid surgery?
60. Why is intraoperative laryngeal nerve monitoring performed during thyroid surgery? What is its impact on the anesthetic plan?
61. What is the embryologic cell of origin of the pheochromocytoma, and what is the difference between it and a paraganglioma?
62. What hormones are produced by pheochromocytoma and paraganglioma tumors, and what are their common signs and symptoms?
63. How common are pheochromocytoma and paraganglioma tumors?
64. How should perioperative hypertension and tachycardia associated with pheochromocytoma and paraganglioma be managed?
65. What is the MEN1 (multiple endocrine neoplasia type 1) syndrome? What is its inheritance pattern?
66. What is the MEN2 (multiple endocrine neoplasia type 2) syndrome? What is its inheritance pattern?
67. What specific tumors are commonly found in patients with MEN1?

68. What are the subtypes of MEN2?
69. What are the anesthetic implications of MEN1 and MEN2?
70. What are carcinoid and neuroendocrine tumors, and what hormones do they produce?
71. Why are midgut carcinoid tumors often asymptomatic? When do they become symptomatic?
72. What is carcinoid syndrome? What is the usual treatment for a carcinoid crisis?
73. What are the perioperative implications of carcinoid and neuroendocrine tumors?
74. What are the principal hormones secreted by the adrenal cortex?
75. What is the mechanism by which stress stimulates the release of cortisol?
76. What is the function of cortisol in the body?
77. What are the symptoms of chronic adrenal insufficiency?
78. What is the difference between primary and secondary (or tertiary) adrenocortical insufficiency?
79. What are the frequent causes of primary adrenocortical insufficiency?
80. What are the frequent causes of secondary or tertiary adrenocortical insufficiency?
81. What is addisonian crisis (acute adrenal failure)? What are its symptoms and causes?
82. What is the treatment for acute adrenal failure?
83. What are the common causes of pituitary apoplexy? What are the signs, symptoms, and treatment of pituitary apoplexy?
84. What is the effect of etomidate on adrenal function?
85. What is the general approach to perioperative steroid replacement in the patient who has steroid-induced adrenal insufficiency?
86. What is critical illness–related corticosteroid insufficiency (CIRCI)?
87. What is Cushing syndrome? What are the signs and symptoms of Cushing syndrome, and how is it diagnosed?
88. What is the difference between primary and secondary (or tertiary) Cushing syndrome?
89. What is the difference between Cushing syndrome and Cushing disease?
90. What are the common causes of secondary Cushing syndrome?
91. What are the anesthetic considerations in a patient with Cushing syndrome?

ANSWERS*

NUTRITIONAL DISORDERS

1. A desirable BMI is generally considered to be 18 to 25. Although a BMI of 30 to 40 is considered obese, morbid obesity is a BMI of 40 or more. Superobese is a BMI of 50 or more, and super-superobese is a BMI of 60 or more. (497)
2. Morbid obesity can impact any organ system of the body. The cardiovascular (hypertension, stroke, right-sided heart failure), endocrine (reproductive hormonal imbalances, impaired fertility, diabetes), and gastrointestinal (hiatal hernias and gastroesophageal reflux from increased intra-abdominal pressure) systems are commonly affected. Involvement of the pulmonary system can be manifested by reduced functional residual capacity, rapid desaturation, restrictive lung disease, and obstructive sleep apnea. Skeletal problems may include back pain and osteoarthritis, particularly of the knees. Some malignancies (colon and breast) are associated with obesity as are some psychological disorders such as depression. (497)
3. Metabolic syndrome applies to the combined complications of obesity. There are six components of the metabolic syndrome: abdominal obesity, atherogenic dyslipidemia, elevated blood pressure, insulin resistance (glucose intolerance), a

---

*Numbers in parentheses refer to pages, figures, boxes, or tables in Pardo MC, Miller RD, eds. *Basics of Anesthesia.* 7th ed. Philadelphia: Elsevier; 2018.

proinflammatory state, and a prothrombotic state. Diagnosis and treatment are important because metabolic syndrome alone predicts approximately 25% of all new-onset cardiovascular disease. (497)

4. Diagnosis of metabolic syndrome is made by the presence of three out of five of the following: abdominal obesity, elevated triglycerides, low high-density lipoprotein (HDL), elevated blood pressure, and elevated fasting blood glucose concentrations. (498)

5. The causes of obesity are multifactorial. They include genetic, environmental, metabolic, and psychosocial factors. Although caloric consumption is important, the urge to eat (or overeat) can be modulated by hormones. Fasting releases several orexigenic (appetite-stimulating) hormones and can cause inflammation. (498)

6. Some considerations in the anesthetic management of the morbidly obese patient include intravenous access, noninvasive blood pressure monitoring, positioning, endotracheal intubation (while preventing hypoxemia), and emergence technique. (498)

7. In the 1970s, it was suggested that fasted obese patients might have larger than normal gastric volumes with a lower than normal pH. This assertion was not supported with strong scientific evidence. More recent studies appear to show that nondiabetic obese patients actually may have less volume at a higher pH than do lean nondiabetic patients. The assertion that obesity increases the risk of the aspiration of gastric contents remains controversial. (498)

8. The most basic tasks may be challenging in the obese patient. Peripheral intravenous line placement may be difficult, and central venous catheterization may be required as an alternative. Blood pressure monitoring may be difficult because of the conical shape of the upper arm. Most blood pressure cuffs are designed for a more cylindrical profile and may not remain in position or function optimally on a cone-shaped arm. Practical options include placing a cuff on the forearm or calf, or inserting an arterial catheter. (498)

9. Positioning an obese patient is difficult because he or she may be wider than the horizontal surface of the operating table. Also, the table must be able to support the patient's weight and move into required positions for surgical access. Extreme positions of tilt demand that the patient be well secured and that potential pressure points be addressed. (498)

10. Obesity is reported to increase the risk of a difficult laryngeal intubation, especially in patients with a higher Mallampati score, obstructive sleep apnea, decreased cervical spine mobility, and large neck circumference. During intubation, diminished functional residual capacity may lead to rapid desaturation. A reverse Trendelenburg position (head up) can reduce atelectasis in dependent lung areas and can help move chest and breast tissue caudally, allowing easier access to the mouth for intubation. (498)

11. No induction or maintenance drug has a distinct advantage in the obese patient. Emergence can be slow because of a reduced rate of elimination of volatile anesthetic agents from adipose tissues. Obese patients are at risk of developing postoperative hypoxemia from atelectasis and hypercarbia due to airway obstruction. (498)

12. Unlike current operations that restrict the gastrointestinal tract, the jejunoileal bypass developed in 1954 was a malabsorptive operation developed for the treatment of hyperlipidemia, atherosclerosis, and obesity. It was abandoned by the 1980s because it caused unacceptable complications, including uveitis, kidney dysfunction, intestinal bacterial overgrowth, and liver damage. (498)

13. Commonly performed weight reduction procedures include the gastric bypass, the gastric sleeve, and the adjustable gastric band. These operations are directed toward restriction of the capacity of the stomach with the goal of early satiety and decreased oral intake. Compared to open bariatric procedures, laparoscopic procedures are associated with lower early postoperative morbidity and mortality rates. (498)

14. Gastric bypass patients generally have improvements in quality of life and comorbid conditions. There is improvement in hypertension, diabetes, and obstructive sleep apnea. The levels of several orexigenic (appetite stimulating) hormones are diminished after bariatric surgery. For example, ghrelin secretion by the gastric fundus and proximal small intestine is increased after nonsurgical weight loss but is unchanged or decreased after bariatric surgical procedures. Other intestinal hormones that regulate appetite and glucose metabolism also are affected favorably by surgery. These hormones include glucagon-like peptide-1, glucose-dependent insulinotropic peptide, and peptide YY. (498)

15. Malnutrition may be present when there is weight loss of 10% to 20% over a short time, when weight is less than 90% of ideal body weight, or when BMI is less than 18.5. Healthy patients may quickly become malnourished after an episode of trauma or acute illness, and critically ill patients develop malnutrition if they are not fed. Malnutrition can occur quickly when caloric requirements exceed intake because of decreased intake, impaired absorption, or an increased metabolic rate. (498)

16. Enteral nutrition is the preferred method of feeding because it is believed to maintain the absorptive gastrointestinal villi and reduce transmucosal bacterial transfer into the bloodstream. It results in improved patient outcomes, less infection, and fewer ventilator and intensive care unit days. Long-term feeding usually requires a gastrostomy or jejunostomy tube. Postpyloric (jejunal) placement is frequently preferred as a means to limit regurgitation and the risk of aspiration, although the risk of aspiration with gastric feeding tubes is low. In patients who have pancreatitis, jejunal placement is favored in order to avoid stimulation of pancreatic enzyme secretion. (499)

17. Intravenous feeding (total parenteral nutrition [TPN]) is preferred for patients who do not have a functioning gastrointestinal tract. TPN is considered acceptable for short-term feedings. Risks of long-term TPN include central venous catheter sepsis, thrombosis, hyperglycemia, iatrogenic hypoglycemia, and development of fatty liver. (499)

18. Refeeding syndrome is caused by rapid acute nutritional replacement in a malnourished patient. It is characterized by increased ATP (adenosine triphosphate) production, a significant fall in plasma phosphate, respiratory failure, and cardiac failure. Metabolic rate is increased, resulting in a significant rise in carbon dioxide (CO_2) production and respiratory acidosis. The syndrome may be prevented by slowly increasing the nutritional intake toward caloric goals. (499)

19. Perioperative considerations for malnourished patients include muscle weakness, immunocompromise, preoperative fasting, and perioperative glucose monitoring. Muscle weakness may lead to respiratory failure, and immunocompromise may predispose patients to infection. Preoperative fasting is often an issue in enterally fed critically ill patients, particularly burn and trauma patients. One must weigh the risk of aspiration on induction against the benefit of keeping nutrition at maintenance levels. In the absence of definitive studies, expert opinion generally supports efforts to continue nutrition as much as possible. However, preliminary data support the safety of a short fast (45 minutes) when the feeding tube is located beyond the ligament of Treitz. Perioperative glucose monitoring is necessary in patients receiving TPN because insulin is typically included in the nutrient mixture. Blood glucose should be monitored during procedures more than 2 hours in duration. (499)

GASTROINTESTINAL DISEASE

20. Inflammatory bowel disease (IBD) is believed to result from an aberrant response to the normal flora by the bowel mucosal immune system. The precise trigger for the activation of the immune system in IBD is unclear and likely multifactorial. Patients typically present with complaints of abdominal pain, fever, and diarrhea. There may be a genetic basis as an increased risk is seen in close family members. Caucasians are more susceptible to IBD, and the

Jewish population is at greater risk for Crohn disease. Environmental factors may include smoking, appendectomy, antibiotics, oral contraceptives, and nonsteroidal anti-inflammatory drugs (NSAIDs). (499)

21. There are two categories of inflammatory bowel disease: ulcerative colitis and Crohn disease. Ulcerative colitis is restricted to the large intestine and manifests itself as inflammation and loss of colonic mucosa. Crohn disease can affect any part of the digestive tract and may cause transmural inflammation, leading to abscesses or granulomatous disease. Although they are distinct entities, differentiating between the two may be difficult when Crohn disease manifests itself by only affecting the colon. (499)

22. Specific anesthetic agents are neither preferred nor contraindicated for patients with IBD. Patients taking steroids should continue these prior to surgery and may require supplementation because of iatrogenic adrenal insufficiency. (499)

23. Certain medications prescribed to treat IBD may have anesthetic implications. Interactions between anesthetic and antineoplastic agents are not fully documented in the literature. Cyclosporine is reported to increase the minimum alveolar concentration of volatile agents. Phosphodiesterase effects of azathioprine may partially antagonize nondepolarizing neuromuscular blockade, although this is controversial. Cyclosporine, infliximab, and aminoglycosides potentiate the nondepolarizing neuromuscular blocking agents. (499)

24. Gastroesophageal reflux disease (GERD) is defined as the retrograde movement of gastric contents through the lower esophageal sphincter (LES) into the esophagus. GERD is an extremely common syndrome with a prevalence of 18% to 28% in the United States. (500)

25. GERD occurs when the LES is incompetent or when LES pressure is less than intra-abdominal (or intragastric) pressure. This may result from impaired esophageal motility, LES tone, or gastric motility. GERD can be due to a hiatal hernia. In a hiatal hernia the LES may be displaced cephalad into the thoracic cavity and thus lose the diaphragmatic contribution to its function or the esophagus can became become obstructed by the diaphragm. If gastric contents also move cephalad past the upper esophageal sphincter into the pharynx, pulmonary aspiration of gastric acid and particulate matter may result. Pulmonary aspiration of gastric contents is a serious, potentially life-threatening complication. (500)

26. GERD is diagnosed by heartburn (the most reliable symptom) or regurgitation at least once per week. Besides heartburn, other symptoms include noncardiac chest pain, dysphagia, pharyngitis, cough, asthma, hoarseness, laryngitis, sinusitis, and dental erosions. (500)

27. Conditions associated with GERD include pregnancy, obesity, obstructive sleep apnea, gastric hypersecretion, gastic outlet obstruction, gastric neuropathy, and increased intra-abdominal pressure. (500)

28. Significant GERD occurs in at least 30% to 50% of pregnant women. The mechanism is primarily a progesterone-mediated relaxation of LES tone, with possible contributions from impaired LES function due to elevated intra-abdominal pressure from the enlarging gravid uterus, delayed gastric emptying, and decreased bowel transit. (500)

29. The risk of pulmonary aspiration of gastric contents on induction of anesthesia in patients with GERD is not well established. Risk factors for the pulmonary aspiration of gastric contents are increased in patients with increased intra-abdominal pressures or who are pregnant. (500)

30. The customary approach to induction in patients at risk for the pulmonary aspiration of gastric contents is rapid-sequence induction (RSI) with cricoid pressure (CP) to obstruct the potential flow of gastric contents into the pharynx and trachea. However, the putative benefits of RSI and CP remain controversial. Cricoid pressure can be ineffective if not properly applied. Some undesired side effects of CP include increased risk of regurgitation and failed intubation. Based on studies of the radiographic anatomy, improperly performed CP may not align the cricoid

and esophagus properly with the solid cervical spine underneath. If the cricoid and esophagus are displaced laterally, they may overlie muscle, and the upper esophagus may not be occluded. Complications are more likely in the elderly, children, pregnant women, patients with cervical injury, patients with difficult airways, and patients in whom there is difficulty palpating the cricoid cartilage. (500)

31. Hypertension, bradycardia, elevated peak airway pressures, and desaturation are common intraoperative complications of the Nissen fundoplication. These complications are usually a consequence of pneumoperitoneum and increased intra-abdominal pressure. Postoperative complications include discomfort from carbon dioxide gas accumulation under the diaphragm and postoperative nausea and vomiting. Subcutaneous air may appear in the neck/chest region and is usually self-limited as the body rapidly reabsorbs CO_2 gas. Nausea and vomiting are more concerning complications because vomiting can lead to esophageal rupture in this setting. (500-501)

ENDOCRINE DISEASE

32. Diabetes mellitus is defined as elevated blood glucose levels due to a relative lack of endogenous insulin. It is the most common endocrine disease and affects 20 million Americans. (501)

33. Long-standing diabetes is associated with complications in most organ systems, resulting largely from microangiopathy and macroangiopathy. Risk of complications of diabetes increases with increasing hemoglobin A_{1c} levels. Large- and small-vessel coronary artery disease is common. Diabetic renal failure in young and middle-aged adults is the leading cause of renal failure requiring hemodialysis. Diabetic retinopathy is the leading cause of blindness among adults aged 20 to 74 years old. Greater than 50% of individuals with diabetes develop neuropathy, with a lifetime risk of one or more lower extremity amputations estimated to be 15%. Autonomic neuropathy occurs in 20% to 40% of patients with long-standing diabetes, particularly those with peripheral sensory neuropathy, renal failure, or systemic hypertension. Cardiac autonomic neuropathy may mask angina pectoris and obscure the presence of coronary artery disease. Gastroparesis, which may cause delayed gastric emptying, is a sign of autonomic neuropathy affecting the vagus nerves. (501)

34. The historical classification of diabetes was made according to the presence or absence of insulin requirement. This was unsatisfactory because nearly all diabetics develop a need for insulin at some point. The current classification divides the disease into type 1 diabetes mellitus (T1DM) and type 2 diabetes mellitus (T2DM). T1DM is typically characterized by the absence of any insulin production by the pancreas. T2DM involves a relative lack of insulin plus resistance to endogenous insulin. (501)

35. Blood glucose control is the major treatment goal in both types of diabetes. T1DM always requires insulin to prevent hyperglycemia and ketoacidosis. It is commonly heralded at an early age by a dramatic episode of ketoacidosis. Type 2 diabetics may require insulin but often only require oral hypoglycemic agents, weight loss, or dietary management. The onset of T2DM usually is more insidious and constitutes the majority of diabetics. They are often overweight, so dietary control and weight loss are important, but the cornerstone of management of both types of diabetes is pharmacologic. (501)

36. Metformin reduces serum glucose by decreasing hepatic production and is the preferred initial pharmacologic therapy for T2DM. Addition of a second oral agent, such as a glucagon-like peptide-1 (GLP-1) receptor agonist, or insulin is recommended when noninsulin monotherapy does not achieve target hemoglobin A_{1c}. (501)

37. Measuring glycated hemoglobin (HbA_{1c}) is the most effective method of monitoring glucose control. Glycated hemoglobin is formed during hyperglycemia when glucose permanently combines with hemoglobin in erythrocytes. Because the erythrocyte life span is 120 days, routine HbA_{1c} levels give an indication of how well the diabetes is being controlled over time. Normal HbA_{1c} levels are less than 6%. (501)

38. A well-controlled diabetic may not require special treatment before and during surgery. It is common in those on insulin treatment to reduce the morning dose by 30% to 50% to prevent hypoglycemia due to fasting while still controlling hyperglycemic risk. Sulfonylurea drugs may be continued until the evening before surgery. However, these drugs may also produce hypoglycemia in the absence of morning caloric intake so the general recommendation is to hold oral hypoglycemic agents the morning of surgery. Biguanides (phenformin and metformin) may be associated with lactic acidosis. On the basis of case reports, the common recommendation in the 1990s was to withhold metformin for 48 hours prior to anesthesia in order to avoid fatal lactic acidosis. This recommendation was based on circumstantial anecdotal evidence and has not been studied scientifically. It was called into question on the basis of a subsequent meta-analysis. (501)

39. The optimal level of glucose control in the perioperative and critical care setting remains controversial. Attempts to maintain glucose levels below 108 mg/dL in critically ill patients may result in excess mortality compared with those patients in whom the level was controlled in the 140 to 180 mg/dL range. There are several formulas for sliding scale insulin administration, maintenance infusions of 5% dextrose, and periodic blood glucose monitoring for the perioperative management of insulin-dependent diabetics. (502)

40. Stress-induced neuroendocrine changes, exogenous glucose administration, and a patient's underlying metabolic state can contribute to perioperative hyperglycemia. Potential complications of severe perioperative hyperglycemia include diabetic ketoacidosis, severe dehydration and coma related to the hyperosmolar hyperglycemic nonketotic secondary effects on neurologic outcome after cerebral ischemia, and the increased risk of surgical wound infection. (502)

41. Hyperthyroidism is the condition caused by elevated circulating levels of the unbound thyroid hormones triiodothyronine (T_3) and tetraiodothyronine (thyroxine, or T_4). (502)

42. Some common causes of hyperthyroidism include Graves disease, toxic multinodular goiter, thyroiditis, elevated β-human chorionic gonadotropin levels (gestational hyperthyroidism, choriocarcinoma, hydatidiform mole), struma ovarii (thyroid tissue in an ovarian teratoma), thyroid-stimulating hormone (TSH) secreting pituitary adenoma, and administration of iodinated contrast dye to a susceptible patient. Amiodarone can lead to either hypothyroidism or hyperthyroidism. (502)

43. Graves disease is the most common cause of hyperthyroidism. It is an autoimmune condition in which thyrotropin receptor antibodies continuously mimic the effect of TSH. (502)

44. Hyperthyroidism is manifested by cardiac, neurologic, constitutional, and gastrointestinal signs and symptoms. Thyroid hormone increases cardiac sensitivity to catecholamines, causing hypertension and tachyarrhythmias. Severe hyperthyroidism can result in high-output congestive heart failure or angina, even in the absence of coronary plaques. Patients may exhibit tremor, hyperreflexia, and irritability. Periodic paralysis characterized by hypokalemia and proximal muscle weakness may also occur. Constitutional signs may include fever and heat intolerance. Gastrointestinal symptoms may include nausea, vomiting, diarrhea, hepatic dysfunction, and jaundice. Hyperthyroidism is diagnosed by demonstrating elevated thyroid hormone levels in blood. (502)

45. The difference between hyperthyroidism (thyrotoxicosis) and thyroid storm is a matter of degree. Thyroid storm is the most severe form of the disorder. It is a life-threatening, emergent clinical syndrome with a mortality rate of approximately 30% despite treatment. (502)

46. Worsening signs and symptoms of thyrotoxicosis characterize thyroid storm, including severe cardiac dysfunction, hyperglycemia, hypercalcemia, hyperbilirubinemia, altered mental status, seizures, and coma. (502)

47. Thyroid storm may be triggered in a thyrotoxic patient by any of several stresses, including infection, stroke, or trauma, especially to the thyroid gland. It may also occur with surgery, diabetic ketoacidosis, incorrect antithyroid drug discontinuation, or metastatic thyroid cancer. The administration of certain drugs including pseudoephedrine, aspirin, excess iodine intake, contrast dye, or amiodarone may also trigger thyroid storm. (502)

48. The initial medical treatment of thyroid storm is to reduce thyroid hormone synthesis. Thionamides, such as propylthiouracil (PTU) and methimazole (MMI), inhibit thyroid peroxidase (TPO), which catalyzes the incorporation of iodide into thyroglobulin to produce T_3 and T_4. At least an hour after giving the thionamide, a large dose of stable iodide is given. This is believed to downregulate intracellular production of TPO. β-Adrenergic blocking drugs are used to reduce adrenergic symptoms. Although propranolol is the traditional choice because it also is believed to inhibit peripheral conversion of T_4 to the more potent hormone T_3, other β-blockers (atenolol, metoprolol, or esmolol) have been used. Corticosteroids should also be administered because these patients usually have relative adrenal insufficiency. Finally, plasmapheresis may be a useful adjunct to reduce circulating thyroid hormone effects by removing T_3 and T_4 from the bloodstream. (502)

49. The Wolff-Chaikoff effect is a paradoxically beneficial effect of large doses of iodide on thyroid hormone production. One would anticipate the iodide administration would increase thyroid hormone production through a stoichiometric effect on the reaction that produces T_3 and T_4 from thyroglobulin and iodide. Instead, however, iodide suppresses gene transcription of thyroid peroxidase. The large doses of iodine thus reduce the gland's capacity to produce and release hormone. This benefit is temporary, lasting about a week. (502)

50. There is limited evidence-based literature for intraoperative anesthetic management of patients with hyperthyroidism and no comparative data. It is usually recommended to favor agents that do not cause increased heart rate or sympathetic activation. It is generally advisable to undertake only that which cannot be delayed until thyroid hormone secretion has been controlled by medical management or by radioiodine ablation. (502)

51. Although thyroid storm associated with surgery can occur intraoperatively, it is most likely to present 6 to 18 hours after the surgical procedure. Perioperative thyroid storm treatment is aimed toward decreasing the amount of circulating thyroid hormone and toward decreasing the increase in sympathetic nervous system stimulation. An esmolol infusion can be started and titrated to the desired hemodynamic and cardiovascular effects. Dexamethasone can also be administered to block the release of thyroid hormone from the thyroid gland and the peripheral conversion of T_4 to T_3. Propylthiouracil may be administered to block the uptake of iodine from the thyroid gland, after which iodine may be administered to inhibit the release of thyroid hormone from the thyroid gland. Treatment should be supportive, with the monitoring and treatment of abnormalities in the patient's intravascular fluid status, electrolytes, glucose, and body temperature. Thyroid storm may be difficult to distinguish from other hypermetabolic states, including malignant hyperthermia, pheochromocytoma, neuroleptic malignant syndrome, and sepsis. Dantrolene can be beneficial and should be considered if there is suspicion of malignant hyperthermia. (502)

52. Hypothyroidism is the condition caused by decreased circulating levels of the unbound thyroid hormones triiodothyronine (T_3) and tetraiodothyronine (thyroxine, or T_4). (503)

53. Hypothyroidism is either congenital (cretinism) or acquired. Acquired hypothyroidism may be due to inflammation or to an absence of dietary iodine (so-called endemic goiter). Hashimoto thyroiditis is a chronic autoimmune disease characterized by progressive destruction of the thyroid gland. Hypothyroidism may also be iatrogenic (from the medical or surgical treatment of hyperthyroidism). At least half of patients who receive radioactive iodine

treatment for hyperthyroidism are hypothyroid 10 years later. Secondary hypothyroidism may also occur after hypothalamic or pituitary disease or surgery. (503)

54. The onset of hypothyroidism is usually insidious, and the symptoms often are nonspecific. There may be easy fatigability, lethargy, cold intolerance, periorbital edema, weakness, weight gain, dry skin, or brittle hair. Myxedema can occur in severe cases. It is characterized by reduced cardiac output, attenuated deep tendon reflexes, and nonpitting pretibial edema. Untreated, hypothyroidism can progress to electrolyte disturbances, hypoventilation, hypothermia, or coma. (503)

55. Primary hypothyroidism is present if there are low T_3 and T_4 levels but an elevated TSH. In secondary hypothyroidism, all three thyroid-related hormones are reduced. Subclinical primary hypothyroidism is present in about 5% to 8% of the American population. It has a prevalence of more than 13% in otherwise healthy elderly patients, especially women. (503)

56. Treatment for hypothyroidism involves administration of oral synthetic levothyroxine, 75 to 150 μg/day. It is important to initiate thyroid replacement slowly because acute cardiac ischemia can develop in patients with coronary artery disease from the sudden increase in myocardial oxygen demand as the metabolism and cardiac output increase. Intravenous thyroid replacement therapy is available, but its use is limited to severe presentations such as myxedema coma. (503)

57. Asymptomatic mild to moderate hypothyroidism does not place a patient at an increased risk of perioperative morbidity. There is no unusual sensitivity to inhaled anesthetics, sedatives, or narcotics. Symptomatic or severe hypothyroidism should necessitate surgical delay for thyroid hormone replacement until resolution of neurologic and cardiovascular abnormalities has occurred. (503)

58. For patients undergoing thyroid surgery, airway management is a primary challenge. Tracheal compression from a goiter or thyroid mass can result in symptoms of dyspnea, wheezing, obstructive sleep apnea, or cough. Patients with thyroid enlargement should be evaluated prior to surgery for evidence of tracheal compression or deviation. Reviewing available computed tomography (CT) scans can be helpful when evaluating size of the goiter and its impact on anatomy. A prospective study reported a 5% incidence of difficult endotracheal intubation in euthyroid patients undergoing a thyroidectomy; however, the causes of airway difficulty in these patients were the usual anatomic factors found in the general population and were not related to the thyroid enlargement. In the presence of a cancerous goiter, however, tracheal invasion and tissue fibrosis may impair the mobility of laryngeal structures and impede visualization of glottis opening during laryngoscopy. In patients with severe tracheal compression causing stridor, an awake intubation may be the method of choice to limit the risk of complete airway obstruction after spontaneous ventilation has been ablated. The surgical team should be prepared and ready to perform an emergent tracheotomy or rigid bronchoscopy. (503)

59. Avoidance of coughing during emergence at the conclusion of thyroid surgery is considered important in order to reduce the risk of postoperative hemorrhage. Various interventions have been proposed to minimize cough during emergence, including performing a deep extubation and intravenous administration of the potent short-acting narcotic remifentanil, the α_2-agonist dexmedetomidine, or lidocaine. Postextubation airway compromise may develop because of an expanding hematoma, tracheomalacia, or vocal cord dysfunction from laryngeal nerve injury. (504)

60. Unilateral laryngeal nerve injuries from thyroid surgery produce voice impairment but are not a threat to airway function. In contrast, bilateral recurrent laryngeal nerve injury compromises function of the posterior cricoarytenoid muscles, which are the muscles responsible for separating the vocal cords during breathing. This can lead to life-threatening inspiratory

airway obstruction necessitating intubation or tracheostomy. In such patients, the paralyzed vocal cords do not abduct during the inspiratory phase of the respiratory cycle and may appear apposed in the midline when seen during direct laryngoscopy. Many surgeons request the use of a laryngeal nerve monitoring endotracheal tube as a safety measure during thyroid surgery. These are specialized endotracheal tubes with electrodes positioned in the immediate vicinity of the vocal cords. They send an electromyographic signal to a receiver whenever the vocal cords contract, so that if the surgeon stimulates a laryngeal nerve an audible signal provides a warning of the potential for nerve injury. With the laryngeal nerve monitoring endotracheal tube, no muscle relaxant should be used. (504)

61. A pheochromocytoma is a catecholamine-secreting adrenal medullary tumor whose embryologic cell of origin is the neural crest cell. Paraganglioma is the name given to these tumors when they occur outside the adrenal gland. (504)

62. Pheochromocytoma tumors typically produce the adrenal medullary hormones dopamine, norepinephrine, and epinephrine. The most common symptoms are headache, palpitations, sweating, and tremulousness. The most common sign is hypertension. Severe hypertension during anesthesia and surgical manipulations is a well-recognized manifestation of pheochromocytoma; 8% to 10% of tumors are asymptomatic. The diagnosis is made by measuring urine or blood levels of catecholamine and catecholamine metabolite. (504)

63. The prevalence of pheochromocytoma and paraganglioma tumors in the general population has been reported to be as high as 1 in 2000. (504)

64. Nearly every available antihypertensive agent has been used for the management of pheochromocytomas and paragangliomas; however, actionable evidence-based recommendations favoring one agent over another are limited. The nonselective α-blocker phenoxybenzamine remains the agent most often recommended by authors of review articles and case series. It is the agent with which there is the greatest clinical experience worldwide; it has a long pharmacologic half-life but is very expensive and has no other clinical application. It is useful for the chronic treatment of patients with unresectable catecholamine-secreting tumors. Although it is frequently recommended, it might not be the agent of choice. Because α_2-agonists generally produce bradycardia, sedation, and lower blood pressure, phenoxybenzamine (with both α_1- and α_2-blocking properties) could increase blood pressure and increase pulse, which would be undesirable. Less costly alternatives prior to adrenalectomy include α_1-selective blockers (prazosin, doxazosin, and terazosin), calcium channel blockers, angiotensin-converting enzyme (ACE) inhibitors, angiotensin receptor blockers, β-blockers, and α_2-agonists. Intraoperative hypertension and tachycardia frequently occur despite maximal preoperative antihypertensive therapy and may still require infusions of vasodilators, esmolol, and magnesium for treatment. Dexmedetomidine may be useful as well because of its α_2-agonist activity. (504)

65. Multiple endocrine neoplasia type 1 (MEN1), described by Wermer in 1954, is characterized by a triad of tumors of the pancreas, parathyroid, and pituitary. Its inheritance is autosomal dominant. (505)

66. Multiple endocrine neoplasia type 2 (MEN2), is characterized by autosomal dominant inherited medullary thyroid carcinoma (MTC) and other associated tumors, including pheochromocytoma and parathyroid tumors. (505)

67. In MEN1, pancreas tumors usually secrete gastrin (40%), insulin, glucagon, vasoactive intestinal polypeptide, or pancreatic polypeptide. Pituitary tumors are usually secreting adenomas (prolactin 60%, growth hormone 25%), although some are nonfunctioning adenomas; 95% of MEN1 patients have a parathyroid adenoma, the most common tumor in the syndrome, which usually presents as hypercalcemia. All four parathyroid glands generally must be removed surgically because all are involved by the disease. Other tumors may include adrenal

cortical adenomas, carcinoids, neuroendocrine tumors, lipomas, angiofibromas, and collagenomas. (505)

68. There are two subtypes of MEN2: MEN2A, described by Sipple in 1961, and MEN2B, described by Williams and associates in 1966. MEN2A accounts for 80% of hereditary MTC syndromes. In addition to MTC, 50% of patients with MEN2A develop pheochromocytomas, and 30% develop hyperparathyroidism. MEN2B accounts for 5% of hereditary MTCs and includes mucosal neuromas, pheochromocytoma, and medullary thyroid carcinoma. (505)

69. There are no specific anesthetic implications of MEN1. Anesthetic implications of MEN2 relate to its components and associated conditions. MEN2 may be associated with pheochromocytomas or with von Hippel-Lindau disease, which in turn may include cerebellar tumors. (505)

70. Carcinoids and neuroendocrine tumors are dispersed cells of neural crest embryologic origin. These tumors produce serotonin or other peptide hormones. When these tumors arise in the midgut, they are called *carcinoid tumors*, but when they arise elsewhere in the body, the current term for them is *neuroendocrine tumors*. (505)

71. Midgut carcinoids are usually asymptomatic until they cause bowel obstruction or appendicitis because their venous drainage is via the portal vein to the liver, which detoxifies the excess serotonin they produce. (505)

72. Carcinoid syndrome is a constellation of systemic symptoms of serotonin excess. These symptoms include diarrhea, flushing, palpitations, and bronchoconstriction. It results from tumors outside the hepatic portal drainage field or when there is extensive metastatic liver disease. Octreotide may help ameliorate these symptoms. (506)

73. Perioperative considerations of carcinoid and neuroendocrine tumors result from the direct hemodynamic effects of serotonin. These usually are not problematic in the context of perioperative anesthetic care, and an escalation of hemodynamic monitoring is seldom required as a consequence of the endocrine activity of the tumor. However, certain medications can trigger mediator release, leading to hypotension and tachycardia. Drugs that may cause mediator release include opioids (particularly meperidine and morphine), neuromuscular blockers (atracurium, mivacurium, and d-tubocurarine), epinephrine, norepinephrine, and dopamine. There should be a high index of suspicion of carcinoid heart disease in the face of right-sided valvular heart disease or right-sided heart failure. Echocardiography should be considered as a diagnostic tool. Right-sided heart failure is due to the sclerosing effect of serotonin on the tricuspid and pulmonary valves. It may be the cause of death in as many as 50% of patients with carcinoid syndrome. (506)

74. The principal hormones secreted by the adrenal cortex are cortisol and aldosterone. (506)

75. Cortisol production in the adrenal cortex is stimulated by adrenocorticotropic hormone (ACTH) released from the pituitary gland. ACTH is secreted in response to hypothalamic corticotropin releasing hormone (CRH). Stress stimulates the hypothalamus to release CRH, which increases blood cortisol levels. Cortisol exerts negative feedback influence on the production of both CRH and ACTH. (506)

76. Cortisol maintains homeostasis of the cardiovascular system, especially in the presence of stress. It preserves vascular tone and endothelial integrity, maintaining intravascular volume by reducing vascular permeability. It also potentiates the vasoconstrictor effects of catecholamines. When cortisol levels are deficient, systemic vascular resistance and myocardial contractility are decreased. Cortisol also plays an important role in gluconeogenesis, sodium retention, potassium excretion, and anti-inflammatory effects. (506)

77. Chronic adrenal insufficiency (Addison syndrome) is defined as chronic insufficient cortisol production and secretion, with or without aldosterone insufficiency. The symptoms of chronic adrenal insufficiency are nonspecific

and include fatigue, malaise, lethargy, weight loss, anorexia, arthralgia, myalgia, nausea, vomiting, abdominal pain, diarrhea, and fever. (506)

78. Primary adrenocortical insufficiency is the nonfunctioning of the adrenal glands. Hyponatremia and hyperkalemia may result from the aldosterone deficiency. Secondary adrenocortical insufficiency is the failure of the pituitary to stimulate adrenal production of cortisol. In secondary adrenocortical insufficiency, aldosterone production, under the stimulus of the renin-angiotensin system, remains intact, so hyponatremia and hyperkalemia are uncommon. Tertiary insufficiency is the failure of the hypothalamus to stimulate the pituitary and thus the adrenals. (506)

79. The cause of primary adrenocortical insufficiency is usually immunologic autoimmune adrenalitis, which can be isolated or part of an autoimmune polyendocrinopathy syndrome. Less common causes include malignancies and infections. Malignant causes are generally metastatic cancer, commonly from lung or breast. Infectious causes include tuberculosis. (506)

80. Secondary or tertiary adrenocortical insufficiency usually results from pituitary or hypothalamic injury, tumor, or suppression due to exogenously administered steroids. (506)

81. Acute adrenal failure (addisonian crisis) is circulatory shock resulting from cortisol deficiency. It generally occurs in patients with primary adrenal insufficiency along with a superimposed acute stress, such as trauma, surgery, or infection. Symptoms include hyponatremia, hyperkalemia, hypovolemic shock, and myocardial and vascular unresponsiveness to catecholamines. (506)

82. The treatment for acute adrenal failure usually requires the intravenous administration of several liters of isotonic saline and corticosteroids. In adults the administration of 100 mg of cortisol, or its equivalent, every 6 to 8 hours usually reverses the pathophysiology within the first day of treatment, and orally administered steroids can be started after 24 hours. (506)

83. Pituitary apoplexy is acute pituitary hemorrhage, swelling, or infarction and is potentially life threatening. Pituitary apoplexy most often occurs after infarction of a large pituitary adenoma or postpartum hypotensive pituitary necrosis (Sheehan syndrome). It has also been reported to occur following cardiopulmonary bypass. It is associated with diabetes, hypertension, sickle cell anemia, and acute shock. Signs and symptoms of pituitary apoplexy may include sudden total loss of all anterior and posterior pituitary hormonal secretion, severe hypoglycemia, severe hypotension, central nervous system hemorrhage, cerebral edema, vision loss (often bitemporal hemianopia), severe headache, meningeal irritation, ophthalmoplegia, cardiovascular collapse, or loss of consciousness. Diagnosis is made by computed tomography or magnetic resonance imaging. Corticosteroid replacement is the first line of treatment for both the resulting adrenal insufficiency and brain swelling. Acute surgical decompression of brain swelling may be necessary when there is significant visual loss and mental status alteration. (507)

84. Etomidate is associated with significant but transient (<24 hours) suppression of adrenal cortical function, even after a single dose of the drug. This is especially clinically significant in the setting of critical illness–related corticosteroid insufficiency. (507)

85. Administration of stress dose steroids during the perioperative period remains controversial. Based upon a recent Cochrane review, it appears that recommendations on the use of additional corticosteroids for surgical patients receiving preoperative steroids have not been adequately investigated. Steroid-induced adrenal suppression is highly variable, and its duration is unpredictable, from days to perhaps years. Because the consequences of a short course of steroids are minimal, anticipatory treatment is generally safe. The dosage for replacement therapy should be adequate but not excessive. The scientific foundation of this recommendation is based on surgical research in primates when administering supplements 10 times the normal cortisol production rates

was not superior to simply replacing the normal daily production of cortisol. The daily cortisol production rate for an average adult is between 20 and 30 mg. Based on this, the recommended approach for surgical patients is to begin at the time of surgery with a dose between one and five times the daily production and administer no more than 100 to 150 mg of cortisol equivalent per day, tapering the dose over 48 to 72 hours. The potential risks of the administration of supplemental doses of corticosteroid to patients in the perioperative period are impaired wound healing and an increased rate of infections. (507)

86. The term critical illness–related corticosteroid insufficiency (CIRCI) recently has been applied to clinical situations in which the adrenal response to critical illness and other stresses is inadequate. Prior steroid treatment may be a potential cause of this condition. The patient may not otherwise meet traditional criteria for adrenocortical dysfunction. Signs and symptoms include unexplained vasopressor-dependent refractory hypotension, a discrepancy between the anticipated severity of the patient's disease and the present state of the patient, or high fever without apparent cause or not responding to antibiotics. There may also be hypoglycemia, hyponatremia, hyperkalemia, neutropenia, or eosinophilia. Empiric administration of 100 to 300 mg/day of IV hydrocortisone typically eliminates a preexisting need for vasopressors and is diagnostic. (507)

87. Cushing syndrome is the presence of elevated serum cortisol levels. Patients with Cushing syndrome have a typical physical appearance characterized by rounding of the face, truncal obesity, thin extremities, an upper thoracic fat pad ("buffalo hump"), purple abdominal striae, and thinning of the skin. Physiologic effects of chronic elevated corticosteroid levels include weight gain, hypertension, hypercoagulability, muscle weakness, glucose intolerance, gonadal dysfunction, and osteoporosis. Diagnosis is confirmed by an elevated 24-hour urinary free cortisol. (507)

88. Primary Cushing syndrome is defined as hypercortisolism independent of the level of pituitary ACTH secretion. It is usually due to a hyperfunctioning adrenal gland or an adrenal adenoma. Secondary and tertiary disease occurs from elevated circulating levels of ACTH or an ACTH-like substance. (507)

89. Cushing disease usually refers to one specific form of secondary Cushing syndrome, that of adrenal cortical hyperfunction due to excess production of ACTH by a pituitary adenoma. This accounts for 80% of patients with Cushing syndrome. (507)

90. After Cushing disease, the remainder of patients with secondary Cushing syndrome have ectopic sources of ACTH. These may include primary cancers of the adrenal or metastatic cancers such as lung (usually small cell), thyroid, prostate, pancreas, or intrathoracic neuroendocrine tumors. Secondary Cushing syndrome may also occur with exogenous administration of cortisol-like medications or synthetic ACTH. (507)

91. Cushing syndrome patients may be more susceptible to the effects of muscle relaxants than normal, leading to prolonged muscle relaxation and weakness. Because of this, Cushing syndrome patients may be subject to unanticipated postoperative respiratory failure. (507)

30 CENTRAL NERVOUS SYSTEM DISEASE

Alana Flexman and Lingzhong Meng

NEUROANATOMY

1. What structures make up the supratentorial and infratentorial compartments of the cranium?
2. What is the arterial blood supply to the brain?
3. In what proportion of humans is the classic depiction of the circle of Willis found?
4. What makes up the blood-brain barrier?
5. Name conditions in which the blood-brain barrier may be disrupted.

NEUROPHYSIOLOGY

6. What is normal cerebral blood flow?
7. Name some factors that influence cerebral blood flow.
8. What is the relationship between cerebral metabolic rate and cerebral blood flow?
9. For every 1° C decrease in temperature below normal body temperature, what is the corresponding decrease in cerebral blood flow?
10. Define cerebral perfusion pressure.
11. Within what range of cerebral perfusion pressures will cerebral blood flow remain relatively constant? What is the mechanism by which this occurs?
12. What is the time course in which there is a cerebral autoregulatory response to changes in cerebral perfusion pressure? What is the clinical implication of this?
13. Name conditions in which the cerebral autoregulation curve may be shifted.
14. Name some conditions in which cerebral autoregulation may be impaired.
15. Describe the relationship between Pa_{CO_2} and cerebral blood flow. What are the mechanism and duration of this effect?
16. How much does cerebral blood flow change for every 1-mm Hg increase or decrease in Pa_{CO_2} from 40 mm Hg?
17. What is a potential risk of prolonged, aggressive hyperventilation to a Pa_{CO_2} of less than 30 mm Hg?
18. Below what Pa_{O_2} will cerebral blood flow increase?
19. What are the effects of volatile anesthetics on cerebral blood flow and intracranial pressure?
20. What are the effects of nitrous oxide on cerebral blood flow and intracranial pressure?
21. What are the effects of ketamine on cerebral blood flow and intracranial pressure?
22. What are the effects of thiopental and propofol on cerebral blood flow and intracranial pressure?

23. What are the effects of dexmedetomidine and clonidine on cerebral blood flow and intracranial pressure?
24. What are the effects of benzodiazepines on cerebral blood flow and intracranial pressure?
25. What are the effects of opioids on cerebral blood flow and intracranial pressure?
26. What are the effects of neuromuscular blocking drugs on cerebral blood flow and intracranial pressure?

INTRACRANIAL PRESSURE

27. What are the components of the intracranial compartments?
28. What is a normal intracranial pressure?
29. How does the body compensate for increasing intracranial pressure? What implications does this have clinically?
30. Name some methods used to decrease elevated intracranial pressure.
31. Name some signs and symptoms that may be noted preoperatively that provide evidence that a patient may have an increased intracranial pressure.
32. What are the effects of intravenous anesthetic agents on intracranial pressure?
33. What are the effects of volatile anesthetics on intracranial pressure?
34. What are the effects of opioids, benzodiazepines, and neuromuscular blocking drugs on intracranial pressure?

NEUROPROTECTION

35. What is the current evidence regarding the use of induced hypothermia for neuroprotection in humans?
36. What is the current evidence regarding the use of intravenous anesthetics for neuroprotection?

ANESTHESIA FOR NEUROSURGERY

37. What monitors are typically used for intracranial neurosurgery?
38. What two devices can be used to measure the intracranial pressure?
39. What measures can an anesthesiologist undertake to attenuate increases in arterial blood pressure and intracranial pressure during direct laryngoscopy?
40. What are the advantages and disadvantages of the sitting position for the resection of intracranial tumors?
41. What are some precautions that should be exercised when a Mayfield head clamp is used for neurosurgery?
42. How is maintenance of anesthesia usually achieved in patients undergoing intracranial neurosurgery?
43. What is the desired range of Pa_{CO_2} to optimize cerebral blood flow intraoperatively?
44. What is a potential problem of the administration of positive end-expiratory pressure (PEEP) during mechanical ventilation of the lungs in patients undergoing intracranial neurosurgery?
45. How do peripheral vasodilators affect cerebral blood flow? What is the recommendation regarding the use of these drugs intraoperatively in patients undergoing intracranial neurosurgery?
46. Why might neuromuscular blockade be maintained throughout intracranial surgical procedures?
47. How can cerebral swelling be treated intraoperatively?
48. What are the advantages and disadvantages of osmotic diuretics during neurosurgery?
49. How should intravenous fluid administration be managed intraoperatively in patients undergoing intracranial neurosurgery?
50. Why should glucose-containing intravenous solutions be avoided in neurosurgical patients?
51. Why should coughing and straining by patients awakening from anesthesia be avoided after intracranial surgery? What are some methods by which these responses by the patient can be avoided?
52. Why is rapid awakening desirable in neurosurgical procedures?
53. How should delayed recovery after intracranial surgery be evaluated?

54. What drug is commonly used to treat hypertension on emergence from anesthesia for intracranial neurosurgery?
55. Why are patients undergoing neurosurgical procedures at an increased risk for venous air embolism?
56. Describe the pathophysiology of a venous air embolism. What percentage of adult patients have a probe-patent foramen ovale?
57. What are methods by which a venous air embolism can be detected? Which of them is the most sensitive?
58. What are some signs of a clinically significant venous air embolism?
59. What is the treatment for a venous air embolism?
60. Why should nitrous oxide administration be discontinued in the presence of a venous air embolism?
61. How efficacious is the use of PEEP in the prevention of a venous air embolism?
62. What typically causes death in a fatal venous air embolism?

INTRACRANIAL MASS LESIONS

63. What are some of the common presenting symptoms of patients with an intracranial tumor?
64. What is the anesthetic goal for patients undergoing surgical resection of an intracranial tumor?
65. Why is it important to limit drug-induced depression of ventilation with preoperative medicines in patients who are scheduled to undergo surgical resection of an intracranial tumor?
66. Name some anesthetic considerations that are unique to posterior fossa tumors.
67. What are some additional considerations for resection of a posterior fossa mass in the *sitting position*?

INTRACRANIAL ANEURYSMS AND ARTERIOVENOUS MALFORMATIONS

68. How do patients with ruptured intracranial aneurysms usually present?
69. What is the goal of the anesthetic management of a patient undergoing resection of an intracranial aneurysm or arteriovenous malformation?
70. What are the major complications of intracranial aneurysm rupture?
71. How might the electrocardiogram of patients with a ruptured intracranial aneurysm appear?
72. When is vasospasm after cerebral aneurysm rupture most likely to occur? How is it diagnosed?
73. What is the treatment for vasospasm after cerebral aneurysm rupture?
74. What are the different treatment options for intracranial aneurysms?
75. What are special considerations during temporary clip placement during resection of intracranial aneurysms?
76. What percentage of patients diagnosed with an arteriovenous malformation have an associated aneurysm?
77. What are the different treatment options for intracranial arteriovenous malformations?

CAROTID DISEASE

78. What are the indications for carotid endarterectomy?
79. How should patients scheduled for a carotid endarterectomy be evaluated preoperatively?
80. What are the anesthetic goals for patients undergoing a carotid endarterectomy? What is the critical period during this surgery?
81. How should the arterial blood pressure be managed during a carotid endarterectomy?
82. How should the Pa_{CO_2} be managed during a carotid endarterectomy?
83. What is the purpose of intraoperative neurologic monitoring during a carotid endarterectomy? What are some methods of intraoperative neurologic monitoring?
84. Does local or general anesthesia have better outcomes for carotid endarterectomy?
85. What are some potential postoperative complications after carotid endarterectomy?
86. What are the consequences of postoperative hypertension after carotid endarterectomy?

ANSWERS*

NEUROANATOMY

1. The supratentorial compartment contains the cerebral hemispheres and diencephalon (thalamus and hypothalamus), whereas the brainstem and cerebellum make up the infratentorial compartment. (511)
2. The arterial blood supply to the brain is through the left and right internal carotid arteries (anterior circulation) and the vertebrobasilar system (posterior circulation). Anastomoses between these vessels form the circle of Willis and create a collateral blood supply to protect against focal ischemia. (512)
3. Approximately 20% of the population has an abnormal circle of Willis, implying that collateralization may not be complete in all people. (512)
4. The blood-brain barrier is composed of capillary endothelial cells with tight junctions that prevent free passage of macromolecules or proteins. In contrast, lipid-soluble substances (carbon dioxide, oxygen, anesthetic agents) cross the blood-brain barrier easily. (512)
5. The blood-brain barrier may be disrupted in conditions such as acute systemic hypertension, head trauma, infection, arterial hypoxemia, severe hypercapnia, tumors, and sustained seizure activity. (512)

NEUROPHYSIOLOGY

6. Normal cerebral blood flow (CBF) is 50 mL/100 g of brain tissue per minute and represents approximately 12% to 15% of cardiac output. The brain, albeit being 2% of the body weight, receives a disproportionately large share of cardiac output because of its high metabolic rate and inability to store energy. (512)
7. Factors that influence CBF include (1) cerebral metabolic rate via neurovascular coupling, (2) cerebral perfusion pressure (CPP) via cerebral autoregulation, (3) arterial blood carbon dioxide and oxygen partial pressure (Pa_{CO_2} and Pa_{O_2}, respectively) via cerebrovascular reactivity, (4) sympathetic nervous activity, (5) cardiac output, and (6) anesthetic agents. (512)
8. The cerebral metabolic rate directly affects CBF through neurovascular coupling or cerebral metabolism flow coupling. Cerebral metabolic rate of oxygen ($CMRO_2$) and CBF are closely related: an increase or decrease in $CMRO_2$ results in a proportional increase or decrease in CBF. (512)
9. CBF decreases 7% for every 1° C decrease in body temperature below 37° C. This effect is due to the decrease in the cerebral metabolic rate caused by the decrease in temperature. (512)
10. CPP is defined as the difference between mean arterial pressure (MAP) and central venous pressure or intracranial pressure (ICP), whichever is greater. (513)
11. In healthy, normotensive individuals CBF remains relatively constant between CPPs of approximately 60 to 150 mm Hg. Within this CPP range (60 to 150 mm Hg) the cerebral vasculature is able to dilate or constrict in response to changes in CPP to maintain a constant CBF (approximately 50 mL/100 g/min). Below the lower limit, CBF decreases linearly with a decreasing CPP. In contrast, above the upper limit, CBF increases linearly with an increasing CPP. The plateau is the CPP range between the lower and upper limits where CBF remains stable. This response of the cerebral vasculature to maintain a constant CBF in the presence of alterations in CPP is termed *autoregulation*. (513)
12. Static cerebral autoregulation takes minutes to take effect. In the interim, a rapid increase or decrease in MAP may be associated with a brief period of cerebral hyperperfusion or hypoperfusion, respectively. (513)
13. The cerebral autoregulation curve shifts to the right in patients with chronic uncontrolled hypertension or sympathetic stimulation, and these patients require a higher minimum CPP to maintain adequate CBF. (513)

---

*Numbers in parentheses refer to pages, figures, boxes, or tables in Pardo MC, Miller RD, eds. *Basics of Anesthesia.* 7th ed. Philadelphia: Elsevier; 2018.

14. Autoregulation of CBF may be impaired following traumatic brain injury, intracranial surgery, or severe hypercapnia, or in the presence of inhaled anesthetics. Patients with impaired cerebral autoregulation need to have their CPP tightly controlled so that CBF is not affected by the loss of autoregulatory capacity. (513)

15. Changes in Pa_{CO_2} produce corresponding and same directional changes in CBF between a Pa_{CO_2} of 20 to 80 mm Hg. Such changes in CBF reflect the effect of carbon dioxide–mediated alterations in perivascular pH that leads to dilation or constriction of cerebral arterioles. The Pa_{CO_2}-related change in CBF only lasts for about 6 to 8 hours because of the compensatory change in bicarbonate (HCO_3^-) concentration. (513)

16. CBF increases or decreases approximately 1 mL/100 g/min or 2% for every 1 mm Hg increase or decrease in Pa_{CO_2} from 40 mm Hg. (513)

17. A potential risk of prolonged, aggressive hyperventilation to a Pa_{CO_2} of less than 30 mm Hg is cerebral ischemia. There is evidence to suggest that prolonged aggressive hyperventilation following traumatic brain injury is associated with poorer neurologic outcome. (513)

18. Decreases in Pa_{O_2} below a threshold value of about 50 mm Hg result in an exponential increase in CBF, likely a compensatory mechanism to maintain cerebral oxygen delivery: cerebral oxygen delivery = arterial blood oxygen content × CBF. (513)

19. Volatile anesthetic agents are potent cerebral vasodilators. When administered during normocapnia at concentrations higher than 0.5 MAC (minimum alveolar concentration), desflurane, sevoflurane, and isoflurane rapidly produce cerebral vasodilation and result in dose-dependent increases in CBF, even though $CMRO_2$ is decreased. Therefore, volatile anesthetic agents produce divergent changes in $CMRO_2$ and CBF that are distinct from intravenous anesthetic agents. Volatile agents produce dose-dependent increases in ICP that parallel the increases in CBF and cerebral blood volume. Hyperventilation to decrease Pa_{CO_2} to less than 35 mm Hg attenuates the tendency for volatile anesthetic agents to increase ICP. (513)

20. When used in isolation, nitrous oxide increases CBF and possibly $CMRO_2$; however, these effects appear to be attenuated by the coadministration of other anesthetic agents. (513)

21. The effects of ketamine on cerebrovascular physiology have been variable, which likely reflects different research study conditions. When ketamine is given on its own without control of ventilation, Pa_{CO_2}, CBF, and ICP all increase, whereas when given in the presence of another sedative/anesthetic drug in patients whose ventilation is controlled, these effects are not noted. Because of this controversy, however, ketamine is usually avoided in patients with known intracranial disease. (513)

22. Intravenously administered anesthetic agents such as propofol and thiopental cause simultaneous reduction of $CMRO_2$, CBF, and ICP. The effect of intravenous anesthetics on CBF is attributed to neurovascular coupling (i.e., the decrease in $CMRO_2$ leads to a corresponding decrease in CBF). (514)

23. α_2-Agonists (clonidine and dexmedetomidine) are unique sedatives in that they do not cause significant respiratory depression. They reduce arterial blood pressure, CPP, and CBF with minimal effects on ICP. (514)

24. Benzodiazepines decrease $CMRO_2$ and CBF, analogous to propofol and thiopental although to a lesser extent. Benzodiazepines reduce ICP through reductions in $CMRO_2$ and CBF, although this benefit will be offset if respiratory depression and increases in Pa_{CO_2} occur. (514)

25. Similar to benzodiazepines, opioids decrease $CMRO_2$, CBF, and ICP, analogous to propofol and thiopental although to a lesser extent. However, associated respiratory depression and elevation of Pa_{CO_2} may produce the opposite effect. Opioids should be used with caution in patients with intracranial disease because of their (1) depressant effects on consciousness, (2) production of miosis, and (3) depression of ventilation with associated increases in ICP from Pa_{CO_2} increases. (514)

26. Succinylcholine may increase ICP through increases in CBF although this phenomenon is inconsistently reported in the literature as a result of differences in study design and patient neurologic status. Nondepolarizing neuromuscular blocking drugs do not generally affect ICP except through the potential release of histamine, leading to cerebral vasodilation. (514)

INTRACRANIAL PRESSURE

27. The intracranial compartment normally contains three components: (1) brain matter, (2) cerebrospinal fluid, and (3) blood. (514)
28. Normal ICP is lower than 15 mm Hg. (514)
29. The compensatory mechanism to restore ICP to normal in the face of an expanding component is via compensatory reduction of other intracranial components, including the translocation of cerebrospinal fluid from intracranial space to extracranial space. At the moment when this compensatory mechanism is exhausted, minimal increases in volume lead to marked increases in ICP, and cerebral blood vessels are eventually compressed. (514)
30. Reductions in elevated ICP are achieved through reductions in cerebral blood volume, cerebrospinal fluid, and cerebral edema. Methods of reducing cerebral blood volume include elevation of the head, avoiding constriction at the neck, avoidance of high ventilatory pressures and PEEP, hyperventilation, reduction in $CMRO_2$ (propofol, barbiturates), and avoidance of hypertension and cerebral vasodilators. Cerebrospinal fluid may be drained through an external ventricular or lumbar drain or its production decreased by acetazolamide. Cerebral edema can be reduced with osmotic drugs such as mannitol or with the diuretic furosemide. Dexamethasone will reduce peritumor edema. It is important to prevent ischemia and secondary edema. Finally, resection of space-occupying lesions and decompressive craniectomy are surgical alternatives. (514)
31. Signs and symptoms of an increased ICP include positional headache, nausea and vomiting, hypertension, bradycardia, altered levels of consciousness, altered patterns of breathing, and papilledema. (514)
32. Most intravenous anesthetic agents reduce $CMRO_2$ and CBF, with an associated decrease in ICP. The administration of propofol and thiopental must be done carefully and in doses to avoid decreases in systemic blood pressure and CPP. The effect of ketamine is controversial, and ketamine is probably best avoided as the sole agent in patients with an increased ICP. Etomidate increases the frequency of excitatory peaks on the electroencephalogram and is best avoided in patients with a history of epilepsy, especially considering that seizure activity can markedly increase $CMRO_2$, CBF, and ICP. (514)
33. Volatile anesthetics are cerebral vasodilators and produce dose-dependent increase in ICP that parallels the increase in CBF. Hyperventilation to decrease Pa_{CO_2} to less than 35 mm Hg can attenuate this effect, but volatile anesthetics may be best avoided if high ICP-compensating mechanisms are exhausted, as evidenced by elevated ICP, abnormal mental status, or imaging studies. (515)
34. Opioids and benzodiazepines reduce ICP through reductions in $CMRO_2$ and CBF, although this benefit will be offset if respiratory depression and increases in Pa_{CO_2} occur. Succinylcholine may increase ICP through increases in CBF, but this phenomenon is inconsistently reported in the literature. Its effects are short-lived and clinically inconsequential. Nondepolarizing neuromuscular blocking drugs do not usually affect ICP unless they induce the release of histamine or systemic hypotension. (515)

NEUROPROTECTION

35. Hypothermia has been investigated extensively as a method of cerebral protection during acute injury. Although numerous animal studies have supported temperature reduction to reduce ischemic injury, several large prospective, randomized trials of hypothermia in aneurysm surgery and traumatic brain injury have failed to reproduce a consistent benefit to date. (515)
36. Many anesthetic agents have been proposed as neuroprotectants given their potential to reduce cerebral metabolic rate and excitotoxicity during periods

of oxygen deprivation. Animal studies have supported the ability of many anesthetic agents, including volatile anesthetic agents, barbiturates, propofol, and xenon, to provide neuroprotection, although convincing data are lacking to recommend their use in humans for this purpose. (515-516)

ANESTHESIA FOR NEUROSURGERY

37. In addition to standard monitors, continuous monitoring of systemic blood pressure via a peripheral arterial catheter is recommended. The advantages of invasive blood pressure monitoring include the ability to continuously assess CPP and intravascular volume via indexes such as systolic pressure variation and pulse pressure variation. In addition, these catheters allow for arterial blood gas sampling and accurate determination of Pa_{CO_2}. Central venous catheters are not routinely used; however, exceptions include difficult peripheral venous access and potential of massive transfusion. Measurement of the exhaled carbon dioxide concentration (capnography) is used to adjust mechanical ventilation or assess spontaneous breathing if the airway is not instrumented. The electrocardiogram (ECG) allows prompt detection of cardiac dysrhythmias caused by surgical stimulation of brainstem or intracranial nerves. Neuromuscular blockade is monitored with a peripheral nerve stimulator. (516)

38. Two types of ICP monitors are inserted by neurosurgeons. The intraventricular catheter or external ventricular device (EVD) permits direct measurement of ICP and drainage of cerebrospinal fluid. The subarachnoid or subdural bolt is placed through a burr hole and can be inserted quickly in an emergency setting, but it does not allow for cerebrospinal fluid drainage. (516)

39. The patient's trachea is intubated ideally after the induction of a sufficient level of anesthesia and a peripheral nerve stimulator confirms the establishment of skeletal muscle paralysis so that coughing is avoided, which may result in marked increases in ICP. Injection of additional intravenous doses of propofol, thiopental, opioids, or lidocaine 1 to 2 minutes before initiating direct laryngoscopy may be effective in attenuating the increase in systemic blood pressure and ICP that can accompany tracheal intubation. (517)

40. The sitting position facilitates surgical exposure of posterior fossa tumors, but because of the high risk of venous air embolism (>25% incidence), the prone position is used instead. Other risks associated with the sitting position include upper airway edema as a result of venous obstruction from excessive cervical flexion and quadriplegia from spinal cord compression and ischemia, especially in the presence of preexisting cervical stenosis. (517)

41. The placement of the Mayfield head clamp can elicit a sympathetic response of tachycardia and hypertension. Blunting of this hemodynamic fluctuation can be achieved through the administration of additional doses of propofol or opioids just prior to head frame placement. While the head frame is being placed and removed, and while the patient is fixed in the frame, movement and bucking must be avoided to prevent injury to the patient. (517)

42. Maintenance of anesthesia is often achieved in patients undergoing intracranial surgery with a combination of opioid (either bolus or infusion), continuous infusion of propofol, and inhalation of a volatile anesthetic with or without nitrous oxide. Volatile anesthetic agents must be used carefully because of their ability to increase ICP. Nevertheless, at low concentrations, volatile anesthetic agents (<0.5 MAC) are useful for blunting the increases in systemic blood pressure evoked by surgical stimulation. The choice of anesthetic agents should also take into account the neurophysiologic monitoring being used because certain agents (e.g., volatile anesthetic agents, nitrous oxide, neuromuscular blockers) will impede neurophysiologic monitors such as motor or somatosensory evoked potentials. (517)

43. After tracheal intubation, ventilation of the lungs is controlled at a rate and tidal volume sufficient to maintain Pa_{CO_2} between 30 and 35 mm Hg. There is no evidence of additional therapeutic benefit when Pa_{CO_2} is decreased below this range. (517)

44. Use of positive end-expiratory pressure is not encouraged in patients undergoing intracranial surgery because it could impair cerebral venous drainage and increase ICP, but it can usually be counteracted by raising the head 10 to 15 cm above the level of the chest. (518)

45. Direct-acting vasodilating drugs (hydralazine, nitroprusside, nitroglycerin, calcium channel blockers) may increase CBF and ICP despite causing simultaneous decreases in systemic blood pressure; therefore, use of these drugs, particularly before the dura is open, is not encouraged. (518)

46. Movement, coughing, or reacting to the presence of the tracheal tube during intracranial procedures is avoided because these responses can lead to increases in ICP, bleeding into the operative site, and a brain that bulges into the operative site and makes surgical exposure difficult. Thus, maintenance of an adequate depth of anesthesia is important. Skeletal muscle paralysis is often used to provide added insurance against movement or coughing. However, continuous administration of muscle relaxants is not possible in cases in which motor function monitoring is applied (e.g., either evoked potential or direct cortical or subcortical stimulation). (518)

47. Cerebral swelling occurring intraoperatively can be treated a number of ways. Mannitol at a dose of 0.25 to 1 g/kg or furosemide at a dose of 0.5 to 1 mg/kg is frequently used for this purpose. Intermittent injections of an intravenous anesthetic such as thiopental or propofol may also be administered. Also important is placing the patient in a head-up position when possible as well as avoiding constriction around the neck that may impair venous drainage. Other useful measures include hyperventilation, discontinuing the administration of volatile anesthetic agents, and cerebrospinal fluid drainage. (518)

48. Osmotic agents such as mannitol (0.25 to 1 g/kg IV) or 3% hypertonic saline are frequently administered to reduce cerebral water content and decrease ICP before craniectomy and to improve brain relaxation after craniectomy. The onset of action is 5 to 10 minutes, maximum effects are seen in 20 to 30 minutes, and its effects last for about 2 to 4 hours. However, if administered rapidly, mannitol can also cause peripheral vasodilation (hypotension) and short-term intravascular volume expansion, which could result in increased ICP and volume overload. Acute mannitol toxicity, as manifested by hyponatremia, high measured serum osmolality, and a gap between the measured and calculated serum osmolality of greater than 10 mOsm/kg, can also occur when large does of the drug (2 to 3 g/kg IV) are given. Furosemide (0.5 to 1 mg/kg IV) is often used to decrease brain water and ICP and is thought to be synergistic with mannitol in decreasing ICP. However, hypovolemia secondary to diuresis can decrease the preload and cardiac output that may do more harm than good in terms of tissue perfusion. (518)

49. Maintaining euvolemia with crystalloid solutions such as normal saline, Plasma-Lyte, and lactated Ringer solution is recommended. Colloids such as 5% albumin are also an acceptable replacement fluid, but no improvement in outcome has been shown. (518)

50. Dextrose solutions are not recommended because they are rapidly distributed throughout body water and, if blood glucose concentrations decrease more rapidly than brain glucose concentrations, water crosses the blood-brain barrier and cerebral edema results. Furthermore, hyperglycemia augments ischemic neuronal cell damage by promoting neuronal lactate production, which worsens cellular injury. (518)

51. On awakening from anesthesia, coughing or straining by the patient should be avoided because these responses could increase the possibility of intracranial hemorrhage or edema formation. A prior intravenous bolus of lidocaine, opioid, or both may help decrease the likelihood of coughing during tracheal extubation. Low rate remifentanil infusion has been recognized to be able to facilitate a smooth emergence. (518)

52. Rapid awakening is desirable in neurosurgical procedures to allow for early and frequent neurologic assessment. (518)

53. Delayed return of consciousness or neurologic deterioration in the postoperative period should be carefully monitored and evaluated by computed tomography or magnetic resonance imaging. It is important to rule out intracranial hemorrhage and stroke as early as possible. Tension pneumocephalus as a cause of neurologic deterioration should also be considered. (518)

54. The postoperative stress response and resulting hyperdynamic events (hypertension, tachycardia) are attenuated with the use of hemodynamically active drugs and opioids. Labetalol is commonly used to treat hypertension based on its ability to reduce MAP without cerebral vasodilation. (518)

55. Neurosurgery that requires significant elevation of the head is associated with an increased risk for venous air embolism. Not only is the operative site above the level of the heart, but the venous sinuses in the cut edge of bone or dura may not collapse when transected, allowing for the entrainment of air. (519)

56. The pathophysiologic effects of a venous air embolism occur when air enters the pulmonary circulation and becomes trapped in the small vessels, thereby causing an acute increase in dead space. Massive air embolism may cause air to enter and be trapped in the right ventricle and lead to acute right ventricular failure. Microvascular bubbles may also cause reflex bronchoconstriction and activate the release of endothelial mediators causing pulmonary edema. Air may reach the coronary and cerebral circulations (paradoxical air embolism) by crossing a patent foramen ovale (a probe-patent foramen ovale is present in 20% to 30% of adults) and result in myocardial infarction or stroke. Furthermore, transpulmonary passage of venous air is possible in the absence of a patent foramen ovale. (519)

57. Transesophageal echocardiography is the most sensitive method to detect air embolism, but it is invasive and cumbersome. A precordial Doppler ultrasound transducer placed over the right side of the heart (over the second or third intercostal space to the right of the sternum to maximize audible signals from the right atrium) is the next most sensitive (detects amounts of air as small as 0.25 mL) and a practical noninvasive indicator of the presence of intracardiac air. A sudden decrease in end-tidal concentrations of carbon dioxide reflects increased dead space secondary to continued ventilation of alveoli no longer being perfused because of obstruction of their vascular supply by air bubbles. An increased end-tidal nitrogen concentration may reflect nitrogen from venous air embolism if the inspired oxygen concentration is higher than room air, but this is rarely available. Aspiration of air through a correctly positioned central venous catheter can also be used to diagnose air embolism. (519)

58. During controlled ventilation of the lungs, sudden attempts (gasps) by patients to initiate spontaneous breaths may be the first indication of the occurrence of venous air embolism. Hypotension, tachycardia, cardiac dysrhythmias, cyanosis, and a "mill wheel" murmur are late signs of venous air embolism. A pulmonary artery catheter may provide additional evidence that venous air embolism has occurred because of abrupt increases in pulmonary artery pressure. Additional signs in awake patients include chest pain and coughing. (519)

59. The surgeon should be notified immediately whenever a venous air embolism is suspected. Venous air embolism is treated by (1) irrigation of the operative site with fluid, as well as the application of occlusive material to all bone edges so that sites of venous air entry are occluded; (2) placement of the patient in a head-down position; (3) gentle compression of the internal jugular veins; (4) 100% of inspired oxygen concentration; and (5) supportive care of hemodynamic derangements. (519)

60. If nitrous oxide is being administered, it should be promptly discontinued to avoid the risk of increasing the size of venous air bubbles because of diffusion of this gas into the air bubbles. (519)

61. Despite the logic of positive end-expiratory pressure to decrease entrainment of air, the efficacy of this maneuver has not been confirmed. Furthermore, positive

end-expiratory pressure could reverse the pressure gradient between the left and right atria and predispose to passage of air across a patent foramen ovale. (519)

62. Massive air embolism may cause air to enter and be trapped in the right ventricle and lead to acute right ventricular failure. Microvascular bubbles may also cause reflex bronchoconstriction and activate the release of endothelial mediators causing pulmonary edema. Death is usually due to cardiovascular collapse and arterial hypoxemia. (519)

INTRACRANIAL MASS LESIONS

63. Intracranial mass lesions, especially primary brain tumors, occur most often in patients 40 to 60 years of age, and the initial signs and symptoms may or may not reflect increases in ICP. Headache and seizures that appear in a previously asymptomatic adult suggest the presence of an intracranial tumor. (519)

64. Avoidance of abrupt increases in ICP is an important anesthetic goal when managing patients with intracranial tumors. (520)

65. Preoperative sedative medications may result in depression of ventilation and increases in Pa_{CO_2} in patients with an intracranial tumor. This in turn could lead to an increase in CBF and a corresponding increase in the ICP. (520)

66. Posterior fossa operations have the potential of stimulating or injuring vital brainstem respiratory and circulatory centers and result in intraoperative hemodynamic fluctuations and postoperative ventilation abnormalities. The cranial nerves can also be stimulated or affected, which can lead to intraoperative dysrhythmias and postoperative impairment of protective airway reflexes. Postoperatively, one needs to assess whether the patient will be able to maintain and protect the airway or whether tracheal intubation and ventilation should be continued in the intensive care unit. (520)

67. Sitting position for posterior fossa masses has several additional considerations. The transducer of the arterial line used to monitor beat-to-beat systemic blood pressure should be positioned no lower than the external ear canal level in order to facilitate the assessment of CPP. A properly positioned central venous catheter and precordial Doppler should be used given the high incidence of venous air embolism. Adequate hydration is warranted to compensate for the intravascular volume pooling in the lower extremities. (520)

INTRACRANIAL ANEURYSMS AND ARTERIOVENOUS MALFORMATIONS

68. Although aneurysms may be found incidentally or appear as a slowly enlarging mass, they are most frequently manifested as hemorrhage together with a sudden, severe headache, nausea, vomiting, focal neurologic signs, and depressed consciousness. (520)

69. The anesthetic care for intracranial aneurysm clipping is designed to (1) prevent sudden increases in systemic arterial blood pressure, which would increase the aneurysm's transmural pressure and could result in rupture or rebleeding and (2) facilitate surgical exposure and access to the aneurysm. (520)

70. Major complications of aneurysmal rupture include death, rebleeding, and vasospasm, and they may be treated with either endovascular coiling or surgical clipping via craniectomy. Early treatment is advocated for prevention of rebleeding, but surgery may be associated with greater technical difficulty because of a swollen inflamed brain, whereas delaying treatment increases the risk for rebleeding. Other complications of aneurysm rupture include seizures (10%), acute and chronic hydrocephalus, intracerebral hematoma, and systemic complications, such as neurogenic pulmonary edema and hyponatremia. (520)

71. Changes on the ECG (T-wave inversions, U waves, ST-segment depressions, prolonged QT interval, and rarely Q waves) and mild elevation of cardiac enzymes are frequent in patients with a ruptured intracranial aneurysm but do not usually correlate with significant myocardial dysfunction or poor outcome. (520)

72. Cerebral vasospasm is generally manifested clinically 3 to 5 days after subarachnoid hemorrhage and is the foremost cause of morbidity and death. Transcranial Doppler and cerebral arteriography can detect cerebral vasospasm before clinical symptoms (worsening headache, neurologic deterioration, loss of consciousness) occur. (521)

73. Treatment of vasospasm includes "triple H" therapy (hypervolemia, hypertension, hemodilution), which consists of intravenous administration of fluids or inotropic drugs, or both. The intravenous administration of a calcium channel blocker, nimodipine, decreases the morbidity and mortality risks from vasospasm. Other treatment modalities include selective intra-arterial injection of vasodilators and balloon dilation (angioplasty) of the affected arterial segments using interventional radiology. (521)

74. Intracranial aneurysms may be treated with either endovascular coiling or surgical clipping via craniectomy. Short- to medium-term outcomes are similar in patients treated surgically versus endovascular insertion of platinum coils, although the long-term benefits of one technique over the other continues to be debated. Some patients are unsuitable candidates for endovascular coiling because of the anatomy and location of their aneurysms; in these cases, surgical clipping is needed. (521)

75. Temporary occlusive clips applied to the major feeding artery of the aneurysm can create regional hypotension without the need for systemic hypotension and its inherent risks on multiple organ systems. As a result, normal or even increased systemic arterial blood pressure should be instituted to facilitate perfusion through collateral circulations. In addition to maintaining collateral cerebral circulations via systemic relative hypertension, drugs such as propofol or thiopental may be administered, via either boluses or high-rate infusion to the point of burst suppression on electroencephalography monitoring, in the hope that they can provide some protection from cerebral ischemia. Occasionally, hypothermic circulatory arrest may be used for very large complex aneurysms. Nonetheless, convincing outcome evidence of these maneuvers is lacking. (521)

76. Up to 10% of patients diagnosed with an arteriovenous malformation have an associated aneurysm. (521)

77. Arteriovenous malformations may be treated several ways: expectantly, open resection, endovascular embolization, or with stereotactic radiosurgery (Gamma Knife). Preoperative embolization is frequently employed to reduce blood loss and facilitate surgical resection. (521)

CAROTID DISEASE

78. Carotid endarterectomy (CEA) remains the "gold standard" in treating symptomatic carotid stenosis. Although the perioperative risk of stroke and death (approximately 4-7%) must be taken into account, CEA may be beneficial in asymptomatic patients as well. Data suggest that early CEA (<30 days after symptom onset) is optimal given the presence of unstable atherosclerotic plaque. (521)

79. Preoperative assessment of patients undergoing CEA should focus on assessment of perioperative risk of cardiac ischemia as these patients typically have atherosclerotic disease. The range of normal blood pressures for the patient should be determined. Neurologic symptoms and deficits should be documented preoperatively to prevent any dysfunction noted postoperatively from being incorrectly attributed to the surgical procedure or intraoperative events. (521)

80. Goals of anesthesia for CEA include (1) prevention of cerebral ischemia through maintenance of adequate CPP and (2) prevention of myocardial ischemia through avoidance of acute peaks in blood pressure and heart rate. Ensuring adequate CPP is especially important during the critical period of intraoperative clamping of the carotid artery. (522)

81. During a CEA procedure, the arterial blood pressure should be maintained in a normal or slightly elevated range specific to that patient. This is especially important during intraoperative clamping of the carotid artery. The anesthesiologist should ensure that the MAP is maintained above the patient's baseline pressure (within 20%) to ensure adequate collateral flow through the circle of Willis, particularly when there is no intraluminal shunt in place. Intraoperative hypotension is often treated with phenylephrine. (522)

82. Hypocarbia should be avoided given the risk of cerebral vasoconstriction and ischemia, and the Pa_{CO_2} should be maintained near normal, between 35 and 40 mm Hg. (522)

83. The purpose of intraoperative neurologic monitoring during a CEA is to detect cerebral ischemia and the potential need for an intraluminal shunt placed for perfusion to the ipsilateral brain while the diseased carotid artery is clamped. Several methods of monitoring for cerebral ischemia have been used, including electroencephalography, evoked potentials, transcranial Doppler, cerebral oximetry, and stump pressure (blood pressure in the carotid artery distal to the placement of the surgical clamp as an indication of adequate collateral flow), although none has been shown to definitively improve outcome. (522)

84. Either general or regional anesthesia (deep and superficial cervical plexus block) may be used for this procedure. Although an awake patient may provide a more accurate intraoperative assessment of the patient's neurologic status and more stable hemodynamic profile, the procedure requires a cooperative and motionless patient. Current evidence suggests that outcomes are similar whether CEA is performed under regional or general anesthesia. (522)

85. Potential postoperative complications after a CEA include recurrent laryngeal nerve injury, hemodynamic instability, airway compression secondary to neck hematoma, loss of carotid body function, myocardial infarction, and neurologic dysfunction. Neurologic dysfunction after CEA is usually due to intraoperative emboli or hypoperfusion during carotid artery clamping. (522)

86. Postoperative hypertension after CEA may lead to neck hematoma with airway compromise and hyperperfusion syndrome and should be avoided. (522)

31 OPHTHALMOLOGY AND OTOLARYNGOLOGY

Steven Gayer and Howard D. Palte

OPHTHALMOLOGY

INTRAOCULAR PRESSURE

1. What is a typical range for intraocular pressure (IOP)?
2. How is IOP created and maintained?
3. What are some potential adverse effects of a sustained increase in IOP during anesthesia?
4. What factors during the course of a general anesthetic increase IOP?
5. How much does IOP increase during coughing or vomiting?
6. What physiologic factors (CO_2, temperature) during the course of a general anesthetic decrease IOP?
7. How does ketamine affect IOP? What other attributes of ketamine make it a less than ideal choice for anesthesia in patients undergoing ophthalmic procedures?
8. How much does IOP increase with the intravenous administration of succinylcholine? What is the duration of this effect?
9. What is the mechanism for the increase in IOP following the administration of succinylcholine?
10. What maneuvers may attenuate the rise in IOP associated with succinylcholine use for laryngoscopy and endotracheal intubation?
11. How do paralyzing doses of nondepolarizing neuromuscular blocking drugs affect IOP?
12. How do inhaled anesthetics affect IOP? What is the effect on IOP of most intravenous anesthetics?
13. How do changes in arterial blood pressure affect IOP?

OPHTHALMIC MEDICATIONS

14. How are topical ophthalmic medicines absorbed into the systemic circulation? What topical ophthalmic medicines may be absorbed sufficiently to exert systemic effects?
15. What systemic effects have been attributed to the use of topical ophthalmic β-adrenergic blocking medications?
16. What are the systemic effects of topical ophthalmic phospholine iodide (echothiophate)?
17. Why is phenylephrine administered as a topical ophthalmic medicine? What systemic effect has been attributed to the topical ophthalmic application of this drug?
18. Why are carbonic anhydrase inhibitors, such as acetazolamide, administered as topical ophthalmic medicines? What systemic effects have been attributed to the topical ophthalmic application of this drug?

OCULOCARDIAC REFLEX

19. What is the oculocardiac reflex? What is its reported incidence?
20. When is the oculocardiac reflex most likely to be encountered?
21. What cardiac dysrhythmias may occur as a result of the oculocardiac reflex?
22. How does arterial hypoxemia or hypercarbia affect the oculocardiac reflex? How does the depth of general anesthesia affect the oculocardiac reflex?
23. What is the first line of treatment of the oculocardiac reflex? What measures may be taken if the reflex persists?
24. Is prophylactic use of anticholinergics fully effective in preventing the oculocardiac reflex? What problems may arise from use of an anticholinergic?

PREOPERATIVE ASSESSMENT

25. What are some important demographic characteristics of patients scheduled for ophthalmic surgery?
26. Should antiplatelet or anticoagulant medications be discontinued prior to ophthalmic surgery?
27. What is a key anesthetic consideration for the patient scheduled for ophthalmic surgery with uncontrolled cough, untreated parkinsonian tremor, severe claustrophobia, or pathologic anxiety?

ANESTHETIC OPTIONS

28. What are the anesthetic options for patients having an ophthalmic procedure?
29. What is the significance of the extraocular muscle cone for ophthalmic blocks?
30. What is the ultimate needle tip position for a retrobulbar (intraconal) block?
31. What is the rationale behind extraconal (peribulbar) anesthesia? Where is the ultimate needle tip position?
32. What are some complications of a retrobulbar block?
33. What is the differential diagnosis of altered physiologic status (blood pressure, heart rate) after a needle-based ophthalmic anesthetic block?
34. What are the clinical signs of brainstem anesthesia following an ophthalmic anesthetic block?
35. How does one differentiate brainstem anesthesia from excessive sedation after an ophthalmic anesthetic block?
36. How does a sub-Tenon block differ from a needle-based ophthalmic block?

ANESTHETIC MANAGEMENT OF SPECIFIC OPHTHALMIC PROCEDURES

37. Which patients are at high risk for retinal detachment?
38. What are the anesthetic considerations for patients undergoing surgery to repair a retinal detachment?
39. When must nitrous oxide be avoided as maintenance anesthetic for patients undergoing surgery to repair a retinal detachment? What is the risk associated with this?
40. What is glaucoma? What are its variants?
41. What are the anesthetic goals in the management of glaucoma patients?
42. What are the anesthetic considerations for children undergoing strabismus surgery?
43. What is the most common reason for an inpatient admission for children following strabismus surgery?
44. What factors must be considered in the anesthetic management of patients with traumatic eye injuries?
45. Why is "awake" endotracheal intubation hazardous for patients with open globe injuries?
46. What anesthetic maneuvers may attenuate increases in IOP in traumatic eye injury?
47. Is regional anesthesia contraindicated in traumatic eye injuries?

POSTOPERATIVE OPHTHALMIC ISSUES

48. What is the most common ocular complication following general anesthesia for nonophthalmic surgery? What other condition can mimic it?
49. What are some potential causes of corneal abrasion in patients who are undergoing a surgical procedure?
50. What are the clinical signs of a corneal abrasion?

51. What are some preventive measures that can be taken to reduce the risk of corneal abrasion in patients under general anesthesia? What are some of the potential problems with routine use of ophthalmic ointment?
52. How does acute glaucoma present, and how is it treated?
53. Which surgical procedures are associated with an increased risk of postoperative visual loss?
54. What action should be taken if the patient complains of postoperative visual loss?
55. What specific risks should be discussed preoperatively with patients scheduled to undergo major cardiac or spine surgery?

OTOLARYNGOLOGY

SPECIAL CONSIDER-ATIONS FOR HEAD AND NECK SURGERY

56. What special airway considerations pertain to ENT (ear, nose, throat) surgery?
57. Why are posterior pharyngeal packs used during ENT surgery, and what precautions are required with their use?
58. What supplemental airway devices may be needed for a difficult airway during ENT surgery?
59. What is laryngospasm? How is the reflex mediated?
60. What maneuvers should be taken in response to laryngospasm?
61. Why are children at particular risk during laryngospasm?
62. Should a scheduled ENT surgery be postponed if the child has an upper respiratory infection (URI)? What are the risks associated with proceeding with anesthesia in a child with an active upper respiratory infection?
63. What risks are associated with general anesthesia in a patient with massive epistaxis?
64. What are some symptoms that may alert the anesthesiologist to the presence of obstructive sleep apnea (OSA)? What is the STOP-BANG questionnaire?
65. What features may be noted in the airway examination of a patient with OSA?
66. What are the anesthetic implications of OSA?
67. What elements are necessary to generate an airway fire?
68. Are airway fires possible with monitored anesthesia care?
69. What steps should be taken in the event of a fire in the operating room?

ANESTHESTHETIC MANAGEMENT OF SPECIFIC OTOLARYNGOLOGIC PROCEDURES

70. What are the main anesthetic considerations for ear surgery?
71. What effects may nitrous oxide (N_2O) exert during ear surgery?
72. How is surgical identification of the facial nerve performed intraoperatively in patients undergoing otologic surgery? How might this affect the anesthetic management?
73. Why do otolaryngologists use epinephrine intraoperatively? What are the anesthetic implications of its use?
74. What concentration of epinephrine is considered safe in ear microsurgery?
75. During otolaryngology surgery how can bleeding in the surgical field be minimized?
76. What is an optimal anesthetic plan for emergence from general anesthesia in the patient who has undergone middle ear surgery?
77. Why are patients who have undergone middle ear surgery at risk for postoperative nausea and vomiting?
78. What anesthetic strategies minimize postoperative nausea and vomiting after ear surgery?
79. What are some perioperative issues seen in patients undergoing tonsillectomy and adenoidectomy?
80. What is negative-pressure pulmonary edema?
81. Why is blood loss often underestimated during and after tonsillectomy and adenoidectomy?

82. What are some considerations for the anesthetic management of patients who return to surgery because of significant bleeding after tonsillectomy and adenoidectomy?
83. What organism is frequently responsible for acute epiglottitis?
84. What are the clinical features of acute epiglottitis?
85. What anesthetic precautions are necessary in acute epiglottitis management?
86. What are the clinical features of foreign body aspiration into the airway?
87. What anesthesia precautions are necessary in addressing the patient with an airway foreign body?
88. What postoperative measures are necessary after the removal of a foreign body from the airway?
89. Why is cocaine used for nasal surgery?
90. What are the disadvantages of using cocaine for nasal surgery? Are there alternatives?
91. What considerations are important for general anesthesia emergence in nasal and sinus surgery?
92. What preoperative investigations may be useful in a patient undergoing endoscopic surgery?
93. What techniques may be used to maintain ventilation and oxygenation during airway endoscopy?
94. What risk is associated with the use of a manual high-pressure jet ventilator (Sanders injector apparatus)?
95. What is a laser? What advantages does it offer for surgical procedures?
96. Name some hazards that are associated with laser surgery.
97. What is the purpose of a smoke evacuator used during laser surgery?
98. What measures can be taken during laser surgery to minimize the risk of an endotracheal tube (ETT) fire?
99. Why should the ETT cuff be filled with saline or an indicator dye during laser surgery?
100. What medical issues are frequently encountered in patients undergoing radical neck dissection?
101. How does a history of radiation to the larynx, pharynx, or oral cavity affect anesthetic management?
102. What arrhythmias may be precipitated during radical neck dissection, and why?
103. What nerve injuries and their corresponding clinical manifestations may be encountered postoperatively after head and neck surgery?
104. What catastrophic postoperative event may occur after neck surgery?
105. How may hypocalcemia present after thyroid or parathyroid surgery?
106. What are the cause and clinical signs of thyroid storm?
107. Why might a patient not be able to symmetrically grimace following parotid surgery? What monitor may help prevent this complication?
108. What is the Le Fort classification of maxillary fractures?

ANSWERS*

OPHTHALMOLOGY

Intraocular Pressure

1. Intraocular pressure (IOP) ranges between 10 and 22 mm Hg. In the intact normal eye there is a typical diurnal variation of 2 to 5 mm Hg. Small changes can occur with each cardiac contraction and with closure of the eyes, mydriasis, and changes in posture. (525)

---

*Numbers in parentheses refer to pages, figures, boxes, or tables in Pardo MC, Miller RD, eds. *Basics of Anesthesia*. 7th ed. Philadelphia: Elsevier; 2018.

2. Intraocular pressure is primarily a balance between the production and drainage of aqueous humor. Aqueous humor is actively secreted from the posterior chamber's ciliary body and flows through the pupil into the anterior chamber where it becomes mixed with aqueous fluids, which are passively produced by blood vessels on the iris's forward surface. It ultimately exits the eye into episcleral veins that flow into the superior vena cava. (525)

3. Potential adverse effects of a sustained increase in IOP during anesthesia include acute glaucoma, retinal ischemia, hemorrhage, and permanent visual loss. (525)

4. During general anesthesia any maneuver that obstructs venous return from the eye to the right side of the heart will increase IOP. These maneuvers include Trendelenburg positioning, tight cervical collar, straining, retching, vomiting, and coughing. A tightly applied face mask, direct laryngoscopy, and intubation also increase IOP, as well as hypoxemia and hypoventilation. (525)

5. Coughing or vomiting can increase IOP by 40 mm Hg or more. (525)

6. During general anesthesia hyperventilation and hypothermia decrease IOP. (525)

7. There is controversy surrounding the effect of ketamine on IOP. Although ketamine may not increase IOP, it can induce a rotatory nystagmus, cycloplegia, and blepharospasm (tight squeezing of the eyelids), making it less than ideal for use in ophthalmic surgical procedures. Additionally, it is proemetic and increases secretions. (525)

8. Succinylcholine can produce an increase in IOP of about 9 mm Hg in 1 to 4 minutes after intravenous administration. This effect can last up to 7 minutes. (525)

9. Increases in IOP secondary to the administration of succinylcholine are due to a number of mechanisms including tonic contraction of the extraocular muscles, relaxation of the orbital smooth muscle, choroidal vascular dilation, and cycloplegia, which impedes aqueous outflow. (525)

10. Pretreatment with a small dose of nondepolarizing neuromuscular blocker, lidocaine, β-blocker, or acetazolamide may attenuate increases in IOP associated with use of succinylcholine for direct laryngoscopy and endotracheal intubation. (525)

11. Nondepolarizing neuromuscular blocking drugs decrease IOP by relaxing the extraocular muscles. (525)

12. Both inhaled and most intravenous anesthetics produce dose-related reductions in IOP. This is probably due to multiple mechanisms including central nervous system depression, decreased production of aqueous humor, enhanced outflow of aqueous humor, and relaxation of the extraocular muscles. The effect of ketamine on IOP is controversial. (525)

13. Arterial hypertension can transiently increase IOP but has minimal influence on IOP. Venous drainage is the key factor affecting IOP. (525)

OPHTHALMIC MEDICATIONS

14. Topical ophthalmic agents can be absorbed systemically via the conjunctiva or drain down the nasolacrimal duct and be absorbed through the nasal mucosa. These agents include acetylcholine, anticholinesterases, cyclopentolate, epinephrine, phenylephrine, and timolol. (525)

15. Topical ophthalmic β-adrenergic blocking medications may produce atropine-resistant bradycardia and bronchospasm and can exacerbate congestive heart failure. (525)

16. Phospholine iodide (echothiophate) is a miosis-inducing anticholinesterase that profoundly interferes with metabolism of succinylcholine. Patients with low levels of plasma cholinesterase are especially at risk for prolonged paralysis. (525)

17. Phenylephrine drops are available in concentrations of 2.5% and 10%, and are administered to cause mydriasis (pupil dilation). Systemic absorption via the nasolacrimal duct of 10% phenylephrine can induce transient malignant hypertension. (525)

18. The topical ophthalmic administration of acetazolamide inhibits the production of aqueous humor. Its systemic effects include diuresis and hypokalemic metabolic acidosis. (525–526)

OCULOCARDIAC REFLEX

19. The oculocardiac reflex is a vagal-mediated response that manifests with an abrupt, profound decrease in heart rate. It occurs in response to extraocular muscle traction or external pressure on the globe. The reported incidence varies widely from 15% to 80%. (526)

20. The oculocardiac reflex is most often encountered during strabismus surgery. However, it can arise during any type of ophthalmic surgery as well as some otolaryngology procedures. A regional anesthetic ophthalmic block can ablate it. Paradoxically, it may be triggered during the administration of this block. (526)

21. The oculocardiac reflex can manifest as a variety of dysrhythmias including junctional or sinus bradycardia, atrioventricular block, ventricular bigeminy, multifocal premature ventricular contractions, ventricular tachycardia, and asystole. (526)

22. Hypercarbia, hypoxemia, and light planes of general anesthesia all augment the incidence and severity of the oculocardiac reflex. (526)

23. Prompt removal of the surgical stimulus causing the oculocardiac reflex often results in rapid recovery. At the first sign of any dysrhythmia, surgery must stop, and all pressure on the eye or traction on extraocular muscles must be discontinued. Other measures that can be taken include the administration of a parasympatholytic such as atropine or glycopyrrolate. Increasing the depth of general anesthesia (provided that the patient is hemodynamically stable) should be considered. Alternatively, infiltration of local anesthetic attenuates recurrence of the reflex. (526)

24. The prophylactic use of an anticholinergic is not 100% effective in preventing the oculocardiac reflex. Side effects that may result from the use of an anticholinergic include persistent tachycardia. This may have serious consequences in geriatric patients and those with a history of heart disease. (526)

PREOPERATIVE ASSESSMENT

25. Ophthalmic surgery patients are often at the extremes of age, ranging from premature newborns to nonagenarians. Age-specific considerations such as altered pharmacokinetics and pharmacodynamics apply. The elderly, syndromic pediatric patients, and premature infants commonly have comorbid conditions that carry important anesthesia implications. (526)

26. The cessation of antiplatelet or anticoagulant drugs prior to ophthalmic surgery is controversial. One must weigh the risks of intraocular bleeding versus the risks of perioperative stroke, myocardial ischemia, or deep venous thrombosis. (526)

27. An important component of the preoperative assessment of patients scheduled to undergo ophthalmic surgery is to gauge the likelihood of patient movement during surgery. An inability to remain supine and relatively still during eye surgery under monitored anesthesia care may result in eye injury with devastating long-term visual consequences. (527)

ANESTHETIC OPTIONS

28. The anesthetic options for ophthalmic procedures include general anesthesia, retrobulbar (intraconal) block, peribulbar (extraconal) anesthesia, sub-Tenon block, and topical analgesia. (527)

29. The extraocular muscle cone separates the intraconal from the extraconal space and determines whether the local anesthetic administered in an ophthalmic block is delivered as a retrobulbar or peribulbar block. (527)

30. A retrobulbar (intraconal) block is accomplished by inserting a steeply angled needle into the muscle cone such that the tip of the needle is behind (retro) the globe (bulbar). Injection of a small volume of local anesthetic into this compartment will produce rapid-onset akinesia and analgesia. (527)

31. The boundary separating the intraconal from extraconal space is porous. Local anesthetics injected outside the muscle cone diffuse inward, resulting in anesthesia of the eye. An extraconal block is achieved by directing a needle with minimal angulation to a shallow depth, such that the tip remains outside the muscle cone. Because in an extraconal block local anesthetics are injected farther from the nerves than in an intraconal block, larger volumes and more time are necessary to allow for diffusion of the local anesthetic to achieve the block. It is also considered to be a theoretically safer block because the needle is not directed at the apex of the orbit. (527)

32. Complications of needle-based ophthalmic regional anesthesia include superficial or retrobulbar hemorrhage, elicitation of the oculocardiac reflex, intraocular injection of local anesthetic, penetration or puncture of the globe, optic nerve trauma, intravenous injection of local anesthetic solution and resultant seizures, central retinal artery occlusion, brainstem anesthesia, and blindness. (527)

33. The differential diagnosis of alterations in a patient's physiologic status following a needle-based ophthalmic anesthetic block include excessive sedation, brainstem anesthesia, and intravascular injection of local anesthetic. Intravenous sedation is the most common cause of altered physiologic status (blood pressure, heart rate, rhythm, ventilation) after a needle-based ophthalmic block. Brainstem anesthesia has a gradual onset and may persist for 10 to 40 minutes, or longer. The intravascular injection of local anesthetic is characterized by an abrupt onset of seizure activity that is of a brief, limited duration. (527)

34. Clinical signs of brainstem anesthesia following an ophthalmic anesthetic block include altered consciousness proceeding to apnea, cardiac instability, and dilation of the contralateral pupil. Brainstem anesthesia usually manifests within 6 to 10 minutes following the block. Seizure activity is typically *not* a feature of brainstem anesthesia. (527)

35. The features of excessive sedation after an ophthalmic anesthetic block may mimic those of brainstem anesthesia. The key difference is that excessive sedation with opiates may induce miosis of the contralateral pupil. Brainstem anesthesia often results in a mydriatic, nonreactive pupil and akinesia of that globe. (528)

36. A sub-Tenon block is performed using a blunt cannula inserted into the space between the globe's sclera and surrounding the Tenon capsule. Local anesthetic injected into this space blocks the optic and ciliary nerves as they penetrate the capsule. (528)

ANESTHETIC MANAGEMENT OF SPECIFIC OPHTHALMIC PROCEDURES

37. Diabetics and patients with severe myopia are at particular risk for retinal detachment. (528)

38. Retinal surgery is often prolonged and associated with greater manipulation of the eye. Patients may require deeper planes of general anesthesia or a dense regional block. One surgical technique involves the intravitreal injection of a perfluorocarbon gas, such as sulfur hexafluoride. This technique limits the use of nitrous oxide for anesthesia. (528)

39. When the surgical technique for repair of a retinal detachment involves the injection of intravitreal perfluorocarbon gas, nitrous oxide should be discontinued 20 minutes prior to gas injection or avoided altogether. Perfluorocarbons are relatively insoluble gases that are surgically instilled in order to tamponade the retina; these may take up to 28 days to resorb. Nitrous oxide is 100 times more diffusible than sulfur hexafluoride and, therefore, can expand the size of a gas bubble. This will raise IOP and may result in retinal ischemia with permanent loss of vision. (528)

40. Glaucoma is a condition characterized by raised IOP, optic nerve injury, and gradual loss of vision. It is thought that a sustained increase in IOP results in diminished perfusion of the optic nerve. Variants include closed angle (acute) glaucoma and open angle (chronic) glaucoma. (528)

41. The key anesthetic goals in the management of glaucoma patients include avoiding mydriasis (by ensuring miotic drops are continued), understanding the interactions between glaucoma medications and anesthetic agents, and preventing increases in IOP associated with the induction, maintenance, and emergence from anesthesia. Of note, the intravenous administration of atropine does not result in mydriasis and should be used if indicated during anesthesia. (528-529)

42. The anesthetic considerations for children undergoing strabismus surgery include an awareness of the high incidence of intraoperative oculocardiac reflex, an increased risk for malignant hyperthermia, and the high incidence of postoperative nausea and vomiting (PONV). Strabismus is a neuromuscular disorder that can be associated with other myopathies. The frequency of masseter muscle spasm after succinylcholine is fourfold greater than baseline. (529)

43. The most common reason for pediatric inpatient admission following strabismus surgery is PONV. (529)

44. The anesthetic management of patients with traumatic eye injuries must balance the specific risks of increasing IOP and exacerbating the ocular insult versus anesthetizing a nonfasted patient at risk for aspiration upon the induction of general anesthesia. Increasing IOP via a tightly applied face mask, laryngoscopy and intubation, or from coughing or bucking may result in extrusion of globe contents and jeopardize the ultimate visual outcome. A rapid sequence induction is indicated for the nonfasted patient. (529)

45. Awake endotracheal intubation may be appropriate in patients with difficult airways. However, in the setting of an open globe increases in IOP can lead to adverse visual outcomes. The risks associated with rises in IOP produced by an awake intubation must be weighed against the inherent dangers of the difficult airway. (529)

46. It is important to avoid maneuvers that increase IOP in patients with a traumatic eye injury. The patient should be positioned in a slight reverse Trendelenburg tilt. If no airway problems are anticipated, consider the rapid sequence induction of anesthesia with a large dose of nondepolarizing neuromuscular blocking agent. If succinylcholine is selected, the systemic hypertension and rise in IOP that follow its administration can be attenuated by the preinduction administration of intravenous medications such as lidocaine and opioids. Also, pretreatment with a small dose of a nondepolarizing neuromuscular blocking agent is useful. (529)

47. Regional anesthesia for patients with traumatic eye injuries may be an option for select injuries and in patients at higher risk for general anesthesia. (530)

POSTOPERATIVE OPHTHALMIC ISSUES

48. The most common ocular complication following general anesthesia for nonophthalmic surgery is corneal abrasion. It is important to remember a painful eye may also be a manifestation of acute glaucoma. (530)

49. Mechanical damage to the cornea can occur during the induction of anesthesia. It can be caused by dangling eye tags, anesthesia masks, drapes, or other objects that come in contact with the open eye. Abrasions can also occur secondary to the loss of the blink reflex with subsequent drying from exposure to the atmosphere and diminished tear production. (530)

50. The clinical signs of a corneal abrasion include conjunctivitis, tearing, and foreign body sensation. (530)

51. Preventive measures to reduce the risk of a corneal abrasion include gently taping the eyelid shut during mask ventilation, intubation, and intraoperatively. Ointments may cause an allergic reaction or blur postemergence vision. Protective goggles may be beneficial. (530)

52. Acute glaucoma is painful, with the presence of a mydriatic pupil. Intravenous mannitol or acetazolamide can decrease IOP and relieve pain. Acute glaucoma calls for urgent consultation with an ophthalmologist. (530)

53. The risk of postoperative visual loss is higher in prolonged spine surgery in the prone position and in cardiac surgery. (530)

54. Early consultation with an ophthalmologist is essential when a patient complains of postoperative visual loss. Funduscopic and visual field examinations may aid in diagnosis. (530)

55. Patients undergoing major cardiac, spine, or head/neck surgery are at risk of experiencing postoperative visual loss. This rare complication should be discussed as a component of the preoperative consent. (530)

OTOLARYNGOLOGY

SPECIAL CONSIDER-ATIONS FOR HEAD AND NECK SURGERY

56. There are multiple airway considerations specific to ENT surgery. Because ENT surgery takes place around the head, the airway becomes relatively inaccessible to the anesthesia provider, termed *field avoidance*. Furthermore, there is a real possibility of encountering a difficult airway because of anatomic factors, surgical issues, or underlying pathologic problems. Attention should be directed to establishing and securing the airway, preferably with an endotracheal tube (ETT). During patient positioning and head movement the endotracheal tube position may advance or dislodge, become occluded, or disconnect from the anesthesia circuit. Also, the airway may become compromised in the perioperative period by undetected bleeding, edema, or surgical manipulation. (530)

57. Posterior pharyngeal packs placed during ENT surgery minimize the risk of aspiration by sealing the larynx from blood that reaches the pharynx. It is vital to alert operating room personnel of their placement and to confirm their removal prior to extubation. (530)

58. Supplemental airway devices that may be needed for a difficult airway during ENT surgery include the videolaryngoscope or fiberoptic bronchoscope. A tracheostomy kit may be necessary for the gravely compromised airway. Ancillary equipment should be readied prior to the commencement of anesthesia. (530)

59. Laryngospasm is an abrupt, intense, and often prolonged closure of the larynx that leads to compromises in ventilation and oxygenation. The ensuing hypercarbia, hypoxia, and acidosis elicit an autonomic sympathetic response producing hypertension and tachycardia. The reflex is mediated through vagal stimulation of the superior laryngeal nerve, which temporally lessens and eventually causes relaxation of the vocal cords. Laryngospasm may be precipitated by instrumentation of the endolarynx, blood or secretions on the vocal cords, and surgical manipulation at inadequate depths of anesthesia. (530)

60. Prompt recognition and intervention are key to the treatment of laryngospasm. Treatment modalities include the administration of 100% oxygen via positive-pressure face mask ventilation, placement of oral or nasal airways, and deepening of anesthesia with intravenous or inhalational agents. In refractory cases, a small dose of succinylcholine may be required. (530)

61. In neonates, infants, and small children even brief laryngospasm is perilous. In this group oxygen saturation drops rapidly because of a small functional residual capacity and relatively high cardiac output. (531)

62. The child with an upper respiratory infection (URI) undergoing ENT surgery is at increased risk of airway issues, notably breath-holding, oxygen desaturation, and postoperative croup. However, not all children with a URI need their ENT surgery postponed. An assessment of the benefits of surgery versus the risk of airway compromise should be made. For example, the performance of a myringotomy with placement of ventilation tubes requires minimal airway manipulation and has a decreased risk of airway hyperreactivity. (531)

63. Massive epistaxis is often associated with ongoing hemorrhage and concealed swallowing of blood. These patients are at high risk for regurgitation and aspiration. Clinically, they are anxious, are hypovolemic, and may have hemodynamic instability. The preoperative placement of a large-bore peripheral intravenous cannula and adequate rehydration are vital. Hypotension and continued hemorrhage should be anticipated intraoperatively. (531)

64. Obstructive sleep apnea (OSA) is characterized by upper airway obstruction and disordered breathing patterns during sleep. Symptoms include snoring, early morning headache, sleep disturbances, daytime somnolence, and personality changes. In children there may be behavioral and growth disturbances as well as poor school performance. The STOP-BANG questionnaire is a tool used to screen patients for OSA. STOP-BANG is an acronym for the questions (Snoring, Tired, Observed, Pressure, BMI, Age, Neck circumference, and Gender). (531)

65. The airway examination of a patient with OSA may reveal a combination of limited mouth opening and a large tongue. This may make visualization of the pharynx difficult. Patients with OSA are often obese, and in adult men the neck circumference is large, often exceeding 17 inches. (531)

66. One must anticipate difficult airway management in the patient with OSA. Mask ventilation, laryngoscopy, and intubation are often challenging. Intraoperative hypertension is common. OSA patients are exquisitely sensitive to the effects of hypnotics and narcotics and may require prolonged recovery room monitoring. Postoperatively the patients may also need to be monitored with continuous pulse oximetry depending on the surgical procedure and need for postoperative systemic narcotics. (531)

67. Three key elements will produce an airway fire:
    a. A heat or source of ignition (laser or electrosurgical unit)
    b. Fuel (paper drapes, gauze swabs)
    c. Oxidizer (O_2, air, N_2O) (531)

68. During monitored anesthesia care the danger of an airway fire exists because heat and fuel elements are still present, particularly in procedures involving the face and neck while administering supplemental oxygen. It is important to drape properly, remove the source of oxidation, and discontinue delivery of supplemental oxygen during electrocautery. (531)

69. In the event of a fire in the operating room, rescue persons in immediate danger, sound the fire alarm, confine the fire by closing doors, and extinguish the flames with the appropriate agent. (531)

ANESTHETIC MANAGEMENT OF SPECIFIC OTOLARYNGOLOGIC PROCEDURES

70. There are many anesthetic considerations for ear surgery. N_2O increases middle ear pressure and causes serous otitis. Facial nerve monitoring may be required, necessitating the avoidance of intraoperative neuromuscular blockade. Epinephrine injection may precipitate acute hypertension and tachyarrhythmia. Smooth emergence is preferable to avoid coughing, bucking, and acute hypertension. PONV occurs with an increased incidence in these procedures, making prophylactic antiemetic measures helpful. (531)

71. Nitrous oxide is more soluble than nitrogen in blood and diffuses into air-filled cavities. The increases in middle ear pressure may disrupt tympanoplasty grafts. Also, the acute discontinuation of N_2O may produce serous otitis. Nitrous oxide, if used at all, should be administered in moderate concentrations (<50%) and discontinued at least 20 to 30 minutes prior to graft application. (531)

72. The surgeon frequently uses a facial nerve monitor to prevent trauma to or accidental incision of the facial nerve and its branches. The use of neuromuscular blocking drugs should be curtailed in order to prevent attenuation of the monitor's twitch response. Succinylcholine or a single small dose of an intermediate-acting nondepolarizing neuromuscular blocking agent is preferred. Absence of full paralysis should be confirmed with a neuromuscular monitor prior to surgical dissection. (531)

73. Epinephrine is injected during ear microsurgery to decrease bleeding and improve visualization within the surgical field. Systemic uptake may precipitate hypertension, tachycardia, and dysrhythmias. (531)

74. Epinephrine concentrations should be limited to 1:200,000 in ear microsurgery. (531)

75. Maneuvers to minimize bleeding in the surgical field during otolaryngology surgery include use of topical or injected epinephrine, moderate reverse Trendelenburg (head-up) positioning, and volatile anesthetics to decrease arterial blood pressure (within an acceptable range). The use of potent vasoactive drugs and controlled hypotension is controversial. (531)

76. The smooth emergence from general anesthesia after middle ear surgery minimizes the risk of graft disruption or acute hemorrhage. Episodic coughing and bucking will produce hypertension that may result in poor surgical outcome. In the uncomplicated airway, extubation of the trachea at a deep plane of anesthesia with spontaneous respiration may be beneficial. (532)

77. PONV is common after middle ear surgery because of manipulation of the vestibular apparatus. Factors that contribute to PONV include anesthesia technique (use of nitrous oxide and narcotics), inadequate hydration, and postoperative movement. (532)

78. The number of agents used to prevent PONV after ear surgery is guided by a relative risk analysis. Prophylactic agents include corticosteroids, 5-HT$_3$-receptor antagonists, neurokinin-1 receptor antagonists, scopolamine patches, and low-dose propofol. Gastric decompression is useful if blood has been swallowed. Scopolamine crosses the blood-brain barrier and may cause confusion, particularly in the elderly. Avoidance of nitrous oxide and narcotics, as well as maintaining adequate hydration, may also be useful to prevent PONV. (532)

79. Perioperative issues seen in patients undergoing tonsillectomy and adenoidectomy include airway obstruction, bleeding, cardiac arrhythmias, and croup (postextubation airway edema). Upper airway obstruction in children may only manifest during sleep. The routine use of premedication prior to tonsillectomy is probably best avoided in patients with OSA, obesity, intermittent airway obstruction, or significant tonsil hypertrophy. Airway obstruction is accelerated by the loss of pharyngeal tone associated with the induction of anesthesia, and manipulation of the airway during light planes of anesthesia may result in acute airway obstruction. Limiting the air leak to 20 cm H$_2$O peak airway pressure as well as intravenous dexamethasone may minimize postoperative edema. (532)

80. Negative-pressure pulmonary edema manifests clinically when the patient inhales forcefully against a closed glottis, as with airway obstruction. This effort generates marked negative intrathoracic pressures that are transmitted to the pulmonary interstitial tissue and promotes fluid transition from the pulmonary circulation into the alveoli. (533)

81. Blood loss during tonsillectomy and adenoidectomy is either overt (into the suction bottle) or covert (swallowed). Blood loss is underestimated because the covert loss is not seen. (533)

82. Considerations for the anesthetic management of post-tonsillectomy bleed include the possibility of undetected and prolonged hemorrhage, concomitant hypovolemia, and regurgitation of blood swallowed into the stomach. Measures required include rehydration, rapid sequence induction of general anesthesia, protection of the airway with a cuffed ETT (minimize risk of aspiration), and drainage of gastric contents. (533)

83. Acute epiglottitis is an infectious disease caused by *Haemophilus influenzae* type b. It most often affects children between the ages of 2 and 7. (533)

84. Clinically, the patient with acute epiglottitis presents with sudden onset of fever and dysphagia. Symptoms progress rapidly and the child may transition from an acute pharyngitis to complete airway obstruction and respiratory failure within a few hours. The clinical picture is of an agitated, drooling child leaning forward and holding the head in an extended position. The

child becomes exhausted from the work of breathing against an almost fully occluded airway. (533)

85. Acute epiglottitis is an airway emergency. Direct visualization of the glottis should not be attempted until in the operating room fully prepared to manage the airway because stimulation and struggling may produce acute airway obstruction. Emergency airway equipment should be readied. A surgeon adept at rigid bronchoscopy and tracheostomy should be present at the bedside. An inhaled induction of anesthesia maintaining spontaneous respiration is preferred. The degree of airway narrowing is unpredictable, so a range of ETT sizes should be available. Atropine may dry secretions and prevent bradycardia. (533)

86. Clinical features of the tracheal aspiration of a foreign body include sudden dyspnea, dry cough, hoarseness, and wheezing. Foreign body aspiration is an airway emergency. (533)

87. A preoperative plan and mutual intraoperative cooperation between the anesthesia provider and surgeon caring for the patient with foreign body airway aspiration are vital in order to avoid inadvertent distal displacement of the foreign body. Removal of the foreign body can be accomplished by either direct laryngoscopy or rigid bronchoscopy without the application of positive airway pressure. The surgeon should be prepared for an emergency cricothyrotomy or tracheostomy in the event of acute airway occlusion. Total intravenous anesthesia with maintenance of spontaneous ventilation can eliminate operating room pollution. (533)

88. After the removal of a foreign body from the airway, postoperatively the patient should receive humidified oxygen and remain under close observation for development of airway edema. (533)

89. Cocaine is used for nasal surgery because it is an effective topical anesthetic agent. Because it is also a potent vasoconstrictor, it reduces bleeding in the surgical field and shrinks the nasal mucosa. (533)

90. The disadvantages of using cocaine for nasal surgery include altered sensorium (euphoria and dysphoria) and untoward cardiac arrhythmias. For these reasons, cocaine can be substituted by a "pseudococaine" solution containing a local anesthetic and a vasoconstrictor. (533)

91. Prior to the emergence from general anesthesia after nasal and sinus surgery the removal of posterior pharyngeal packs should be confirmed. Protective airway reflexes should be present prior to extubation because of possible airway edema and ongoing bleeding. (533)

92. Endoscopic surgery includes bronchoscopy, laryngoscopy, and microlaryngoscopy, which all involve direct manipulation of the airway. In these procedures, the airway should be assessed, carefully paying special attention to the presence of stridor (indicator of compromise). Preoperative investigations such as blood gas analysis, flow-volume loops, radiographic studies, and magnetic resonance imaging may be useful. (533)

93. A variety of techniques can be employed to provide oxygenation and ventilation during airway endoscopy. The trachea may be intubated with a small-diameter pediatric ETT, but this may impair visualization of the posterior commissure. An alternative technique, jet ventilation, utilizes high-flow oxygen insufflation through a small-gauge catheter placed in the trachea. (534)

94. The use of the manual high-pressure jet ventilator carries risks of pneumothorax and pneumomediastinum. (534)

95. Laser is an acronym for *light amplification by stimulated emission of radiation*. It produces an intense focused light beam that allows for precise and controlled coagulation, incision, and vaporization of tissues. Advantages of laser surgery include its ability to target lesions, provide hemostasis, produce minimal edema, and promote rapid healing. (534)

96. Hazards associated with laser surgery include atmospheric contamination by fine particles of vaporized tissues, misdirected laser energy, venous gas embolism, and ocular (retina) injury. There is also risk of ETT fire during airway surgery. (534)

97. During laser surgery an efficient smoke evacuator, as well as special masks, is necessary because small, vaporized particles are easily inhaled. (534)

98. During laser surgery certain preoperative and intraoperative measures should be taken to minimize the risk of ETT fire. Preoperatively, one must arrange surgical drapes to avoid accumulation of combustible gases, use an appropriate laser-resistant ETT, and moisten gauze and sponges in the vicinity of the laser. Intraoperatively one must alert the surgeon and operating room personnel to risk, assign specific roles to each operating room member in case of fire, reduce inspired O_2 to minimal values, replace N_2O with air, and wait a few minutes after changes in gas concentration before activating the laser. (534)

99. The purpose of filling the ETT cuff with saline or an indicator dye during laser surgery is to help dissipate laser heat. Furthermore, leaking dye is an indicator of cuff rupture. (534)

100. Radical neck dissection is indicated for removal of a malignancy. These patients frequently have a history of tobacco and alcohol abuse. An extensive preoperative workup is necessary because pulmonary and cardiac disease is prevalent. (534)

101. A history of prior radiation therapy to the larynx, pharynx, or oral cavity may produce marked tissue indurations, scarring, and limitation of mobility. These may cause difficulties with airway management, particularly endotracheal intubation. (534)

102. During radical neck dissection traction or pressure on the carotid sinus may provoke acute arrhythmias. These include prolongation of the QT interval, bradydysrhythmias, and asystole. Treatment includes early detection, cessation of the surgical stimulus, and administration of an anticholinergic agent. Another option is local anesthetic infiltration of the carotid sinus. (534)

103. Injuries to the facial nerve, recurrent laryngeal nerve, and phrenic nerve may all be encountered postoperatively after head and neck surgery. Injury to the facial nerve results in the inability to symmetrically grimace. Injury to the recurrent laryngeal nerve can cause vocal cord dysfunction and, if bilateral, results in airway obstruction after extubation. Injury to the phrenic nerve can result in paralysis to the ipsilateral diaphragm. (534)

104. After neck surgery hematoma formation in the neck may compress the airway and lead to acute obstruction and a surgical emergency. If tracheotomy is not performed during the initial surgery, then the patient requires close monitoring (for laryngeal or upper airway obstruction) in the postoperative phase. Complete airway obstruction from postoperative hematoma formation should be promptly treated by incision and opening of the wound to release the accumulated hematoma. (534)

105. Hypocalcemia after thyroid or parathyroid surgery may present in many forms. Clinical signs may include tetany (carpal spasm), peripheral and circumoral paresthesia, QT interval prolongation, and laryngospasm. (535)

106. Thyroid storm is the excessive release of thyroid hormone in a patient who has inadequately controlled hyperthyroidism. This may occur in the intraoperative or postoperative period following thyroid surgery. Clinical manifestations include tachycardia, hypertension, and diaphoresis. (535)

107. The inability to perform a symmetric grimace after parotid surgery is indicative of facial nerve injury or traction. Because the parotid gland is traversed by the facial nerve, it is customary to monitor the facial nerve function with a facial nerve monitor. Occasionally, the facial nerve may need to be sacrificed. It is then reconstructed with a graft from the greater auricular nerve. Following parotid surgery, a delayed inability to grimace in the recovery room may be an indication of facial nerve compression that needs timely surgical intervention. The surgeon should be alerted to assess the patient in the recovery room. (535)

108. The Le Fort I classification of maxillary fracture extends across the lower maxilla, the Le Fort II fracture is more cephalad and involves the medial canthal area, and the Le Fort III fracture is a high transverse fracture above the malar bone that extends into the orbit. (535)

32 ORTHOPEDIC SURGERY

Andrew D. Rosenberg and Mitchell H. Marshall

RHEUMATOLOGIC DISORDERS

1. Is rheumatoid arthritis (RA) just a disease of the joints and adjacent connective tissue?
2. What are some of the clinical manifestations of RA?
3. What are some airway abnormalities that can occur in patients with RA?
4. Why might the normal mouth opening be decreased in patients with RA?
5. What occurs to the developing mandible in patients with juvenile RA that makes it more difficult to intubate the trachea in this patient population?
6. What are some of the clinical manifestations of cricoarytenoid arthritis?
7. Can neck movement in patients with RA result in cervical spine injury? What is the clinical implication of this?
8. What percent of patients with RA have involvement of their cervical spine?
9. What are three abnormal movements of the cervical spine that may be manifest in patients with RA?
10. What is atlantoaxial subluxation?
11. What pathologic change in RA patients can lead to atlantoaxial subluxation?
12. How is the degree of atlantoaxial subluxation measured? What is this measurement called?
13. What test can be used to determine the atlas-dens interval?
14. What degree of motion between the atlas and dens, or at what atlas-dens interval, is the patient considered to be at risk for spinal cord injury?
15. In the case of pure transverse axial ligament disruption, does flexion or extension increase the atlas-dens interval?
16. If a patient is asymptomatic with neck flexion and extension preoperatively, can the anesthesiologist be reassured of an atlas-dens interval of less than 4 mm?
17. What is subaxial subluxation? What is its clinical significance?
18. What is superior migration of the odontoid? What are the potential clinical manifestations?
19. What is the surgical treatment for superior migration of the odontoid?
20. What effect does RA have on the trachea?
21. What are the pathologic features of ankylosing spondylitis?
22. What is the hallmark neck position in patients with ankylosing spondylitis?
23. Ankylosing spondylitis is associated with which HLA type?
24. What are some considerations for the anesthetic management of patients with ankylosing spondylitis?

SPINE SURGERY

25. What are some considerations for the anesthetic management of patients undergoing spine surgery?
26. What are the various surgical approaches to spine surgery? What are the clinical implications of them?

27. What kinds of endotracheal tubes can be employed to provide one-lung ventilation for thoracic spine surgery?
28. What is an advantage of a bronchial blocker to provide one-lung ventilation for thoracic spine surgery?
29. What newer technique do surgeons employ during thoracoscopic spine surgery to move the lung from the operative field that does not require one-lung ventilation?
30. Why is intraoperative awareness a possible complication of spine surgery?
31. Is it mandatory to employ a monitor for intraoperative awareness in patients undergoing spine surgery?
32. Name some methods to help decrease blood loss in patients undergoing spine surgery.
33. What pharmacologic methods exist to diminish blood loss in patients undergoing spine surgery? Why is aprotinin not used?
34. What are some considerations for patients placed in the prone position?
35. Why is spinal cord integrity monitored during spine surgery?
36. What are various methods used to monitor the spinal cord during spine surgery?
37. What are somatosensory evoked potentials (SSEPs)? What part of the spinal cord do they monitor?
38. What changes in latency and amplitude are considered abnormal when monitoring SSEPs during spine surgery?
39. What anesthetic technique should be employed in patients being monitored with somatosensory or motor evoked potentials?
40. What are some surgically related conditions that can interfere with spinal cord monitoring waveform acquisition?
41. Why are some areas of the spinal cord more prone to ischemia?
42. What are some factors that can affect intraoperative spinal cord monitoring waveform acquisition?
43. During spine surgery, what is the time course in which changes in the SSEP waveforms manifest after the loss of spinal cord integrity?
44. What is the appropriate management of a patient during spine surgery once significant changes are noted in the spinal cord monitoring waveforms?
45. What area of the spinal cord is monitored by transcranial motor evoked potentials?
46. How does paralysis with neuromuscular blocking drugs affect transcranial motor evoked potentials?
47. Why might masseter muscle contraction occur during transcranial motor evoked potential monitoring? What is the clinical implication of this?
48. What special precautions should be taken for patients undergoing transcranial motor evoked potential monitoring during spine surgery?
49. How are intraoperative electromyelograms used to determine if a pedicle screw has been placed too close to a nerve root?
50. Can neuromuscular blockade be in effect when electromyelograms are being obtained?
51. What is the role of the intraoperative wake-up test?
52. How is an intraoperative wake-up test performed?
53. Name potential complications of the intraoperative wake-up test.
54. What considerations are important at the conclusion of a spine procedure?
55. How can postoperative pain be managed in the patient after spine surgery?
56. What are some oral medications that may be useful for pain management in the preoperative and postoperative period for patients undergoing spine surgery?
57. What are some intravenous medicines that may be useful for pain management in the postoperative period for patients undergoing spine surgery?
58. For what types of spine surgeries should the use of nonsteroidal anti-inflammatory drugs be avoided?

59. Which patients are at the greatest risk of postoperative visual loss after spine surgery? What are some other possible factors that contribute to postoperative visual loss?

60. What are the two most common types of injuries that result in postoperative visual loss in patients undergoing spine surgery?

61. What are the determinants of the ocular perfusion pressure? What is the clinical implication of this?

62. What are some aspects associated with the prone position that may contribute to postoperative visual loss?

63. According to a recently published study comparing patients who had postoperative visual loss to matched control subjects, what are the risk factors for visual loss due to ischemic optic neuropathy?

64. What are some potential causes of postoperative visual loss due to central retina artery occlusion?

65. According to the American Society of Anesthesiologists (ASA) practice advisory regarding patients at high risk for postoperative visual loss during spine surgery, is the use of deliberate hypotension associated with postoperative visual loss?

66. According to the ASA practice advisory regarding patients at high risk for postoperative visual loss during spine surgery, what type of fluid should be administered with crystalloid in these cases?

67. According to the ASA practice advisory regarding patients at high risk for postoperative visual loss during spine surgery, is there a defined transfusion trigger at which the risk of postoperative visual loss is eliminated?

68. According to the ASA practice advisory regarding patients at high risk for postoperative visual loss during spine surgery, how should the patient's head and the operating room table be positioned when the patient is prone?

SURGERY IN THE SITTING POSITION

69. What neurologic postoperative complications have been noted in patients who undergo surgery in the sitting position?

70. When devastating neurologic postoperative complications occur after surgery in the sitting position, what is the implicated cause?

71. Is the systemic arterial blood pressure at the level of the heart the same as that at the level of the circle of Willis when patients are anesthetized and placed in the sitting position?

72. What calculation more accurately determines the arterial blood pressure at the level of the circle of Willis when patients are anesthetized and placed in the sitting position?

73. What superficial landmark correlates with the circle of Willis?

74. What is the potential risk of hypotension in patients who are anesthetized and placed in the sitting position?

FRACTURED HIP

75. Name several factors that predispose a person to a hip fracture.

76. What is the mortality rate associated with a hip fracture?

77. How do comorbid conditions in the patient with a fractured hip affect the postoperative outcome?

78. Does it make sense to delay surgery in a patient with a fractured hip and a significant comorbid condition in order to improve the patient's medical status prior to surgery?

79. When should patients with a recent myocardial infarction and a fractured hip be scheduled for surgery?

80. What are some considerations for the anesthetic management of patients undergoing hip surgery?

81. Does choice of anesthetic technique—regional or general anesthesia—play a role in the outcome of patients who have fractured a hip?

82. Based on a retrospective study involving over 18,000 hip fracture patients, what type of hip fracture may benefit from regional anesthesia?

83. What are some advantages of regional anesthesia for patients undergoing repair of a hip fracture?

84. What are some advantages of general anesthesia for patients undergoing repair of a hip fracture?

85. What are some peripheral nerve blocks that may be useful in patients undergoing repair of a hip fracture?

86. How are the elderly affected by the use of narcotics in the perioperative period?

TOTAL JOINT REPLACEMENT

87. What are some anesthetic considerations for patients undergoing total joint replacement?

88. What are some considerations regarding positioning of patients undergoing total joint replacement?

89. Use of methylmethacrylate cement is associated with what side effects?

90. What is the cause of the systemic reaction to methylmethacrylate cement?

91. Which patients are at high risk for a systemic reaction to methylmethacrylate cement?

92. What is an appropriate tourniquet inflation pressure for lower extremity surgery?

93. What is the upper limit of tourniquet time before it should be deflated?

94. If tourniquet time exceeds 2 hours and the procedure is not completed, then the tourniquet should be deflated for how long before it is reinflated and why?

95. What are some physiologic signs noted by the anesthesiologist with increasing duration of the tourniquet on an ischemic limb?

96. What are some physiologic signs noted by the anesthesiologist with release of the tourniquet on an ischemic limb?

97. What are some complications associated with tourniquet use?

98. What can result from kinking of the tourniquet tubing?

99. When does the major amount of blood loss occur during total knee replacement surgery?

100. What are some approaches to postoperative pain management in the patient undergoing total knee replacement?

101. What are some concerns regarding regional anesthesia in patients receiving deep venous thrombosis prophylaxis?

102. What are current recommendations for performing a neuraxial block in patients who received enoxaparin?

103. When can redosing of enoxaparin occur after removal of an epidural catheter?

104. What are current recommendations for removal of an epidural catheter in patients on warfarin?

105. What are current recommendations for performing a neuraxial block in patients taking clopidogrel and ticlopidine?

ANSWERS*

RHEUMATOLOGIC DISORDERS

1. Rheumatoid arthritis (RA) is a chronic inflammatory disease that initially destroys joints and adjacent connective tissue and then progresses to a systemic disease affecting major organ systems. (537)

2. Systemic manifestations of RA are widespread beyond the joints and adjacent connective tissue. They may include pulmonary involvement with interstitial fibrosis and cysts with honeycombing, gastritis and ulcers from aspirin and other analgesics, neuropathy, nephropathy, muscle wasting, vasculitis, and anemia. Ultimately the anatomy of the airway is damaged and altered in patients with RA. (537)

---

*Numbers in parentheses refer to pages, figures, boxes, or tables in Pardo MC, Miller RD, eds. *Basics of Anesthesia.* 7th ed. Philadelphia: Elsevier; 2018.

3. Some airway abnormalities that can occur in patients with RA include decreased mouth opening, a hypoplastic mandible, cricoarytenoid arthritis, and cervical spine abnormalities. (538)

4. Normal mouth opening may be decreased in patients with RA as a result of temporomandibular arthritis. (538)

5. The patient with juvenile RA often has a hypoplastic mandible as a result of early fusion. This results in the noticeable overbite in some patients with RA. (538)

6. As with other joints, the cricoarytenoid joint may be affected by RA. Cricoarytenoid arthritis may result in shortness of breath and snoring. RA patients have been misdiagnosed as having sleep apnea when in fact they have cricoarytenoid arthritis. Patients with cricoarytenoid arthritis may present with stridor on inspiration, and stridor may occur in the postanesthesia care unit (PACU) while the patient is recovering from anesthesia. Acute subluxation of the cricoarytenoid joint as a result of tracheal intubation can cause stridor that is not responsive to racemic epinephrine. (538)

7. Yes, movement of the neck in patients with RA can result in cervical spine injury. The RA patient must be carefully evaluated for both the complexity and the risk of endotracheal intubation. Many cervical spine abnormalities may occur in patients with RA, making visualization of the airway difficult and placing the cervical spinal cord at risk. Normal endotracheal intubation maneuvers with neck movement may result in an increased risk of cervical spine injury because of destruction of the bones and ligaments of the cervical spine. (538)

8. The cervical spine is affected in up to 80% of patients with RA. (538)

9. Three abnormal movements of the cervical spine that may be manifest in patients with RA include atlantoaxial subluxation, subaxial subluxation, and superior migration of the odontoid. (538)

10. Atlantoaxial subluxation is the abnormal movement of the C1 cervical vertebra (the atlas) on C2 (the axis). (538)

11. Normally, the transverse axial ligament holds the odontoid process (also referred to as the *dens*), which is the superior projection of the vertebra of C2, in place directly behind the anterior arch of C1. With destruction of the transverse axial ligament by RA, movement of the odontoid process is no longer restricted. As the neck is flexed and extended, the C1 vertebra can sublux on the C2 vertebra. This can result in impingement of the spinal cord, placing it at risk for damage. (538)

12. Subluxation of C1 on C2, referred to as *atlantoaxial subluxation*, can be quantified by a measuring the distance between the back of the anterior arch of C1 and the front of the dens or odontoid. This distance is referred to as the *atlas-dens interval*. (538)

13. Flexion and extension radiographs of the cervical spine are obtained to determine the distance between the atlas and dens, or the atlas-dens interval, and thus the degree of subluxation. (539)

14. If the atlas-dens interval is 4 mm or more atlantoaxial instability is present, the amount of subluxation is considered significant, and the patient is considered to be at risk for spinal cord injury. (539)

15. In a situation in which the transverse axial ligament is disrupted, extension of the neck minimizes the atlas-dens interval and increases the safe area for the spinal cord. Conversely, flexion of the neck increases the atlas-dens interval and decreases the safe area for the spinal cord, making flexion a more frequent risk position. Still, RA affects more than just the transverse axial ligament; therefore, all neck movements in patients with RA have to be evaluated carefully because extension of the neck can also lead to problems. (539)

16. Patients with RA can be asymptomatic with neck flexion and extension preoperatively while awake and still have an atlas-dens interval of greater than 4 mm and be at risk for cervical spine injury. These patients are able to compensate for their cervical spine instability through local muscle. Once

anesthetized and the muscles are relaxed, atlantoaxial subluxation may occur. Therefore, the anesthesiologist should not be falsely reassured by asymptomatic flexion and extension in the awake patient. (539)

17. Subaxial subluxation is the subluxation of 15% or more of one cervical vertebra on another at any level below C2. Subaxial subluxation most commonly occurs at the C5-C6 level. Patients with subaxial subluxation are at risk for spinal cord impingement with neck movement. Minimal neck movement is recommended in these patients. (539)

18. Superior migration of the odontoid is a condition when an intact odontoid process projects up through the foramen magnum and into the skull. This occurs because of inflammation and bone destruction that results in cervical spine collapse with sparing of the odontoid process. This can occur because not all areas of the cervical spine are equally affected in any given patient. If the odontoid is spared, the intact odontoid can impinge on the brainstem, and patients may suffer neurologic symptoms including quadriparesis or paralysis. (539)

19. Surgical treatment for superior migration of the odontoid involves removal of the odontoid to decompress the spinal cord and brainstem. A complicated surgical procedure, referred to as a *transoral odontoidectomy*, may be performed to accomplish this and involves an incision in the posterior pharyngeal wall, followed by removal of the arch of C1 and then removal of the odontoid and pannus, to relieve neurologic symptoms. With completion of the transoral portion of the procedure, the cervical spine is very unstable, necessitating a posterior spinal fusion. (539)

20. Although the cervical spine is affected by RA and may collapse from bone destruction, the trachea is usually spared. This results in the trachea twisting in a characteristic manner as the cervical spine collapses, only serving to increase the difficulty of intubating the trachea of these patients. Tracheal intubation aids such as a fiberoptic bronchoscope, GlideScope, Airtraq, or intubating laryngeal mask airway (LMA) should be available for assistance in endotracheal intubation of these patients should it be required. (539)

21. Ankylosing spondylitis is a rheumatologic disorder in which the process of repetitive minute bone fractures followed by healing results in the characteristic bamboo spine, disease of the sacroiliac joint, fusion of the posterior elements of the spinal column, and fixed neck flexion that is characteristic of this patient population. (540)

22. The hallmark of patients with ankylosing spondylitis is a fused neck in flexion. (540)

23. There is an association between ankylosing spondylitis and HLA-B27, although not all HLA-B27–positive patients are affected with ankylosing spondylitis. (541)

24. Patients with ankylosing spondylitis typically have a rigid cervical spine and neck fused in flexion, which makes endotracheal intubation difficult. Airway manipulation should be performed only after careful assessment, and an intubation assist device can help secure the airway. Patients with ankylosing spondylitis may also develop thoracic and costochondral involvement, which may result in a rapid shallow breathing pattern. (541)

SPINE SURGERY

25. There are several considerations for the anesthetic management of patients undergoing spine surgery, and much depends on the level of the spine in which the surgery will take place, as well as the surgical approach. Preoperative assessment of the patient for underlying neurologic deficits and chronic pain issues is important. For patients in whom the approach may be thoracic, pulmonary function tests may be indicated. In general, spine surgery can be long and complex, with significant blood loss and hemodynamic alterations. Intravascular access and intraoperative monitoring should be adjusted accordingly, and blood products may need to be ordered. In the event that there will be intraoperative monitoring of the spinal cord with evoked potentials, the anesthesia administered for the surgery may need to be modified so as not to interfere with the acquisition of waveforms. (541)

26. Spine surgery may have anterior, posterior, lateral, and thoracic approaches. In some cases, two approaches may be used during the same surgery. Preoperative discussion with the surgeon is crucial (1) to determine the surgical approach as it may influence the location of intravascular access and monitoring placement, (2) to ensure proper positioning and padding accessories, and (3) because there may be a need to provide lung isolation and one-lung ventilation. A thoracic surgical approach may involve open thoracotomy or thoracoscopic techniques. High thoracic and thoracoscopic procedures frequently require one-lung ventilation to ensure adequate visualization. (541)

27. A double-lumen endotracheal tube or a bronchial blocker can be employed to provide one-lung ventilation for thoracic spine surgery. (541)

28. A double-lumen endotracheal tube or a bronchial blocker can be used with a single-lumen endotracheal tube to provide one-lung ventilation for thoracic spine surgery. An advantage of the bronchial blocker is the avoidance of the need to change the tube between different stages of the procedure or at the end of the operation. With the bronchial blocker, deflating the cuff and withdrawing the catheter back into its casing and recapping the proximal end returns the endotracheal tube to its single-lumen tube characteristics. If extubation of the trachea at the end of the surgical procedure is not indicated, the endotracheal tube does not have to be changed, thereby avoiding the issue of changing an endotracheal tube in the presence of potentially significant airway edema. Make certain that the PACU staff is properly educated as to the various ports of the bronchial blocker. (541)

29. Some surgeons are using carbon dioxide insufflation as the sole means of moving the lung away from the surgical field even in high thoracic spine surgical procedures. This obviates the need for one-lung ventilation and allows for the use of a single-lumen endotracheal tube for the entire procedure. (542)

30. Patients undergoing spine surgery appear to be at an increased risk for intraoperative awareness as a result of the requirement that the anesthetic technique administered to them be modified to allow for obtaining adequate intraoperative neurophysiologic monitoring waveforms to assess spinal cord integrity. Therefore, some advocate the use of brain function monitoring in these patients to help avoid intraoperative awareness. (542)

31. Awareness monitoring is not a standard in anesthesia and, as noted in the Practice Advisory for Intraoperative Awareness and Brain Function Monitoring, a decision should be made on a case-by-case basis by the individual practitioner for selected patients (e.g., light anesthesia). There was a consensus in the advisory that brain function monitoring is not routinely indicated for patients undergoing general anesthesia as the "general applicability of these monitors in the prevention of intraoperative awareness had not been established." In fact, Avidan and associates demonstrated that awareness is not decreased with use of brain function monitoring. (542)

32. Methods to decrease blood loss in spine surgery patients include predonation, hemodilution, wound infusion with a dilute epinephrine solution, hypotensive anesthesia techniques, red blood cell salvage, positioning to diminish venous pressure, careful surgical hemostasis, and the administration of antifibrinolytics. (542)

33. Medications to decrease blood loss during surgery include the antifibrinolytics aprotinin, tranexamic acid, and ε-aminocaproic acid. Aprotinin, a serine protease inhibitor, effectively decreased blood loss in cardiac patients and has been demonstrated to be efficacious in patients undergoing spine surgery as well. The negative side effects of aprotinin in cardiac patients include an increased risk of myocardial infarction (MI) or heart failure by approximately 55%, nearly double the risk of stroke, increased risk of long-term mortality, and a higher death rate in patients receiving aprotinin as demonstrated in a study over a 5-year period comparing aprotinin and lysine analogs in high-risk cardiac surgery. The study was terminated early and resulted in relabeling

and ultimately withdrawing aprotinin from the market so that it is no longer available. The synthetic lysine analogs, tranexamic acid and ε-aminocaproic acid, have also been employed in spine surgery as well as in patients undergoing orthopedic surgery. Tranexamic acid can be administered by an initial bolus injection of 10 mg/kg over 30 minutes followed by a continuous infusion of 1 mg/kg/h, although other regimens may be utilized. (542)

34. Spine surgery is often performed with the patient in the prone position, and careful positioning avoids injury. Movement to the prone position should be performed in a carefully coordinated manner with the surgical team. The neck should not be hyperextended or hyperflexed but placed in the neutral position. The endotracheal tube is positioned so it is not kinked, contact areas are padded, and the face and eyes are protected. Pressure and stretch on nerves are avoided by proper padding and preventing any extension over 90 degrees. The abdomen needs to be hanging free to avoid increased venous pressure and thereby increased venous bleeding. The prone position alters pulmonary dynamics, so pulmonary function must be reassessed in this position. (543)

35. Monitoring spinal cord integrity is an important component of major surgical procedures involving distraction and rotation of the spine such as occurs with major anteroposterior spinal fusions and scoliosis surgery. Spinal cord monitoring is employed to detect, and hopefully reverse in a timely manner, any adverse effects on the spinal cord noted during the operative period. (543)

36. There are a variety of methods to monitor the spinal cord during spine surgery. They include SSEPs, motor evoked potentials, including transcranial motor evoked potentials, electromyograms (EMGs), or a wake-up test. (543)

37. SSEPs are sensory evoked potential waves generated in the extremities by repetitive stimulation that propagate up through the dorsum or sensory portion of the spinal cord and into the brain, where these signals or waveforms are detected via electrodes placed over the scalp. Specific areas on the scalp coincide with the brain's sensory areas for the upper and lower extremities, and proper signal acquisition obtained over these sites indicates an intact sensory or dorsal portion of the spinal cord. The SSEP waveform generated from multiple repetitive stimulations is analyzed for its latency and amplitude. (543)

38. An increase in latency of greater than 10% or a decrease in amplitude of 60% or more, as well as the inability to obtain a proper waveform or signal, may be indicative of spinal cord dysfunction or disruption. (543)

39. If SSEPs alone are being monitored, an inhaled anesthetic, equivalent to a small percentage (<50%) of 1 MAC, can be administered. Volatile anesthetics may interfere with signal acquisition in patients monitored with transcranial motor evoked potentials and may have to be discontinued, if used at all, if adequate signals cannot be obtained. Intravenous anesthetics will need to be administered in these surgical cases. Although neuromuscular blockade may be used to facilitate tracheal intubation, paralysis should not be maintained if transcranial motor evoked potentials are being continuously monitored. If the patient is having pedicle screws placed, then the neuromuscular blockade needs to be terminated before the EMGs are obtained so that testing can be properly performed. A small dose of ketamine can be given in the perioperative period as an additional pain relief modality to provide analgesia for major surgery including spine surgery. (543)

40. Surgically related conditions that can result in interference of waveform acquisition during spinal cord monitoring include direct injury or trauma to the cord or impairment of the blood supply. Distraction, rotation, excessive bleeding, and severing or clamping of arterial blood supply can result in ischemia to the cord and neurologic injury. (543)

41. Some areas of the spinal cord are more vulnerable and therefore more prone to ischemia because their blood supply is dependent on watershed blood flow. (543)

42. Many factors can alter intraoperative spinal cord monitoring waveforms unrelated to surgery. They should be properly detected and eliminated. These factors may include hypotension, hypothermia, high concentrations of volatile anesthetics, benzodiazepines, hypercarbia or hypocarbia, and anemia. Only a small concentration of volatile anesthetic should be employed when SSEP monitoring is used. Midazolam and other benzodiazepines are avoided because they may interfere with obtaining a waveform. Some anesthesiologists even avoid nitrous oxide and use a combination of air in oxygen. (543)

43. Direct injury to the spinal cord results in immediate changes in SSEP waveforms. In contrast, if surgery impairs blood supply and thus renders the spinal cord ischemic, the change in SSEP waveforms may take up to half an hour to manifest. (543)

44. Once a significant change in intraoperative spinal cord monitoring waveforms is noted, specific maneuvers should be used to restore spinal cord blood flow, such as releasing the rotation and distraction of the spine if applicable. Because there may be insufficient blood supply to the spine as a result of spinal cord manipulation, the mean arterial blood pressure should be increased in an effort to restore adequate blood flow to the spine. All variables such as hemoglobin, temperature, arterial carbon dioxide concentration, and arterial blood pressure should be considered. Once these are all evaluated, a wake-up test may be necessary if the waveforms do not improve. (544)

45. Transcranial motor evoked potentials allow for monitoring the patient's spinal cord motor pathways throughout the entire procedure. Stimulation over the motor cortex of the brain generates a waveform, which is propagated down the motor pathways and detected distally in the arm or leg. This stimulation results in a characteristic waveform. (544)

46. To generate transcranial motor evoked potentials, the patient cannot have residual neuromuscular blockade. (544)

47. The electrical current causing the stimulus over the motor cortex during transcranial motor evoked potential monitoring also stimulates muscles directly in the area of the electrodes placed in the scalp—the masseter muscle and muscles of mastication. This muscle contraction may result in a strong bite, which can potentially injure the tongue, lip, and endotracheal tube. Instances of significant tongue lacerations and damage to endotracheal tubes can occur, and this can develop into emergency situations, especially with the patient in the prone position. (545)

48. Special precautions should be taken for patients undergoing transcranial motor evoked potential monitoring during spine surgery. The tongue should not protrude through the teeth. Placing a bite block made of tongue depressors and gauze in the back of the mouth along the teeth line bilaterally will help prevent injury. In the prone position, any motion may allow for the tongue to slip and fall between the teeth, rendering it vulnerable to laceration. Each stimulus is associated with a masseter muscle contraction, so the patient is at risk as long as waveforms are being generated. (545)

49. Intraoperative electromyelograms are used to determine if a pedicle screw has been placed too close to a nerve root by sending an electric current through the screw and measuring the electromyelogram distally. If a low milliamp current can stimulate the nerve root, then the screw is too close to the nerve root. In general, a current greater than 7 mA is considered safe enough to know that the pedicle screw is not too close to the nerve root. (545)

50. For accurate electromyelogram testing, residual neuromuscular blockade must be terminated or reversed. (545)

51. The intraoperative wake-up test was traditionally used to assess spinal cord integrity in many scoliosis cases. Development of sophisticated spinal cord monitoring is now standard in many hospitals, and the wake-up test is generally reserved for those situations in which monitoring is unobtainable or a significant intraoperative change in spinal cord monitoring waveforms is noted. (545)

52. The intraoperative wake-up test is performed as follows: turn off all inhaled anesthetics, reverse any neuromuscular blocking drug present, and stop infusions such as dexmedetomidine, propofol, narcotics, or ketamine. If spontaneous respirations do not begin, inject naloxone, 0.04 mg at a time, to reverse any residual narcotic effect. The patient's head should be held to reduce the risk of self-extubation. Patient compliance with a command denotes adequate recovery from general anesthesia. Prior to assessing lower extremity function, there should be confirmation of upper extremity function. Then, while someone is observing the feet, ask the patient to wiggle his or her toes. A rapid-acting anesthetic such as propofol should be ready to be administered as soon as the assessment is complete, so the patient can rapidly be reanesthetized. If the wake-up test is not successful in demonstrating adequate motor movement, further surgical intervention may be warranted, and the patient may require transport to the radiology suite for additional imaging studies. (545)

53. Potential complications of an intraoperative wake-up test include increased bleeding, venous air embolism, and even inadvertent extubation of the trachea in the prone position with the wound exposed. (545)

54. At the conclusion of a spine procedure, the patient is placed in the supine position. All lines and tubes are secured so that intravenous line, arterial line, and airway access are not lost at this crucial time. Carefully reassess the patient for hemodynamic status, intravascular fluid volume status, hematocrit, blood loss, degree of fluid and blood replacement, temperature, and the potential for airway edema. Premature extubation must be avoided. Also, facial edema, respiratory effort, the amount of pain medication, and the presence of splinting and pain should be evaluated before extubating the trachea. After tracheal extubation, the supplemental oxygen should be administered and the patient transported to the PACU. Electrolytes, hemoglobin, and clotting studies should be ordered as indicated. (545)

55. Postoperative pain management may prove complicated after spine surgery as some patients may be taking significant amounts of pain medications, particularly opioids, prior to surgery. For these patients, as well as for narcotic-naive patients, a perioperative pain management plan can be developed and incorporated in the patient's care plan. In fact, the pain management pathway should consider utilizing preoperative oral pain medications, intraoperative infusion of pain medications, and postoperative medications to supply a multimodal pain regimen, with the goal of maximizing pain relief while considering methods to decrease narcotic-related respiratory depression. (545)

56. Oral medications that may be useful for pain management in the preoperative and postoperative period for patients undergoing spine surgery include acetaminophen, anticonvulsants (e.g., gabapentin and pregabalin), antispasmodics that work at the spinal cord level (e.g., baclofen, tizanidine), anti-inflammatory medications, and opioids. (545)

57. Following spine surgery, patient-controlled analgesia (PCA) may be effective, with the dose tailored to the patient's needs. Some centers utilize ketamine as an analgesic adjunct postoperatively. Intravenous acetaminophen is an excellent addition to the pain management regimen in patients who are NPO (nothing by mouth). (545)

58. The use of the nonsteroidal anti-inflammatory drugs (NSAIDs), such as ketorolac, needs careful consideration as they will interfere with bone formation and therefore should be avoided in patients who just underwent spinal fusion. NSAIDs can be considered on an individual basis when bone healing is not a factor, with cautionary consideration of cardiac-related issues resulting from their administration. (545)

59. Although the cause is unclear, patients undergoing prolonged spine surgery (>6 hours) in the prone position who have large blood loss (>1 L) are particularly at risk for postoperative visual loss. In fact, in the ASA visual loss registry blood loss of more than 1 L and procedures of 6 hours or longer were present

in 96% of cases. Yet patients with small blood loss and short procedures also have had visual loss. Other possible etiologic perioperative factors include anemia, hypotension, and prone positioning as well as systemic diseases such as diabetes, hypertension, and vascular disease. (546)

60. The ASA visual loss registry points to ischemic optic neuropathy as a major cause of postoperative visual loss. Of the 93 cases reported in the registry, 83 resulted from ischemic optic neuropathy, with the remainder attributed to central retinal artery occlusion. Variations in the blood supply to the optic nerve may play a role in the development of ischemic optic neuropathy, including reliance on a watershed blood supply to critical areas of the optic nerve. (546)

61. The ocular perfusion pressure (OPP), or the blood pressure supplying blood flow to the optic nerve, is a function of the mean arterial pressure (MAP) and intraocular pressure (IOP) such that OPP = MAP − IOP. Increases in IOP or decreases in MAP can have a negative impact on the ocular perfusion pressure. (546)

62. Several aspects of the prone position may contribute to postoperative visual loss. They include increased intraocular and venous pressure from positioning in the prone position, edema, a compartment syndrome within the orbit, and resistance to arterial blood flow such as from direct pressure on the eye. (546)

63. A recent study entitled Risk Factors Associated with Ischemic Optic Neuropathy compared 80 patients reported in the registry who suffered ischemic optic neuropathy to matched control subjects. In this study male sex, obesity, use of a Wilson frame, longer cases, greater estimated blood loss, and a decreased percentage of colloid are associated with an increased incidence of postoperative visual loss from ischemic optic neuropathy. (546)

64. Central retinal artery occlusion may be embolic in nature, or the result of direct pressure on the eyeball, and tends to be unilateral. (546)

65. According to the ASA practice advisory regarding patients at high risk for postoperative visual loss during spine surgery, the use of deliberate hypotension has not been shown to be associated with postoperative visual loss. (546)

66. According to the ASA practice advisory regarding patients at high risk for postoperative visual loss during spine surgery, colloid should be administered in addition to crystalloid to maintain intravascular volume. (546)

67. According to the ASA practice advisory regarding patients at high risk for postoperative visual loss during spine surgery, there is no defined transfusion trigger at which the risk of postoperative visual loss is eliminated. (546)

68. According to the ASA practice advisory regarding patients at high risk for postoperative visual loss during spine surgery, when in the prone position the patient's head should be positioned level with or higher than the heart when possible. Also, when possible, maintain the head in a neutral forward position without significant neck flexion, extension, lateral flexion, or rotation. (546)

SURGERY IN THE SITTING POSITION

69. Postoperative complications that have been noted in the patient undergoing surgery in the sitting position are rare but significant and devastating. These neurologic complications include stroke, ischemic brain injury, and vegetative states. (546)

70. When devastating neurologic postoperative complications occur after surgery in the sitting position, the implicated cause is a decrease in cerebral perfusion pressure resulting in insufficient blood supply to the brain. (546)

71. No, the systemic arterial blood pressure is not the same at the level of the heart as it is at the level of the circle of Willis when patients are anesthetized and placed in the sitting position. This is due to the arterial blood pressure gradient that develops between the heart and brain in this position. (547)

72. When patients are anesthetized and placed in the sitting position, one can more accurately determine the arterial blood pressure at the circle of Willis through the following calculation: for each centimeter of head elevation above the level of the heart there is a decrease in arterial blood pressure of 0.77 mm Hg. Therefore, arterial blood pressure measured at the level of the heart is not the blood and perfusion pressure at the brain. Indeed, a 20-cm difference in height between the heart and the circle of Willis calculates to approximately a 15- to 16-mm Hg gradient. (547)

73. A convenient point for measuring height difference between the heart and brain is the external auditory meatus, which is at the same level as the circle of Willis. Even so, there is still a significant amount of brain tissue above this level. (547)

74. When patients are anesthetized and placed in the sitting position, the mean arterial blood pressure should be maintained to avoid decreases in the cerebral perfusion pressure and to potentially avoid devastating neurologic injury. Thus, hypotension in these patients should be avoided. This is particularly true in the elderly or in patients with chronic hypertension in whom the cerebral autoregulatory curve is altered. (547)

FRACTURED HIP

75. Factors predisposing a person to a hip fracture include medical comorbid conditions, osteoporosis, lower limb dysfunction, visual impairment, increasing age, Parkinson disease, previous fracture, stroke, female gender, dementia, institutionalized patients, excess alcohol or caffeine consumption, cold climate, and use of psychotropic medications. (547)

76. Mortality rates can range up to 14% to 36% in the first year after fracture. (547)

77. Multiple studies have shown that patients with a hip fracture suffering from comorbid conditions do more poorly postoperatively than healthier patients. In one study the presence of four to six comorbid conditions is associated with increased mortality rate when compared to patients with fewer comorbid conditions. Roche and associates, in studying 2448 patients, reported that the presence of three or more comorbid conditions was a strong preoperative risk factor, with the postoperative development of chest infection or heart failure being associated with a high mortality rate. White and associates reported that ASA I and II patients had mortality rates equal to age-matched control subjects, but ASA III and IV patients had higher mortality rates (49% vs. 8%) after a hip fracture. Moran and colleagues, in a study of 2660 hip fracture patients with an overall mortality rate of 9% at 30 days, 19% at 90 days, and 30% at 12 months, noted that healthy patients did well as long as surgery was performed within 4 days. Patients with comorbid conditions had a nearly 2.5 times increased mortality rate at 30 days as compared with healthy patients. (547)

78. Generally, when significant comorbid conditions that need correction exist, patients benefit from a delay in surgery while their medical status improves. The mortality rate in high-risk patients in one study decreased from 29% to 2.9% when time was taken to correct physiologic abnormalities. This was also demonstrated by Kenzora and co-workers, who noted a higher mortality rate (34% vs. 6.9%) in patients who went immediately into surgery as compared to those who were delayed 2 to 5 days to improve their medical status. Also, patients admitted to the hospital immediately after fracture did better than those admitted more than a day later. (547)

79. Previously, hip surgery was delayed up to 6 months following a myocardial infarction (MI), but now the tendency is to risk-stratify patients based on the severity of their myocardial infarction to determine wait time until surgery. The recent MI needs to be evaluated on a risk-benefit ratio comparing the risk of surgery after a recent MI with the negative side effects of keeping a patient bed bound with its attendant risks of pneumonia, pulmonary embolism, pain, loss of ability to walk, and decubitus ulcers. Factors to consider are the extent of the MI, additional myocardium that may be at risk, if the patient suffers

from postinfarct angina, and the presence of congestive heart failure (CHF). Although ongoing angina or the presence of CHF may preclude early surgery, a small subendocardial MI with a minimal increase in cardiac enzymes and normal echocardiogram and stress test would allow consideration for an earlier intervention. A fractured hip usually prevents the patient from undergoing a normal exercise stress test, requiring a pharmacologic stress test if needed. (547)

80. Considerations for the anesthetic management of patients undergoing hip surgery include the patient's intravascular fluid volume status and the potential for significant perioperative blood loss, patient positioning and proper padding on the fracture table, maintaining normothermia, and whatever additional comorbid conditions may be present as these patients are typically elderly. (547)

81. A long-standing issue has been whether one anesthetic technique, regional or general, is associated with better outcomes in patients undergoing hip fracture repair. In general, the data accumulated over many years and many different studies have not documented a clear advantage of one technique over another. Choice of anesthesia technique should be made on a case-by-case basis. (547)

82. A 2012 retrospective study involving 18,158 hip fracture patients revealed that use of regional anesthesia resulted in lower mortality rates and fewer pulmonary complications in patients with intertrochanteric hip fractures but not in those patients suffering femoral neck fractures. (547)

83. Advantages of regional anesthesia for patients undergoing repair of a hip fracture are that (1) it avoids endotracheal intubation and airway manipulation and the medications that need to be administered to accomplish this, (2) it decreases the total amount of systemic medication the patient receives throughout the procedure, and (3) it may play a role in decreasing the risk of thromboembolism. The vasodilatory effect of the spinal anesthetic may help the patient with CHF. However, intravascular fluid still should be given cautiously because CHF may worsen as the intravascular vasodilatory effect of the spinal anesthesia recedes. (548)

84. An advantage of general anesthesia for patients undergoing repair of a hip fracture is that it is easy to administer, particularly in patients in whom movement and positioning for a regional anesthetic may be painful. In addition, in a patient who may be hypovolemic, general anesthesia may be preferred to avoid a precipitous decrease in arterial blood pressure that may occur as a result of the decrease in systemic vascular resistance that accompanies regional anesthesia. (548)

85. Lumbar plexus, femoral, and lateral femoral cutaneous nerve blocks may be used in selected situations for patients undergoing hip fracture repair. Combined femoral and lateral femoral cutaneous nerve blocks can be used for anesthesia in patients undergoing hip fracture repair requiring only cannulated pins. (548)

86. The dose and frequency of pain medication given to elderly patients in the perioperative period may need to be decreased. Pain medicines should be given cautiously because of an increased circulation time, and the cumulative effect of administered opioids may become evident when not expected. (548)

TOTAL JOINT REPLACEMENT

87. Anesthetic considerations for patients undergoing total joint replacement include the patient's age, concurrent medical conditions, blood loss, proper positioning and padding, hemodynamic variations during the procedure, the use of methylmethacrylate, and the risk of fat and pulmonary emboli. (548)

88. Patients undergoing total joint replacement may be positioned either supine or lateral. If supine, the arm on the ipsilateral side of surgery will need to be flexed away from the patient's side, which may have implications for intravenous catheter placement. If the patient is to be placed in the lateral position, an axillary roll and lateral positioners to stabilize the pelvis are required. Lateral positioners can compress abdominal contents and interfere with respiratory function. (548)

89. The use of methylmethacrylate cement is associated with cardiopulmonary side effects such as hypoxia, bronchoconstriction, hypotension, cardiovascular collapse, and even death. (548)

90. The systemic reaction to methylmethacrylate cement may result from the liquid methylmethacrylate cement monomer itself, which is used in producing the cement for cementing the prosthesis, or may be due to air, fat, or bone marrow elements being forced into the circulation. In fact, transesophageal echocardiography during reaming and cementing does indicate methylmethacrylate and fat emboli flow to the heart from the surgical site. The higher the liquid content of the liquid monomer in the mix with the polymer methylmethacrylate cement at the time of insertion, which occurs from not adequately mixing or not waiting long enough for mixing to occur, the more frequently side effects are noted. (548)

91. Patients who are at high risk for a reaction to methylmethacrylate cement include those who are hypovolemic at the time of cementing, hypertensive patients, and patients with significant preexisting cardiac disease. (549)

92. In the lower extremity surgery, the tourniquet is inflated to approximately 100 mm Hg above the systolic blood pressure, as this will prevent arterial blood from entering the exsanguinated limb. (549)

93. As tourniquets render the limb ischemic, there is a limit to inflation time before the ischemia can result in permanent limb damage. The safe upper limit of ischemia time is considered to be 2 hours. The surgeon should be informed of tourniquet inflation time at 1 hour and then as the tourniquet approaches the 2-hour limit so it can be deflated in a timely manner. (549)

94. If the total tourniquet time will exceed the 2-hour limit, the tourniquet should be deflated at 2 hours for a period of at least 15 to 20 minutes before it is reinflated. This will allow for the wash-out of acidic metabolites from the ischemic limb as the limb is reperfused with oxygenated blood. (549)

95. With increasing duration of the tourniquet on an ischemic limb the sympathetic response to increasing pain manifests as increasing arterial blood pressure and heart rate. These reverse with deflation of the tourniquet such that aggressive management of the blood pressure and heart rate during tourniquet inflation can result in hypotension when the tourniquet is deflated. (549)

96. Recirculation of the ischemic limb with release of the tourniquet is noted by a decrease in blood pressure and an increase in end-tidal carbon dioxide as the acid products recirculate. The hypotension usually responds to intravascular fluid administration and vasopressors if necessary. (549)

97. Complications associated with tourniquet use include nerve damage; vessel damage, especially in patients with atherosclerosis; and skin damage. One source of skin damage is the antiseptic prep solution, if it is allowed to seep under the tourniquet and tourniquet padding at the time of skin prep, causing a chemical burn. Additional concerns at the time of tourniquet deflation are pulmonary embolism and a decrease in core temperature as the isolated extremity is reperfused. (549)

98. If the tourniquet tubing is kinked and not noticed, deflation of the tourniquet at the box may not effectively deflate the tourniquet, placing the patient at risk for prolonged tourniquet inflation time, limb ischemia, and associated complications. (549)

99. Because of the use of a tourniquet during total knee replacement surgery, operating room blood loss is usually not significant. Some surgeons do not deflate the tourniquet until the wound is closed and the dressing is on the patient. In this situation blood loss is usually less, but there is a risk of postoperative bleeding. If much blood loss occurs into drains in the PACU, hypotension may result. (549)

100. Patients undergoing total knee replacement experience more postoperative pain than patients undergoing a total hip replacement. A postoperative pain management plan may include oral and intravenous pain medications, as well

as nerve blocks. Preoperative oral pain medications such as acetaminophen, gabapentin, or NSAIDs (with cardiovascular risk considered) are employed by some as part of a total knee pain pathway. With postoperative ambulation as early as the PACU becoming popular, there is a need to provide adequate pain relief for mobilization. Peripheral nerve blocks such as a femoral or an adductor canal block can supply such pain relief. The adductor canal block potentially spares motor components of the femoral nerve, preserving motor strength in the femoral nerve distribution; it is not clear that use of femoral or adductor canal blocks results in a higher incidence of falls. Postoperative pain relief may also include patient-controlled anesthesia, continuous infusions through catheters, individual nerve blocks of the lower extremities, and intravenous or oral medications. (550)

101. The concerns regarding regional anesthesia in patients receiving deep venous thrombosis prophylaxis are bleeding in the epidural space, epidural hematoma formation, and paralysis. The signs of epidural hematoma formation (pain, numbness, and weakness) can be masked by the infusion of epidural local anesthetics, which can delay diagnosis and increase risk. (550)

102. The American Society of Regional Anesthesia and Pain Medicine (ASRA) recommends waiting at least 12 hours before neuraxial needle placement in a patient who received a preoperative dose of enoxaparin. (550)

103. The ASRA recommends waiting 4 hours prior to dosing enoxaparin after an epidural catheter is removed. (550)

104. The ASRA recommends patients on warfarin should have their catheter removed only when the international normalized ratio (INR) is less than 1.5. (550)

105. Current recommendations in the ASRA Practice Advisory, Anticoagulation, 3rd edition, 2010, suggest that clopidogrel be discontinued for 7 days prior to performing a neuraxial block. However, the article quotes labeling as recommending this, whereas the PDR section for clopidogrel actually recommends that for elective surgery it be discontinued for only 5 days. The executive summary for the Anesthetic Management of the Patient Receiving Antiplatelet Medication, as part of the third edition, states, "On the basis of labeling and surgical reviews, the suggested time interval between discontinuation of thienopyridine therapy and neuraxial blockade is 14 days for ticlopidine and 7 days for clopidogrel. If a neuraxial block is indicated between 5 and 7 days of discontinuation of clopidogrel, normalization of platelet function should be documented." In patients who need to be maintained on clopidogrel or who have not discontinued it for an adequate time period, other anesthetic techniques should be considered. The guidelines for some of the antiplatelet medications will probably undergo revision as physicians gain experience with the use of medications such as clopidogrel in the perioperative period. (550)

33 OBSTETRICS

Jennifer M. Lucero and Mark D. Rollins

PHYSIOLOGIC CHANGES IN PREGNANT WOMEN

1. How do the maternal intravascular fluid, plasma, and erythrocyte volumes change during pregnancy?
2. How does the coagulation status change during pregnancy?
3. What is the average maternal blood loss during the vaginal delivery of a newborn? What is the average maternal blood loss during cesarean delivery?
4. How does the maternal cardiac output change from nonpregnant levels?
5. In an uncomplicated pregnancy, what changes occur in blood pressure, the systemic vascular resistance, and central venous pressure?
6. What is the supine hypotension syndrome? What symptoms accompany the syndrome?
7. What compensatory mechanisms do most women have that prevent them from experiencing supine hypotension syndrome?
8. How can the maternal hypotension be minimized by the clinician caring for the pregnant patient?
9. What are some echocardiographic changes during pregnancy?
10. What are some aspects of the upper airway that undergo physiologic changes in pregnancy? What are the clinical implications of these changes?
11. How does minute ventilation change during pregnancy from nonpregnant levels? How does maternal Pa_{CO_2} change as a result of the change in minute ventilation?
12. How does maternal Pa_{O_2} change during pregnancy?
13. How do the binding characteristics of hemoglobin change during pregnancy?
14. How does oxygen consumption change during pregnancy and labor?
15. What are the changes in lung volumes that occur with pregnancy?
16. Why does the pregnant patient desaturate rapidly with apnea?
17. What are the gastrointestinal changes in pregnancy that render the woman vulnerable to gastric reflux?
18. How should the pregnant patient be managed clinically with regard to her risk of gastric reflux?
19. How does the MAC (minimum alveolar concentration) of anesthesia with volatile anesthetics change in pregnancy?
20. How do the epidural and subarachnoid spaces change in pregnancy? How is the sensitivity to local anesthetics different in the pregnant versus nonpregnant patient? How are the dosing requirements for neuraxial anesthesia affected by these changes?
21. How do renal blood flow and glomerular filtration rate change in pregnancy? How does this affect the normal upper limits of creatinine and blood urea nitrogen in pregnant patients?
22. Does hepatic blood flow change during pregnancy? How are plasma protein concentrations and plasma cholinesterase activity altered by pregnancy?

PHYSIOLOGY OF THE UTEROPLACENTAL CIRCULATION

23. How are maternal and fetal blood delivered to the placenta?
24. What is the uterine blood flow rate at term?
25. What are the determinants of uterine blood flow?
26. What factors affect the transfer of oxygen between the mother and fetus?
27. How are the fetal and maternal hemoglobin dissociation curves shifted? What is the effect of this?
28. What is normal fetal Pa_{O_2}?
29. What factors affect placental exchange of drugs and other substances? What is the most reliable way to minimize fetal transfer of a drug?
30. Which drugs commonly used in anesthesia have limited ability to cross the placenta? Which readily cross the placenta?
31. How does the pH of fetal blood affect the transfer drugs? What is ion trapping?
32. What characteristics of the fetal circulation are protective against the distribution of large doses of drugs to vital organs?

STAGES OF LABOR

33. Name the stages of labor and the events that define each stage.
34. What is an "active-phase arrest"? What is an "arrest of descent"?

ANATOMY OF LABOR PAIN

35. In the first stage of labor, from which organs do afferent nerve impulses originate, and what are the associated sensory levels?
36. In the second stage of labor, from which organs do afferent nerve impulses originate, and what are the associated sensory levels?
37. Describe which analgesic techniques benefit the pregnant woman for each stage of labor.
38. What are some physiologic effects of labor pain on the mother?

METHODS OF LABOR ANALGESIA

39. Describe the different nonpharmacologic techniques used for labor.
40. What are some limitations of systemic medications for labor pain?
41. What are some effects of opioids on the mother and the fetus that limit their use in labor analgesia?
42. List the different opioid medications used for labor analgesia, their active metabolites, and what limits their utility. Which opioid is used most frequently?
43. What is "morphine sleep"?
44. How is remifentanil used as a labor analgesic, and what are the indications for its use?
45. Can inhaled nitrous oxide be administered safely for labor and delivery analgesia?
46. When is ketamine used in labor and delivery, and what additional benefits does it provide for pain control?

NEURAXIAL TECHNIQUES

47. What are the different types of neuraxial techniques used for labor analgesia?
48. What are some local anesthetics used for neuraxial labor analgesia and their potential complications?
49. What are some advantages and disadvantages of the coadministration of an opioid for neuraxial labor analgesia?
50. What are some advantages and disadvantages of the coadministration of clonidine and epinephrine for neuraxial labor analgesia?
51. What are the benefits of neuraxial techniques for labor analgesia?
52. During what stage of labor should neuraxial labor analgesia be administered?
53. Does neuraxial analgesia affect the progress of labor or the rate of cesarean delivery?
54. What preparations should be made prior to the administration of neuraxial labor analgesia?
55. Should laboring women remain NPO ("nothing by mouth") after placement of an epidural or combined spinal-epidural?

56. What is a walking epidural, and what are the associated risks?
57. Name the tissue layers and ligaments encountered when placing an epidural, and in what order the anesthesiologist encounters each.
58. American Society of Anesthesiologists (ASA) recommendations regarding aseptic technique for placement of neuraxial block include what specific precautions?
59. What are the interspaces where the neuraxial block for labor analgesia is placed? What are the risks of placing the neuraxial block higher or lower than this range of interspaces?
60. What is a "test dose," and what does it assess?
61. What is the combined spinal-epidural (CSE) technique, and what are some benefits of this technique?
62. Can a test dose be used with a CSE?
63. What is patient-controlled epidural analgesia (PCEA) and some advantages of its use?
64. What is programmed intermittent epidural boluses (PIEB) and some advantages of its use?
65. What is a "saddle block," and when is it utilized during labor and delivery?

CONTRAINDICATIONS AND COMPLICATIONS OF NEURAXIAL ANESTHESIA

66. What are the contraindications to neuraxial procedures?
67. Is known infection with human immunodeficiency virus (HIV) a contraindication to epidural placement?
68. List the potential complications of a neuraxial block.
69. What is the rate of post–dural puncture headache (PDPH)? What are the treatment options for PDPH?
70. What are some effects of an unintended intravascular injection of local anesthetic?
71. What is the treatment for systemic bupivacaine toxicity?
72. What physiologic effects do you expect to see with a high spinal or high epidural?
73. What are the important differences in performing ACLS (advanced cardiac life support) for the pregnant woman compared to a nonpregnant patient?
74. What is the rate of hypotension after neuraxial blockade?
75. What is the first-line pharmacologic treatment of hypotension after a neuraxial block?
76. How does epidural analgesia affect maternal body temperature?

OTHER NERVE BLOCKS FOR LABOR ANALGESIA

77. Where is local anesthetic injected to achieve a paracervical block? When is a paracervical block useful, and what are its disadvantages?
78. When is a pudendal block useful? What are the disadvantages of this type of block?

ANESTHESIA FOR CESAREAN DELIVERY

79. What are some benefits of regional anesthesia over general anesthesia for cesarean delivery?
80. What are benefits of general anesthesia over regional anesthesia for cesarean delivery?
81. What are some advantages and disadvantages of spinal anesthesia for cesarean delivery compared to epidural anesthesia?
82. What dermatome level of spinal anesthesia ensures patient comfort adequate for cesarean delivery? How can this be achieved with a spinal anesthetic?
83. What are some advantages and disadvantages of epidural anesthesia for cesarean delivery compared to spinal anesthesia?
84. Which local anesthetics and dose are typically administered to achieve an adequate density and dermatomal level of epidural anesthesia for cesarean delivery?

85. What is the advantage of the administration of preservative-free morphine into the epidural space for cesarean delivery? What are some of the negative side effects that may accompany epidural morphine administration?

86. What are some indications for general anesthesia for cesarean delivery? What are some benefits of general anesthesia for cesarean delivery?

87. What are the main causes of increased morbidity and mortality associated with general anesthesia during pregnancy?

88. How should difficulty with endotracheal intubation be managed by the anesthesiologist?

89. What is the approach to general anesthesia for cesarean delivery with respect to preparation, induction, maintenance, and emergence?

90. What is the level of exposure of the fetus to propofol after the administration of induction doses for general anesthesia?

91. What are some of the advantages and disadvantages of etomidate for the induction of general anesthesia for cesarean delivery?

92. What are some of the advantages and disadvantages of ketamine for the induction of general anesthesia for cesarean delivery?

93. How readily do benzodiazepines such as diazepam and midazolam cross the placenta? How can they affect the neonate?

94. What are the effects of using volatile anesthetics for cesarean delivery on the fetus and newborn?

95. What neuromuscular agents are typically used for cesarean deliver with general anesthesia? Do they result in neuromuscular blockade of the fetus or relaxation of the uterus?

ABNORMAL PRESENTATIONS AND MULTIPLE BIRTHS

96. What percent of live births are twins, and why is the number increasing? What are the complications that develop with multiple gestations?

97. What are the modes of delivery for twin pregnancies? What anesthetic techniques can be used to optimize delivery?

98. What is external cephalic version, and what are the associated risks?

99. What is a shoulder dystocia? What are the risk factors associated with the development of a shoulder dystocia? What are the risks to the fetus during a shoulder dystocia?

HYPERTENSIVE DISORDERS OF PREGNANCY

100. What are the four classifications of hypertensive disorders in pregnancy? What distinguishes gestational hypertension from chronic hypertension?

101. What is the percent of preeclampsia in the general population? What are the risk factors associated with developing preeclampsia?

102. What are new the criteria for the diagnosis of preeclampsia?

103. What is preeclampsia with severe features?

104. What is HELLP syndrome?

105. What is the mechanism of preeclampsia?

106. Does preeclampsia always result in immediate delivery?

107. What is the clinical use of magnesium sulfate in the treatment of preeclampsia? What are some considerations when using this treatment?

108. What are the clinical signs of magnesium sulfate toxicity? What is the treatment?

109. Which antihypertensive drugs are commonly used in preeclampsia?

110. What are some anesthetic considerations for neuraxial analgesia for patients with preeclampsia?

111. What are some anesthetic considerations in the urgent or emergent delivery in patients with preeclampsia?

HEMORRHAGE IN PREGNANT WOMEN

112. What are some causes of hemorrhage in the pregnant patient? When do these typically manifest?

113. What is placenta previa? What are the associated risk factors?

114. What are some anesthetic considerations and surgical treatments for patients with placenta previa?
115. What is abruptio placentae? What are some risk factors for abruptio placentae?
116. What are the clinical presentation and anesthetic considerations for the management of abruptio placentae?
117. What are some risk factors for uterine rupture? What is the incidence of uterine rupture associated with vaginal birth after a previous cesarean delivery?
118. What approximate percent of vaginal deliveries are associated with some amount of retained placenta? What are some options for the anesthetic management of patients with retained placenta?
119. What are some risk factors for uterine atony?
120. Which medications are used to manage uterine atony? What are their side effects?
121. Define placenta accreta, increta, and percreta.
122. In a patient with known placenta previa, how does the risk of placenta accreta change with the number of prior cesarean deliveries?

AMNIOTIC FLUID EMBOLISM

123. What is the clinical presentation of an amniotic fluid embolism? What are some conditions that may mimic amniotic fluid embolism?
124. How is the definitive diagnosis of an amniotic fluid embolism made?

ANESTHESIA FOR NONOBSTETRIC SURGERY DURING PREGNANCY

125. What are common nonobstetric surgeries that occur during pregnancy?
126. When should nonobstetric surgeries be performed during pregnancy?
127. What are some considerations for the anesthetic management of pregnant patients undergoing nonobstetric surgery?
128. Should routine pregnancy testing be done in women of childbearing age prior to undergoing surgery?
129. Which anesthetics are teratogenic?
130. How can intrauterine fetal hypoxia and acidosis be prevented during nonobstetric surgery?
131. When should fetal heart rate monitoring be done during nonobstetric surgery?
132. What is the usual cause of premature labor that presents in the pregnant patient after having undergone nonobstetric surgery? How can premature labor be treated?
133. Can laparoscopic surgery be performed safely during the third trimester?

DIAGNOSIS AND MANAGEMENT OF FETAL DISTRESS

134. Describe the frequency of normal uterine contractions and tachysystole. What is the treatment for tachysystole?
135. What was fetal heart rate monitoring designed to assess?
136. What is the normal baseline fetal heart rate (FHR)?
137. Define FHR variability in terms of absent, minimal, moderate, and marked.
138. What is the definition of an FHR acceleration?
139. What is a late deceleration indicative of in the fetus?
140. What is a variable deceleration indicative of in the fetus?
141. What are the three categories in the three-tier FHR classification system for general fetal assessment?
142. How should category III FHR tracings be managed?

EVALUATION OF THE NEONATE AND NEONATAL RESUSCITATION

143. Define the values of each Apgar score category.
144. What are normal blood gas values for the umbilical artery and vein?
145. During neonatal evaluation and resuscitation, when is it appropriate to give positive-pressure ventilation and chest compressions?
146. What is the dose of epinephrine given for neonatal resuscitation?
147. Should naloxone be given in the delivery room for neonatal resuscitation?
148. In neonates delivered with meconium-stained amniotic fluid, when should suctioning below the cords be instituted?

ANSWERS*

1. The maternal intravascular fluid volume increases beginning in the first trimester of pregnancy. By term, the intravascular fluid volume has increased by about 1000 mL to 1500 mL above the nonpregnant state. The plasma volume increases by approximately 50% at term, whereas the erythrocyte volume increases by approximately 25%. Because the plasma volume increases by twice as much as the erythrocyte volume, the woman has a relative physiologic anemia. That is, the hematocrit of the pregnant woman is relatively less than her nonpregnant state. This is termed the *physiologic anemia of pregnancy*. (554)

2. The pregnant woman at term is in a hypercoagulable state secondary to increases in factors I, VII, VIII, IX, X, and XII and decreases in factors XI and XIII and antithrombin III. This results in an approximately 20% decrease in prothrombin time (PT) and partial thromboplastin time (PTT). Platelet count may remain normal or decrease 10% by term. (555)

3. The average maternal blood loss during the vaginal delivery of a newborn is 300 to 500 mL. The average maternal blood loss during the delivery of a newborn by cesarean delivery is 800 to 1000 mL, but blood loss during a cesarean delivery is greatly variable. The increase in intravascular fluid volume and the hypercoagulable state of the mother help to counter the blood losses incurred during this time. The contracted uterus after either type of delivery creates an autotransfusion of approximately 500 mL of blood, which decreases the overall effect of the blood loss on the mother. (555)

4. Cardiac output increases by about 35% by the end of the first trimester, and at term it increases by approximately 50% from its baseline. This increase in cardiac output at term is due to increases in both stroke volume (25% to 30%) and heart rate (15% to 25%). Labor further increases in cardiac output by 10% to 25% during the first stage and 40% in the second stage. The largest increase in cardiac output occurs just after delivery, when it increases as much as 80% above prelabor values. This is the maximal change in cardiac output in the woman. Cardiac output decreases to prelabor values about 48 hours after delivery and has substantial further decreases toward prepregnant values by 2 weeks post partum. (555)

5. Despite increases in both cardiac output and plasma volume, the systolic blood pressure of the woman having an uncomplicated pregnancy typically decreases secondary to a 20% reduction in systemic vascular resistance at term. Systolic, mean and diastolic blood pressures may all decrease 5% to 15% by 20 weeks of gestational age and gradually increase toward prepregnant values as the pregnancy progresses toward term. Central venous pressure does not change during pregnancy despite the increased plasma volume because venous capacitance increases. (555)

6. Supine hypotension syndrome, as the name implies, is the decrease in blood pressure seen when the pregnant patient lies in the supine position. The supine hypotension syndrome occurs because of a decrease in cardiac output of approximately 10% to 20% when the gravid uterus compresses the inferior vena cava. This results in decreased venous return and preload for the heart. Compression of the vena cava may contribute to venous stasis and potentially ankle edema, varices, and increased risk of venous thrombosis. The gravid uterus can also compress the lower abdominal aorta and lead to arterial hypotension in the lower extremities, but maternal symptoms or decreases in systemic blood pressure as measured in the arms are often not reflective of this decrease. The major clinical significance of the aortoiliac artery compression is the decrease in placental and uterine blood flow that results.

---

*Numbers in parentheses refer to pages, figures, boxes, or tables in Pardo MC, Miller RD, eds. *Basics of Anesthesia*. 7th ed. Philadelphia: Elsevier; 2018.

The decrease in blood flow through the uteroplacental unit leads to fetal compromise. Symptoms that accompany the hypotension include diaphoresis, nausea, vomiting, and possible changes in cerebration. (555)

7. Most pregnant women, when lying in the supine position, are able to compensate for the possible decrease in blood pressure that results from the compression of the inferior vena cava by the gravid uterus. One compensatory mechanism includes maintaining venous return by diverting blood flow from the inferior vena cava to the paravertebral venous plexus. The blood then goes to the azygos vein and returns to the heart via the superior vena cava. Dilation of the epidural veins may make unintentional intravascular placement of an epidural catheter more likely. A "test dose" is given before dosing an epidural catheter in order to decrease the likelihood of an unrecognized intravascular placement before initiating neuraxial blockade. Another compensatory mechanism is an increase in peripheral sympathetic nervous system activity. This increases peripheral vascular tone and helps to maintain venous return to the heart. Regional anesthesia, however, can interfere with these compensatory mechanisms by causing sympathetic nervous system blockade, rendering the pregnant woman at term more susceptible to decreases in blood pressure. (556)

8. The aortocaval compression, and thus maternal hypotension, can be minimized by having the woman lie in the lateral position. Uterine displacement can also be used, typically with displacement being to the left because the inferior vena cava sits just to the right of and anterior to the spine. Left uterine displacement is accomplished by table tilt or the placement of a wedge or folded blanket under the right hip, elevating the hip by 10 to 15 cm. (556)

9. Echocardiographic changes during pregnancy include anterior and leftward displacement of the heart, increases in right (20%) and left (10%) heart chamber sizes, and associated left ventricular hypertrophy and increase in ejection fraction. About 1 in 4 women have mitral regurgitation. In addition, small pericardial effusions may be present. (556)

10. There is significant capillary engorgement of the mucosal layer of the upper airway and increased tissue friability during pregnancy. This results in increased risk of obstruction from tissue edema and bleeding with instrumentation of the upper airway. Additional care is needed during suctioning, placement of airways (avoid nasal instrumentation if possible), direct laryngoscopy, and intubation. In addition, because the vocal cords and arytenoids are often edematous, smaller cuffed endotracheal tubes (6.0- to 6.5-mm internal diameter) may be a better selection for intubation of the trachea for pregnant patients. The presence of preeclampsia, upper respiratory tract infections, and active pushing with associated increased venous pressure further exacerbate airway tissue edema, making both intubation and ventilation more challenging. (556)

11. Minute ventilation increases during pregnancy to about 50% above prepregnancy levels, likely due to increases in circulating progesterone and CO_2 production. This change occurs in the first trimester of pregnancy and remains elevated for the duration of the pregnancy. An increase in tidal volume is the main contributor to increase in minute ventilation, with only a small contribution from minimal increases in respiratory rate. During the first trimester, as a result of the increase in minute ventilation, the resting maternal Pa_{CO_2} decreases from 40 mm Hg to about 30 mm Hg. Arterial pH, however, remains only slightly alkalotic (7.42 to 7.44) secondary to increased renal excretion of bicarbonate ions. (556)

12. Maternal Pa_{O_2} changes during the progression from early gestation to term. Early in gestation the Pa_{O_2} in the mother is slightly increased above prepregnancy values to over 100 mm Hg while breathing room air. This is secondary to maternal hyperventilation and subsequent decreased Pa_{CO_2}. As the pregnancy progresses the Pa_{O_2} is normal or even slightly decreased. The decrease in Pa_{O_2} during the course of pregnancy likely results from airway closure and associated intrapulmonary shunt. (556)

13. Maternal hemoglobin is right shifted, with the P_{50} increasing from 27 to approximately 30 mm Hg. A rightward shift lowers hemoglobin's affinity for oxygen, thus displacing oxygen from hemoglobin and releasing it to the tissues (556)

14. Oxygen consumption increases by 20% from prepregnancy rates at term. During labor, oxygen consumption increases by 40% above prelabor rates during the first stage and 75% during the second stage. (556)

15. Maternal lung volumes start to change in the second trimester. This change is a result of mechanical compression by the gravid uterus as it enlarges and forces the diaphragm cephalad. This leads to a decrease in the woman's functional residual capacity (FRC) by approximately 20% at term. This is the result of approximately equal decreases in both the expiratory reserve volume (ERV) and residual lung volume (RV). This can result in an FRC less than closing capacity and increased atelectasis in the supine position. There is no significant change in vital capacity seen during pregnancy. The rapid rates of change in the alveolar concentration of inhaled anesthetics during induction and emergence from anesthesia occur secondary to the combination of increased minute ventilation and decreased functional residual capacity. Apnea in the pregnant woman rapidly leads to arterial hypoxemia. (556)

16. There are at least three physiologic contributions for more rapid desaturation observed during pregnancy. First, a decreased FRC leads to subsequent decreased oxygen reserve. Second, maternal oxygen consumption is increased by 20% at term, with further increases noted during labor. Third, the aortocaval compression and decreased venous return lead to decreases in cardiac output in the supine intubating position. This decrease in cardiac output would lead to an increase in overall oxygen extraction and therefore decrease the level of oxygenation of blood returning to the heart. Because of the rapid decrease in maternal Pa_{O_2} with apnea or hypoventilation, preoxygenation with 100% O_2 for 3 minutes or four maximal breaths over the 30 seconds just prior to induction of emergent general anesthesia is recommended. (557)

17. Multiple gastrointestinal changes render the pregnant woman significantly vulnerable to the regurgitation of gastric contents beyond 20 weeks of gestation. The enlarged uterus acts to displace the stomach and pylorus cephalad from its usual position. This repositions the intra-abdominal portion of the esophagus into the thorax and leads to relative incompetence of the physiologic gastroesophageal sphincter. The tone of the gastroesophageal sphincter is further reduced by the higher progesterone and estrogen levels of pregnancy. Gastric pressure is increased by the gravid uterus. Gastrin secreted by the placenta stimulates gastric hydrogen ion secretion. The pH of the woman's gastric fluid is predictably low as a result. Reflux and subsequent esophagitis are common during pregnancy. During labor, gastric emptying is delayed, and intragastric fluid volume tends to be increased as a result. Anxiety, pain, and the administration of opioids can further decrease gastric emptying. (557)

18. Clinically, the pregnant patient must always be treated as if she has a full stomach. Regardless of what amount of time has elapsed since her last ingestion of solids, she is at increased risk of regurgitation and aspiration of gastric contents. This includes the routine use of nonparticulate antacids, rapid-sequence induction, cricoid pressure, and cuffed intubation as part of general anesthesia induction sequence in a pregnant woman after approximately 20 weeks of gestational age. Pharmacologic interventions that are recommended in the woman to help minimize the risks of pulmonary aspiration are aimed at decreasing the severity of acid pneumonitis should aspiration occur. The administration of antacids to pregnant women before the induction of anesthesia is common practice. This is as an attempt to increase the pH of gastric contents. ASA guidelines recommend the "timely administration

of oral nonparticulate antacids, intravenous (IV) H_2-receptor antagonists, and/or metoclopramide for aspiration prophylaxis" prior to the induction of anesthesia in pregnant women. Nonparticulate antacids such as 30 mL sodium citrate work rapidly. Metoclopramide can significantly decrease gastric volume in as little as 15 minutes in the absence of prior opioid administration, and H_2-receptor antagonists can increase gastric fluid pH in approximately 1 hour. (557)

19. The MAC (minimum alveolar concentration) of anesthesia with volatile anesthetics is decreased within the first trimester of pregnancy by up to 40% in animal studies and 28% in human studies. However, electroencephalographic monitoring studies did not reflect these results, but rather showed the effects of sevoflurane on the brain are similar in pregnant and nonpregnant patients. (557)

20. During pregnancy, both the epidural and intrathecal spaces are decreased in volume from their prepregnancy state because of the engorgement of epidural veins and the increased intra-abdominal pressure resulting from the progressive enlargement of the uterus. However, cerebrospinal fluid pressure does not increase with pregnancy. The decrease in the epidural space decreases the required volume of local anesthetic necessary to achieve a particular level of anesthesia by facilitating its spread in the epidural space. The decreased intrathecal space also facilitates the spread of spinal anesthetic and decreases the dose required from prepregnancy values. There also seems to be an increased sensitivity to local anesthetics by women who are pregnant. The decreased local anesthetic requirement in pregnant women appears to have a biochemical component to it as well as a mechanical one. This is based on the observation of decreased required neuraxial local anesthetic doses as early as the first trimester, prior to significant uterine enlargement. (557)

21. Renal blood flow and glomerular filtration rate in the pregnant woman are both increased. By the third month of pregnancy the increase is about 50% to 60%. This results in a decrease in what is considered the normal upper limit of both the blood urea nitrogen and serum creatinine concentrations during pregnancy to about 50% of what it was in the prepregnancy state. Renal blood flow and glomerular filtration rate return to prepregnancy levels around 3 months post partum. (558)

22. Hepatic blood flow does not change significantly with pregnancy. Plasma protein concentrations are reduced in pregnancy secondary to dilution. The decreased albumin levels can create increased blood levels of highly protein-bound drugs. Plasma cholinesterase, or pseudocholinesterase, decreases in activity by about 25% to 30% during pregnancy. This decrease in activity is first noted by about the 10th week of gestation and persists for as long as 6 weeks post partum. There is no clinical manifestation from this change in plasma cholinesterase activity and no significant change in the duration of action of succinylcholine. (558)

PHYSIOLOGY OF THE UTEROPLACENTAL CIRCULATION

23. The function of the placenta is to unite maternal and fetal circulations. This union allows for the physiologic exchange of nutrients and waste. Maternal blood is delivered to the placenta by the uterine arteries. Fetal blood is delivered to the placenta by the two umbilical arteries. Nutrient-rich blood is transferred from the placenta to the fetus via a single umbilical vein. The two most important determinants of placental function are uterine blood flow and the relative concentrations and characteristics of the substances to be exchanged across the placenta. (558)

24. Uterine blood flow increases during gestation from approximately 100 mL/min before pregnancy to 700 mL/min at term. Adequate uterine blood flow must be maintained to ensure the placental circulation is sufficient and therefore guarantee fetal well-being. About 80% of the uterine blood flow perfuses the placenta, and 20% supports the myometrium. Uterine blood flow at term is about 10% of cardiac output. (558)

25. During pregnancy uterine blood flow has limited autoregulation, and the uterine vasculature is essentially maximally dilated under normal pregnancy conditions. Uterine blood flow is proportional to the mean blood perfusion pressure to the uterus and inversely proportional to the resistance of the uterine vasculature. Decreased perfusion pressure can result from systemic hypotension secondary to hypovolemia, aortocaval compression, or decreased systemic resistance from either general or neuraxial anesthesia. Uterine blood flow also decreases with increased uterine venous pressure. This can result from vena caval compression (supine position), uterine contractions (particularly uterine tachysystole as may occur with oxytocin administration), or significant abdominal musculature contraction (Valsalva maneuver during pushing). Additionally, extreme hypocapnia (Pa_{CO_2} <20 mm Hg) associated with hyperventilation secondary to labor pain can reduce uterine blood flow to the point of fetal hypoxemia and acidosis. Epidural or spinal anesthesia does not alter uterine blood flow as long as maternal hypotension is avoided. Endogenous catecholamines induced by stress or pain and exogenous vasopressors have the capability of increasing uterine arterial resistance and decreasing uterine blood flow. The use of phenylephrine to correct maternal hypotension does not influence fetal well-being. Although ephedrine is also safe to use in moderate amounts to treat maternal hypotension, phenylephrine administration results in less fetal acidosis and base deficit as shown in clinical trials. (558)

26. Transfer of oxygen between the mother and the fetus is dependent on a variety of factors including the ratio of maternal to fetal umbilical blood flow, the oxygen partial pressure gradient, the respective hemoglobin concentrations and affinities, the placental diffusing capacity, and the acid-base status of the fetal and maternal blood (Bohr effect). (558)

27. The fetal oxyhemoglobin dissociation curve is left-shifted (greater oxygen affinity), whereas the maternal hemoglobin dissociation curve is right-shifted (decreased oxygen affinity), resulting in facilitated oxygen transfer to the fetus. (558)

28. The fetal Pa_{O_2} is normally 40 mm Hg and never more than 60 mm Hg, even if the mother is breathing 100% oxygen. Placental exchange from the mother to the fetus represents venous rather than arterial blood. (558)

29. The relative transfer of drugs and other substances less than 1000 Da from the maternal circulation to the fetal circulation and vice versa is determined primarily by diffusion. Factors that affect the exchange of substances from the maternal circulation to the fetus include the concentration gradient of the substance across the placenta, maternal protein binding, molecular weight, lipid solubility, and degree of ionization of the substance. The most reliable way to minimize the amount of drug that reaches the fetus is by minimizing the concentration of the drug in the maternal blood. (559)

30. Nondepolarizing neuromuscular blocking drugs have a high molecular weight and low lipid solubility. These two characteristics together limit the ability of nondepolarizing neuromuscular blocking drugs to cross the placenta. Succinylcholine is highly ionized, preventing it from diffusing across the placenta despite its low molecular weight. Additionally, both heparin and glycopyrrolate have significantly limited placental transfer. Placental transfer of local anesthetics and opioids is facilitated by the relatively low molecular weights of these substances. (559)

31. Fetal blood is slightly more acidic than maternal blood, with a pH about 0.1 unit less than maternal blood pH. The lower pH of fetal blood facilitates the fetal uptake of drugs that are basic. Weakly basic drugs, such as local anesthetics and opioids, that cross the placenta in the nonionized state become ionized in the fetal circulation. This results in an accumulated concentration of drug in the fetus for two reasons. First, once the drug becomes ionized it cannot readily diffuse back across the placenta. This is known as *ion trapping*. Second, a concentration gradient of nonionized drug

is maintained between the mother and the fetus. In the case of lidocaine administration, this may mean that if the fetus was distressed and acidotic and lidocaine was maternally administered in sufficient doses, lidocaine may accumulate in the fetus. This can be particularly harmful to the fetus if direct maternal intravascular local anesthetic injection occurs. Decreased neonatal tone and potential bradycardia can result from significant fetal local anesthetic toxicity. (559)

32. The fetal circulation protects against the distribution of large doses of drugs to vital organs in two ways. First, about 75% of the blood that is coming to the fetus via the umbilical vein first passes through the fetal liver. Despite decreased liver enzyme activity in comparison to adults, fetal/neonatal enzyme systems are adequately developed to metabolize most drugs. This allows for a significant amount of drug metabolism to take place before entering the fetal arterial circulation and delivery to the heart and brain. Second, drug within umbilical vein blood enters the inferior vena cava via the ductus venosus. This blood is diluted by drug-free blood returning from the lower extremities and pelvic viscera of the fetus, resulting in a decrease in the concentration of drug in the inferior vena cava. (559)

STAGES OF LABOR

33. Labor is a continuous process divided into three stages. The first stage is the onset of labor until the cervix is fully dilated. This first stage is further divided into latent and active phases. The latent phase can persist for many hours. The active phase begins at the point when the rate of cervical dilation increases (often between 5- and 6-cm dilation). The second stage of labor begins when the cervix is fully dilated and ends when the neonate is born. This stage is referred to as the "pushing and expulsion" stage. The third and final stage begins with birth of the neonate and is completed when the placenta is delivered. (559)

34. If a woman fails to dilate adequately in the active phase despite pharmacologic interventions, this is considered *active phase arrest* and will result in a cesarean delivery. During the second stage of labor, the patient may not be able to push the neonate out of the pelvis. This is termed *arrest of descent*. If the neonate is low enough in the pelvis, the obstetrician can perform an instrumented vaginal delivery via vacuum or forceps; otherwise, a cesarean delivery is needed. (559)

ANATOMY OF LABOR PAIN

35. During the first stage of labor (cervical dilation) the majority of painful stimuli results from afferent nerve impulses from the lower uterine segment and cervix. This pain is typically visceral in nature (dull, aching, poorly localized). The nerve cell bodies are located at the dorsal root ganglia of the T10 to L1 levels. (560)

36. In the second stage of labor afferents originating from the vagina, perineum, and pelvic floor travel primarily via the pudendal nerve to the dorsal root ganglia of the S2 to S4 levels. This pain is typically somatic in nature (sharp and well localized). (560)

37. During the first and second stages of labor the pregnant woman may benefit from neuraxial techniques such as an epidural or combined spinal-epidural (CSE). Although used infrequently, a paracervical block can also be administered during the first stage of labor to block transmission of pain at the paracervical ganglion. A single-shot spinal block can be used for the second stage of labor but is limited by duration. A pudendal block provides pain relief to the lower vagina and perineum and is infrequently used for labor analgesia during the second stage of labor. Typically, the obstetrician performs both the paracervical and pudendal block. (560)

38. Labor pain stimulates the maternal sympathetic nervous system, increasing plasma catecholamine levels, which can lead to maternal tachycardia, hypertension, and reduced uterine blood flow. (560)

METHODS OF LABOR ANALGESIA

39. A variety of nonpharmacologic techniques for labor analgesia exist. They include hypnosis, the breathing techniques described by Lamaze, acupuncture, acupressure, the LeBoyer method, transcutaneous nerve stimulation, massage, hydrotherapy, vertical positioning, the presence of a support person, intradermal water injections, biofeedback, and many others. A meta-analysis reviewing the effectiveness of a support individual (e.g., doula, family member) noted that women with a support individual used less pharmacologic analgesia, had a decreased length of labor, and had a lower incidence of cesarean delivery. In a 2006 retrospective survey, nonpharmacologic methods of tub immersion and massage were rated more or equally effective in relieving pain compared to the use of opioids in labor. (560)

40. Systemic medications for labor pain are dose-limited secondary to their potential effects of maternal sedation, respiratory compromise, loss of airway protection, and effects on the fetus. Sedatives, anxiolytics, and dissociative drugs are rarely used for labor pain. Systemic opioid use is common, particularly in the early stages of labor, but must be administered judiciously. (560)

41. Effects of opioids on the mother that limit their use in labor analgesia include nausea, vomiting, pruritus, decreased stomach emptying, and sedation. All opioids readily cross the placental barrier and can cause decreased fetal heart rate (FHR) variability and dose-related respiratory depression. (561)

42. Fentanyl is commonly used for labor analgesia. It has a short duration with no active metabolites. Given in small IV doses of 50 to 100 µg per hour, there are no significant differences in neonatal Apgar scores and respiratory effort compared to mothers who have not received fentanyl. Morphine was used more frequently in the past but currently is rarely used. Its active metabolite (morphine-6-glucuronide) has a prolonged duration of analgesia, the half-life is longer in neonates compared to adults, and it produces significant maternal sedation. Meperidine is still one of the most frequently used opioids worldwide. The maternal half-life of meperidine is 2 to 3 hours, with half-life in the fetus and newborn significantly greater (13 to 23 hours) and more variable. In addition, meperidine is metabolized to an active metabolite (normeperidine) that can significantly accumulate after repeated doses. With increased dosing and shortened time between doses there are increased neonatal risks of decreased Apgar scores, lowered oxygen saturation, and prolonged time to sustained respiration. (561)

43. In latent labor, obstetric providers may use intramuscular (IM) morphine combined with phenergan for analgesia, sedation, and rest termed *morphine sleep*. This produces analgesia for approximately 2.5 to 6 hours with an onset of 10 to 20 minutes. (561)

44. Remifentanil patient-controlled analgesia (PCA) has been considered for women who have contraindications to neuraxial blockade. Although labor pain lessened with remifentanil, a randomized controlled trial comparing epidural analgesia to remifentanil PCA had overall pain scores that were decreased in the epidural group. A more recent equivalence trial performed between remifentanil PCA and epidural analgesia found remifentanil was inferior to epidural analgesia for satisfaction of pain relief and pain relief scores. More sedation and hemoglobin desaturation were noted during remifentanil analgesia, but there was no difference between groups in fetal and neonatal outcome measures. (561)

45. An inhaled anesthetic of 50% nitrous oxide blended with 50% oxygen may be used for labor analgesia. The inhalation of nitrous oxide for analgesia during labor and delivery should be self-administered after appropriate patient instruction. Opioids should not be coadministered in order to provide a safe analgesic method not associated with hypoxia or loss of consciousness. Optimal

results from the administration of nitrous oxide during labor are obtained by having the woman inhale the nitrous oxide between contractions, so that an effective concentration of nitrous oxide is achieved for the uterine contraction. About 45 seconds of continuous breathing of the nitrous oxide is necessary in order for optimal labor analgesia with contractions. Side effects are mild, with nausea, dizziness, and drowsiness most common. Maternal cardiovascular and respiratory depression is minimal, uterine contractility is not affected, and neonatal depression does not occur regardless of the duration of nitrous oxide administration. (561)

46. During labor, ketamine can be administered to provide rapid analgesia in acute urgent situations associated with severe pain in divided IV doses (10 to 20 mg) totaling less than 1 mg/kg. It has a quick onset (30 seconds) and minimal duration of action (<5 minutes). It has been associated with undesirable psychomimetic side effects (bad dreams), which can be lessened by the coadministration of benzodiazepines. (561–562)

NEURAXIAL TECHNIQUES

47. Epidural, spinal, and combined spinal-epidural (CSE) are the neuraxial techniques typically used for labor analgesia. Neuraxial analgesia involves the administration of local anesthetics, often with the coadministration of an opioid or other adjunctive agents. (562)

48. The local anesthetics most commonly used for neuraxial labor analgesia are bupivacaine and ropivacaine. These are both amide-linked and are degraded by the P-450 enzymes in the liver. When administered appropriately they are safe, but an accidental intravascular injection can result in significant maternal morbidity (seizures, loss of consciousness, severe arrhythmias, and cardiovascular collapse), maternal fatality, and the potential for fetal accumulation (ion trapping). (562)

49. The coadministration of an opioid augments the neuraxial labor analgesia provided by local anesthetics by improving the quality and duration of the analgesia with local anesthetic–sparing effects. Neuraxial opioids alone can be administered but are not as effective. Disadvantages of neuraxial opioids include maternal side effects of pruritus, sedation, and nausea. In addition, administration of intrathecal opioids can result in fetal bradycardia independent of hypotension. (562)

50. Clonidine is an epidural adjuvant to local anesthetics used in neuraxial blockade for analgesia. Clonidine inhibits the release of substance P in the dorsal horn and produces analgesia. It also increases the level of acetylcholine in the cerebrospinal fluid. Neuraxial clonidine can augment analgesia, but sedation and hypotension are associated with its use. The Food and Drug Administration (FDA) has issued a "black box" warning regarding the possibility of significant hypotension with neuraxial clonidine in obstetrics, and caution should be used. Epidural epinephrine has been shown to decrease the dose of local anesthetic required for labor analgesia. (562)

51. Benefits of neuraxial techniques for labor analgesia include the most effective labor analgesia, the highest rates of maternal satisfaction, minimal sedative side effects, reduced maternal catecholamine concentrations, the facilitation of maternal active participation during labor, and the avoidance of hyperventilation. (562)

52. Any time a woman in labor without contraindications requests neuraxial analgesia, regardless of the stage of her labor, a neuraxial blockade may be placed. The timing of placement does not depend on an arbitrary cervical dilation. A single-shot spinal analgesic has a finite analgesic time depending on the local anesthetic and should be taken into account when utilizing this technique (e.g., it is ideal if the obstetrician is performing an instrumented vaginal delivery in a woman without previous neuraxial block). Epidural catheter delivery techniques can be extended throughout the length of the labor. (562)

53. Neuraxial analgesia is associated with a prolonged second stage of labor with an approximate increased duration of 20 minutes or longer. This prolonged duration is not harmful to the fetus provided that fetal status is reassuring. Women with neuraxial analgesia did have an increased rate of instrumented vaginal delivery when compared to women receiving systemic opioid labor analgesia in one retrospective review. Randomized controlled clinical trials comparing women receiving either systemic opioids or neuraxial analgesia in early labor demonstrated no difference in rates of cesarean delivery. (562)

54. Prior to the administration of neuraxial labor analgesia the pregnant patient's history and physical examination should be performed, the airway assessed, informed consent obtained, and the confirmation of the availability of resuscitative equipment should be established. Mother and fetus should be closely monitored with maternal vital signs and FHR during the imitation of neuraxial blockade. (562)

55. Otherwise healthy laboring women may have modest amounts of clear liquids throughout labor. However, in complicated labors (e.g., by morbid obesity, difficult airway, concerning fetal status), the decision to restrict oral intake should be individualized. (562)

56. Placing opioids alone in the epidural or intrathecal space (if placing a CSE) is considered a walking epidural (the term may also include any epidural analgesic technique that allows safe ambulation and may occasionally contain extremely dilute concentrations of local anesthetic). The opioid-based solution, while providing analgesia, has minimal effects on sympathetic or motor nerves. This allows the woman to ambulate after tests for motor blockade indicate that she is not at risk of falling. Even so, the woman should be closely monitored and ideally should only ambulate when accompanied because proprioception and balance may be impaired. (562)

57. The Tuohy needle (specialized epidural placement needle) traverses the skin and subcutaneous tissues, supraspinous ligament, interspinous ligament, and the ligamentum flavum before it is advanced into the epidural space as confirmed by the "loss of resistance" technique. (562)

58. Aseptic technique should be used during neuraxial procedures, including (1) jewelry removal (e.g., rings and watches), handwashing and use of caps, masks, and sterile gloves; (2) use of individually packaged chlorhexidine (preferred) or povidone-iodine (preferably with alcohol) for skin preparation, allowing for adequate drying time; (3) sterile draping; and (4) use of sterile occlusive dressings at the catheter insertion site. (562)

59. The needle is normally inserted between the L2 and L4 interspaces. If the needle is placed too high there is a risk of puncturing the conus medullaris if the needle inadvertently punctures the dura. In addition, coverage of sacral roots needed during the second stage may be inadequate. If the catheter is placed lower than L4 the neuraxial block may not adequately cover the nerves that innervate the uterus and cervix and may not provide the necessary labor analgesia for uterine contractions and cervical dilation. (563)

60. Prior to infusion of local anesthetic through an epidural catheter a test dose typically composed of 3 mL of 1.5% lidocaine containing 1:200,000 epinephrine is infused. The anesthesia provider waits 3 minutes to confirm no increase in heart rate or blood pressure and no systemic symptoms of lidocaine infusion have resulted such as tinnitus or perioral tingling. Additionally, the patient is asked to move her lower extremities to confirm that the bolus was not placed in the intrathecal space, which would result in motor blockade. (563)

61. In the CSE technique a spinal needle is placed through the epidural needle and an intrathecal dose of local anesthetic or opioid is administered. A 24- to 27-gauge pencil-point spinal needle is commonly selected to reduce the risk of post–dural puncture headache (PDPH). Benefits of this technique are its quicker onset of analgesia and no motor blockade if opioids (e.g., 10 to 20 μg fentanyl) are used alone in the intrathecal space. One disadvantage of a CSE is the delay in verification of a functioning epidural catheter. (563)

62. A test dose can be and should be utilized with the CSE technique. The test will confirm whether the catheter is intravascular by changes in heart rate and blood pressure, and unintended intrathecal catheter placement can still be assessed as the patient should still be able to move her lower extremities after typical spinal local anesthetic doses (e.g., 2.5 mg bupivacaine) in the spinal portion of the CSE. (563)

63. Patient-controlled epidural analgesia (PCEA) allows the patient to deliver a chosen anesthetic mixture with or without a background infusion through programmable infusion pumps. Advantages of PCEA include reduced need for medical personnel, decreased motor block, improved patient satisfaction, and lower local anesthetic consumption. This method of epidural analgesia does not result in increased maternal or neonatal adverse events. (563)

64. The programmed intermittent epidural boluses (PIEB) technique administers fixed epidural boluses at scheduled intervals. This technique can be used alone or with a PCEA technique. The PIEB technique may slightly reduce local anesthetic usage, improve maternal satisfaction, and decrease the need for rescue boluses. (563)

65. If primarily perineal anesthesia is needed (i.e., forceps delivery, perineal laceration repair), the patient may be left in the sitting position for 2 to 3 minutes and hyperbaric local anesthetic used in order to concentrate the sensory block toward the sacral fibers ("saddle block"). A true saddle block anesthetic (requiring more time in the sitting position) does not produce complete uterine pain relief because the afferent fibers (extending to T10) from the uterus are not blocked. (565)

CONTRAINDICATIONS AND COMPLICATIONS OF NEURAXIAL ANESTHESIA

66. Certain conditions contraindicate neuraxial procedures, including (1) patient refusal, (2) infection at the needle insertion site, (3) significant coagulopathy, (4) hypovolemic shock, (5) increased intracranial pressure from mass lesion, and (6) inadequate provider expertise. Other conditions such as systemic infection, neurologic disease, and mild coagulopathies are relative contraindications and should be evaluated on a case-by-case basis. (565)

67. Neither HIV nor hepatitis infection is a contraindication to placement of neuraxial anesthesia. (565)

68. Possible complications of neuraxial analgesia include inadequate block, hypotension, intravascular catheter placement, systemic toxicity of local anesthetic, unintentional intrathecal catheter placement, excessive blockade, post–dural puncture headache (PDPH), epidural hematoma, epidural abscesses, meningitis, and nerve or spinal cord injury. Other side effects include pruritus, nausea, shivering, urinary retention, motor weakness, low back soreness, and a prolonged block. (565)

69. The rate of accidental dural puncture during epidural catheter placement is approximately 1% to 2%, and approximately half of these will result in a severe headache. PDPHs are typically managed with analgesics, hydration, rest, caffeine, and blood patch if necessary. (565)

70. If accidental intravascular injection of local anesthetic occurs, dose-dependent effects can be mild (tinnitus, perioral tingling, mild arterial blood pressure and heart rate changes) or major (seizures, loss of consciousness, severe arrhythmias, cardiovascular collapse). (565)

71. If systemic bupivacaine local anesthetic overdose occurs, in addition to following standard ACLS algorithms for pregnancy, consider use of a 20% IV lipid emulsion to bind the drug and decrease toxicity. (566)

72. A high spinal (total spinal) can result from an unrecognized epidural catheter placed subdural, migration of the catheter during its use, or an overdose of local anesthetic in the epidural space (i.e., high epidural). Both high spinals and high epidurals can result in severe maternal hypotension, bradycardia, loss of consciousness, and blockade of the motor nerves to the respiratory muscles. (566)

73. ACLS guidelines for pregnancy include use of left uterine displacement, avoidance of lower extremity vessels for drug delivery, chest compressions positioned slightly higher on the sternum, and no modifications to the defibrillation protocol except removal of fetal and uterine monitors prior to shock, unless it would result in a significant delay. In any situation of maternal cardiac arrest with unsuccessful resuscitation, the fetus should be emergently delivered if the mother does not have return of spontaneous circulation (ROSC) within 4 minutes of the arrest. This guideline for emergent cesarean delivery increases the chances of survival for both the mother and neonate. The use of checklists and prior simulation can improve health care provider performance in these rare but critical events. (566)

74. Hypotension (decrease in systolic blood pressure >20%) secondary to sympathetic blockade is the most common complication of neuraxial blockade for labor analgesia, with rates of approximately 14%. Left uterine displacement and hydration are used to decrease hypotension with initiation of neuraxial blockade. (566)

75. Small vasopressor boluses of either phenylephrine or ephedrine can be used to treat hypotension. Although ephedrine was historically used primarily, phenylephrine is now the preferred treatment as it is associated with less placental transfer and fetal acidosis. However, because significant decreases in maternal heart rate are associated with a decreased cardiac output, both heart rate and blood pressure should be considered when determining vasopressor management. If treated promptly, maternal hypotension does not lead to fetal depression or neonatal morbidity. (566)

76. Labor epidural anesthesia can be associated with a rise in maternal body temperature. Interestingly, only about 20% of women with labor epidurals develop a fever, and the remaining 80% have no body temperature increase. The cause of the temperature increase remains uncertain but appears associated with noninfectious proinflammatory cytokines. The temperature rise is not associated with an increase in maternal white blood cell count or the incidence of neonatal sepsis. (566)

OTHER NERVE BLOCKS FOR LABOR ANALGESIA

77. For a paracervical block, local anesthetic must be injected submucosal, lateral, and posterior to the uterocervical junction bilaterally. Sensory fibers originating from the uterus, cervix, and upper vagina travel through this area. Therefore, this block is most effective to help provide analgesia during the first stage of labor and is usually not effective for the second stage of labor. The major disadvantage of a paracervical block is potential fetal bradycardia. In approximately 15% of laboring women who receive this block, fetal bradycardia develops 2 to 10 minutes after the local anesthetic solution is injected. Although the definitive cause of the bradycardia is not known, it is often associated with fetal acidosis. The bradycardia is normally limited to less than 15 minutes with supportive treatment as needed. (566)

78. A pudendal nerve block is useful for anesthesia of the lower vagina and perineum needed for delivery with an episiotomy or low forceps delivery. This technique can be used when neuraxial anesthesia is unavailable. The obstetrician typically performs this block, which is done transvaginally with the woman in the lithotomy position. The failure rate is high and complications include local anesthetic toxicity, ischiorectal or vaginal hematoma, and rarely, fetal injection of local anesthetic. (567)

ANESTHESIA FOR CESAREAN DELIVERY

79. Benefits of regional anesthesia over general anesthesia for cesarean delivery include avoidance of the risks of general anesthesia, including the decreased risk of pulmonary aspiration, difficult airway, decreased fetal depression from exposure to anesthetic agents, placement of neuraxial opioids for postoperative pain, and the maintenance of maternal awareness. No clinically significant differences in neonatal outcome after cesarean delivery with regional anesthesia or general anesthesia have been shown. (567)

80. Benefits of general anesthesia over regional anesthesia for cesarean delivery include rapid and dependable onset, secure airway, controlled ventilation, and potential for less hemodynamic instability. (567)

81. Advantages of spinal anesthesia compared to epidural anesthesia for cesarean delivery include its technical ease of administration, low levels of systemic medication that decrease the risk of systemic toxicity and fetal drug levels, its low failure rate, and its rapid onset time. Disadvantages of spinal anesthesia for cesarean delivery include the finite time of anesthesia provided and its higher incidence of hypotension. It can be safely used in preeclamptic patients. (567)

82. Spinal anesthesia with a sensory level of T4 is usually sufficient for patient comfort during cesarean delivery. Exteriorization of the uterus or traction of the abdominal viscera may still lead to discomfort in the woman. A T4 sensory level can be achieved with the administration of hyperbaric bupivacaine 10 to 15 mg. The medication will flow with the spinal curvature to a position near T4. (567)

83. Advantages of epidural anesthesia for cesarean delivery include the ability to extend the duration of anesthesia if necessary, to control block height, and to slowly titrate the dose to avoid precipitous maternal hypotension. Disadvantages of epidural anesthesia for cesarean delivery include the potential for intravascular injection of toxic levels of local anesthetic and its technical difficulty, longer onset time, less reliability, and increased perception of visceral pain with peritoneal manipulation. (567)

84. An approximate volume of 15 to 20 mL of local anesthetic solution must be delivered in the epidural space to achieve the T4 to sacrum sensory level of anesthesia necessary for cesarean delivery. Before the administration of such high volumes of local anesthetics a test dose for epidural catheter placement should be administered. Local anesthetics typically administered for cesarean delivery by epidural catheter placement include 2% lidocaine and 3% 2-chloroprocaine. Each of these should be administered in increments to further minimize the risk of accidental IV administration of toxic levels of local anesthetic. Addition of epinephrine (1:200,000) or fentanyl (50 to 100 µg) can enhance the intensity and duration of the block. For the rapid onset of analgesia with a lumbar epidural catheter, as in an urgent cesarean delivery, 3% 2-chloroprocaine has the quickest onset. (567)

85. The epidural administration of preservative-free morphine during cesarean delivery decreases postoperative pain requirements up to 24 hours after the operation. The dose of epidural morphine commonly administered is 1.5 to 3 mg. Side effects of epidural morphine include pruritus, nausea and vomiting, and, on rare occasions, delayed respiratory depression. (568)

86. Indications for general anesthesia for cesarean delivery include fetal distress and required emergent delivery to prevent poor fetal outcome, maternal hemorrhage, and contraindications to regional anesthesia such as maternal coagulopathy or maternal refusal. Benefits of general anesthesia for cesarean delivery include a more reliable and rapid onset of anesthesia, less hypotension and hemodynamic instability than regional anesthesia, and control of the airway and ventilation. (568)

87. The relative risk of general anesthesia for cesarean delivery is 1.7 times that of neuraxial anesthesia. The majority of the mortality risk is associated with failed intubation or issues surrounding the induction period. Appropriate airway examination, preparation, familiarity with various airway techniques, and an algorithm for the difficult airway are critical for providing a safe anesthetic. (568)

88. Contributing factors associated with a difficult intubation during pregnancy include inadequate time for preoperative evaluation of the airway, unpredicted airway edema, and emergency situations. If a difficult airway is suspected preoperatively, an awake fiberoptic intubation of the trachea should be considered. The anesthesiologist must have a difficult airway algorithm readily available

to follow should she or he be confronted with a difficult or failed intubation. There should be equipment immediately available for the difficult airway, such as a variety of functioning laryngoscope blades, several sizes of endotracheal tubes, laryngeal mask airways, a fiberoptic bronchoscope, and the means to perform a cricothyrotomy. Extra help should be solicited. Numerous attempts at laryngoscopy should be avoided to prevent increasing airway edema and bleeding. If hypoxia should occur during attempted laryngoscopy, the patient should be hand ventilated with bag and mask while cricoid pressure is maintained. If intubation attempts fail, the cesarean delivery may proceed if the anesthesiologist communicates that she or he can reliably ventilate the mother with either face mask or laryngeal mask airway (LMA). Other options may include allowing the patient to resume spontaneous ventilation, waking the patient and fiberoptically intubating the trachea, or in dire circumstances of inadequate ventilation and hypoxemia, a surgical airway. (568)

89. Prior to the induction of general anesthesia for cesarean delivery a nonparticulate antacid should be administered, adequate preoxygenation is performed, and surgical readiness is confirmed. A rapid-sequence induction is typically performed. Maintenance of anesthesia is achieved with a combination of a volatile anesthetic, propofol, nitrous oxide, and additional muscle relaxant if needed. Opioid and benzodiazepine administration is usually delayed until after delivery of the baby to avoid placental transfer of these drugs. Following delivery, halogenated anesthetics should be partially or completely replaced with other anesthetics to decrease uterine atony. Extubation of the trachea is done once the patient is awake and airway reflexes have returned. (568)

90. The level of exposure of the fetus to propofol after its administration to the pregnant patient for the induction of general anesthesia is generally low. No significant effects on the newborn behavior scores and markers of well-being are noted with typical induction doses of 2.5 mg/kg, but large doses of 9 mg/kg are associated with neonatal depression. (568)

91. Like propofol, etomidate has a quick onset because of its high lipid solubility. The rapid redistribution results in a relatively short duration of action. At typical induction doses (0.3 mg/kg), unlike propofol, etomidate has minimal cardiovascular effects, making it a suitable choice in for the induction of anesthesia in the pregnant patient who is actively hemorrhaging, has uncertain intravascular fluid volume status, and is at risk for hypotension. Etomidate is painful on injection, can cause muscle tremors, has higher rates of nausea and vomiting, and has increased risk of seizures in patients with decreased thresholds. (568)

92. Ketamine induction (1 to 1.5 mg/kg) produces a rapid onset of anesthesia, but unlike propofol, ketamine increases arterial pressures, heart rate, and cardiac output through central stimulation of the sympathetic nervous system. This makes it advantageous in pregnant women with hemodynamic compromise, such as the pregnant patient who is actively hemorrhaging. If administered in an amount greater than a typical induction dose, ketamine can increase uterine tone, reduce uterine arterial perfusion, and lower seizure threshold. (568)

93. Benzodiazepines such as diazepam and midazolam readily cross the placenta and yield roughly equal maternal and fetal blood levels. Diazepam has active metabolites that can accumulate in the neonate and lead to respiratory depression. Induction doses of midazolam have been associated with profound neonatal hypotonia. (569)

94. Maintenance of anesthesia for cesarean delivery often includes the inhalation of a low concentration (<0.75 MAC) of halogenated anesthetic in combination with either nitrous oxide or propofol. The volatile anesthetic is an important component to decrease the incidence of maternal recall. Uterine tone after delivery is maintained when the concentration of volatile anesthetic used is low. Maternal blood loss is minimized, the uterine response to oxytocin is not altered, and little neonatal depression is seen. Placental transfer of

volatile anesthetics is rapid because they are nonionized, highly lipid-soluble substances of low molecular weight. Fetal concentrations depend on the concentration and duration of anesthetic administered to the mother. There is no evidence to show that neuraxial anesthesia is superior to general anesthesia for neonatal outcome. However, emergent delivery of a depressed fetus often results in a depressed neonate. A long time from induction to delivery may result in a lightly anesthetized, but not an asphyxiated, neonate. If excessive concentrations of volatile anesthetics are administered for prolonged periods, neonatal effects of these drugs, as evidenced by flaccidity, cardiorespiratory depression, and decreased tone, may be anticipated. It is important to recognize that if neonatal depression is due to transfer of anesthetic drugs, the infant is merely anesthetized and should respond easily to simple treatment measures such as assisted ventilation of the lungs to facilitate excretion of the volatile anesthetic. Rapid improvement of the infant should be expected, and if it does not occur, it is important to search for other causes of depression. (569–570)

95. Succinylcholine (1 to 1.5 mg/kg IV) remains the neuromuscular blocking drug of choice for obstetric anesthesia because of its rapid onset and short duration of action. Because it is highly ionized and poorly lipid-soluble, only small amounts cross the placenta. It is normally hydrolyzed in maternal blood by the enzyme pseudocholinesterase and does not generally interfere with fetal neuromuscular activity. If large doses are given (2 to 3 mg/kg) it results in detectable levels in umbilical cord blood, and extreme doses (10 mg/kg) are needed for the transfer to result in neonatal neuromuscular blockade. Rocuronium is an acceptable alternative. It provides adequate intubating conditions in approximately 60 seconds at doses of 1.2 mg/kg. Unlike succinylcholine it has a much longer duration of action, potentially decreasing maternal safety in the event the anesthesiologist is unable to intubate or ventilate the patient. Under normal circumstances, the poorly lipid-soluble, highly ionized, nondepolarizing neuromuscular blockers do not cross the placenta in amounts significant enough to cause neonatal muscle weakness. This placental impermeability is only relative, and when large doses are given over long periods, neonatal neuromuscular blockade can occur. Uterine smooth muscle is not affected by neuromuscular blockade. (570)

ABNORMAL PRESENTATIONS AND MULTIPLE BIRTHS

96. In 2013 twin pregnancy accounted for 3.4% of the live births. The vast majority of multiple gestations are twin (97% to 98%). Higher order multiples account for only 0.1% to 0.2% of births. Multiple pregnancies pose a significant risk to both the mother and the fetuses, with a higher rate of preterm labor, preeclampsia, gestational diabetes, preterm premature rupture of membranes, intrauterine growth restriction, and intrauterine fetal demise. The United States is seeing an increase in multiple gestations with the expanded use of artificial reproductive technologies. (571)

97. The majority of twin pregnancies are vertex-vertex positioning of the fetuses and can be delivered vaginally. If the second twin is breech, it is important to discuss the mode of delivery with the obstetricians and perinatologists. If a vaginal delivery is attempted, an emergent cesarean delivery might be required if the second twin changes position after delivery of the first or develops fetal bradycardia. Placement of an epidural can facilitate delivery and extraction of the second twin if it becomes necessary for the obstetrician to perform an instrumented delivery of the second twin. At the late second stage of delivery a more concentrated local anesthetic will optimize the perineal anesthesia. Drugs that provide quick uterine relaxation (IV nitroglycerin) also improve delivery conditions. At this time, the potential for head entrapment or fetal bradycardia is highest, and a denser block allows for possible transition to cesarean delivery. (571)

98. Singleton breech presentation occurs in about 3% to 4% of all pregnancies. External cephalic version (ECV) has a mean success rate of approximately 60%. The procedure involves rotating the fetus via external palpation and pressure of the fetal parts. Neuraxial analgesia may improve success of the ECV. The risks of ECV include placental abruption, fetal bradycardia, and rupture of membranes. The anesthesia provider should be immediately available if an ECV is being performed in case an urgent or emergent cesarean delivery is needed. (571)

99. A shoulder dystocia occurs when, after delivery of the fetal head, further expulsion of the infant is prevented by impaction of the fetal shoulders with the maternal pelvis. Shoulder dystocia occurs in approximately 1% to 1.5% of all deliveries and is an obstetric surgical emergency. Risk factors include macrosomia, diabetes, obesity, history of dystocia, labor induction, and instrumented delivery. Fetal pH declines 0.04 unit/min between delivery of the head and trunk. Once shoulder dystocia is diagnosed, a set of maneuvers is performed to deliver the infant, with the final maneuver being pushing the fetus back up and proceeding to emergent cesarean delivery. Cases of shoulder dystocia 7 minutes or longer have a significant increase in risk of neonatal brain injury. Among the fetal injuries and sequelae of shoulder dystocia are brachial plexus injury, neurologic injury from asphyxia, and broken clavicle. Often these neurologic injuries improve over time with roughly less than 10% permanent Erb palsy. (571)

HYPERTENSIVE DISORDERS OF PREGNANCY

100. The four classifications of hypertensive disorders in pregnancy are preeclampsia-eclampsia, chronic hypertension, chronic hypertension with superimposed preeclampsia, and gestational hypertension. Gestational hypertension is diagnosed in previously normotensive women who develop elevated blood pressure (SBP >140 mm Hg or DBP >90 mm Hg) after 20 weeks of gestational age. Chronic hypertension is elevated blood pressures predating pregnancy, occurring prior to 20 weeks of gestation, or persisting for more than 12 weeks post partum. (572)

101. Preeclampsia affects 7.5% of pregnant women worldwide. Risk factors include primigravida, chronic hypertension, gestational/preexisting diabetes, obesity, preeclamptic family history, multiple gestation, and use of assisted reproductive technology. (572)

102. The criteria for the diagnosis of preeclampsia is SBP higher than 140 mm Hg or DBP higher than 90 mm Hg that occurs after 20 weeks of gestation or during the postpartum period in a previously normotensive woman. This increase in blood pressure is either associated with excess protein in the urine or the new development of thrombocytopenia (platelets less than 100,000), renal insufficiency, impaired liver function, cerebral or visual disturbances, or pulmonary edema. Proteinuria is defined as urinary excretion of 0.3 g protein or higher in a 24-hour urine specimen. (572)

103. Preeclampsia with severe features is diagnosed if one or more of the following criteria are present:
    - SBP higher than 160 mm Hg or DBP higher than 110 mm Hg on two occasions at least 4 hours apart while the patient is on bed rest
    - Thrombocytopenia (platelet count less than 100,000/µL)
    - Impaired liver function as indicated by abnormally elevated blood concentrations of liver enzymes (to twice normal concentration), severe persistent right upper quadrant or epigastric pain unresponsive to medication and not accounted for by alternative diagnoses, or both
    - Progressive renal insufficiency (serum creatinine concentration greater than 1.1 mg/dL or a doubling of the serum creatinine concentration in the absence of other renal disease)
    - Pulmonary edema
    - New-onset cerebral or visual disturbances (572)

104. A subcategory of severe preeclampsia is HELLP syndrome, which is a constellation of Hemolysis, Elevated Liver enzymes, and Low Platelet count. (572)

105. Although the exact cause remains unknown, preeclampsia begins with the pathogenic maternal/fetal interface. During placental formation there is failure of complete trophoblast cell invasion of the uterine spiral arteries, creating decreased placental perfusion. This may ultimately lead to early placental hypoxia. Ultimately there is upregulation of cytokines and inflammatory factors as seen in sepsis. (572)

106. Currently, the definitive treatment of preeclampsia is delivery. If the pregnancy is remote from term in the presence of severe preeclampsia, a determination must be made whether to deliver or expectantly manage. This requires repeated evaluation of the mother and fetus. It is critical for the anesthesiologist on labor and delivery to be aware of these patients and their clinical course, as they can rapidly deteriorate and require urgent or emergent delivery. (572)

107. Magnesium sulfate is used for seizure prophylaxis in preeclamptic women. The infusion is usually performed by loading 4 to 6 g over 20 to 30 minutes, then a continued magnesium sulfate infusion of 1 to 2 g/h until 12 to 24 hours after delivery. Considerations of the use of magnesium sulfate infusions in this patient population include its potentiation of neuromuscular blockade of both depolarizing and nondepolarizing muscle relaxants, its effect of uterine and smooth muscle relaxation, and that magnesium sulfate is excreted renally and may have prolonged effects in patients with decreased renal function. (573)

108. Magnesium sulfate toxicity can be seen clinically as loss of deep tendon reflexes, respiratory depression, and neurologic compromise. The therapeutic blood level range for seizure prophylaxis is between 6 and 8 mg/dL. Loss of deep tendon reflexes occurs at 10 mg/dL with prolonged PQ intervals and widening QRS complex on the electrocardiogram. Respiratory arrest occurs at 15 to 20 mg/dL, and asystole occurs when the level exceeds 20 to 25 mg/dL. If toxicity occurs, IV calcium chloride (500 mg) or calcium gluconate (1 g) should be administered. (573)

109. Current guidelines recommend treating women with preeclampsia with an SBP higher than 160 mm Hg to prevent intracerebral hemorrhage. Initial therapy normally includes IV labetalol and hydralazine. However, without IV access oral nifedipine can be considered. In refractory severe hypertension, nitroglycerin and sodium nitroprusside may be used in the acute situation with appropriate invasive monitoring. (573)

110. Neuraxial analgesia is the preferred analgesic for preeclamptic patients, but there are several anesthetic considerations related to its administration. Hemoglobin and platelet levels should be evaluated, the risk-benefit ratio should be discussed with the patient, including the risk of epidural hematoma, platelet levels may need to be reevaluated prior to removal of an epidural catheter, and hypotension should be cautiously treated to avoid rebound hypertension due to catecholamine sensitivity. (573)

111. Anesthetic considerations in the urgent or emergent delivery in patients with preeclampsia include their increased risk for upper airway edema and difficult intubation, the potential for exaggerated hypertension associated with laryngoscopy, possible uterine atony secondary to magnesium sulfate in combination with an inhaled anesthetic, and the relative contraindication of methylergonovine for the treatment of uterine atony as its administration can precipitate a hypertensive crisis in this patient population. (573)

HEMORRHAGE IN PREGNANT WOMEN

112. Placenta previa, abruptio placentae, and uterine rupture are major causes of bleeding in the third trimester and during labor. Postpartum hemorrhage occurs in 3% to 5% of all vaginal deliveries and is typically due to uterine atony, retained placenta, placenta accreta, or lacerations involving the cervix or vagina. Morbidity can be reduced through recognition of the risk of hemorrhage, quantification of blood loss, preparation, and prompt treatment. (574)

113. Placenta previa is an abnormal uterine implantation of the placenta in front of the presenting fetus. The incidence is approximately 1 in 200 pregnancies. Risk factors include advanced age, multiparity, assisted reproductive techniques, prior hysterotomy, and prior placenta previa. Placenta previa classically presents as painless vaginal bleeding that usually occurs preterm in the third trimester, although most previas are now diagnosed antenatally by ultrasonography. (574)

114. A trial of labor may be acceptable in some patients with placenta previa based on the distance of the previa edge from the cervical os. In these situations, neuraxial analgesia can be appropriate in the absence of active bleeding. For cesarean section large-bore IV lines, fluid warmers, invasive monitoring, and the availability of blood products are indicated. In an emergent situation, induction of anesthesia with ketamine or etomidate may be useful. Massive transfusion protocol may be instituted. If hemorrhage is not controlled with standard measures, the obstetric team can consider (1) uterine artery ligation, (2) B-Lynch sutures, (3) an intrauterine balloon, (4) use of arterial embolization by interventional radiology if the patient is stable for transport, or (5) hysterectomy. (574)

115. Abruptio placentae is separation of the placenta after 20 weeks of gestation, but before delivery. The incidence is approximately 1 in 100 pregnancies and is associated with a seven times increase in maternal mortality. Risk factors include advanced age, hypertension, trauma, smoking, cocaine use, chorioamnionitis, premature rupture of membranes, and history of prior abruption. (574)

116. The patient with abruptio placentae often has painful, frequent uterine contractions. When the separation involves the placental margin, it can present as vaginal bleeding with associated uterine tenderness. Abruptio placentae can also occur without vaginal bleeding in which blood can accumulate in large volumes (>2 L) and be entirely concealed within the uterus. Therefore, the degree of vaginal bleeding may not reflect the total amount of blood loss from the placenta. Chronic bleeding and clotting between the uterus and placenta can cause maternal disseminated intravascular coagulopathy (DIC). Severe hemorrhage necessitates emergent cesarean delivery and the use of general anesthesia. (574)

117. Risk factors for uterine rupture include prior uterine scar, rapid spontaneous delivery, motor vehicle trauma, trauma from instrumented vaginal delivery, large or malpositioned fetus, and excessive oxytocin stimulation. After previous cesarean delivery, vaginal birth is associated with a 1% or less incidence of uterine rupture. The presentation of uterine rupture is variable but may include vaginal bleeding, cessation of contractions, fetal bradycardia, loss of station, and persistent abdominal pain normally not masked by neuraxial analgesia. Unfortunately, none of these findings is 100% sensitive. An abnormal FHR pattern represents the most common associated sign of uterine rupture. Although persistent abdominal pain between contractions is highly correlated with uterine rupture, it is not always present. (575)

118. Retained placenta occurs when some portion of the placenta has not been spontaneously delivered within 1 hour of delivery of the fetus. Uterine bleeding continues as a result of the inability of the uterus to contract around adherent placenta. Approximately 2% to 3% of all vaginal deliveries are associated with some retained placenta. The treatment involves manual exploration of the uterus for the removal of retained placental parts. The anesthetic management of patients with retained placenta has as its goal uterine relaxation as well as decreasing the pain and anxiety of the patient. Anesthetic methods that may be used to initially accomplish this typically include IV sedation (keeping airway reflexes intact) or dosing of a preexisting epidural catheter. If uterine relaxation is necessary for assisted placental removal, nitroglycerin (given in 200-μg IV boluses) is normally effective. Additionally, relocation to the operating

room and placement of neuraxial analgesia may be beneficial for thorough evaluation. Rarely, induction of general anesthesia with tracheal intubation and administration of a volatile anesthetic to provide uterine relaxation will be necessary. (575)

119. Risk factors for postpartum uterine atony include retained products, long labor, high parity, macrosomia, polyhydramnios, excessive oxytocin augmentation, and chorioamnionitis. Uterine atony can occur immediately after delivery or several hours later. (575)

120. The treatment of uterine atony is by the administration of agents that increase uterine tone. Oxytocin (20 to 40 IU/L wide-open IV infusion or with algorithms that bolus 3 IU at a time) is normally the initial treatment. This dilute solution of oxytocin exerts minimal cardiovascular effects, but rapid IV injection is associated with tachycardia, vasodilation, and hypotension. Methylergonovine (0.2 mg IM) is an ergot derivative. Because of the significant vasoconstriction, it is relatively contraindicated in preeclamptics and patients with cardiac disease. The prostaglandin $F_{2\alpha}$ (0.25 mg IM) is associated with nausea, tachycardia, pulmonary hypertension, desaturation, and bronchospasm. It should be avoided in asthmatics. Prostaglandin E_1 (600 μg oral/sublingual/rectal) has no significant cardiac effects but may cause hyperthermia. (575)

121. Placental implantation beyond the endometrium gives rise to (1) placenta accreta vera, which is implantation and adherence onto the myometrium; (2) placenta increta, which is implantation into the myometrium; and (3) placenta percreta, which is penetration through the full thickness of the myometrium. With placenta percreta, implantations may occur onto bowel, bladder, ovaries, or other pelvic organs and vessels. (575)

122. In patients with placenta previa and no previous cesarean delivery, the incidence of accreta is approximately 3%. However, the risk of placenta accreta associated with placenta previa increases with the number of previous cesarean deliveries. With one previous uterine incision, the incidence of placenta accreta has been reported to be 11%, with two previous uterine incisions the rate is 40%, and with three or more prior uterine incisions the incidence rises to above 60%. Patients with both placenta previa and accreta can have rapid and massive intraoperative blood loss, with a reported median of blood loss ranging from 2000 mL to 5000 mL. (575–576)

AMNIOTIC FLUID EMBOLISM

123. The incidence of amniotic fluid embolism (AFE) is estimated between 1 and 6 cases per 100,000 deliveries. Clinical features of AFE include the sudden onset of hypotension, respiratory distress, hypoxia, disseminated intravascular coagulopathy, altered mental status, and eventual maternal collapse. These signs must be differentiated from other more common morbidities of pregnancy and delivery, such as acute hemorrhage, inhalation of gastric contents, air embolism, pulmonary thromboembolism, high spinal, anaphylaxis, peripartum cardiomyopathy, and local anesthetic toxicity. (576)

124. The diagnosis of AFE is a clinical diagnosis of exclusion because no diagnostic laboratory test for AFE currently exists. Although in the past it had been believed that aspirating amniotic fluid debris such as fetal squamous cells from the maternal pulmonary circulation was diagnostic, the presence of fetal squames has been demonstrated in asymptomatic pregnant women. Definitive diagnosis is extremely difficult or impossible, even with postmortem examination. (576)

ANESTHESIA FOR NONOBSTETRIC SURGERY DURING PREGNANCY

125. The most common causes of nonobstetric surgeries that occur during pregnancy are trauma, appendicitis, and cholecystitis. The incidence is as high as 1% to 2% of pregnancies. (576)

126. Elective procedures for the pregnant patient should be delayed until at least 6 weeks post partum. When possible, nonurgent operations should be delayed

until after the first trimester in order to minimize teratogenic effects on the fetus or spontaneous abortion. The second trimester is considered the optimal time for surgical intervention, as the risk of preterm labor is higher in the third trimester. In the case of acutely urgent surgical procedures, their timing should mimic that of nonpregnant patients. (577)

127. Considerations for the anesthetic management of pregnant patients undergoing nonobstetric surgery include maternal awareness, hemodynamics, respiration, deep venous thrombus prophylaxis, postoperative analgesia, the prevention of intrauterine fetal hypoxia and acidosis, the concern for spontaneous abortion or preterm labor, and monitoring of FHR and uterine activity often for 24 hours postoperatively. For these reasons the anesthesia provider should consult with an obstetrician and perinatologist to determine a plan for unexpected events, determine if FHR monitoring is appropriate, and discuss a plan for cesarean delivery should it become necessary for a maternal or fetal indication. There is no evidence that regional techniques provided better outcomes to either mother or fetus compared to general anesthesia for these patients. (577)

128. Routine pregnancy testing for women of childbearing age prior to undergoing surgery remains controversial. Because there is a possibility that anesthesia will unknowingly be administered to women in early pregnancy, ASA guidelines recommend "pregnancy testing may be offered to female patients of childbearing age and for whom the result would alter the patient's management." (577)

129. Because the critical gestational period for organogenesis occurs between 15 and 56 days of gestation, teratogenic drugs administered during this time will exert their most disastrous effects. In animal studies most drugs, including anesthetics, have been demonstrated to be teratogenic in at least one animal species. Most data regarding the administration of anesthetics to pregnant women in the first trimester are retrospective. There is no evidence that any of the currently used local or systemic anesthetics are teratogenic (with the exception of cocaine) when administered during pregnancy. Neurodegeneration and widespread apoptosis following exposure to anesthetics has been clearly established in developing animals, and a few studies demonstrate cognitive impairment in adult animals after neonatal anesthetic exposure. Similar to the fetus, the long-term effects of anesthetic exposure in young children remain unknown. Some, but not all, studies suggest neurocognitive deficits could occur following anesthetic exposure in infants and toddlers. (577)

130. Intrauterine fetal hypoxia and acidosis has been associated with maternal hypotension, arterial hypoxemia, and excessive changes in the $Paco_2$. During surgery, the goals are maintenance of normocarbia and adequate uterine perfusion pressure using fluids, vasopressors, and uterine displacement if after 20 weeks of gestational age. It is recommended that the maternal inhaled concentration of oxygen should be at least 50%. High oxygen consumption of the placenta, uneven distribution of maternal and fetal blood flow in the placenta, and specific hemoglobin binding characteristics prevent fetal Pao_2 from exceeding about 60 mm Hg even with high maternal arterial oxygen levels. (577)

131. FHR monitoring via Doppler is possible at 16 to 18 weeks of gestational age, but variability as a marker of fetal well-being is not established until 25 to 27 weeks. Fetal monitoring can display fetal compromise and allows further optimization of the maternal and fetal condition with in utero resuscitation maneuvers. Currently there is no evidence for the efficacy of FHR monitoring. In addition, interpretation is difficult as most anesthetics reduce FHR variability, placement and signal acquisition may be challenging, and a trained person is needed for interpretation. The decision of whether or not to monitor the FHR during nonobstetric surgery should be individualized case by case in discussion with an obstetrician and other perioperative team members. (577)

132. The usual cause of premature labor that presents in the pregnant woman after having nonobstetric surgery is the underlying pathologic process that led to the need for surgery and not the anesthetic technique. Intra-abdominal procedures have more risk than minor peripheral procedures. Postoperative monitors should include continuous FHR monitoring and monitoring of maternal uterine activity. Premature labor can be treated through the administration of tocolytics in consultation with an obstetrician. Common tocolytics include terbutaline, indomethacin, and nifedipine. (577)

133. Laparoscopic surgery is as safe as an open approach during any trimester, and the indications for its use are the same as for nonpregnant patients. Trimester does not influence the complication rate, and the conversion to open is low (1%). There is a slightly higher fetal loss rate, but a lower preterm delivery rate is noted compared to open approaches. Most studies comparing laparoscopic to open techniques note no difference in fetal or maternal outcomes. (578)

DIAGNOSIS AND MANAGEMENT OF FETAL DISTRESS

134. Normal uterine activity is 5 contractions or less in 10 minutes, averaged over a 30-minute window, whereas tachysystole is defined as more than 5 contractions in 10 minutes, averaged over a 30-minute window. If a tonic contraction or period of tachysystole occurs during labor, treatment with either sublingual or IV nitroglycerin can briefly relax the uterus and restore fetal perfusion. In addition, the obstetrician can administer subcutaneous terbutaline. (578)

135. Intrapartum FHR monitoring was designed to detect hypoxia in labor and allow the clinicians to intervene prior to acidosis and long-term fetal central nervous system (CNS) damage. The fetal brain responds to peripheral and central stimuli: (1) chemoreceptors, (2) baroreceptors, and (3) direct effects of metabolic changes within the CNS. FHR monitoring was developed as a crude, nonspecific method of tracking fetal oxygenation and distress. (578)

136. The normal baseline FHR is between 110 and 160 beats per minute. (578)

137. Baseline variability is determined by examining fluctuations that are irregular in amplitude and frequency during a 10-minute window excluding accelerations and decelerations. Variability is classified as follows:
    a. Absent FHR variability: amplitude range undetectable
    b. Minimal FHR variability: amplitude range greater than undetectable and 5 beats/min or less
    c. Moderate FHR variability: amplitude range 6 beats/minute to 25 beats/min
    d. Marked FHR variability: amplitude range above 25 beats/min (579)

138. An FHR acceleration is an abrupt increase in FHR defined as an increase from the acceleration onset to the peak in less than 30 seconds. In addition, the peak must be 15 beats/min or more and last 15 seconds or longer from the onset to return. Before 32 weeks of gestation, accelerations are defined as having a peak 10 beats/min and duration of 10 seconds or longer. (579)

139. Late decelerations are a result of uteroplacental insufficiency causing relative fetal brain hypoxia during a contraction. The change results in sympathetic response and increased peripheral vascular resistance in the fetus, elevating the fetal blood pressure, which is detected by the fetal baroreceptors and results in a slowing in the FHR. In addition, the relative hyperemia causes a chemoreceptor-mediated stimulation of the vagus nerve and decrease in FHR. Another type of late deceleration is decompensation of the myocardial circulation and fetal myocardial failure in the presence of worsening hypoxia. (579)

140. Variable decelerations are generally synonymous with umbilical cord compression. (579)

141. A three-tiered FHR classification system is currently used for a more general fetal assessment. To qualify as normal, or category I, all of the following apply: baseline FHR between 110 and 160 beats/min, moderate baseline

FHR variability, no late or variable decelerations, early decelerations may be present or absent, and accelerations may be present or absent. Category II FHR tracing is considered indeterminate. FHR tracings in category II include fetal tachycardia, prolonged decelerations more than 2 minutes but less than 10 minutes, and recurrent late decelerations with moderate baseline variability. Category III FHR tracings are abnormal and associated with abnormal fetal acid-base state. These tracings may include a sinusoidal FHR pattern or absent FHR variability with recurrent late decelerations, recurrent variable decelerations, or bradycardia. (579)

142. Category III FHR tracings require prompt patient evaluation and efforts to improve the fetal condition. Interventions may include change in the maternal position, treatment of hypotension, use of supplemental oxygen, and treatment of tachysystole if present. If the FHR tracing doesn't improve, expeditious delivery of the fetus should proceed. (580)

EVALUATION OF THE NEONATE AND NEONATAL RESUSCITATION

143. Apgar scoring system:

Characteristic	Score = 0	Score = 1	Score = 2
Heart rate (bpm)	Absent	<100	>100
Breathing	Absent	Slow	Irregular, crying
Reflex irritability	No response	Grimace	Cry
Muscle tone	Limp	Flexion of the extremities	Active
Color	Cyanotic	Body pink, extremities cyanotic	Pink

(581)

144. Normal umbilical cord blood gas values:

Parameter	Mean Artery	Mean Vein
pH	7.27	7.34
P_{CO_2} (mm Hg)	50	40
P_{O_2} (mm Hg)	20	30
Bicarbonate (mEq/L)	23	21
Base excess (mEq/L)	−3.6	−2.6

(581)

145. During neonatal evaluation, if breathing and crying do not occur, then clearing of the airway (mouth then nose) and repeated stimulation should be performed. Following this, the 1-minute Apgar score is determined with evaluation of the respirations, heart rate, and color. In the event of apnea or heart rate less than 100 beats/min, positive-pressure hand ventilation should be provided with 21% oxygen or up to 100% oxygen using a properly fitted face mask (avoiding excessive inspiratory pressure >30 cm H_2O). Based on the current 2015 neonatal resuscitation guidelines, if the clinician begins with room air it is recommended that supplemental oxygen be titrated to achieve appropriate preductal oxygen saturation values that would be seen in a healthy infant. The guidelines note that 100% oxygen should be used if chest compressions are required. Chest compressions, intubation, and positive-pressure ventilation with 100% oxygen become indicated in the event the heart rate drops below 60 beats/min. (581)

146. The dose of epinephrine for neonatal resuscitation is 0.1 to 0.3 mL/kg of a 1:10,000 solution given rapidly intravenously through an umbilical artery catheter inserted just below the abdominal skin (preferred) or other IV access point. The dose may be repeated every 3 to 5 minutes, if necessary. (583)

147. Naloxone is no longer recommended for use in newborns in the delivery room. Should the newborn manifest respiratory depression in the delivery room, appropriate ventilation should be maintained until the neonate is transported to the intensive care nursery, where naloxone can be given if determined to be necessary. (583)

148. Currently, neonates at delivery with meconium-stained amniotic fluid (MSAF) who are at term and do not require intubation. However, if poor muscle tone, inadequate breathing efforts, or heart rate less than 100 beats/min are present after birth, resuscitation with positive-pressure ventilation should be initiated. Although a provider skilled in tracheal intubation should be present at all MSAF deliveries, routine intubation for tracheal suction below the cords in this setting is no longer suggested. Instead emphasis is on initiating ventilation within the first minute of life in nonbreathing or ineffectively breathing infants by clearing the airway and use of positive-pressure ventilation. (583)

34 PEDIATRICS

Erin A. Gottlieb and Dean B. Andropoulos

1. How do intercostal muscle tone and chest wall compliance in neonates compare with those of adults?
2. How does alveolar ventilation in neonates compare with that of adults?
3. How does the tidal volume per weight in neonates compare with that of adults?
4. How does the respiratory rate in neonates compare with that of adults?
5. How does carbon dioxide production in neonates compare with that of adults? How does the $Paco_2$ in neonates compare with that of adults?
6. How does the Pao_2 change in the first few days of life?
7. How does total lung capacity in neonates compare with that of adults?
8. How does the normal newborn breathing pattern compare with that of adults?
9. How do systemic vascular resistance and pulmonary vascular resistance change at birth?
10. At what ages do the ductus arteriosus, ductus venosus, and foramen ovale close? What percent of adults have a probe patent foramen ovale?
11. How does the oxygen consumption of a neonate compare with that of an adult?
12. How does the cardiac output of a neonate compare with that of an adult?
13. Are changes in the cardiac output of a neonate more dependent on changes in the heart rate or stroke volume?
14. How does autonomic innervation of the heart in neonates or infants compare with that of adults? What is the clinical significance of this?
15. How effective is kidney function at birth? When does kidney function become approximately equivalent to that of an adult?
16. At what age are adult levels of urine-concentrating abilities achieved?
17. How does the position of the oxyhemoglobin dissociation curve in a neonate compare with that of an adult? Describe how this affects the affinity of oxygen for hemoglobin. At what age does the curve approximate that of an adult?
18. How does the hemoglobin level of a neonate compare with that of an adult? How does the hemoglobin level change as the infant progresses to 2 years old?
19. What hemoglobin level is worrisome in the newborn? What hemoglobin level is worrisome in infants older than 6 months of age?
20. How well do neonates reflexively respond to hemorrhage as compared with adults?
21. What percent body weight in neonates is contributed by the extracellular fluid volume? How does this compare with an adult?
22. Why is intramuscular vitamin K given to all newborns?
23. What are some ways in which infants and children maintain normal body temperature? Why is maintenance of normal body temperature more difficult in neonates and children than in an adult?

PHARMACOLOGIC DIFFERENCES

24. What are some physiologic characteristics of neonates that explain the pharmacokinetic differences between infant and adult responses to drugs?
25. How does the hepatic metabolism of drugs in infants compare to that of adults?
26. How does the renal excretion of drugs in infants compare to that of adults?
27. How are the uptake and distribution of inhaled anesthetics different in neonates and infants when compared with those of adults?
28. What is the effect of intracardiac shunting on the rapidity of anesthesia induction with halogenated anesthetic gases?
29. How does the minimum alveolar concentration (MAC) of inhaled anesthetics change from birth to puberty?
30. What physiologic factors increase the sensitivity of neonates to the effects of intravenous anesthetics?
31. How does the dose of propofol change between neonates and adults?
32. How does the rate of plasma clearance of opioids differ between neonates and adults?
33. Are neonates more or less sensitive to nondepolarizing neuromuscular blocking drugs than adults? How does the initial drug dose differ between these two groups?
34. How does the duration of action of nondepolarizing neuromuscular blocking drugs differ between neonates and adults?
35. How does the dose of neostigmine necessary to antagonize neuromuscular blockade in the neonate compare with the dose necessary in the adult? How does this affect clinical practice?
36. How does the dose of succinylcholine necessary to produce neuromuscular blockade in the infant and neonate compare with the dose necessary in the adult?

FLUIDS AND ELECTROLYTES

37. What is the preferred crystalloid fluid to replace intraoperative losses and compensate for any preoperative fluid deficit?
38. What is a reasonable approach to replace preoperative fluid deficits in pediatric patients?
39. What is the recommendation for fluid maintenance and replacement in the pediatric population?
40. How are third-space losses and fluid replacement estimated according to the degree of invasiveness of the surgery? How does this contribute to an overall fluid management strategy for pediatric patients?
41. What is the goal for urine output when monitoring the intraoperative volume status of the pediatric patient?
42. When should glucose administration be considered in the pediatric population?

TRANSFUSION THERAPY

43. What formula can be used to help guide the anesthesiologist with blood loss replacement?
44. What is the transfusion threshold for packed red blood cells (PRBCs) in pediatric patients? What is the expected hemoglobin increase with PRBC transfusion?
45. What patients should have leukocyte reduction and irradiation of PRBC processing prior to transfusion?
46. What is the indication for a platelet transfusion in pediatric patients, and what is the expected response to platelet transfusion?
47. What is the usual indication for transfusion of fresh frozen plasma (FFP) in pediatric patients? What is the expected response to FFP administration?
48. What is the usual indication for administration of cryoprecipitate in pediatric patients? What factors are present in cryoprecipitate? What is the expected response to cryoprecipitate administration?

49. What is the indication for the administration of fibrinogen concentrate in pediatric patients? What are examples of pediatric cases in which fibrinogen replacement might be indicated?
50. What are some other pharmacologic agents that will either reduce blood loss or help achieve hemostasis with major blood loss surgery in pediatric patients?

THE PEDIATRIC AIRWAY

51. What are some aspects of the pediatric preoperative airway assessment?
52. What are some physiologic characteristics of the pediatric airway that differ from the adult airway?
53. Are supraglottic airways used for routine airway or difficult airway management in children? Is the use of the laryngeal mask associated with an increase in respiratory complications compared with tracheal intubation?
54. Why has the classic teaching that uncuffed endotracheal tubes should be used for intubating the trachea of pediatric patients under the age of 8 years changed?
55. What are some indications for cuffed endotracheal tubes in infants and small children?
56. What is the general approach to the difficult pediatric airway, and how does it differ from the adult difficult airway?
57. What is the leading cause of difficult airway management in infants and young children? What are some genetic syndromes that cause this condition?

ANESTHETIC CONSIDERATIONS

58. What history should be obtained from a preoperative evaluation of a pediatric patient? What are some considerations that are specific to the pediatric population with regard to the history and physical examination?
59. How can the preoperative evaluation help to identify patients at risk for malignant hyperthermia (MH) and anesthesia-induced rhabdomyolysis (AIR)?
60. What does a history of snoring, pauses in breathing, and gasping during sleep suggest? How does a history of obstructive sleep apnea alter the anesthetic plan for tonsillectomy and adenoidectomy?
61. What are the potential risks of anesthetizing a child with an upper respiratory infection (URI)?
62. What preoperative laboratory data may be important in the pediatric population?
63. What are the recommendations for the preoperative ingestion of solids and clear liquids for pediatric patients?
64. What are the common options for premedication in children?
65. What types of nonpharmacologic techniques can be used for allaying anxiety and assisting anesthetic induction in children?
66. What are some methods of maintaining intraoperative normothermia in the pediatric patient? Why is it important that these preparations are done in advance of bringing the patient into the operating room?
67. How can the induction of anesthesia be achieved in pediatric patients without an intravenous catheter in place?
68. What is a potential risk that can occur during stage 2 (the excitement phase) of an inhaled induction, and how can it be managed?
69. What is the indication for the placement of an intravenous catheter in the pediatric patient undergoing a surgical procedure?
70. When should an intravenous catheter be placed in the pediatric patient undergoing an inhaled induction?
71. How can the induction of anesthesia be achieved in pediatric patients with an intravenous catheter in place?
72. When is the intramuscular induction of anesthesia most commonly used? What drugs and doses are most often used?
73. How can the anesthesiologist regulate the intravenous fluids to be administered in the pediatric patient?

74. What is the concern regarding the use of succinylcholine in pediatric patients? What are some alternatives that may be used?

75. Under what circumstances is succinylcholine accepted for use for neuromuscular blockade in the pediatric population?

76. What are some signs the clinician may use to determine the adequacy of the depth of anesthesia for surgery in the pediatric population?

77. When hypotension accompanies the administration of volatile anesthetics to neonates, what is it likely to be indicative of?

78. How does intraoperative monitoring in the pediatric population differ from intraoperative monitoring in the adult population?

79. What problem may be encountered with the monitoring of end-tidal carbon dioxide concentrations in pediatric patients?

80. How should the size of a blood pressure cuff be selected? What errors in blood pressure measurement may be encountered with an erroneously sized cuff?

81. What veins may be used to monitor the central venous pressure in the neonate? In infants? In children?

82. Are most pediatric patients extubated "awake" or "deep"? What are some of the clinical implications of awake and deep extubation techniques? What are the potential benefits and risks of a deep extubation?

83. What are the potential benefits and risks of intravenous acetaminophen?

84. What are some regional anesthetic blocks that can be administered in the pediatric population?

85. Which local anesthetic and what dose are commonly used in a caudal anesthetic? What is the approximate duration of the postoperative pain relief obtained from this caudal anesthetic? How is the length of the dural sac different in children and adults?

86. What are some postoperative airway issues that may arise in the postanesthesia care unit (PACU) in the pediatric population?

87. What are some risk factors for postoperative nausea and vomiting in the pediatric population?

88. How can the risk of postoperative nausea and vomiting be decreased in pediatric patients?

89. What is emergence delirium?

90. What scales and methods are used for assessing pain in children in the postanesthesia care unit?

91. What are some examples of maladaptive behavioral changes that can occur for the first few days after surgery in the pediatric patient? What are some perioperative factors that have been shown to influence the incidence of these behavioral changes?

MEDICAL AND SURGICAL DISEASES AFFECTING THE NEONATE

92. What is necrotizing enterocolitis, and which patients are at risk?

93. What are the clinical manifestations of necrotizing enterocolitis?

94. How is necrotizing enterocolitis treated?

95. What are some of the anesthetic considerations for surgery for neonates with necrotizing enterocolitis?

96. What are gastroschisis and omphalocele? What are the similarities and differences between these conditions?

97. How are gastroschisis and omphalocele treated surgically in the modern era? What are some of the anesthetic considerations for these conditions?

98. What clinical circumstance leads to suspicion of a tracheoesophageal fistula in a neonate?

99. What are some other congenital anomalies associated with a tracheoesophageal fistula? What are the components of the VACTERL association?

100. How is tracheoesophageal fistula treated surgically in the modern era?

101. How should neonates with a tracheoesophageal fistula be managed?

102. What are some of the risk factors for morbidity and mortality in a neonate undergoing repair of a tracheoesophageal fistula?

103. What side is most commonly affected by a congenital diaphragmatic hernia (CDH)? If not detected prenatally, what are the most common physical examination findings that suggest the presence of a CDH?

104. What are some comorbid conditions associated with CDHs?

105. How is the diagnosis of a CDH made?

106. What is the immediate treatment for the neonate with a CDH? What is the risk of hand ventilation with bag and mask in these neonates?

107. What strategies can be used to improve oxygenation and treat pulmonary hypertension in patients with a CDH?

108. What is the risk of positive-pressure ventilation of the lungs of the neonate with a CDH?

109. What are some strategies for the anesthetic management of neonates with a CDH?

110. What is the significance of a patent ductus arteriosus (PDA) in the premature infant? What is a medical approach to treatment?

111. What are some anesthetic considerations and pitfalls for PDA closure in the premature neonate?

112. What patients require maintaining a PDA after birth? What options are available for maintaining a PDA?

113. What is retinopathy of prematurity? What is another name for this pathologic finding?

114. What is a risk factor for retinopathy of prematurity? At what age does the risk of retinopathy of prematurity become negligible?

115. What Pa_{O_2} value should be maintained during anesthesia in the premature neonate to minimize the risk of retinopathy of prematurity?

116. What is the surgical treatment for the neonate undergoing surgery for retinopathy of prematurity? What are the anesthetic considerations?

117. What is myelomeningocele, and how is it managed surgically? What are some of the anesthetic considerations?

118. What is pyloric stenosis? What is the incidence of pyloric stenosis per live birth?

119. How does the neonate with pyloric stenosis typically present?

120. What electrolyte imbalances are seen in infants with pyloric stenosis?

121. Is the surgical correction of pyloric stenosis in infants an elective or emergent procedure?

122. How should the induction of anesthesia in infants with pyloric stenosis proceed?

123. What is respiratory distress syndrome?

124. What are some physiologic complications that result from respiratory distress syndrome?

125. How should neonates with respiratory distress syndrome be managed intraoperatively?

126. What is bronchopulmonary dysplasia? What are some characteristic findings in these patients?

127. Which pediatric patients are at risk of hypoglycemia?

128. What are some manifestations of hypoglycemia in neonates? How do these manifestations change with general anesthesia? What is the immediate treatment of hypoglycemia in these patients?

129. Which pediatric patients are at risk of hypocalcemia?

130. When might hypocalcemia occur intraoperatively? How might intraoperative hypocalcemia manifest?

131. What is the incidence of malignant hyperthermia (MH) in the pediatric population? What is the incidence in the adult populations?

132. What is the association between malignant hyperthermia and the calcium ion channel?

133. What are some anesthetic triggering drugs for malignant hyperthermia?

134. What are some clinical signs of malignant hyperthermia?

135. What is the treatment for malignant hyperthermia?

136. How can the patient at risk for malignant hyperthermia be identified preoperatively?
137. Which anesthetic regimen is reliably safe for patients susceptible to malignant hyperthermia? Name some drugs used in anesthesia that have not been shown to trigger malignant hyperthermia.
138. What preparations must take place before the administration of anesthesia to patients susceptible to malignant hyperthermia?
139. Is regional anesthesia considered safe for patients at risk for malignant hyperthermia?

SPECIAL ANESTHETIC CONSIDERATIONS

140. Patients of what age are at risk of apnea spells in the postoperative period? How should these infants be managed postoperatively?
141. In what remote locations are pediatric anesthetics commonly performed? Are the requirements for preanesthetic evaluation, monitoring, and recovery the same for these anesthetics?
142. What is the ex utero intrapartum therapy (EXIT) procedure, and what are the indications for this procedure? What are some of the anesthetic considerations?
143. What are some indications for fetal surgery, and what are some anesthetic considerations? What conditions have been addressed via fetal interventions? What are the approaches that can be taken to intervene on the fetus? What are some resuscitative strategies for the fetus that can be performed on the mother and the fetus?
144. What anesthetic and sedative agents have been implicated in developmental neurotoxicity in animal models? Is there clinical evidence to change the practice of pediatric anesthesia?
145. Prolonged anesthesia in neonatal rodent studies is associated with neurotoxicity in the developing brain. What changes should be made to the current approach to anesthesia in the infant? What current studies are being done to investigate the effects of anesthetic exposure early in human life?

ANSWERS*

DEVELOPMENTAL PHYSIOLOGY

1. Intercostal muscle tone is decreased and chest wall compliance is increased in infants compared to adults. (588)
2. Alveolar ventilation in neonates is four to five times higher than that of adults. (588)
3. Tidal volume per weight in neonates is similar to that of adults. (588)
4. The respiratory rate in neonates is three to four times higher than that of adults. (588)
5. Carbon dioxide production in neonates is higher than that of adults. The Pa_{CO_2} in neonates is similar to that of adults, despite the increase in production. This is due to the increase in alveolar ventilation in neonates when compared with adults. (588)
6. The Pa_{O_2} in the first few days after birth increases rapidly. The initially low Pa_{O_2} is due to a decrease in the functional residual capacity and to the perfusion of alveoli filled with fluid. The functional residual capacity of neonates increases over the first few days of life until it reaches adult levels at about 4 days of age. (588)
7. The total lung capacity in infants is much less than that of adults owing to the decrease in muscle tone. (588)

---

*Numbers in parentheses refer to pages, figures, boxes, or tables in Pardo MC, Miller RD, eds. *Basics of Anesthesia.* 7th ed. Philadelphia: Elsevier; 2018.

8. The normal newborn has periodic breathing, with pauses less than 10 seconds and periods of increased respiratory activity. This differs from apnea, which is associated with desaturation and bradycardia. Apnea is associated with prematurity. (588)

9. The fetal circulation is characterized by high pulmonary vascular resistance (PVR) and very little blood flow and low systemic vascular resistance (SVR), with the placenta as the major low-resistance vascular bed. Right-to-left shunted blood flows through the ductus arteriosus and the foramen ovale. At birth, increased alveolar oxygenation and lung expansion decrease PVR, removing the placenta increases SVR, and increased left atrial pressure functionally closes the foramen ovale. (589)

10. The ductus arteriosus is functionally closed in 98% of neonates at 4 days of life. The ductus venosus closes with clamping of the umbilical vein. The foramen ovale closes between 3 and 12 months of age. About 30% of adults have a probe patent foramen ovale. (590)

11. The oxygen consumption of a neonate is about twice that of an adult. In neonates the oxygen consumption increases from 5 mL/kg per minute at birth to about 7 mL/kg per minute at 10 days of life and 8 mL/kg per minute at 4 weeks of life. Oxygen consumption gradually declines over the subsequent months. (590)

12. The cardiac output of a neonate is 30% to 60% higher than that of adults. This helps to meet the increase in oxygen demand neonates have as compared with adults. (590)

13. Changes in the cardiac output of a neonate or infant are dependent on changes in the heart rate, because stroke volume is relatively fixed by the lack of distensibility of the left ventricle in this age group. The neonate's myocardium depends heavily on the concentration of ionized calcium, such that hypocalcemia can significantly depress myocardial function. (590)

14. The parasympathetic innervation to the heart predominates early in life, while the sympathetic nervous system is still developing. This is manifest clinically by the increased propensity of neonates and infants to respond to laryngeal stimulation with bradycardia and even asystole. Many anesthesia providers will pretreat their patients with an anticholinergic prior to airway instrumentation. (591)

15. Kidney function at birth is immature. There is a decreased glomerular filtration rate, decreased sodium excretion, and decreased concentrating ability relative to that of an adult. Kidney function progressively matures over the first 2 years of life. Initially, in the first 3 months of life, kidney function increases rapidly to double or triple the glomerular filtration rate possible at birth. Kidney function then matures more slowly from 3 months to 24 months, when adult levels of kidney function are reached. (591)

16. Adult levels of urine concentrating ability are achieved by 6 to 12 months of age. (591)

17. In neonates, the oxyhemoglobin dissociation curve is shifted to the left. This reflects a P_{50} lower than 26 mm Hg, meaning that less of a Pao_2 is required for a 50% saturation of hemoglobin. Conversely, the oxygen is more tightly bound to hemoglobin in neonates, necessitating a lower Pao_2 for release of oxygen to the tissues. This occurs as a result of fetal hemoglobin. The position of the oxyhemoglobin dissociation curve becomes equal to that of adults by 4 to 6 months of age. (591)

18. The hemoglobin level of a neonate is approximately 17 g/dL. This, along with the increase in cardiac output, helps to offset the increase in oxygen requirements characteristic of neonates. At 9 to 12 weeks of life the hemoglobin of term infants decreases to about 11 g/dL during the time period when fetal hemoglobin is being replaced by adult hemoglobin. This is termed the *physiologic anemia of infancy*, which may persist for a few months. During the remainder of the first year of life the hemoglobin level gradually increases and continues to do so until puberty, when hemoglobin levels approach adult hemoglobin levels. (591)

19. A hemoglobin level of 13 g/dL or less is worrisome in the newborn. In infants older than 6 months of age, a hemoglobin level less than 10 g/dL is worrisome. (591)

20. Because of the decreased ability of neonates to vasoconstrict in response to hypovolemia, neonates are less able to tolerate hemorrhage with vasoconstrictive responses. (591)

21. Extracellular fluid volume accounts for approximately 40% of the body weight of the neonate at birth. This compares with approximately 20% of body weight in adults being accounted for by extracellular fluid volume. The proportion of extracellular fluid volume to body weight in neonates approaches the adult proportion by 18 to 24 months of age. (591)

22. All newborns are given intramuscular vitamin K because at birth the vitamin K–dependent coagulation factors are present only at 20% to 60% of adult levels, leading to a prolonged prothrombin time. Without the administration of vitamin K it can take several weeks for the factors to reach normal levels because of synthesis in an immature liver. (591)

23. Some ways in which infants and children maintain normal body temperature include the metabolism of brown fat, crying, and vigorous movements. The metabolism of brown fat is stimulated by circulating norepinephrine. Children and infants, unlike adults, do not shiver to maintain their body temperature. Maintenance of normal body temperature is more difficult in neonates and infants than in adults because of their larger body surface area/volume ratio, as well as the relative lack of fat for insulation. (591)

PHARMACOLOGIC DIFFERENCES

24. There are several physiologic characteristics of neonates that explain the pharmacokinetic differences between infant and adult responses to drugs. Infants have a lower concentration of circulating proteins and a lower affinity of circulating proteins to bind to drugs. This results in an increased concentration of circulating free drug that normally binds to proteins and an increased drug effect. In infants there is increased extracellular fluid volume and increased volume of distribution necessitating a larger initial dose of drug to achieve a given effect. This is true for such drugs as succinylcholine and fentanyl. There is also decreased percentage of body fat and muscle in small infants compared to adults so that drugs that rely on redistribution for termination of a clinical effect (e.g., thiopental, propofol) may have a prolonged clinical effect. (592)

25. Because of reduced hepatic enzyme activity and decreased hepatic blood flow, the hepatic metabolism of drugs is about 50% of adult values at birth in a full-term infant. The hepatic metabolism of drugs increases rapidly in the first month of life to near adult values and is fully mature by 1 to 2 years of age. (592)

26. Because of immature glomerular and tubular function, the renal excretion of drugs is prolonged in infants, resulting in prolonged elimination half-times. Glomerular and tubular function is nearly mature at 20 weeks after birth and is fully mature at 2 years. (592)

27. The uptake and distribution of inhaled anesthetics are more rapid in neonates than in adults. This is most likely due to a smaller functional residual capacity per body weight in neonates, as well as to greater tissue blood flow to the vessel-rich group. The vessel-rich group of tissues includes the brain, heart, kidneys, and liver. This group comprises approximately 22% of total body volume in neonates, as compared with the 10% of total body volume in adults. (592)

28. Patients with right-to-left intracardiac shunting have a slower inhaled induction of anesthesia, owing to the volume of blood bypassing the lungs and not increasing its anesthetic level. This results in a slower rise in the arterial level of the anesthetic and a slower induction. This effect is most pronounced with less soluble anesthetics, such as desflurane and sevoflurane, and less pronounced

with more soluble anesthetics, such as halothane and isoflurane. Left-to-right intracardiac shunts have little or no effect on the rapidity of induction. (592)

29. The minimum alveolar concentration (MAC) of inhaled anesthetics changes from birth to puberty. The MAC of inhaled anesthetic agents is highest in infants 1 to 6 months old. The MAC is 30% less in full-term neonates for isoflurane and desflurane. Sevoflurane MAC at term is the same as at age 1 month. Preterm neonates have a lower MAC than term neonates. Cerebral palsy and developmental delay also reduce MAC by 25%. (593)

30. Physiologic factors that make neonates more sensitive to the effects of intravenous anesthetics include an immature blood-brain barrier and a decreased ability to metabolize drugs. They are more sensitive to highly protein-bound drugs because of the lower serum albumin and protein concentrations in neonates. In many cases the increased extracellular fluid volume and volume of distribution present in neonates offsets the increased sensitivity to intravenous drugs when compared with adults, thereby approximately equalizing the dose of initial intravenous injection of drug to achieve a given result. (593)

31. The dose of propofol required to produce loss of lid reflex is higher in neonates and children, compared with adults. (593)

32. The rate of plasma clearance of opioids is decreased in neonates when compared with adults. (593)

33. Neonates are more sensitive than adults to nondepolarizing neuromuscular blocking drugs. This means that a lower plasma concentration of drug is required to produce similar pharmacologic results. Because of an increased extracellular fluid volume and increased volume of distribution in neonates when compared with adults, the initial dose of nondepolarizing neuromuscular blocking drug in these two age groups is similar. This is true despite the increased sensitivity to the drug for neonates. (593)

34. The duration of action of nondepolarizing neuromuscular blocking drugs in neonates may be prolonged while the mechanisms for clearance are still immature in the neonate. For example, the clearance of *d*-tubocurarine parallels the glomerular filtration rate at various ages. There exists a great deal of variability among pediatric patients with regard to the duration of effect of nondepolarizing neuromuscular blocking drugs. Monitoring of the neuromuscular junction with a peripheral nerve stimulator is recommended when nondepolarizing neuromuscular blocking drugs are administered to this population. (593)

35. The dose of neostigmine necessary to antagonize neuromuscular blocking drugs in the neonate is less than that of adults, although clinically the same dose may be used. (593)

36. The dose of succinylcholine per body weight necessary to produce neuromuscular blockade in the neonate and infant is increased from the adult dose. This is presumed to be due to the increase in extracellular fluid volume and increase in volume of distribution in neonates and infants. (593)

FLUIDS AND ELECTROLYTES

37. Non–glucose-containing isotonic fluids are most appropriate to replace losses. These fluids include lactated Ringer solution and Plasma-Lyte A, which both contain physiologic levels of sodium and potassium. Normal saline can be used, but with supraphysiologic levels of sodium and chloride, a hyperchloremic, hypernatremic metabolic acidosis can occur with the administration of large volumes. (593)

38. Preoperative fluid deficits in the pediatric patient can be estimated by multiplying the number of hours the patient has been NPO (taking nothing by mouth) by the hourly maintenance fluid requirement based on the 4-2-1 rule. Replace 50% of this deficit in the first hour and the remaining 50% in the second hour. Patients presenting for emergency surgery may have larger fluid deficits

owing to vomiting, fever, third-space fluid loss, or blood loss. For elective surgery, minimizing preoperative fluid deficits by allowing clear liquids to be ingested orally up to 2 hours before surgery is an effective strategy to minimize preoperative deficits. (593)

39. Fluid maintenance and replacement in the pediatric population are based on the patient's age and metabolic rate, underlying disease process, type and extent of surgery, and anticipated fluid translocation. The maintenance rate of pediatric patients is related to their metabolic demand, which in turn is related to the ratio of body surface to weight. Hourly fluid requirements are estimated to be 4 mL/kg for children up to 10 kg, an additional 2 mL/kg for each kilogram of body weight between 10 kg and 20 kg, and an additional 1 mL/kg for each kilogram of body weight above 20 kg. Additional fluid replacement may be required for the patient's third-space losses or other losses such as evaporative losses. Fluid replacement can be guided by the patient's systemic blood pressure, tissue perfusion, and urine output. (593)

40. For minimally invasive surgery, third-space losses are estimated to be 0 to 2 mL/kg/h. This includes superficial surgery such as strabismus repair. For mildly invasive surgery such as ureteral reimplantation, these losses are estimated at 2 to 4 mL/kg/h. For moderately invasive surgery such as elective bowel reanastomosis, fluid losses are estimated at 4 to 8 mL/kg/h, and for maximally invasive surgery such as bowel resection for necrotizing enterocolitis, fluid losses are estimated to be 8 to 10 mL/kg/h or greater. To this hourly fluid administration is added the maintenance fluid requirement according to the 4-2-1 rule, the preoperative fluid deficit as noted previously, and replacement for blood loss. The latter is replaced with 3 mL of isotonic crystalloid for each milliliter of estimated blood loss, or 1 mL of colloid such as 5% albumin for each milliliter blood loss, or milliliter for milliliter of blood product such as packed red blood cells. (593)

41. A goal for urine output when monitoring the intraoperative volume status in the pediatric patient is 0.5 to 1 mL/kg/h. (593)

42. In children older than 1 year of age, the stress and catecholamine release associated with surgery usually prevent hypoglycemia. Glucose is commonly given to patients who are younger than 1 year of age or less than 10 kg. Pediatric patients at a high risk for hypoglycemia include newborns of diabetic mothers, or neonates whose hyperalimentation has been discontinued. Maintenance fluids of 5% dextrose in 0.45 normal saline can be administered to these patients intraoperatively as a piggy-back infusion by pump with care not to bolus glucose-containing solutions. (594)

TRANSFUSION THERAPY

43. The following formula may be used by the anesthesiologist to help guide blood loss replacement:

$$\text{MABL (mL)} = \text{EBV (mL)} \times (\text{patient Hct} - \text{minimum acceptable Hct})/\text{patient Hct}$$

where MABL is maximum allowable blood loss, EBV is estimated blood volume, and Hct is hematocrit. The estimated blood volume is between 70 mL/kg at about 5 years of age and 100 mL/kg in the premature newborn. This formula should be applied to the pediatric patient prior to surgery so that when the threshold is reached, it is immediately recognized and the transfusion is initiated. (594)

44. The pediatric patient's transfusion threshold varies greatly according to the patient's underlying physiology, age, nature of the surgery, and anticipated ongoing blood loss and must be individualized. For patients with cyanotic heart disease, a hemoglobin threshold of 12 to 13 g/dL is often used. For otherwise healthy acyanotic patients, a lower threshold of 7 to 8 g/dL is often used. The

transfusion of 10 to 15 mL/kg of packed red blood cells (PRBCs) should increase hemoglobin by 2 to 3 g/dL. (594)

45. Leukocyte reduction and irradiation of PRBCs should be done for infants younger than 4 months of age, immunocompromised patients, and transplant or potential transplant recipients. This special processing minimizes the risk of febrile, nonhemolytic transfusion reactions, human leukocyte antigen (HLA) allosensitization, cytomegalovirus transmission, and graft-versus-host disease. (594)

46. The indication for platelet transfusion in a pediatric patient is dependent on platelet number, function, and the presence or absence of bleeding. The administration of 5 to 10 mL/kg of platelet concentrate transfusion should increase platelet count by 50,000/dL to 100,000/dL. (594)

47. The indication for fresh frozen plasma (FFP) administration in pediatric patients is to correct coagulopathy due to insufficient coagulation factors. The administration of 10 to 15 mL/kg will increase most coagulation factors by 15% to 20%, which is often sufficient to improve hemostasis. (594)

48. Indications for cryoprecipitate administration in pediatric patients most often are low fibrinogen concentrations from massive hemorrhage or dilution from cardiopulmonary bypass. Cryoprecipitate is also a source of factor VIII and factor XIII, in addition to fibrinogen. One unit of cryoprecipitate administered per 5 kg of patient weight to a maximum of 4 units is usually sufficient to restore adequate fibrinogen levels. (594)

49. Fibrinogen can be replaced by administration of either cryoprecipitate or human fibrinogen concentrate. Fibrinogen replacement is often required in pediatric cardiac surgery, and its use is increasing in complex pediatric surgery, including craniofacial and scoliosis surgery. (594)

50. The lysine analogs ε-aminocaproic acid and tranexamic acid reduce fibrinolysis by inhibiting plasmin. Recombinant factor VIIa is used for patients with factor VII deficiency or hemophiliacs with inhibitors to factors VIII and IX. It is also used in cases of massive hemorrhage such as cardiac surgery or trauma, as a lifesaving measure to reduce bleeding. This agent causes a "thrombin burst" when exposed to tissue factor, resulting in massive activation of the coagulation cascade. Thrombotic complications have been reported with recombinant factor VIIa. (595)

THE PEDIATRIC AIRWAY

51. The preoperative airway assessment in children should involve visual inspection for micrognathia, midface hypoplasia, limited mouth opening or cervical mobility, or other craniofacial abnormalities. The patient and parents should be asked about the presence of loose teeth or orthodontic appliances. (595)

52. There are multiple physiologic differences between the pediatric airway and the adult airway. Pediatric patients tend to have a larger tongue relative to the size of their mouths. Particularly true in neonates is that the occiput is larger, so that placing the head in the neutral position naturally places the head in a position favorable for direct laryngoscopy. Extending the head can make direct laryngoscopy difficult. The larynx is more cephalad in pediatric patients, with the cricoid cartilage opposing the C4 vertebra rather than the C6 vertebra as in adults. The larynx is also more anterior. The epiglottis is longer, floppier, and U-shaped and has more of a horizontal lie. The narrowest point of the airway is at the level of the cricoid cartilage in the presence of neuromuscular blockade. These differences between the pediatric airway and the adult airway are present until about the age of 8 years, after which the difference between the pediatric airway and the adult airway is mainly just a difference in size. (595)

53. Supraglottic airway devices can be used for routine cases, but they are also an important part of the difficult airway algorithm in pediatric patients, providing a means to oxygenate and ventilate and a conduit for endotracheal tube placement using a fiberoptic scope. The use of the laryngeal mask airway has actually been associated with a decreased risk of respiratory complications compared with an endotracheal tube in pediatric patients. (595)

54. Because the narrowest point of the pediatric airway is at the level of the cricoid cartilage, it was believed that an endotracheal tube that passes easily through the larynx may cause ischemia or damage to the trachea distally. However, recent imaging studies challenge this notion, and the difference in diameter between the larynx and subglottis in younger children is minimal. Historically, uncuffed tubes were the standard of care in children younger than 8 years of age owing to concerns about subglottic stenosis and postextubation stridor. However, with the introduction of tubes with high-volume–low-pressure cuffs, recent studies suggest that there is no increased risk of airway edema with cuffed endotracheal tubes and that the use of cuffed endotracheal tubes may decrease the number of laryngoscopies and intubations due to inappropriate tube size. The risk of postintubation tracheal edema is greatest in children between 1 and 4 years of age, whether a cuffed or uncuffed endotracheal tube is used. Postintubation tracheal edema/croup can be treated with humidified gases and aerosolized racemic epinephrine. Dexamethasone has also been administered intravenously for the treatment of postintubation tracheal edema. (595)

55. Cuffed endotracheal tubes are especially useful when poor ventilatory compliance exists or a change in ventilatory compliance is expected. In patients with chronic lung disease, a cuffed tube may be the most efficient way to deliver breaths requiring high pressures on the ventilator. If an uncuffed tube is used, the leak around the tube may be excessive. Cuffed tubes may also be indicated in cases in which compliance may change, such as complete reduction of gastroschisis or omphalocele. With the increase in intra-abdominal pressure, higher pressures may be needed to ventilate, and a large leak can develop. If a cuffed tube is in place, the cuff can be inflated until the leak disappears. Cuffed tubes are also useful when transesophageal echocardiography is planned, as compliance often changes with probe placement. Cuffed tubes are often advised when reliable oxygenation and ventilation are absolutely critical, as when caring for a patient with severe pulmonary hypertension or when separating from cardiopulmonary bypass with high pulmonary artery pressures; trying to manage a leak in this situation can negatively affect hemodynamic status. (595)

56. The approach to the difficult pediatric and adult airway is generally similar: maintain spontaneous respiration; use adjuncts such as the laryngeal mask airway, video laryngoscope, or fiberoptic bronchoscope to secure the airway; awaken the patient if possible if the airway cannot be secured; avoid neuromuscular blockade until the airway is secured; and have surgical backup for emergency tracheostomy for particularly difficult cases. The major difference between managing the pediatric versus adult airway is that young pediatric patients will not tolerate an "awake" intubation with topical anesthesia of the airway; they must have some level of moderate to deep sedation or general anesthesia. Also, cricothyrotomy is technically difficult in small patients and ventilation via this method ineffective. Thus, this method cannot be used in young pediatric patients. (595)

57. Micrognathia is the single most common cause of difficult mask ventilation and tracheal intubation in young pediatric patients. Pierre-Robin sequence, Goldenhar syndrome, and Treacher-Collins syndrome are the most commonly encountered conditions resulting in micrognathia. (595)

ANESTHETIC CONSIDERATIONS

58. The preoperative history in the pediatric patient often comes from a parent. The patient's age and weight help to guide selection of appropriate equipment, airway supplies, and drug dosing. The history obtained should include such things as premature birth, congenital anomalies, sleep-disordered breathing, allergies, bleeding tendencies, and any recent exposure to communicable diseases. A special consideration for the pediatric population is whether the patient has had any recent upper respiratory tract infection, which makes it more likely that the patient will have increased secretions and airway hyperreactivity with anesthesia. Elective surgeries may be delayed in the presence of an upper airway infection. With regard to the airway examination,

the presence of loose teeth should be evaluated, and removal of the loose tooth or teeth before airway manipulation should be considered. (596)

59. The patient at risk for malignant hyperthermia (MH) may be identified preoperatively by a detailed medical history and family history of problems with anesthesia. The diagnosis of definitive susceptibility to MH required skeletal muscle biopsy and in vitro caffeine halothane muscle contracture testing. Genetic testing for the ryanodine receptor abnormalities has also become available. Disorders associated with MH susceptibility are King-Denborough syndrome, central core disease, and multiminicore disease. Succinylcholine and volatile anesthestics should not be given to patients at risk for MH. Anesthesia-induced rhabdomyolysis (AIR) is different from MH. AIR is characterized by muscle breakdown leading to acute renal insufficiency, hyperkalemia, and possible cardiac arrest. Patients with dystrophinopathies and myopathies are at risk for AIR. AIR is usually attributed to succinylcholine administration, but volatile anesthetics have also been implicated. (596)

60. Snoring, breathing pauses, and gasping all suggest obstructive sleep apnea (OSA) in pediatric patients. These patients may or may not have had a formal sleep study. They are often scheduled for tonsillectomy and adenoidectomy. One should maintain a high index of suspicion that OSA is present. Patients may be exquisitely sensitive to narcotics and may require an extended stay in the postanesthesia care unit or inpatient admission with monitoring of pulse oximetry, especially in younger patients. (597)

61. The risks of anesthetizing a child with an upper respiratory tract infection (URI) are largely manageable, but they include laryngospasm, bronchospasm, and the need for oxygen postoperatively to treat hypoxemia from atelectasis. Although it is preferable to avoid anesthetizing children with an active URI, patients for otolaryngologic procedures are often ill, and it can be very difficult to find a window to schedule surgery when the patient is well. (597)

62. Laboratory data are typically unnecessary in the routine pediatric patient. Laboratory data should be ordered based on abnormalities in the history and physical examination. Urine pregnancy testing is practiced for menstruating females in many institutions. (597)

63. Children should stop eating solid food 6 to 8 hours before a procedure. Milk, fortified breast milk, and formula should be discontinued 6 hours before a procedure. Unfortified breast milk should be discontinued 4 hours before a procedure, and clear liquids should be discontinued 2 hours before a procedure. Care should be taken with scheduling and parental communication such that a pediatric patient is not without fluids for longer than necessary, both for patient comfort and safety. (597)

64. Premedication of the pediatric patient should take into consideration the age of the patient, the patient's underlying medical condition, the length of surgery, the mode of induction of anesthesia, and whether the patient will be staying in the hospital after the procedure. Infants younger than 6 months old typically do not require premedication, whereas patients between 9 months and 5 or 6 years old may benefit from premedication before separation from their parents. Common options for premedication include midazolam, ketamine, clonidine, and dexmedetomidine. Midazolam can be administered via oral, intranasal, rectal, and intramuscular routes. Oral midazolam is the most widely used premedication in North America. Ketamine can also be delivered via oral, intranasal, rectal, and intramuscular routes. Ketamine preserves airway tone while producing sedation, amnesia, and analgesia but is also associated with excessive salivation, nystagmus, postoperative nausea and vomiting, and hallucinations. Both clonidine and dexmedetomidine are α_2-agonists. Clonidine is given orally but must be given at least 1 hour prior to the anesthetic. Dexmedetomidine is usually given intranasally, and the onset

time is approximately 30 minutes. Both clonidine and dexmedetomidine have the benefit of decreasing anesthetic requirements intraoperatively. (597)

65. Nonpharmacologic techniques for allaying anxiety and assisting anesthetic induction include parental presence, assistance of child life specialists, and distraction techniques such as a hand-held video game. Parental presence at the induction of anesthesia may increase parental anxiety and even syncope in the parent. The temperament of the parents must be assessed prior to this technique. No technique works for every child, and learning to read the patient and the family can be helpful in choosing a patient-specific strategy. (597)

66. Because of their larger body surface area/weight ratio, infants tend to lose body heat much more rapidly than adults, by both radiation and convection. This is particularly true in a cold operating room environment so preparations to maintain normothermia should be done in advance of bringing the patient to the operating room. Warming the operating room and using radiant warmers, warmed intravenous fluids, airway humidification, and forced air warming are all methods of maintaining normothermia. (598)

67. In the pediatric patient without an intravenous catheter, anesthesia can be induced via inhalation. An inhalation induction can be achieved by initially having the child breathe sevoflurane with or without nitrous oxide, with incremental increases in the concentration of sevoflurane. The only volatile anesthetic available for inhalation induction in the United States is sevoflurane, because it is much less pungent than the other volatile anesthetics. It is critical to recognize that while the pediatric patient is being induced, the anesthesiologist often increases concentrations of the volatile anesthetic to dangerous inspired concentrations of volatile anesthetic if maintained. Once anesthesia is induced, it is important to reduce the inspired concentrations of volatile anesthetic to routine maintenance levels. This is especially true just before intubating the trachea, because connection of the circuit and ventilating the intubated patient with high inspired concentrations of volatile anesthetic while potentially distracted with endotracheal tube positioning are risks. High inspired concentrations of volatile anesthetic, if continued, can lead to myocardial depression that is difficult to reverse. (598)

68. Laryngospasm, along with coughing, vomiting, and involuntary movement, can occur in stage 2 (the excitement phase) of induction of anesthesia. Laryngospasm is accompanied by a rocking-boat motion of the chest and abdomen as the patient attempts to inspire against a closed glottis. Laryngospasm should be treated by closing the pop-off valve and creating positive pressure of about 10 cm H_2O against the glottis. If necessary, positive-pressure ventilation can be attempted. In most circumstances these measures will reverse the laryngospasm, and the patient will spontaneously ventilate. Should these two interventions not reverse the laryngospasm, succinylcholine can be administered intravenously or intramuscularly. Succinylcholine is the neuromuscular blocking drug of choice under these circumstances. (598)

69. The placement of an intravenous catheter should be done in every pediatric patient undergoing a surgical procedure other than for very short surgical procedures. (598)

70. After an inhaled induction of anesthesia, the intravenous catheter should be placed after the patient has already passed through stage 2 of anesthesia. (598)

71. In the pediatric patient with an intravenous catheter, the induction of anesthesia can be achieved by the intravenous administration of an induction agent such as propofol 2 to 3 mg/kg, ketamine, or etomidate. An intravenous induction is the induction method of choice in patients at risk for the aspiration of gastric contents or with significant cardiopulmonary compromise. (598)

72. The intramuscular induction of anesthesia is most commonly used in children who are severely uncooperative or developmentally delayed. Ketamine is most commonly used at a dose of 5 mg/kg. Intramuscular atropine or glycopyrrolate

can be added to decrease excess salivation. If the patient will not accept oral premedication or the mask, intramuscular induction may be the safest option for both the patient and the anesthesia care team. Intramuscular induction with ketamine has also been used safely in children with congenital heart disease for whom a drop in systemic vascular resistance may be poorly tolerated and for patients with burns who may have hemodynamic instability, airway compromise, and difficult intravenous access. (598)

73. The administration of intravenous fluids in pediatric patients can be regulated by the use of a calibrated drip chamber yielding 60 drops/mL, and filled with only 50 to 100 mL of intravenous fluid, so as to minimize the risk that excessive amounts of fluid are accidentally administered. (598)

74. There are multiple concerns regarding the use of succinylcholine in pediatric patients. First, the administration of succinylcholine can result in cardiac arrhythmias, including bradycardia and, rarely, cardiac sinus arrest. The pretreatment of pediatric patients with atropine may reduce succinylcholine-induced bradycardia. Second, it is believed that in patients who have been administered succinylcholine and have subsequent masseter muscle rigidity, there may be impending malignant hyperthermia. Finally, there have been reports of pediatric patients who were otherwise healthy and went into irreversible cardiac arrest after the administration of succinylcholine. Many of these patients had hyperkalemia, rhabdomyolysis, and acidosis. It is postulated that these pediatric patients may have had undiagnosed myopathies. Postmortem muscle biopsies have shown many of them to have muscular dystrophy. The group at highest risk of this catastrophic event are males 8 years of age or younger. Because of these concerns, there is now a "black box warning" by the U.S. Food and Drug Administration prohibiting routine use of succinylcholine in pediatric patients. It is only indicated for airway emergencies, such as laryngospasm or rapid-sequence induction. Some alternatives that may be used are the nondepolarizing neuromuscular blocking drugs, such as larger doses of vecuronium or rocuronium. (598)

75. Succinylcholine is accepted for use for rapid onset neuromuscular blockade in pediatric patients for the treatment of laryngospasm and in patients at high risk for aspiration of gastric contents in whom rapid sequence induction/intubation is indicated. (598)

76. Signs for the adequacy of depth of anesthesia for surgery are the same for neonates, infants, and children as they are in adults. Those signs include blood pressure, heart rate, and skeletal muscle movement. Processed electroencephalographic technologies may be used as in the adult population but are less reliable in younger children. (598)

77. Hypotension in the neonate that accompanies the administration of volatile anesthetics is likely to be indicative of hypovolemia. (598)

78. Intraoperative monitoring in the pediatric population is not any different from intraoperative monitoring in the adult population undergoing comparable surgical procedures. Routine monitors should include blood pressure, heart rate, electrocardiogram, peripheral oxygen saturation, capnography, anesthetic gas concentration, and temperature monitoring. (598)

79. The monitoring of end-tidal carbon dioxide concentrations in small children, infants, and neonates may be complicated by large dead space introduced between the CO_2 sampling line and the trachea by endotracheal tube connectors, condenser humidifiers, and elbow connectors at the end of the Y-piece of the anesthesia circuit. The small tidal volumes of these patients exacerbate the problem and can result in falsely low end-tidal CO_2 readings. In addition, congenital heart disease patients with right-to-left shunting will have a falsely low end-tidal CO_2 because of the blood bypassing the lungs. (598)

80. An appropriately sized blood pressure cuff is one that is greater than one third of the circumference of the limb. A blood pressure cuff that is too small will

result in artificially high blood pressures. The opposite is also true, that a blood pressure cuff that is too large will result in artificially low blood pressures. (598)

81. Central venous pressure can be monitored in the neonate via an umbilical vein catheter. The internal jugular vein, femoral vein, or subclavian vein can be used for central venous pressure monitoring in neonates, infants, and children. (598)

82. It is common practice in pediatric anesthesia to extubate the trachea of the patient during deep anesthesia. The advantage of extubating the trachea during deep anesthesia is that emergence from anesthesia without a tracheal tube in place avoids coughing and straining on surgical suture lines, as removal of the endotracheal tube is prior to the return of airway reactivity. The decision of when to extubate the trachea is made on a case-by-case basis, however. Potential risks of deep extubation are associated with an unprotected, anesthetized airway. The patient may aspirate blood or secretions, vomit, have laryngospasm, hypoventilate, or experience airway obstruction. For this reason, the patient who has undergone a deep extubation should be monitored closely. A face mask and device for delivering positive pressure should be at the bedside, and anesthesia and recovery room personnel should be ready to intervene. (599)

83. Intravenous acetaminophen is a useful addition to the available options for perioperative pain control in children. Intravenous administration has more predictable bioavailability than rectal or oral forms of the drug, and compared with narcotic pain medication, it does not depress respiration. Because of concern about acetaminophen overdose and hepatotoxicity, careful communication between caregivers and parents about dosing times and amounts of acetaminophen and acetaminophen-containing medications is critical. (599)

84. There are several procedures in which regional anesthetic techniques can be considered in the pediatric population. For circumcision or hypospadias repair, a penile block may be used. For inguinal hernia repair an ilioinguinal and iliohypogastric block may be used. For femur surgery, a fascia iliaca compartment block may be used. For arm and wrist surgery a brachial plexus block may be used. Intravenous regional anesthesia may also be used in the pediatric patient for tendon laceration repairs or extremity fractures. Caudal anesthesia is a common form of anesthesia and is used for postoperative pain relief in the pediatric population in whom the surgical site is below the level of the diaphragm. Conversely, a lumbar epidural anesthetic may also be used in the pediatric patient. Children who undergo regional blocks commonly receive sedation to the extent that they are unable to communicate pain or paresthesia sensations during the course of the block. For this reason, ultrasound guidance is believed to increase the safety profile of performing peripheral nerve blocks in children. (599)

85. For caudal epidural anesthesia, the local anesthetic most commonly used is bupivacaine at a concentration of 0.125% to 0.25%, and ropivacaine at 0.1% to 0.2%. The volume is 0.5 to 1 mL/kg, up to a maximum of 20 mL. The duration of pain relief provided by this dose of local anesthetic in the caudal epidural space is 4 to 6 hours, therefore possibly providing some postoperative pain relief. The dural sac extends more caudad in children than in adults, making inadvertent intrathecal injection a possibility. The risks of caudal epidural anesthesia are minimal. (599)

86. Postoperative airway issues that may arise in the recovery room include apnea, obstruction, laryngospasm, hypoventilation, hypoxemia, and stridor/postintubation croup due to swelling. The airway must be continuously monitored and treatment rendered, if necessary. (599)

87. Risk factors for postoperative nausea and vomiting in the pediatric patient population include age 3 years or older, strabismus surgery, prolonged duration of surgery, and previous history of postoperative nausea and vomiting in the patient or in a parent or sibling. (599)

88. The risk of postoperative nausea and vomiting can be decreased in pediatric patients through the avoidance of narcotics and nitrous oxide administration. Additionally, two-drug pharmacologic prophylaxis with ondansetron and dexamethasone has an expected relative risk reduction for postoperative nausea and vomiting of approximately 80%. (599)

89. Emergence delirium refers to a dissociated state of consciousness that occurs while waking from anesthesia. It occurs more frequently in the pediatric population after anesthesia with sevoflurane or desflurane. During this time the pediatric patient is inconsolable, irritable, incoherent, or uncooperative. The patient may be crying, moaning, kicking, and restless, and there can be accidental removal of intravenous catheters, surgical bandages, and drains. During emergence delirium, children usually do not recognize or identify familiar and known objects or people. Emergence delirium is generally self-limiting and typically lasts only about 5 to 15 minutes. (600)

90. Scales for assessing pain in children include the FLACC (face, legs, activity, cry, consolability) Scale and the Wong-Baker Faces Pain Scale. These tools are helpful in children, as it can be difficult to differentiate pain from anxiety, disorientation, anger, and emergence delirium. (600)

91. Examples of maladaptive behavioral changes that can occur after surgery in the pediatric patient include sleeping and eating disturbances, separation anxiety, and new-onset enuresis. Parental anxiety, parental presence at induction, parental presence in the postanesthesia care unit, and the use of premedication have all been shown to influence the incidence of these behavioral changes. (600)

MEDICAL AND SURGICAL DISEASES AFFECTING THE NEONATE

92. Necrotizing enterocolitis (NEC) is an intestinal mucosal ischemic injury sometimes resulting in bowel necrosis and intestinal perforation. Reduced mesenteric blood flow from a patent ductus arteriosus, bacterial infection, and the institution of enteral feeding all have a role in the cause of necrotizing enterocolitis. NEC is a common surgical emergency in the neonate, primarily in premature newborns; over 90% of affected patients are born before 36 weeks of gestation. From 20% to 40% of NEC patients will require surgery, with a surgical mortality rate of 23% to 36%. (600)

93. Because patients with NEC are often premature, they may have other complications of prematurity. Clinical signs may include abdominal distention, bloody stools, dilated intestinal loops, and pneumatosis intestinalis. Patients with NEC with a bowel perforation are often unstable and critically ill with sepsis and hemodynamic instability, acidosis, coagulopathy, and pulmonary morbidity. (600)

94. Medical treatment of NEC without evidence of bowel necrosis or intestinal perforation includes bowel rest, gastric decompression, broad-spectrum antibiotics, and serial abdominal examinations and radiographs. NEC with perforation may require emergent laparotomy, with drainage, bowel resection, and reanastomosis or creation of ostomies. In more recent years treatment by primary peritoneal drainage via a small incision and surgical drain placement has gained popularity for smaller, sicker patients. (600)

95. Surgery for NEC is most often emergent. Invasive monitoring often includes a peripheral arterial catheter for frequent arterial blood gas analysis; umbilical artery catheters are often removed because of concern over further mesenteric ischemia. Central venous access is desirable, but surgery should not be delayed by attempts to secure invasive monitors. The neonate should be assessed for presence of and correction of intravascular fluid, electrolyte and coagulation abnormalities, hemodynamics, respiratory instability, and broad-spectrum antibiotics. In the critically ill neonate this usually requires large volumes of intravenous fluids, 5% albumin, PRBCs (to maintain hemoglobin at 10 to 15 g/dL), FFP and platelets for DIC and blood loss, inotropic support with dopamine or epinephrine, calcium administration and other electrolyte and glucose

corrections, and mechanical ventilation, maintaining the Pao_2 50 to 70 mm Hg or higher, and maintaining core temperature at 36° C or higher. Postoperatively mechanical, inotropic, fluid, and mechanical ventilatory support is continued and report given to the neonatal intensive care unit team. (601)

96. Gastroschisis and omphalocele are both abdominal wall defects. Gastroschisis is usually to the right of the umbilical cord, and intestines protrude. It is not covered by a sac and is usually an isolated defect. An omphalocele is a midline defect. It is covered by a peritoneal sac and is frequently associated with other midline anomalies. (601)

97. Large or giant defects are now managed with a staged approach, whereby the intestines are partially reduced into the peritoneal cavity, and the edges of the defect are sutured to a synthetic "silo." The intestines are then reduced into the peritoneal cavity in several steps over days to weeks. This is followed by final surgical closure of the defect. The former approach of one-stage repair has been abandoned because of the high incidence of intestinal ischemia and respiratory morbidity associated with this strategy. Anesthetic considerations include awareness of associated defects with omphalocele patients, especially congenital heart disease. Covering the defect with moist gauze, administering adequate intravenous fluid to account for very large third-space losses with exposed viscera, providing appropriate muscle relaxation, and careful attention to ventilator status as the intestines are reduced are important anesthetic considerations. During surgical reduction of abdominal contents, ventilatory compliance may change, resulting in higher peak pressure during volume control ventilation or decreased tidal volumes during pressure control ventilation. Careful monitoring of ventilation is critical, and changes in settings should be expected. (602)

98. A tracheoesophageal fistula (TEF) should be suspected when soon after birth a neonate develops cyanosis, choking, and coughing during oral feedings. The clinician should also suspect the presence of a TEF when an oral catheter cannot be passed into the stomach. The severity of illness in these patients can range from mild to severe. (602)

99. From 30% to 40% of neonates with a TEF have associated congenital heart disease, including ventricular septal defect, tetralogy of Fallot, and coarctation of the aorta. TEF is also a component of the VACTERL association (Vertebral defects, imperforate Anus, Cardiac defects, TE fistula, Renal anomalies, and Limb anomalies). Prematurity accompanies TEFs about 40% of the time. (602)

100. Although early approaches to TEF repair were often staged, the preferred strategy for repair in about 80% to 90% of patients is a one-stage ligation of the TEF with primary esophageal repair, without a gastrostomy. Critically ill premature infants may still require gastrostomy before thoracotomy and TEF ligation. If the critically ill neonate has high ventilation pressures and gastric distention, emergent right thoracotomy and ligation of the TEF are indicated. (603)

101. Neonates with a TEF are at risk for pulmonary aspiration, gastric distention, and difficulty with ventilation. These neonates should have a catheter placed in the esophagus to drain secretions and prevent the accumulation of fluids in the esophageal pouch. Manual positive-pressure ventilation of the lungs with a mask should be kept at a minimum to lessen the risk of gastric distention and pulmonary aspiration. When intubating the trachea of an infant with a TEF, the anesthesiologist must be careful to place the endotracheal tube distal to the level of the fistula. This placement can be confirmed through the auscultation of decreased breath sounds over the stomach. Some surgeons or anesthesiologists will perform a rigid or flexible bronchoscopy to diagnose the location of the fistula to aid in endotracheal tube placement. Care should be taken to avoid endobronchial intubation as well. Attention to breath sounds, chest movement with ventilation, peak inspiratory pressures, and oxygen saturation should continue throughout the

surgical procedure because small movements in the endotracheal tube can lead to its malposition. (603)

102. Risk factors for perioperative morbidity and mortality in neonates undergoing repair of a TEF include complex congenital heart disease, low birth weight (<2 kg), poor pulmonary compliance, large pericarinal fistula, and planned thoracoscopic repair. (603)

103. Congenital diaphragmatic hernia (CDH) usually affects the left side, and abdominal contents usually herniate into the left chest through the posterolateral foramen of Bochdalek. Almost all the abdominal viscera can be in the chest, including the liver and spleen. CDH results from the incomplete closure of the diaphragm in an embryologic stage of development of the fetus. Lung development is restricted on this side, and the degree of hypoplasia depends on the gestational age at which the herniation occurred. Physical findings associated with CDH include scaphoid abdomen, bowel sounds in the chest, cyanosis, and respiratory distress. The incidence of CDH is about 1 in every 2500 live births. (604)

104. Some comorbid conditions associated with CDHs include polyhydramnios, congenital heart disease, and pulmonary hypertension. (604)

105. The diagnosis of a CDH can be made in utero during ultrasonography of the fetus. The diagnosis at birth is confirmed by the clinical manifestations of the anomaly, by auscultation of intestines and decreased breath sounds over the affected lung area, and by chest radiograph. On the chest radiograph, loops of intestine are seen in the affected thorax, as well as a shift of the mediastinum to the opposite side. (604)

106. The immediate treatment of a CDH in a neonate involves decompression of the stomach with a nasogastric tube, endotracheal intubation minimizing hand ventilation of the lungs, and the administration of oxygen. Positive pressure when ventilating by hand with bag and mask can increase the volume of the gastrointestinal tract with air, further compromising pulmonary function by direct mechanical compression. This can lead to hypotension as well as worsening hypoxemia. The lungs should be ventilated with small tidal volumes at a rate of 60 to 150 breaths/min. (604)

107. In patients with CDH, hyperventilation of the lungs with oxygen can improve pulmonary blood flow by reversing the hypoxia and acidosis. High-frequency oscillatory ventilation and inhaled nitric oxide are frequently used to improve gas exchange and reduce pulmonary artery pressures. The neonate with a CDH in whom arterial oxygenation is difficult may require extracorporeal membrane oxygenation (ECMO) for stabilization before surgical intervention. ECMO support of these neonates has led to a decrease in the mortality rate of neonates with CDH. Surgery is often delayed in the critically ill neonate with a CDH while the pulmonary vascular resistance decreases. Surgery may be accomplished while on ECMO or on high-frequency oscillatory ventilation. (604)

108. Positive-pressure ventilation of the lungs of a neonate with a CDH can result in a pneumothorax on the contralateral side of the affected lung if peak airway pressures exceed 25 to 30 cm H_2O. Expansion of the hypoplastic lung after surgical correction of the CDH should not be attempted because of the risk of pneumothorax or other damage to the normal lung. (604)

109. The anesthetic management of neonates with a CDH should include monitoring of arterial and central venous pressures and analysis of arterial blood gases to maximize oxygenation, reducing Pa_{CO_2} to lower pulmonary artery pressures, and increasing pH. Inotropic support may be necessary. Volatile anesthetics may not be tolerated, so analgesia and blunting of the pulmonary hypertensive response to painful stimuli is provided with opioids such as fentanyl and possibly small doses of benzodiazepines or ketamine. Nitrous oxide should be avoided because it can diffuse into the loops of

intestine in the chest and expand the intestines further, leading to more pulmonary compromise. (605)

110. A patent ductus arteriosus (PDA) is most often seen in premature infants and can result in pulmonary edema, which complicates respiratory distress syndrome and prevents weaning from mechanical ventilator support. It also may "steal" systemic blood flow, resulting in mesenteric ischemia and increasing the risk for necrotizing enterocolitis, hypotension, and cardiac failure from the large left-to-right shunt. Indomethacin treatment is often attempted but may result in platelet and renal dysfunction. (605)

111. PDA ligation is often performed at the bedside in the neonatal intensive care unit, and full monitoring including capnography must be provided. Transport to a distant operating room has a significant risk for cardiopulmonary instability. Anesthesia is usually provided with fentanyl, 25 to 50 µg/kg, with an intravenous amnestic agent or low-dose volatile anesthetic. Temperature, glucose levels, and blood loss must all be monitored, and PRBCs must be available. Because the PDA is so large, it can be mistaken for the descending thoracic aorta, and the aorta may be inadvertently ligated. The anesthesiologist must monitor lower extremity perfusion, most commonly via pulse oximeter on the foot, to detect this problem. (605)

112. Patients with congenital heart disease may require a PDA to either provide a source of pulmonary blood flow (e.g., pulmonary atresia) or to provide systemic blood flow (e.g., coarctation of the aorta, hypoplastic left heart syndrome). Closure of the PDA results in profound cyanosis if the ductus is needed to provide pulmonary blood flow, and it results in poor systemic cardiac output and shock if the ductus is needed to provide systemic blood flow. The infusion of prostaglandin E_1 or the transcatheter placement of a ductal stent are both strategies for maintaining a PDA. (605)

113. Retinopathy of prematurity, also referred to as retrolental fibroplasia, is a condition in which the retinal vasculature becomes neovascularized and scarred. Permanent visual impairment can result. (605)

114. The pathophysiology of retinopathy of prematurity is complex, but the cause is related to excessive oxygen tension in the vessels of the retina. A risk factor for retinopathy of prematurity is a Pao_2 greater than 80 mm Hg or an oxygen saturation greater than 94% in the presence of prematurity. Retinopathy of prematurity has occurred in neonates whose Pao_2 was maintained at about 150 mm Hg for 2 to 4 hours. Wide swings in oxygen tension as seen in ventilated premature infants with cardiopulmonary instability such as those with respiratory distress syndrome, PDA, sepsis, and apnea/bradycardia increase risk. Neonates whose birth weights are lower than 1500 g are especially at risk. The risk of retinopathy of prematurity becomes negligible 44 weeks after conception. (605)

115. A Pao_2 between 50 and 70 mm Hg or an oxygen saturation between 88% and 93% should be maintained during anesthesia in the premature neonate to minimize the risk of retinopathy of prematurity. (605)

116. The surgical treatment for retinopathy of prematurity is usually urgent or emergent, as premature infants in the neonatal intensive care unit receive regular retinal examinations and the findings may lead to the need for immediate surgical intervention. Treatment is through retinal ablative therapy with indirect laser photocoagulation, and these cases may last several hours. The length of surgery, the risk of postanesthetic apnea in the premature infant, and eye discomfort after the procedure all support the maintenance of postoperative mechanical ventilation for 12 to 24 hours following the procedure. (605)

117. Myelomeningocele is a defect in the development of the neural tube, resulting in an open neural placode covered only by a thin membrane and cerebrospinal fluid. It is diagnosed in utero with ultrasound and ranges from small lumbosacral defects with minimal neurologic sequelae to large thoracolumbar defects with high paraplegia. After birth, the infant is managed prone so as not to rupture

the sac. Anesthesia induction involves either intubation in the lateral decubitus position or brief supine positioning on a padded gel doughnut to protect the sac. A nonlatex environment, including surgical gloves, is crucial to avoid latex sensitization. Muscle relaxants are avoided so the surgeon can evaluate motor function during the repair. The patient is managed prone during the initial days after surgery. (606)

118. Pyloric stenosis occurs as a result of hypertrophy of the pyloric smooth muscle. This muscle hypertrophy, in combination with edema of the pyloric mucosa, results in progressive obstruction of the pylorus. The incidence of pyloric stenosis is 1 in every 500 live births. (606)

119. The usual clinical scenario of an infant with pyloric stenosis is one of persistent vomiting in a male infant at 2 to 8 weeks of age. These infants present with weight loss, dehydration, lethargy, poor skin turgor, sunken eyes and fontanel, poor urine output, and electrolyte abnormalities. (606)

120. The electrolyte imbalances that are commonly seen in infants with pyloric stenosis occur as a result of the loss of hydrogen and chloride ions that is associated with persistent vomiting. These electrolyte imbalances include hyponatremia, hypokalemia, hypochloremia, and metabolic alkalosis. There is often a compensatory respiratory acidosis. (606)

121. Concerns for the anesthesiologist caring for the patient with pyloric stenosis include the metabolic abnormalities, severe dehydration, and full stomach, often with barium after a radiologic study. These all place the infant at an increased risk for morbidity perioperatively. Although pyloric stenosis is a medical emergency, surgical correction of pyloric stenosis is an elective procedure. The corrective procedure for these infants can be done after 24 to 48 hours of intravenous fluid rehydration, the correction of their electrolyte abnormalities, and suctioning on a catheter placed in the stomach. (606)

122. The induction of anesthesia in infants with pyloric stenosis should be preceded by the emptying of stomach contents with a catheter to minimize the risk of the pulmonary aspiration of gastric contents. Induction should then be done in a rapid-sequence fashion with cricoid pressure. Alternatively, an awake intubation may be performed, although this is rarely practiced in the modern era. Extubation of the trachea after the procedure should only be performed when the infant is awake and vigorous because postoperative depression of ventilation is frequently seen in these infants. This may be partially due to an increase in cerebrospinal fluid pH, which decreases the respiratory drive. In fact, these patients should be monitored for 12 to 24 hours postoperatively for apnea. (606)

123. Respiratory distress syndrome, also referred to as hyaline membrane disease, is a syndrome affecting preterm neonates who at birth have a deficiency of surfactant. Surfactant is necessary to maintain alveolar stability, so without it alveoli collapse. Surfactant is a surface active phospholipid in the alveoli that can now be administered into the lungs of neonates for the treatment or prevention of respiratory distress syndrome. The compliance of the lung and arterial oxygenation often improve rapidly after its administration. The administration of surfactant has decreased the morbidity and mortality risks from this syndrome. (606)

124. With the alveolar collapse associated with respiratory distress syndrome, there is resultant right-to-left intrapulmonary shunting, arterial hypoxemia, and metabolic acidosis. (606)

125. Neonates with respiratory distress syndrome should have their arterial oxygenation closely monitored intraoperatively. The Pa_{O_2} the anesthesiologist should try to maintain in these patients is the Pa_{O_2} level the patient had before surgery. This may require high inspired concentrations of oxygen and positive end-expiratory pressure. The Pa_{O_2} should ideally be monitored from a preductal artery. If the surgical procedure is short and intra-arterial monitoring is not

feasible, oxygenation may be monitored by pulse oximetry. These neonates are at an increased risk for pneumothorax with positive-pressure ventilation. Neonates with respiratory distress syndrome should be well hydrated. It may be prudent to maintain the hematocrit near 40% to optimize the delivery of oxygen to the tissues. (606)

126. Bronchopulmonary dysplasia is a chronic pulmonary disorder in infants and children who had prolonged respiratory disease at birth, defined as the need for supplemental oxygen beyond 30 days of life after a diagnosis of respiratory distress syndrome. It is thought to result from the required high inspired concentrations of oxygen and mechanical ventilation with high peak airway pressures for a prolonged period of time as treatment for the respiratory disease. Some characteristic findings in patients with bronchopulmonary dysplasia are increased airway resistance, increased airway reactivity, decreased arterial oxygenation due to ventilation-to-perfusion mismatch, and recurrent pulmonary infections. A chest radiograph in these patients may show large lung volumes, fibrosis, and atelectasis. These patients may have chronic hypercarbia as well. The incidence of bronchopulmonary dysplasia has decreased since the advent of surfactant therapy in neonates at risk. (606)

127. Neonates are at risk of developing hypoglycemia, particularly neonates of diabetic mothers. Hypoglycemia is defined by a plasma glucose concentration less than 40 mg/dL in the preterm neonate, less than 50 mg/dL for the term neonate younger than 3 days old, and less than 60 mg/dL in the term neonate older than 3 days of age. Neonates are at risk of hypoglycemia secondary to their poorly developed system for the maintenance of adequate plasma glucose concentrations. In addition, patients receiving total parenteral nutrition with high dextrose concentrations are at risk for hypoglycemia if the infusion is interrupted. Also, patients with poor nutritional status or liver disease often have inadequate hepatic glycogen stores and are also at risk. (606)

128. Manifestations of hypoglycemia in neonates include irritability, seizures, bradycardia, hypotension, and apnea. These clinical manifestations may be masked by general anesthesia, making perioperative vigilance very important; frequent analysis of blood glucose is important in patients at risk. The immediate treatment of hypoglycemia in neonates is the intravenous administration of 0.5 to 1 g/kg of glucose. (606)

129. Preterm neonates are at risk of developing hypocalcemia. Hypocalcemia in the neonate is defined by a plasma ionized calcium concentration less than about 1.1 mEq/dL. Fetuses develop their calcium stores during the third trimester, so the preterm neonate has inadequate calcium stores at birth. (606)

130. Hypocalcemia might occur intraoperatively as a result of citrated blood transfusions or during an exchange transfusion. The rapid infusion of citrate that occurs with citrated blood or fresh frozen plasma transfusions can result in hypotension secondary to hypocalcemia. The hypotension can be minimized by the administration of calcium gluconate, 1 to 2 mg intravenously for every 1 mL of blood transfused. (606)

131. The incidence of malignant hyperthermia in the pediatric population has been reported to be as high as 1 in 12,000 pediatric anesthetics. However, with the virtual disappearance of the use of two of the most potent triggering agents, halothane and succinylcholine, in the pediatric population, this incidence is now believed to be significantly lower. The incidence of malignant hyperthermia in the adult population is approximately 1 in 40,000 adult anesthetics. (606)

132. The calcium channel is important in the pathophysiology of malignant hyperthermia. There is a defect in the calcium release channel in the sarcoplasmic reticulum of the skeletal muscle, specifically the ryanodine receptor (RYR1 gene mutation is the leading cause). This defect allows for

higher concentrations of calcium to be sustained in the myoplasm, resulting in persistent skeletal muscle contractions when a patient at risk for developing malignant hyperthermia is exposed to inciting anesthetic agents of drugs. The genetic coding site for malignant hyperthermia is the ryanodine receptor. (606)

133. Anesthetic triggering drugs for malignant hyperthermia include succinylcholine and volatile anesthetics, halothane being by far the most potent agent. (606)

134. Clinical signs of malignant hyperthermia are related to some of the consequences of sustained skeletal muscle contraction. These include tachycardia, arterial hypoxemia, metabolic acidosis, respiratory acidosis, and increases in body temperature. Early signs of malignant hyperthermia include tachycardia and an increase in the exhaled concentration of carbon dioxide that are otherwise unexplained. A late sign of malignant hyperthermia is the increase in body temperature. (606)

135. The primary treatment for malignant hyperthermia is dantrolene. Dantrolene inhibits the release of calcium from the sarcoplasmic reticulum. The dose of dantrolene to be administered is 2-3 mg/kg intravenously and repeated every 5 to 10 minutes until the symptoms are controlled. Other treatment interventions for malignant hyperthermia are directed toward supportive management. First, the inhaled anesthetic being administered should be immediately discontinued. The lungs should be hyperventilated with oxygen. For the hyperthermia, active cooling should be initiated. Active cooling may include 15 mL/kg of cold saline, given intravenously every 10 minutes. Gastric lavage with cold saline and surface cooling may also be used. For the severely acidotic patient, sodium bicarbonate may be administered at a dose of 1-2 mEq/kg intravenously and guided by arterial pH. Diuresis of the patient should also be considered, either by hydration, mannitol, or furosemide. (606)

136. The patient at risk for malignant hyperthermia may be identified preoperatively by a detailed preoperative medical history and by a family history that especially notes any problems with anesthesia. Preoperative testing of the level of creatine kinase is not always useful because only about 70% of patients who are susceptible to malignant hyperthermia have increased resting levels of creatine kinase. The definitive diagnosis of a patient's susceptibility to malignant hyperthermia requires a skeletal muscle biopsy. The skeletal muscle is then tested in vitro for isometric contracture in response to exposure to caffeine or halothane or both. This test has the highest sensitivity and specificity for MH. Recently, genetic testing for the ryanodine receptor abnormality (RYR1 mutation) has become available. This test is not as sensitive as the contracture test but is highly specific. (606)

137. No anesthetic regimen is known to be reliably safe for administration to patients who are susceptible to malignant hyperthermia. Some drugs that are used in anesthesia that have not been shown to trigger malignant hyperthermia include barbiturates, opioids, benzodiazepines, propofol, etomidate, nitrous oxide, local anesthetics, and nondepolarizing neuromuscular blocking drugs. (606)

138. It is now the consensus of many that preoperative dantrolene is not necessary in susceptible patients because general anesthesia with nontriggering agents has proven to be mostly uneventful. There are multiple preparations for the operating room before anesthetizing a patient at risk for malignant hyperthermia. The vaporizers may be removed or sealed. The soda lime should be changed, and the fresh gas outlet hose may be changed. High fresh gas flows should be maintained for at least 20 minutes prior to the induction of anesthesia, and an expired gas analyzer should be confirm that traces of anesthetic gases have been purged. (606)

139. Regional anesthesia is considered safe for patients at risk for malignant hyperthermia. However, the operating room and anesthesia machine should be prepared as if the patient were to receive a general anesthetic. (606)

140. Former premature infants who present for surgery are at an increased risk for postanesthetic apnea. This risk increases with increased prematurity at birth and younger age at the time of the anesthesia. Apnea spells that result in the cessation of breathing for 20 seconds or longer can lead to cyanosis and bradycardia. Especially at risk are preterm infants younger than 50 weeks' postconception. It is estimated that 20% to 30% of preterm infants have apnea spells during their first month of life. Apnea spells may be increased in the neonate in the postoperative period secondary to the residual effects of inhaled and injected anesthetics that affect the control of breathing. The recommendation for these patients is that apnea and bradycardia monitors be used after surgery that will sound an alarm if apnea or bradycardia is detected in the patient. These patients are not candidates for outpatient surgery because of the risk of apnea occurring at home where health care providers are not available to respond. Treating anemia and administering a single dose of intravenous caffeine citrate will reduce the incidence and severity of postanesthetic apnea in this population. The current recommendation is that former premature infants should have their elective surgery delayed until 50 weeks' postconceptual age or greater to minimize this risk. Prior to this, and on a case-by-case basis, infants may need to be admitted postoperatively for 24 hours of apnea monitoring. (607)

141. Anesthesia and sedation are delivered in the cardiac catheterization laboratories, magnetic resonance imaging (MRI) and computed tomography scanners, gastrointestinal and pulmonary procedure suites, interventional radiology, radiation therapy, dental clinics, and many other locations. MRI scanning in particular has undergone explosive growth and greatly increased the need for remote sedation and anesthesia services. Requirements for preanesthetic evaluation, monitoring, and recovery are identical to those for operating room surgical anesthesia. MRI-compatible anesthesia machines and monitors are available, and full monitoring must be used. In particular, capnography for nonintubated, sedated patients via divided nasal cannula should be used for all sedation cases. (607)

142. The ex utero intrapartum therapy (EXIT) procedure involves partial delivery of the head, chest, and arms of the fetus to manage a severe airway or pulmonary anomaly. The fetus remains connected to the placental circulation to provide oxygenation and carbon dioxide removal during the procedure to secure the airway or manage the airway or lung mass. Indications include large airway, neck, or chest masses such as cystic hygroma, teratoma, and congenital adenomatoid malformation. Two anesthesiologists are required, one for the mother and one for the fetus. The mother requires deep inhalational general anesthesia to reduce uterine tone during the fetal procedure to prevent placental separation. The fetus receives intravenous or intramuscular fentanyl or morphine for analgesia. Resection of the mass or securing the airway by rigid bronchoscopy or tracheostomy is the primary goal. Then the fetus is delivered. (607)

143. Fetal intervention has been used to address a number of conditions with varied success. These conditions include myelomeningocele, congenital cystic adenomatoid malformation, sacrococcygeal teratoma, congenital diaphragmatic hernia, bladder outlet obstruction, hypoplastic left heart syndrome, and twin-twin transfusion syndrome. Approaches to the fetus include a minimally invasive approach assisted by fetoscopy, echocardiography, and ultrasound and an open approach through a hysterotomy. Resuscitative strategies for the fetus include maternal interventions such as left uterine displacement, oxygen delivery, and augmentation of blood pressure by volume or vasopressor administration. Medications such as atropine, epinephrine, calcium gluconate and sodium bicarbonate can be given directly to the fetus as well. Packed red blood cells can be administered, cardiac compressions can be performed, and pericardial effusions can be drained in an effort to stabilize and resuscitate the fetus. (607)

144. In animal models, agents that bind to γ-aminobutyric acid (GABA) receptors as agonists and to *N*-methyl-D-aspartate (NMDA) receptors as antagonists have been implicated in neuronal cell death caused by apoptosis. GABA agonists include volatile anesthetics, propofol, and benzodiazepines. NMDA antagonists include ketamine. There is currently no existing data that should change the existing approach to anesthesia in the infant. (607-608)

145. The GAS (General Anaesthesia and Awake-Regional Anesthesia in Infancy), PANDA (Pediatric Anesthesia & Neurodevelopment Assessment), and MASK (Mayo Anesthesia Safety in Kids) studies are current studies investigating the effects of anesthetic exposure early in life. The recently reported results of the GAS trial found that there was no evidence that a short exposure to sevoflurane anesthesia in infancy increased the risk of adverse neurodevelopmental outcome at 2 years of age compared with awake-spinal anesthesia. There are currently no existing data that should change the existing approach to anesthesia in the infant. (608)

35 ELDERLY PATIENTS

Sheila R. Barnett

WHY GERIATRIC ANESTHESIOLOGY IS IMPORTANT

1. What are some of the challenges encountered when taking care of elderly patients?
2. Is advanced chronologic age a risk factor?

MORBIDITY AND MORTALITY RATES

3. What are some of the factors influencing mortality rates in the geriatric patient population?
4. How does a postoperative complication impact outcome in very old patients?

AGE-RELATED PHYSIOLOGIC CHANGES

5. How is organ function affected by aging? How might this affect the elderly patient in the perioperative period?
6. What age-related changes in systolic blood pressure, heart rate, cardiac output, stroke volume, and cardiac conduction occur in the elderly?
7. Why are elderly patients more susceptible to congestive heart failure when subjected to fluid overload than younger counterparts?
8. How do drug-induced heart rate changes in the elderly compare with the heart rate response seen in younger patients administered the same drugs?
9. How do reflex-mediated heart rate increases in response to hypotension differ between elderly and younger patients?
10. In an awake, elderly patient, what is the significance of orthostatic hypotension without an associated increase in heart rate?
11. What age-related changes in gas exchange, the alveolar-to-arterial oxygen gradient, and the ventilation-to-perfusion ratio occur in the elderly?
12. What age-related changes in vital capacity, forced exhaled volume in 1 second, residual volume, and functional residual capacity occur in the elderly?
13. How do ventilatory responses to hypoxia and hypercapnia change with age? Why is this particularly important to the anesthesiologist?
14. Why does pneumonia occur with an increased frequency in elderly patients?
15. What age-related changes in renal blood flow, glomerular filtration rate, and urine-concentrating ability occur in the elderly? What clinical implications do these have?
16. How do plasma concentrations of creatinine change with age?
17. What age-related change in hepatic blood flow occurs in the elderly? What clinical implication does this have?
18. How does the production of albumin change with age? What clinical implication does this have?
19. What age-related changes in esophageal and intestinal motility and gastroesophageal sphincter tone occur in the elderly? What clinical implications do these have?

20. What physiologic changes occur with aging that predispose the elderly patient to hypothermia? What clinical implication does this have?
21. What age-related changes in the central and peripheral nervous systems occur in the elderly?
22. How do age-related changes in the central and peripheral nervous systems affect the minimum alveolar concentration (MAC) of anesthesia in the elderly patient?
23. What age-related change in neurotransmitter levels occurs in the elderly?
24. What age-related changes in cognition occur in the elderly? What clinical implication do these changes have?
25. What clinical relevance do osteoporosis, osteoarthritis, and rheumatoid arthritis have for the anesthesiologist caring for the elderly patient?
26. What is the potential significance of mental status changes that occur with extension and rotation of the head?
27. What clinical relevance do the age-related loss of collagen and decreases in skin elasticity have for the anesthesiologist caring for the elderly patient?

PERIOPERATIVE CARE IN THE ELDERLY

28. Why is it important to inquire about functional status in the elderly patient?
29. What are some elements of the preoperative evaluation that are of particular relevance to elderly patients?
30. What are some examples of activities of daily living (ADLs) and instrumental ADLs (IADLs)?
31. What preoperative laboratory testing should be done routinely based on the advanced age of the patient?
32. Should preoperative testing include a routine electrocardiogram (ECG) based on an age cutoff in elderly patients?
33. What are some of the challenges when obtaining a preoperative assessment in an institutionalized patient?
34. What are some recommended strategies to evaluate nutrition in older patients?
35. What is meant by the term *frailty*? What is its clinical relevance?
36. What are the five observable conditions that are common frailty characteristics identified in the phenotype frailty screen? What are some additional adaptations that supplement this screen?
37. What are the Frailty Index and Comprehensive Geriatric Assessment tools?
38. What is a simple tool that can be used to evaluate cognitive function preoperatively?
39. Why should certain antihypertensive medications be held on the morning of surgery?
40. What are some preoperative laboratory abnormalities that might be observed in elderly patients taking diuretic medications?
41. How are pharmacodynamic changes in the elderly reflected with regard to inhaled anesthetics and opioids?
42. How are pharmacodynamic changes in the elderly reflected with regard to nondepolarizing neuromuscular blocking drugs? How does aging affect the sensitivity of elderly patients to muscle relaxants?
43. What pharmacokinetic changes in the elderly make them susceptible to cumulative drug effects and adverse drug reactions?
44. What age-related changes in the elderly result in a decreased clearance of drugs? Give some examples of drugs for which elimination times may be affected.
45. What age-related changes in the elderly result in changes in the volume of distribution? Give some examples of drugs for which pharmacokinetic properties may be altered.
46. Why should preoperative anxiolytics be used sparingly in the elderly population? What can be used as a substitute?

47. How should the induction dose of anesthetic be altered in the elderly patient?
48. How should the dose of opioids be altered in the elderly patient?
49. What is the concern regarding the administration of meperidine in elderly patients?
50. Why might hand ventilation by bag and mask be difficult in the edentulous patient?
51. Why might endotracheal intubation be difficult in a patient with poor dentition or cervical arthritis?
52. Are there any unique risks to the elderly with the reversal of nondepolarizing neuromuscular blocking drugs with anticholinesterase drugs?
53. What are some postoperative risks that elderly patients are more prone to than younger patients?
54. What are some considerations regarding monitored anesthesia care in the elderly patient?
55. What are some medicines that can be used for monitored anesthesia care in the elderly patient?
56. What types of procedures that elderly patients are likely to undergo might warrant regional anesthesia as an alternative to general anesthesia?
57. What is an advantage that regional anesthesia may have over general anesthesia for hip surgery in elderly patients?
58. What is the advantage to maintaining consciousness in the elderly patient during a regional anesthetic for a surgical procedure?
59. What are some reasons why elderly patients may be more sensitive to regional anesthesia than younger patients?
60. How might the hypotensive effects of a sympathectomy resulting from regional anesthesia be attenuated?
61. What advantage does epidural anesthesia have over spinal anesthesia that can be of particular benefit in the elderly population?

POSTOPERATIVE CARE

62. What are some of the consequences of untreated postoperative pain in the elderly patient?
63. What are some methods of assessing and treating pain in patients with significant dementia or delirium?
64. What are some examples of adjuvant nonopioid medication that can be used to treat pain in the elderly patient?
65. What are some of the advantages of postoperative epidural analgesia in elderly patients?
66. How should the dose of local anesthetic used in a regional technique be altered in an elderly patient?
67. What are the most common postoperative neurologic events in elderly patients?
68. When is postoperative delirium in the elderly patient most likely to present?
69. What are some possible clinical manifestations of postoperative delirium in the elderly patient?
70. What are some causes of postoperative delirium in elderly patients?
71. What are some of the consequences of delirium in elderly patients?
72. How should postoperative delirium be managed?
73. How is postoperative cognitive dysfunction different from delirium?
74. What are some patient clinical factors and surgical procedures that are associated with an increased risk of perioperative stroke?

MEDICATIONS TO AVOID IN THE GERIATRIC POPULATION

75. What are some medications that should be avoided in elderly patients?

ANSWERS*

WHY GERIATRIC ANESTHESIOLOGY IS IMPORTANT

1. The elderly population represents a heterogeneous group of individuals with widely varying functional and reserve capacity. In the United States over 30% of inpatient surgeries are performed in patients over 65 years. Although, there may be a wide disparity between the chronologic and physiologic age in all individuals, aging is associated with a gradual deterioration of organ function, and some age-related changes are inevitable. Elderly patients may also exhibit atypical symptoms leading to delays in diagnosis and more advanced disease at presentation. Other challenges encountered include polypharmacy, the high prevalence of dementia and cognitive dysfunction in the very elderly, and the difficulty in estimating functional reserve in patients with limited mobility and multiple comorbid conditions. (610)

2. Advanced chronologic age is a risk factor for surgical morbidity and mortality. Elderly patients who require surgery are at a greater risk of perioperative complications than their younger counterparts, and the development of complications in themselves increases the risk of a negative outcome including increased length of stay, institutionalization, and even death. This is due to a combination of the effects of chronic disease and generalized age-related decreases in organ function leading to diminished functional reserve. Overall, the comorbid conditions found in elderly patients are the most significant contributors to the development of perioperative complications or perioperative death, rather than the age of the patient. (611)

MORBIDITY AND MORTALITY RATES

3. The need for emergency surgery is one of the most important predictors for mortality rate following surgery in older patients. The circumstances of the emergency itself may be compromising the patient's physiologic status, such as with hemorrhage or dehydration. In these circumstances the older patient with poor baseline function and organ reserve may not be able to respond rapidly to this acute alteration in physiologic state. In addition, emergency cases preclude the preoperative time necessary to control coexisting diseases and maximize organ function. The lack of optimization impacts the ability to withstand the stress imposed by surgery. Other important factors influencing the postoperative outcomes in elderly patients include delayed presentation of a condition, high American Society of Anesthesiologists (ASA) physical status, partial or complete immobility, intracavitary surgery, and congestive heart failure. Older patients tend to present later with more advanced disease and thus be more compromised physiologically at presentation. (611)

4. Complications may be poorly tolerated in very old patients. Patients over 80 years old who developed a postsurgical complication had a fourfold increase in mortality rate. Complications are also associated with an increase in length of hospital stay and morbidity. The most significant complications include cardiac arrest, renal failure, and myocardial infarction. Avoiding even minor complications is one of the cornerstones of management of geriatric patients undergoing anesthesia and surgery. (611–612)

AGE-RELATED PHYSIOLOGIC CHANGES

5. Organ function, in general, declines with age. The decline in organ function associated with aging in the elderly has been characterized as a decline in the ability of the elderly patient's organs to adapt, or compensate, in response to acute stressors. The perioperative period is associated with stressors on numerous organs, leaving elderly patients vulnerable to develop worsening organ dysfunction in the perioperative period. Underappreciated age-related

*Numbers in parentheses refer to pages, figures, boxes, or tables in Pardo MC, Miller RD, eds. *Basics of Anesthesia.* 7th ed. Philadelphia: Elsevier; 2018.

declines in organ function and difficult-to-measure functional reserve may account for why elderly patients unexpectedly develop postoperative complications. For example, the presence of mild renal insufficiency may be missed owing to seemingly normal creatinine levels in a frail older patient with low muscle mass, predisposing the patient to perioperative renal failure. Similarly, previously asymptomatic diastolic dysfunction may predispose the elderly patient to postoperative congestive heart failure following rehydration. (612)

6. Age-related changes in the cardiovascular system of elderly people include an increase in stiffness of the vasculature and an increase in the presence of diastolic dysfunction. In the absence of cardiac disease per se, the cardiac output and stroke volume are largely preserved. Alterations in the conduction system are common, and older patients are predisposed to developing arrhythmias and heart block. Systemic blood pressure steadily increases with age as a result of the decrease in compliance of arterial walls. Alterations in the cardiac sympathetic nervous system result in a diminished ability to increase heart rate in response to stress. In elderly patients a sedentary lifestyle and deconditioning may lead to diminished cardiac output and reserve capacity. The decrease in cardiac output does not appear to occur in elderly patients who have maintained physical fitness. (613)

7. Aging is associated with increased ventricular stiffening that contributes to delayed left ventricular relaxation during diastole. This is referred to as diastolic dysfunction and leads to a decrease in diastolic filling. Approximately one third of older individuals with normal left ventricular function have diastolic dysfunction. Diastolic dysfunction limits a patient's capacity to handle excess intravascular fluid, and thus excess fluid loading can lead to the rapid development of congestive heart failure. (613)

8. The plasma concentration of adrenergic agents required to produce a specific cardiovascular response is increased in the elderly. When adrenergic drugs such as isoproterenol are administered to elderly patients, the change in heart rate is less prominent than the changes in heart rate seen when isoproterenol is administered to younger patients. This is believed to be due to a decrease in the elderly patient's responsiveness at the β-adrenergic receptor. The decrease in responsiveness may occur secondary to a reduced affinity of β-adrenergic agents for the receptor and the impairment of adenylate cyclase activation. This same effect of decreased cardiovascular response has also been noted with the administration of atropine and α-adrenergic agonists. The reduction in parasympathetic tone is also reflected in the reduction in beat-to-beat variability. The levels of circulating norepinephrine rise steadily with aging, supporting a reduction in the sensitivity of the receptor. (613)

9. When hypotension occurs in younger patients, there is a baroreflex-mediated increase in heart rate that occurs to help offset the physiologic effects of the hypotension. In the elderly patient, the reflex-mediated increase in heart rate in response to hypotension is much less pronounced, and as a result elderly patients are prone to develop orthostatic hypotension. The decline in baroreceptor sensitivity and cardiac autonomic function has been termed the *dysautonomia of aging*. It appears to be due to a combination of a decrease in sensitivity of the baroreflexes themselves and a decrease in the ability of the adrenergic receptors to respond, limiting the reflex increase in heart rate. (613)

10. In an awake elderly patient being evaluated for orthostatic hypotension, the lack of an increase in heart rate upon assuming the upright position in the presence of hypotension may reflect autonomic dysfunction. Other signs of autonomic dysfunction include a lack of beat-to-beat heart rate variability or an absence of sinus arrhythmia with respiration. Autonomic dysfunction may occur secondary to aging and vascular stiffening, coexisting diseases such as diabetes or renal failure, or drug effects. (613)

11. There is an age-related decrease in gas exchange in the elderly patient. The most significant age-related change in the lung of the elderly patient is a deterioration of lung elastin. As a result of the degenerative changes in the lungs, there is a breakdown of alveolar septa. This is accompanied by an increase in both anatomic and alveolar dead space and an increase in ventilation-to-perfusion mismatch. These changes are reflected by an increase in the alveolar oxygen pressure and a decrease in the Pa_{O_2} by about 0.5 mm Hg per year after 20 years of age. There are no age-related changes in the Pa_{CO_2}. (613)

12. Age-related changes in the pulmonary system of elderly people include a decrease in vital capacity, a decrease in the forced exhaled volume in 1 second, an increase in residual volume, and an increase in functional residual capacity. These occur as a result of the decreased elasticity of the lungs and increased stiffness of the thorax. (613)

13. Elderly patients have a decreased ventilatory response to hypercapnia and hypoxia. When compared with younger patients, this response can be decreased by about one half. It is important that the anesthesiologist be cognizant of this, because this response is further decreased by the administration of opioids and inhaled anesthetics. (614)

14. Postoperative pneumonia is associated with increased mortality rate, and postoperative pulmonary complications account for 40% of perioperative deaths in older patients. Elderly patients are predisposed to pulmonary complications for several reasons; they have decreases in pulmonary reserves; a decreased level of laryngeal, pharyngeal, and airway cough reflexes; and an increased propensity to aspirate pharyngeal secretions. Elderly patients also have depressed immune function, probably due to involution of the thymus gland and altered function of T lymphocytes. Together, these may explain the increased risk of pulmonary aspiration and an increased incidence of pneumonia in elderly patients when compared with younger patients. (614)

15. Decreases in renal blood flow, glomerular filtration rates, and urine-concentrating abilities accompany aging. These changes are due to alterations in the renal vasculature and may be at least partially due to the age-related decrease in cardiac output. There are also progressive decreases in the total number of nephrons and glomeruli units with age. Clinically, this has some implications for the anesthesiologist caring for the elderly patient. First, elderly patients may be more sensitive to, and less able to adapt to, fluid deprivation or fluid overload. Second, the elderly may be at an increased risk for renal ischemia in the perioperative period. Third, elderly patients have limited ability to concentrate urine and are therefore predisposed to hyponatremia. Finally, drugs that are cleared renally may have a prolonged duration of effect, thereby decreasing the dose requirements of these drugs in the elderly patient. Acute renal failure in elderly patients in the postoperative period has a significant mortality rate. (614)

16. Although renal function decreases with age, in the absence of concomitant renal disease, plasma creatinine concentrations do not change with age. This is because the increase in creatinine that would be expected to accompany the age-related decline observed in the glomerular filtration rate (GFR) is offset by the decrease in muscle mass. There is a decreased production of creatinine secondary to this decrease in muscle mass. (614)

17. Decreases in hepatic blood flow are seen in the elderly as a direct result of decreases in hepatic tissue mass and decreases in cardiac output. Clinically, a delayed clearance of hepatically cleared drugs may result from the decrease in hepatic blood flow in elderly patients. Drugs that may be affected include opiates, barbiturates, benzodiazepines, propofol, etomidate, and most nondepolarizing neuromuscular blocking drugs. (614)

18. The production of albumin is decreased in the elderly, and this may be exacerbated by poor nutrition. Clinically, the reduced albumin may result in a decrease in the binding of drugs administered to elderly patients and an increase

in the free, active portion of the drug. A low preoperative albumin level has been associated with increased mortality rate after surgery. (614)

19. Esophageal and intestinal motility decrease with age, as does gastroesophageal sphincter tone. Clinically, these age-related changes in gastrointestinal function may lead to an increased risk of pulmonary aspiration in elderly patients undergoing general anesthesia. (614)

20. There are several factors that together predispose the elderly to hypothermia in the perioperative period. The reduction in metabolic rate that occurs with aging results in a reduction in heat production. Peripheral vasoconstriction is also less efficient in the elderly person, leading to a diminished ability to conserve heat through redistribution. Shivering is also diminished, and when it occurs it may lead to increased oxygen consumption that may not be tolerated in patients with significant cardiac disease. Hypothermia can have additional negative effects of slowed metabolism of medications and impaired coagulation. (614)

21. Age-related changes occur in both the central and peripheral nervous systems of elderly people. In the central nervous system there is a progressive decline in central nervous system activity and a loss of neurons. This is especially marked in the cerebral cortex and is reflected as a reduction of brain size in radiographic studies. Cerebral blood flow decreases in proportion to decreases in cerebral mass. The autoregulation of cerebral blood flow remains intact. In the peripheral nervous system, there is a decrease in the conduction velocity of peripheral nerves and possibly a decrease in the number of fibers in the spinal cord tracts as well. This is reflected in the increase in the thresholds for the perception of stimuli from virtually all the senses, including pain. (614)

22. The physiologic changes in the central and peripheral nervous systems of elderly people result in a decrease in the minimum alveolar concentration (MAC) by as much as 30% from young adult values. This corresponds to a decreased dose of volatile anesthetic required to achieve a given physiologic central nervous system response in elderly patients. (614)

23. Aging is associated with changes in neurotransmitter levels, and this may be exaggerated in certain dementias. Most significant declines occur in acetylcholine and serotonin receptors in the cortex and dopamine receptors and levels in the substantia nigra and neostriata. (614)

24. Cognitive deficits such as memory difficulty and decreases in processing speed accompany normal aging, the degree of which varies greatly. Mild cognitive impairment can be a precursor to Alzheimer dementia, which is estimated to affect 45% of people over 85 years of age. Other types of dementias include vascular dementia, dementia associated with Parkinson disease, dementia with Lewy bodies, and frontotemporal dementia. Cognitive impairment, whether or not classified as dementia, is a major risk factor for postoperative cognitive complications. (614)

25. Osteoporosis, osteoarthritis, and rheumatoid arthritis occur most frequently in elderly people. These diseases must be considered while positioning the patient for a surgical procedure, as well as while positioning the head and neck for intubation of the trachea. Intubation of the trachea may be more difficult as a result of these diseases. (614)

26. The elderly patient who experiences changes in mental status with extension and rotation of the head may have vertebrobasilar insufficiency or cervical osteoarthritis. In the case of vertebrobasilar insufficiency, cerebral ischemia may result. It is therefore useful to evaluate the elderly patient for symptoms with extension and rotation of the head should this position be necessary for the surgical procedure. (614)

27. A loss of collagen and decreases in the elasticity of the skin of elderly people put them at an increased risk of sustaining injury to their skin during surgical procedures, particularly during prolonged procedures. Elderly patients are

vulnerable to sustaining decubitus ulcers and injury during the removal of adhesive electrocardiogram (ECG) pads or tape. (614)

PERIOPERATIVE CARE IN THE ELDERLY

28. Establishing baseline functional status is one of the most important aspects of the preoperative evaluation of elderly patients. Elderly patients with an excellent functional capacity have a reduced risk of postoperative complications. (614)

29. The preoperative evaluation of the elderly patient scheduled should include the routine preoperative elements for any other patients. An additional goal of the preoperative evaluation of elderly patients is to stratify and minimize risk. The preoperative evaluation should include some key elements that are more relevant to patients in this age group in order to achieve this goal. The patient's functional capacity is one of the most important aspects of the elderly patient's preoperative assessment. This includes an evaluation of the patient's physical fitness, as well as the ability to perform activities of daily living (ADLs). In addition, a brief assessment of cognition can be used to identify if a patient is at increased risk for developing postoperative cognitive problems such as delirium. A careful inventory of all medications, including over-the-counter drugs, should be documented. For patients on multiple medications it can be helpful to have the patient bring the vials to the hospital on the day of surgery or admission. Polypharmacy is common in the older population and can lead to negative drug interactions perioperatively. Malnutrition, as well as drug and alcohol dependence, must also be considered in the elderly patient scheduled for surgery. Finally, the preoperative visit provides an opportunity to begin a discussion on advance health care directives. (615)

30. ADLs describe common behaviors that allow an assessment of an elderly person's function within the living situations. The basic five ADLs are bathing, dressing, toileting, transferring, and eating. Instrumental ADLs (IADLs) describe more advanced activities that would be expected in persons living independently. They include the ability to use the telephone and public transport, do shopping, prepare a meal, do basic housekeeping and budgeting, and manage one's own medications. (616)

31. No preoperative laboratory testing is indicated routinely based on a patient's advanced age. Preoperative laboratory testing should be based on the patient's medical history and the invasiveness of the scheduled procedure. Routine preoperative testing based on age cutoffs leads to unnecessary testing and the risk of false positive and unchecked results. (615)

32. Although it has been popular in the past to use an age cutoff for preoperative ECGs, this approach is not recommended. The preoperative ECG should be ordered when the patient's history or symptoms suggest significant cardiac disease. Because cardiovascular disease is common in older patients, ECGs will probably remain one of the most commonly ordered preoperative tests. Elderly patients frequently have abnormal baseline ECGs, and part of the preoperative evaluation will need to include comparisons to prior ECGs to establish if the observed changes are new findings. (615)

33. Chronically institutionalized patients can present a unique challenge with regard to their preoperative assessment. These patients frequently have complex medical and medication histories and in addition may have limited ability to communicate. It may not be practical to request a separate visit to a preoperative clinic for these patients. In these cases, a thorough review of the medical record may be performed before the surgery. In all cases, it is important to establish who will be providing consent for the surgery and anesthesia prior to the surgery date. (615)

34. Poor nutrition is associated with worse outcomes in older patients. Calculating the body mass index and measuring albumin, prealbumin, and transferrin levels can provide some information about baseline nutritional status. This should

be accompanied by an inquiry about recent weight loss and gastrointestinal symptoms or anorexia. (616)

35. Frailty is a characterized by a generalized decrease in physiologic reserve across multiple systems that is out of proportion to what might be expected during "normal" aging. Frailty is independently associated with an increase in perioperative complications, morbidity, mortality, delirium, length of stay, and postoperative institutionalization. (616)

36. Clinically, frailty is associated with a history of unintended weight loss, weakness (e.g., poor hand grip strength), self-reported exhaustion, slow walking speed, and low physical activity. These are described in the clinical phenotype model. The phenotype frailty screen may be supplemented with other traits including measures of daily function such as ADLs or IADLs, a Timed Up and Go test of gait and mobility, a cognitive function assessment, a measure of comorbid burden, evaluation for anemia, a nutritional assessment, and a history of falls. (616)

37. The Frailty Index is a multidimensional score that measures the number of predetermined deficits—including comorbid conditions, abnormal laboratory tests, assessment of function, and traits such as weakness and cognitive function. It is a calculated score; the higher the score the more frail the individual is considered. The Comprehensive Geriatric Assessment (CGA) is a systematic multidimensional assessment that includes a medical evaluation (usually by a geriatrician), an assessment of the patient's cognitive and functional status, social support, and disability. This screen includes a screen for frailty. The CGA also provides recommendations for preoperative optimization and postoperative management of the elderly patient. (616)

38. The Mini-Cog is a simple test that can be used to evaluate cognitive function preoperatively. The Mini-Cog test assesses several cognitive domains including language, memory, visual motor skills, and executive function. It includes a three-item recall and a clock drawing test. (617)

39. Although most antihypertensive medications are recommended to be taken on the morning of surgery, persistent and difficult to treat postinduction hypotension has been observed in elderly patients treated with angiotensin-converting enzyme (ACE) inhibitors. For that reason it is recommended that ACE inhibitors be withheld the morning of surgery or for 10 to 12 hours preoperatively. Other antihypertensive medications should generally be continued on the day of surgery. (618)

40. Diuretic medications, in combination with decreases in organ function, may result in electrolyte abnormalities in elderly patients. Common laboratory abnormalities include hypokalemia, mild hyponatremia, and contraction alkalosis. These abnormalities can be detected in preoperative laboratory tests. (618)

41. Pharmacodynamic changes in the elderly lead to an increase in sensitivity to certain medications and necessitate a decrease in recommended doses in these patients. The plasma concentration of inhaled anesthetics, opioids, and the benzodiazepine midazolam that is required to produce a specific effect in an elderly person is decreased compared to younger counterparts. For example, the dose of fentanyl and alfentanil required to achieve a given effect in an elderly patient may be decreased by as much as 50% compared to a young adult. The increased sensitivity to anesthetics seen in elderly patients parallels the decrease in cerebral cortex tissue mass and cerebral metabolic rate. This is subsequently reflected as a decrease in the MAC of anesthesia in elderly patients. (618)

42. The plasma concentration of nondepolarizing neuromuscular blocking drugs required to produce a specific twitch response effect is similar in both elderly and younger people. This implies that the sensitivity of elderly patients to nondepolarizing neuromuscular blocking drugs does not change with age. (618)

43. Pharmacokinetics (the absorption, distribution, metabolism, clearance, and excretion of a drug) accounts for the concentration of a drug at the end-organ

site or receptor level. Pharmacokinetic changes in the elderly include decreases in drug clearance and changes in the volume of distribution, making the elderly more susceptible to cumulative drug effects and adverse drug reactions. The plasma concentrations of thiopental, propofol, and etomidate required to produce a specific response are similar in both elderly people and younger people. However, age-related pharmacokinetic changes, especially with respect to distribution, may necessitate a reduction in the initial dose of these medications. (618)

44. A decreased clearance of drugs in the elderly can be attributed to decreases in renal blood flow, decreases in the glomerular filtration rate, decreases in hepatic blood flow, and decreases in hepatic microsomal enzyme activity. Decreases in renal blood flow and decreases in the glomerular filtration rate together may result in the prolongation of the effects of pancuronium, digoxin, and several antibiotics in elderly patients. Likewise, decreases in hepatic blood flow and decreases in hepatic microsomal enzyme activity together may result in the prolongation of the effects of vecuronium, lidocaine, and propofol in elderly patients. (618)

45. The volume of distribution can be divided into the central volume of distribution and the peripheral volume of distribution. The central volume of distribution refers to the volume of the heart and great vessels and the venous volume. A decreased central volume of distribution in the elderly produces an increased initial concentration of drug in the plasma after a bolus injection. The decrease in the central volume of distribution has been thought to be due to decreases in total body water in elderly patients. More recently, this theory has come under scrutiny. Nevertheless, higher initial plasma concentrations of drug after the initial bolus of conventional doses of the drug are seen in elderly patients. Drugs that are affected in this manner include thiopental, propofol, and etomidate when administered for the induction of anesthesia, as well as the initial bolus of opioids. The peripheral volume of distribution includes additional volumes of distribution attached to the central volume. The peripheral volume of distribution in elderly patients is increased owing to a relative increase in body fat and a decrease in the amount of drug bound by protein. The increased peripheral volume of distribution may also be reflected as a delay in the rate of elimination of lipid-soluble drugs that are stored in fat, such as opioids and the volatile anesthetics. (619)

46. Preoperative anxiolytics should be used sparingly in the elderly population because they can cause undesirable levels of sedation and confusion in these patients. In addition, the residual effects of these medicines may persist even after the surgical case has been completed. In lieu of the preoperative anxiolytic medicines, a detailed explanation of the events that will occur before and after the surgical procedure may be a useful anxiolytic substitute. (619)

47. The induction dose of an anesthetic should be reduced for an older patient compared to a younger patient. The reduction appears to be mostly due to pharmacokinetic changes. The drug administered for induction exerts its pharmacologic effects in the circulation for a longer amount of time, and the receptors are exposed to a larger initial concentration. The induction dose of anesthetic in the elderly patient is not decreased for pharmacodynamic reasons, because the plasma concentration of induction drug required to produce a desired effect is equal in elderly and younger patients. (620)

48. There is great interindividual variability in the response to opioids in elderly patients, and as such the dose administered should be titrated to its desired effect. The dose of opioid may need to be reduced by as much as 50% from that administered to younger patients, mostly due to pharmacodynamic changes in elderly patients. In addition, decreases in clearance and the potential accumulation of active metabolites may warrant longer intervals before redosing. (620)

49. Meperidine can cause delirium in older patients, possibly due to its anticholinergic effects and through accumulation of its active metabolite normeperidine. For this reason it is not recommended for sedation or analgesia in older patients. (620)

50. Hand ventilation by bag and mask may be difficult in the edentulous patient secondary to a poor mask-to-face fit. It is often easier to hand ventilate by bag and mask when the edentulous patient's dentures are left in place or an oral airway is used. (620)

51. Endotracheal intubation may be difficult in a patient with poor dentition or cervical arthritis. Difficulty in patients with poor dentition arises because of the need to avoid loose teeth during direct laryngoscopy to avoid dislodgment of the teeth. Patients with cervical arthritis may be difficult to endotracheally intubate because of the decreased range of motion, especially extension, of the neck. (620)

52. The reversal of nondepolarizing neuromuscular blocking drugs in the elderly patient does not warrant any special considerations for the anesthesiologist, because there are no unique risks of this in the elderly patient population. The incidence of cardiac dysrhythmias after the administration of glycopyrrolate or neostigmine may be increased in elderly patients who have cardiovascular disease. (620)

53. Several postoperative complications are more common in older patients compared to younger patients. These include cardiovascular events such as myocardial infarction and congestive heart failure, especially from diastolic dysfunction. This is most likely related to the frequency of cardiovascular disease in the elderly population and underlying age-related changes. Central nervous system complications are the next most commonly encountered postoperative complication in the elderly patient. Although cerebrovascular accidents are more common in older patients than in younger patients, they are still uncommon and usually occur in a patient with preexisting cardiac or vascular disease. More common central nervous system events are postoperative delirium and postoperative cognitive dysfunction. These are especially common in older patients with preexisting dementia, depression, and cognitive impairment—for example, in patients who have had a cerebrovascular accident in the past. Pulmonary complications include postoperative hypoxia and pneumonia. It is possible that early ambulation may minimize some of the pulmonary risks. (620)

54. Considerations regarding monitored anesthesia care in elderly patients include their sensitivity to medications, pulmonary changes, and their decreased ventilatory responses to hypercapnia and hypoxemia. Thus, elderly patients are more susceptible to developing hypoxemia and hypoventilation during procedures. Supplemental oxygen and end-tidal CO_2 monitoring are recommended. (620)

55. Standard medicines that can be used for monitored anesthesia care in the elderly patient include propofol, midazolam, short-acting opioids (e.g., fentanyl, remifentanil), small doses of ketamine (especially for painful procedures), and dexmedetomidine. The dose of dexmedetomidine may be limited by its side effects of prolonged sedation, bradycardia, and hypotension. (620)

56. Regional anesthesia is an alternative to general anesthesia for elderly patients undergoing surgical procedures such as transurethral resection of the prostate, gynecologic procedures, inguinal hernia repair, or the treatment of hip fractures. Regional techniques such as peripheral nerve blocks are becoming increasingly popular and may be a valuable adjuvant to general anesthesia in elderly patients. They may reduce the amount of anesthesia needed and improve postoperative pain control. (620)

57. Regional anesthesia may be advantageous over general anesthesia for hip surgery in elderly patients. Regional anesthesia may be associated with decreases in perioperative blood loss and decreases in the incidence of deep venous

thrombosis. There is no evidence, however, that one method of anesthesia is safer than the other. (620)

58. An advantage to maintaining consciousness in the elderly patient during a regional anesthetic for a surgical procedure is that the anesthesiologist is able to communicate with the patient during the procedure. Changes in mental status can herald the onset of a developing adverse event. For example, confusion during a transurethral resection of the prostate may be an early warning sign of the development of hyponatremia or fluid overload. Similarly, a patient may complain of chest pain or shortness of breath signaling the presence of myocardial ischemia. Additionally, there may be decreased immediate postoperative confusion in elderly patients after having received a regional anesthetic as compared with a general anesthetic. (620)

59. Elderly patients may be more sensitive than younger patients to regional anesthesia, especially spinal anesthesia. Possible reasons why this may be true include decreased vascular absorption from the spinal space, decreases in vertebral column length, and a decreased reflex compensatory sympathetic nervous system response. Together, these may manifest as a prolonged duration of action, increased anesthesia level, and exaggerated decreases in blood pressure following a spinal anesthetic. (620)

60. Attenuation of the hypotensive effects of a regional anesthetic may be achieved by the prophylactic administration of an intramuscular dose of ephedrine before administering the spinal anesthetic. Adequate hydration minimizes the effects of a sympathectomy on blood pressure but does not consistently eliminate the hypotensive effects of spinal anesthesia in elderly patients. (620)

61. Epidural anesthesia is advantageous over spinal anesthesia in that it may be administered more slowly than a spinal anesthetic, with the onset of the resulting sympathectomy being more gradual. This may result in a more gradual decrease in the elderly patient's blood pressure than that seen with a spinal anesthetic. (620)

POSTOPERATIVE CARE

62. Untreated postoperative pain in elderly patients is associated with serious consequences in elderly patients. These include increased length of hospital stay, morbidity, pulmonary complications, and delirium. (620)

63. To assess pain in a patient with dementia or delirium a nonverbal pain scale can be used, such as the Pain Assessment IN Advanced Dementia (PAIND). This pain scale involves the observation of five items: breathing, vocalization, facial expression, body language, and consolability. Treatment of pain in these patients may involve the administration of pain medicines at regularly scheduled intervals rather than on an as-needed basis. (621)

64. Adjuvant nonopioid medicines that can be used to treat pain include acetaminophen, nonsteroidal anti-inflammatory drugs (NSAIDs), and gabapentin. Acetaminophen can be used to reduce opioid requirements in elderly patients. NSAIDs can also lead to lower narcotic requirements, but the dose must be adjusted to reduce the risk of renal insufficiency or gastrointestinal side effects such as bleeding. For example, the dose of ketorolac should be reduced to 15 mg intravenously every 6 hours in the elderly patient. Gabapentin is another medication that can be used in the perioperative period to reduce opioid use. It is renally excreted, and the dose should be reduced in older patients. It can also cause sedation in large doses. (621)

65. Postoperative epidural analgesia in elderly patients has been associated with improved pulmonary function, reduced atelectasis, easier extubation of the trachea, and shorter intensive care unit stays in patients who have had thoracic and upper abdominal surgeries. (621)

66. The metabolism and excretion of local anesthetic drugs is reduced in the elderly. When administering a regional anesthetic in elderly patients, the overall dose should be reduced. (621)

67. The most commonly encountered postoperative neurologic events in elderly patients are delirium and cognitive dysfunction. Postoperative delirium has been estimated to occur in at least 10% to 15% of elderly patients undergoing surgical procedures. It may occur in as many as 60% of patients undergoing repair of an acute hip fracture. (621)

68. Postoperative delirium is most likely to present one or more days after surgery in elderly patients. This type of delirium is termed *interval delirium*. This is in contrast to emergence delirium commonly seen in pediatric patients that occurs within minutes after the emergence from anesthesia. (621)

69. Clinical manifestations of postoperative delirium in elderly patients may include alterations in attention, cognition, and sleep-wake cycles; a reduced level of consciousness; and increases or decreases in psychomotor behavior. These patients are often disoriented to time, place, and person. Close monitoring of these patients is essential to prevent patients from harming themselves by attempting to get out of bed or by pulling out catheters. (621)

70. Causes of postoperative delirium in the elderly patient include drug toxicity, fluid and electrolyte imbalances, hypoxemia, anemia, uremia, myocardial ischemia, congestive heart failure, infection, pain, or depression. Antiparkinsonian drugs, antihypertensives, and anticholinergic and psychotropic medications tend to increase the risk of drug interactions with anesthetics and postoperative analgesics to produce postoperative delirium. A deficiency of neurotransmitters such as acetylcholine and dopamine is hypothesized to be the underlying physiologic cause of postoperative delirium. (621)

71. Delirium in elderly patients has been associated with increased mortality rate, length of hospital stay, and loss of independence evidenced by an increased risk of transfer to an assisted living and nursing home. Delirium can persist for weeks or even months in elderly hospitalized patients. (621)

72. Postoperative delirium should prompt a search for an underlying cause, such as hypoxemia or pain. If necessary, agitated patients may benefit from small doses of intravenous haloperidol. (621)

73. Postoperative cognitive decline is a subtle alteration in cognitive function and mental ability. Unlike delirium, postoperative cognitive dysfunction is not associated with acute confusion or agitation. Neuropsychological testing is required for its diagnosis. (621)

74. Some patient clinical factors and surgical procedures that are associated with an increased risk of perioperative stroke include advanced age, hypertension, reduced ejection fraction of less than 40%, cardiac, vascular, and head and neck surgery. Most perioperative strokes are embolic and ischemic. (621)

MEDICATIONS TO AVOID IN THE GERIATRIC POPULATION

75. Aging is associated with changes in drug metabolism that may alter the half-life of a medication and also physiologic receptor changes that may change the impact of a given medication. For example, many elderly patients, especially with dementia, have decreased central cholinergic reserve. This is important when these patients are administered drugs with high cholinergic potency—for example, atropine or scopolamine. The antiemetic scopolamine is a tertiary quaternary amine that crosses the blood-brain barrier. The central anticholinergic effects of scopolamine may lead to significant delirium in elderly patients and should be avoided. Other medications that can similarly cause delirium through central anticholinergic effects include atropine, chlorpheniramine, diphenhydramine, and promethazine. (622)

36 ORGAN TRANSPLANTATION

Randolph H. Steadman and Victor W. Xia

CONSIDERATIONS FOR ORGAN TRANSPLANTATION

1. What conditions preclude transplantation?
2. Most transplant candidates are screened for comorbid conditions prior to being waitlisted. What additional beneficial preoperative measures can be undertaken once a donor is identified?
3. Describe the difference between donation after brain death (DBD) and donation after cardiac death (DCD) organ donation.

KIDNEY TRANSPLANTATION

4. Who is a candidate for renal transplantation?
5. What is the most common cause of end-stage renal disease?
6. Why should the preoperative assessment of potential renal transplant recipients focus on screening for ischemic heart disease?
7. What is the kidney donor risk index?
8. What are the preoperative considerations for the patient scheduled to undergo renal transplantation?
9. What laboratory values for potassium and hemoglobin are acceptable in patients scheduled to undergo a renal transplantation?
10. Where is the donor kidney transplanted in the recipient patient? From where does it derive its vascular supply? Where is the ureter anastomosed?
11. What are some intraoperative considerations for the anesthetic management of patients undergoing renal transplantation?
12. What considerations must be made when selecting a neuromuscular blocking drug (NMB) and an opioid for patients undergoing renal transplantation?
13. What effect do volatile anesthetics have on renal function?
14. Why should intravascular fluid balance be maintained in patients undergoing renal transplantation? Which crystalloid and colloid are preferred?
15. What are common diuretics used during renal transplantation?
16. What intraoperative monitoring is appropriate during renal transplantation?
17. How is maintenance of renal perfusion best accomplished postoperatively?

LIVER TRANSPLANTATION

18. Name the four most common indications for liver transplantation in the United States.
19. What is the MELD (model for end-stage liver disease) score? What is its clinical application?
20. What are the preoperative considerations for the patient scheduled to undergo liver transplantation?
21. What characterizes the hyperdynamic circulation seen in over two thirds of liver transplant recipients?

22. What is the best screening test for portopulmonary hypertension? What is its clinical significance?
23. What is hepatopulmonary syndrome? What is its clinical significance?
24. What is the most common cause of death in acute liver failure?
25. What are the goals of the anesthetic plan for liver transplantation?
26. What are the three stages of liver transplant procedures?
27. What are the characteristic physiologic derangements of the preanhepatic stage of liver transplant procedures?
28. What are the characteristic physiologic derangements of the anhepatic stage of liver transplant procedures?
29. What is the "piggy-back" technique, and why is it used in some patients?
30. Why is venovenous bypass used in some centers?
31. What are the characteristic physiologic derangements that occur with reperfusion of the donor graft (neohepatic stage) during liver transplant procedures?
32. What is reperfusion syndrome?
33. What signs of liver function can be assessed intraoperatively after graft reperfusion?

HEART TRANSPLANTATION

34. Who is a candidate for heart transplantation?
35. What are some preoperative considerations when assessing the patient undergoing heart transplantation?
36. What are some perioperative goals for the anesthetic management of heart transplant patients?
37. What vessels are transected and anastomosed during heart transplant surgery? What does this mean with regard to a central venous or pulmonary artery catheter?
38. Why might bradycardia be seen after reperfusion, and how is it treated?
39. Does the transplanted heart respond to catecholamines that are direct or indirect acting?
40. Why might right-sided heart failure be seen in patients during reperfusion, and how is it treated?
41. What are some possible causes of pulmonary hypertension during heart transplantation, and how is it treated?
42. Name the physiologic conditions that should be optimized prior to weaning from cardiopulmonary bypass.
43. What are some postoperative considerations in the management of heart transplant patients?

LUNG TRANSPLANTATION

44. What are some indications for lung transplantation?
45. What are some preoperative considerations for the patient undergoing a lung transplant procedure?
46. In addition to standard monitors and transesophageal echocardiography (TEE), why is endobronchoscopy necessary during lung transplant surgery?
47. Why are double-lumen endotracheal tubes used for intubation of the trachea during lung transplant procedures?
48. What are some challenges and strategies in the anesthetic management of patients undergoing a lung transplant procedure?
49. What are some postoperative management considerations in the lung transplant patient?
50. Why are lung transplant patients predisposed to developing pneumonia in the transplanted lung?

PANCREAS TRANSPLANTATION

51. Who is a candidate for pancreas transplantation?
52. What are some preoperative considerations in patients undergoing pancreas transplantation?
53. Why should intraoperative hyperglycemia be avoided in patients undergoing pancreas transplant surgery?
54. What other organ is often transplanted simultaneously along with the pancreas?

ANSWERS*

CONSIDERATIONS FOR ORGAN TRANSPLANTATION

1. Untreated systemic infection, incurable malignancy, untreated substance abuse, and lack of sufficient social support to comply with posttransplant care can preclude transplantation. (625)
2. Because of the long wait times between listing and transplantation, once a donor is identified preoperative screening tests may need to be repeated. Most important are tests for ischemic heart disease (postoperative cardiovascular fatality is second in frequency to infection), assessment of laboratory results such as electrolytes and hemoglobin, and if needed, preoperative dialysis. (625)
3. Most commonly deceased donor organ procurement occurs after brain death (DBD). Because of organ shortages, the number of grafts from donation after cardiac death (DCD) is increasing, although it remains a minority of donors. Candidates for DCD are patients who have irreversible brain injury but don't meet brain death criteria, and who are not expected to survive once life-preserving measures such as mechanical ventilation are withdrawn. In DCD, the patient is brought to the operating room, life support is withdrawn, cardiac death is confirmed, and then the organs are procured. For DCD there is a period of warm ischemia that does not occur in DBD. (625)

KIDNEY TRANSPLANTATION

4. Kidneys are the most commonly transplanted major organ. Patients who have end-stage renal disease and are being considered for, or are currently receiving, dialysis are candidates for renal transplantation. Transplantation has led to lower overall morbidity and mortality rates compared to dialysis. (626)
5. The most common cause of end-stage renal disease leading to chronic dialysis dependence is diabetes mellitus, followed by hypertension and glomerulonephritis. These three causes account for over two thirds of the cases of renal failure. (626)
6. Patients who are potential renal transplant recipients should have a preoperative assessment for ischemic heart disease because the cardiovascular risk in patients requiring dialysis is increased tenfold compared to that of normal patients. In addition, ischemic heart disease may be silent, particularly in diabetic patients. As a result of preexisting vasodilation, stress echocardiography is probably better than thallium imaging in predicting postoperative cardiac events. Coronary angiography should be considered in high-risk patients. (626)
7. The kidney donor risk index (KDRI) provides an assessment of risk associated with donor kidneys. Donor factors in the KDRI include older, hypertensive, and diabetic donors and grafts with a prolonged duration of cold ischemia (long preservation times) or warm ischemia (DCD). (626)
8. Preoperative considerations for the patient scheduled to undergo a renal transplant procedure are similar to those for any other surgical procedure in which the patient has chronic renal failure. This includes scheduling of hemodialysis prior to surgery to optimize the patient's volume status, electrolytes, and acid-base balance. The serum glucose levels of the patient with diabetes mellitus should also be evaluated before and during surgery. (626)
9. Potassium levels of 5.0 to 5.5 mEq/L are acceptable in patients scheduled to undergo renal transplantation because mild increases in potassium may reflect normal homeostasis for renal failure. Anemia is common in renal failure patients but may increase cardiovascular risk in patients with ischemic heart disease. Hemoglobin concentrations greater than 12 g/dL may increase the risk of thrombotic events, however. (626)
10. The donor kidney is transplanted on one side of the recipient's iliac fossa. The vascular supply for the transplanted kidney is derived from the iliac vessels. The

*Numbers in parentheses refer to pages, figures, boxes, or tables in Pardo MC, Miller RD, eds. *Basics of Anesthesia.* 7th ed. Philadelphia: Elsevier; 2018.

ureter of the transplanted kidney is anastomosed directly to the recipient's bladder. (626)

11. Some intraoperative considerations for the anesthetic management of patients undergoing renal transplantation include drug excretion, management of intravascular volume and adequate hemodynamics, appropriate monitoring, and minimizing the risk of renal dysfunction in the transplanted kidney. (627)

12. Choice of neuromuscular blocking (NMB) drug or opioid during anesthesia for renal transplantation should take into account drug metabolism and duration of action, and the potential for the buildup of toxic metabolites. An NMB drug that does not rely primarily on renal clearance should be selected. Cisatracurium is particularly attractive because its metabolism is independent of both the kidney and liver. Pancuronium, vecuronium, and rocuronium all have a prolonged duration of action in renal failure patients. Morphine may have a prolonged duration of action in renal failure patients secondary to its active metabolite, which is cleared by the kidneys. Meperidine should also be avoided because its metabolite has seizure-inducing potential. (627)

13. Volatile anesthetics all produce a dose-dependent decrease in renal blood flow and glomerular filtration rate. They are all acceptable for use, however, in patients undergoing renal transplantation. Although sevoflurane in rats produces a nephrotoxic metabolite (compound A), similar effects have not been seen in humans, making it an acceptable choice for anesthesia. Additionally, the fluoride levels produced through the metabolism of sevoflurane and isoflurane are negligible, making their administration acceptable in these patients. (627)

14. Intravascular fluid balance should be maintained during renal transplantation to improve renal perfusion; adequate intravascular fluid balance has been shown to reduce the incidence of acute tubular necrosis in the transplanted kidney. In an intensive care unit (ICU) population, balanced salt solutions (e.g., Ringer lactate, Plasma-Lyte) are preferred over hyperchloremic crystalloid such as normal saline because they are associated with a lower incidence of acute kidney injury. Paradoxically, they elevate serum potassium levels less than potassium-free crystalloids, because the potassium-free crystalloids elevate potassium levels by generating a hyperchloremic state. Albumin is the colloid of choice in these patients. (627)

15. The diuretics mannitol and furosemide are often administered intraoperatively during renal transplant procedures to facilitate diuresis. However, controlled studies supporting an improved outcome in graft function are lacking. (627)

16. Arterial line monitoring during renal transplantation is avoided in some centers in order to preserve arterial access for dialysis but are used routinely in other centers. Central intravenous lines may be placed for the administration of immunosuppression induction medicines. (627)

17. Maintaining renal perfusion in the postoperative period is best accomplished by maintaining intravascular volume status. Dopamine, large-dose diuretics, and osmotic diuretics provide no proven benefit. (628)

LIVER TRANSPLANTATION

18. The most common indications for liver transplantation in the United States are hepatitis C, alcoholic liver disease, cholestatic disease, and malignancy. Combined, these diagnoses account for 70% of waiting list candidates. Patients with acute hepatic failure, chronic end-stage liver disease, tumors (in the absence of extrahepatic spread), and metabolic abnormalities affecting their liver are candidates for liver transplantation. Newer antiviral agents may decrease the future need for transplantation for hepatitis C, and nonalcoholic steatohepatitis (NASH) is expected to become an increasingly prevalent cause leading to transplantation in the coming years. (628)

19. Patient acuity, as determined by the MELD score, is used to allocate organs. The MELD score predicts 90-day mortality rate in the absence of liver transplantation. The international normalized ratio of prothrombin time (INR), creatinine, and bilirubin are used to derive the MELD score. (628)

20. Preoperative considerations for the patient undergoing liver transplantation include screening for ischemic heart disease, portopulmonary hypertension, hepatopulmonary syndrome, variceal bleeding, ascites, renal disease, acid-base abnormalities, coagulopathy, anemia, and encephalopathy. Encephalopathy, even if not clinically overt, can lead to sensitivity to sedative and analgesic medications. (628)

21. The hyperdynamic circulation seen in over two thirds of liver transplant recipients is characterized by a high cardiac output and low systemic vascular resistance. Circulating vasoactive substances, which are normally cleared by the liver, are responsible for the low systemic vascular resistance. The decreased afterload results in an elevated cardiac output. This hyperdynamic state can be confused with sepsis. (628)

22. Resting echocardiography is a highly sensitive screening test for portopulmonary hypertension; however, it is not specific. Therefore, patients with an estimated right ventricular systolic pressure greater than 50 mm Hg should undergo right-sided heart catheterization to confirm or rule out the diagnosis. Mean pulmonary artery pressures higher than 35 mm Hg are associated with a perioperative mortality rate of 50%, and treatment prior to transplantation should be considered. (628)

23. Hepatopulmonary syndrome (HPS) consists of arterial hypoxemia ($Pa_{O_2} < 70$ mm Hg on room air) in the presence of an intrapulmonary shunt. Liver transplantation cures HPS, albeit over a variable time course. A preoperative $Pa_{O_2} < 50$ mm Hg is associated with greater postoperative morbidity and, in some studies, postoperative fatality. (629)

24. Cerebral edema is the most common cause of death in acute liver failure. Acute liver failure accounts for approximately 5% of liver transplantations. (629)

25. The goals of the anesthetic plan for liver transplantation are to maintain systemic vascular resistance and avoid intravenous agents that undergo extensive hepatic metabolism. In addition, rapid transfusion of fluids and products should be possible as well as the availability of vasopressors, laboratory analysis, and intraoperative monitoring with lines and possibly transesophageal echocardiography (TEE). (629)

26. The preanhepatic, anhepatic, and neohepatic stages make up the liver transplant procedure. The preanhepatic stage involves the dissection of the portal venous structures and mobilization of the native liver. The anhepatic stage begins when the native liver's blood supply is interrupted by clamping of the suprahepatic and infrahepatic inferior vena cava and the portal vein. The neohepatic stage begins with the return of vascular supply to the graft, usually via the vena cava and portal vein. (629)

27. The preanhepatic stage of liver transplant procedures is characterized by cardiovascular instability because of sudden decreases in the intra-abdominal pressure and the exacerbation of chronic hypovolemia owing to loss of ascites and hemorrhage. Metabolic and electrolyte abnormalities can occur during this stage, including metabolic acidosis, and hypocalcemia results from citrate toxicity. Hemorrhage, often requiring the rapid infusion of fluids and blood products, is related to the degree of portal hypertension and adhesions from prior abdominal surgery. (629)

28. The anhepatic stage of liver transplant procedures is characterized by decreases in venous return and cardiac output. For this reason, sympathomimetic drugs are often administered during this portion of the liver transplant procedure to maintain cardiac output. Hypocalcemia and metabolic acidosis commonly occur during this stage as a result of citrate toxicity and decreased renal perfusion pressure, respectively. The anhepatic stage is the most hemodynamically quiescent stage of liver transplantation. (629)

29. The "piggy-back" technique, an alternative to the classic caval-interruption technique, involves the anastomosis of the donor hepatic veins to the recipient vena cava. The piggy-back technique is preferred by some centers because it avoids transection of the inferior vena cava, which may preserve venous return. (629)

30. Extracorporeal venovenous bypass is used in some centers in conjunction with the classic caval-interruption technique to reroute blood from the inferior vena cava to the superior vena cava in order to augment venous return. It is not universally used because it prolongs surgery and has potential complications, including air embolism. (629)

31. The neohepatic stage of liver transplant procedures is characterized by the potential for precipitous hyperkalemia, acidosis, and hypothermia due to the cold ischemic effluent from the graft and lower extremities entering the central circulation. The systemic vascular resistance drops, and emboli of blood or air can occur. Hyperkalemia is exacerbated by the washout of the potassium-containing solution used to preserve the liver, in addition to unclamping of the inferior vena cava and portal vein. Fibrinolysis can also occur, leading to ongoing oozing due to microvascular bleeding. Antifibrinolytic drugs may need to be administered if the fibrinolysis is not self-limited. Hypotension, arrhythmias, and cardiac arrest may potentially occur during this time. (629)

32. Reperfusion syndrome is characterized by decreases in systemic blood pressure and systemic vascular resistance during the neohepatic phase of liver transplantation. Insulin (effective if given in advance), calcium, adrenergic agonists, and alkalizing agents are often administered to treat hyperkalemia and maintain systemic vascular resistance and pH during this period. (629)

33. Signs of liver function after graft reperfusion include improvement in metabolic acidosis (due to metabolism of citrate to bicarbonate), a reduced calcium requirement (due to the metabolism of citrate), and a rising body temperature (due to exothermic reactions in the liver). In some cases an increase in urine output may reflect the resolution of hepatorenal syndrome. (630)

HEART TRANSPLANTATION

34. Patients with end-stage heart disease are candidates for heart transplantation. The most common indications for heart transplantation are idiopathic dilated cardiomyopathy, ischemic heart disease, and congenital heart disease, which combined account for more than 90% of heart transplants. (630)

35. Preoperative considerations when assessing the patient undergoing heart transplantation include current cardiac status, inotropic and anticoagulant drugs, and what mechanical support is required, such as an intra-aortic balloon pump or ventricular assist device. Patients should not have severe, irreversible pulmonary hypertension or active infection. Monitors are selected including arterial and central intravenous lines and TEE. Finally, because of the urgency of the procedure, heart transplant patients often have a full stomach. (630)

36. Perioperative goals for the anesthetic management of heart transplant patients include maintaining systemic blood pressure and coronary filling, optimizing preload, reducing afterload to improve ejection fraction, supporting contractility, correcting acid-base abnormalities, and avoiding pulmonary vasoconstriction, hypercapnia, and high tidal volumes. The induction and maintenance of anesthesia should provide good endotracheal intubating conditions while preserving cardiac function. Selection of drugs is dictated by underlying heart condition and assessment of benefits and risks of each drug. (630)

37. Vessels and structures that are transected and anastomosed during heart transplant procedures include the aorta, pulmonary artery, and left and right atria. These steps are done during cardiopulmonary bypass. A central venous or pulmonary artery catheter that is in place at the onset of surgery must be pulled back into the internal jugular vein when the patient's heart is excised. (630)

38. Bradycardia may be seen after reperfusion in the donor heart because it is denervated and not responsive to hemodynamic changes. Bradycardia can be treated by pacing (usually 90 to 110 beats/min) or chronotropic drugs such as isoproterenol. Isoproterenol maintains myocardial contractility and heart rate in the denervated donor heart and decreases pulmonary vasculature resistance. (631)

39. The transplanted heart reacts better to direct-acting catecholamines. Indirect-acting drugs including atropine, which work via the autonomic nervous system, are ineffective because of denervation of the graft. (631)

40. Right-sided heart failure may be seen in patients during reperfusion because of pulmonary hypertension or ischemia of the right ventricle on reperfusion. The primary treatment goals of right-sided heart failure during heart transplantation are to increase contractility of the right ventricle and decrease pulmonary artery resistance. Failure to respond to treatment may necessitate mechanical right ventricular support. (631)

41. Pulmonary hypertension during heart transplantation can be due to an increase in cardiac output, pulmonary vessel spasm, and emboli. It is exacerbated by hypoxemia and hypercarbia. Treatment of pulmonary hypertension can be with nonselective vasodilators such as nitroglycerin and sodium nitroprusside, but these drugs can also decrease systemic vascular resistance and result in systemic hypotension. Selective drugs such as inhaled nitric oxide, aerosolized iloprost, and sildenafil may be helpful. (631)

42. Prior to weaning from cardiopulmonary bypass, patients should be normothermic and free from acid-base and electrolyte disturbances. The lungs are ventilated and the cardiac chambers are free from air. (631)

43. Postoperative considerations in heart transplant patients include management of oxygenation, ventilation, intravascular volume, pulmonary and systemic pressures, coagulation, and body temperature. Inotropic and chronotropic support is often required in the few days following heart transplant. Permanent pacemaker implantation may be necessary because of the loss of sinus node function. Patients should be monitored for postoperative bleeding and graft function, which can require emergent intervention. (631)

LUNG TRANSPLANTATION

44. Indications for lung transplantation include chronic obstructive lung disease and interstitial lung disease in adults and cystic fibrosis in children. (631)

45. Preoperative considerations for the patient undergoing lung transplant include the severity of the disease, controlling anxiety without oversedation, cautious use of supplemental oxygen so as not to abolish the hypoxic drive, and possible epidural placement for postoperative pain management. (632)

46. Endobronchoscopy is necessary during lung transplant surgery not only to assess the position of the double-lumen endotracheal tube but also to examine airway anastomoses for stenosis, bleeding, and obstruction secondary to blood or sputum. (632)

47. Double-lumen endotracheal tubes are used for intubation of the trachea for lung transplant surgery to allow for isolated ventilation of either the left or right lung. One lung may be ventilated while the other is being transplanted. (632)

48. Challenges in the anesthetic management of patients undergoing lung transplant include the onset of positive-pressure ventilation causing a precipitous decrease in venous return and potential cardiac arrest in patients with severe pulmonary hypertension, positive-pressure ventilation further damaging diseased lungs and worsening hypoxemia and hypercarbia, air trapping, barotrauma, ventilation-perfusion mismatch during one-lung ventilation, and increased pulmonary hypertension during pulmonary artery clamping, particularly in patients with preexisting elevation of pulmonary artery pressure. Strategies for the management of patients undergoing lung transplant include preparation for emergent cardiopulmonary bypass during the induction of anesthesia, ventilation with low tidal volumes, intravascular fluid volume restriction, and the use of nonselective and selective pulmonary vasodilators. (632)

49. Some postoperative management considerations in the lung transplant patient include the avoidance of barotrauma, volutrauma, and anastomotic dehiscence during positive-pressure ventilation. (632)

50. Lung transplant patients are predisposed to pneumonia in the transplanted lung due to disruption of lymphatic drainage, poor mucociliary function, obstruction of bronchi from clots in the bronchial suture lines, and loss of the cough reflex. Immunosuppression exacerbates the risk of infection. (632)

PANCREAS TRANSPLANTATION

51. Patients with diabetes mellitus are candidates for pancreas transplantation. The most common indication for pancreas transplantation is type 1 diabetes. However, more transplants are performed in patients with type 2 diabetes in recent years. (632)

52. Preoperative considerations in patients undergoing pancreas transplantation are similar to those undergoing kidney transplant for end-stage renal disease secondary to diabetes. They include assessment of the effects of diabetes on cardiovascular, autonomic, nervous, renal, gastrointestinal, and metabolic systems. (632)

53. Intraoperative hyperglycemia should be avoided in patients undergoing pancreas transplantation because it may adversely affect islet function and promote posttransplant infection. (632)

54. Pancreas transplant procedures are often performed simultaneously with kidney transplantation because of the advanced nature of the diabetes, which is associated with renal failure. Simultaneous pancreas-kidney transplant recipients experience the best graft survival rates. The success of a pancreas transplant is measured by monitoring blood glucose levels after surgery; blood glucose concentrations may return to normal within hours. (632)

37 OUTPATIENT ANESTHESIA

David M. Dickerson and Jeffrey L. Apfelbaum

1. When and where was the first outpatient surgery clinic opened?
2. What were the primary goals of Dr. Wallace Reed and Dr. John Ford in opening the Phoenix Surgicenter in 1970?

3. What subspecialty society sought to define the field of outpatient anesthesia? What specific contributions did the society bring to the field?

4. What are the expectations of the patient undergoing outpatient surgery?
5. What benefits do the office-based procedures provide patients?
6. What are several specific aims of an outpatient care facility?

7. What are the various venues for outpatient surgery?
8. Who are potential owners of ambulatory surgery centers (ASCs)?
9. What factors contribute to the exceptionally low mortality rate of outpatient surgery?

10. Is there a list of acceptable patients or case types for all outpatient venues?
11. What defines an ambulatory anesthesiologist?
12. What are some responsibilities of an ASC medical director that are often fulfilled by an anesthesia provider?
13. What is the relationship between practice variation, hierarchical culture, patient safety, and health care costs?
14. What procedures are the most frequently performed in the ambulatory surgical setting?
15. What patient characteristics predict unanticipated admission after surgery lasting longer than 1 hour?
16. What quality metrics have been historically tracked by the Agency for Healthcare Research and Quality (AHRQ)?
17. Although unanticipated admission is low, what postdischarge phenomenon was nearly 30-fold higher in incidence than hospital transfer?
18. Is office-based anesthesia as safe as anesthesia for hospital- and ASC-based procedures?
19. What factors have led to the improved track record of office-based anesthesia?
20. Although poor patient selection can result in injury, what is the more common cause of anesthesia-related injury in office-based anesthesia?
21. What factors increase risk in the office-based surgery setting?

THE PERIOPERATIVE JOURNEY OF AN AMBULATORY SURGICAL PATIENT

22. What social factors are essential for successful ambulatory surgery?
23. What percentage of Medicare beneficiaries undergoing cataract surgery had a preoperative evaluation in 2011, and how much did this evaluation cost?
24. Does routine testing before cataract surgery increase safety?
25. What do published guidelines recommend for testing and preoperative optimization of medical issues?
26. As the risk of major adverse cardiac events is both procedure- and patient-specific, what do the 2014 American College of Cardiology/American Heart Association (ACC/AHA) guidelines recommend for assessing this risk?
27. What are some cardiovascular patient clinical factors that are associated with an increased risk of perioperative complications that may preclude a patient from undergoing ambulatory surgery?
28. What are some pulmonary patient clinical factors that are associated with an increased risk of perioperative complications that may preclude a patient from undergoing ambulatory surgery?
29. What are some renal, endocrine, and neurologic patient clinical factors that are associated with an increased risk of perioperative complications that may preclude a patient from undergoing ambulatory surgery?
30. As a part of a thorough preoperative assessment, a STOP-BANG question can screen for what?
31. What factors contribute to increased risk in a patient with an elevated STOP-BANG score?
32. What perioperative risks are associated with obstructive sleep apnea?
33. Is a preoperative assessment required prior to every anesthetic?
34. Can anesthesiologists impact a patient's decision to continue smoking cigarettes after his or her surgery?
35. What are the risks of general anesthesia in patients with an upper respiratory infection?
36. Is routine preoperative pregnancy testing mandatory? As an unanticipated positive pregnancy test result is infrequent, what is the cost of each positive result when the total cost of all negative and positive results is considered?
37. What is monitored anesthesia care (MAC)? Can general anesthesia occur during a MAC?
38. What regional anesthetic techniques can be applied for breast surgery?
39. Does nitrous oxide exposure always cause postoperative nausea and vomiting (PONV)?
40. What techniques can reduce nausea and vomiting after general anesthesia?
41. What defines early (phase I), intermediate (phase II), and late (phase III) recovery?
42. As communication failures frequently contribute to preventable medical errors and adverse events, what techniques for patient handoffs from anesthesia personnel to the recovery team may improve the fidelity of information transfer and retention?
43. What is fast-tracking?
44. What are the benefits of fast-tracking?
45. The success of fast-tracking may be predicted by what key preoperative patient characteristics?
46. What is the result of inappropriate phase I bypass or fast-tracking?
47. Whether coming from the operating room or recovering from phase I, what formal criteria define patient readiness for phase II recovery? What clinical patient characteristics are assessed by these criteria?
48. What are the benefits of not administering opioids before the postoperative period?
49. What are the benefits of multimodal analgesia?
50. What nonopioid therapies can be utilized for pain relief in the outpatient setting?
51. What dose of dexamethasone is sufficient for PONV prophylaxis?
52. How might persistent PONV after an initial 4-mg dose of ondansetron be treated?

53. What criteria are utilized for assessing readiness for postanesthesia care unit (PACU) discharge, and what are the benefits of using a standardized scoring system?
54. How should the outpatient surgical patient who does not meet discharge criteria be managed?
55. What common challenges are present for the patient after discharge from an outpatient surgical facility?
56. What are the challenges to the caregiver after discharge from the outpatient surgical facility?
57. Are newer, long-acting, antiemetic agents superior to traditional, less expensive options?
58. What are some predictors of postdischarge nausea and vomiting 3 to 7 days after ambulatory surgery?
59. Should all patients be contacted after outpatient regional anesthesia?
60. Should all patients be contacted after ambulatory anesthesia?

ANSWERS*

INTRODUCTION

1. Dr. Ralph Waters opened the Downtown Anesthesia Clinic, the first modern ambulatory surgery center, in Sioux City, Iowa, in 1919. (634)
2. As inpatient surgery became more expensive, Dr. Reed and Dr. Ford sought to decrease the cost of surgery while maintaining high quality and safety, all the while creating an environment that was comforting to and convenient for the patient. (634)

OUTPATIENT ANESTHESIA IS DIFFERENT

3. The Society for Ambulatory Anesthesia (SAMBA) developed guidelines that shape clinical care, research, and education. The activities of the Society and a shifting of the majority of surgeries to the outpatient setting forged the practice patterns of today's ambulatory anesthesiologist. (635)

OUTPATIENT ANESTHESIA IS PATIENT-CENTERED

4. Expectations of patients undergoing outpatient surgery include safety during the procedure, relief of pain, freedom from nausea, and a rapid return to normal daily function and routine. They also expect minimal burden and convenience for patient caretakers, who may include friends or family. (635)
5. Convenience, privacy, and cost-efficiency are the primary patient benefits of office-based procedures. (635)
6. The specific aims of an outpatient care facility are as follows: maintain a predictable environment through selectivity of procedure, place, provider, and patient; promote a culture of vigilance and patient safety; maintain best practices through continued evaluation of peer-reviewed literature and site performance; standardize workflow to ensure "best practices"; and achieve rapid and smooth induction, maintenance, and emergence from anesthesia with minimal if any side effects and maximal patient safety. (635)

DEFINING THE VALUE OF AMBULATORY CARE

7. The various venues for outpatient surgery are a freestanding ambulatory surgery center (ASC), freestanding hospital outpatient department, a proceduralist's office, or a hospital-based outpatient department. (635)
8. Potential owners of ASCs include hospitals, investment groups, physician groups, and individual physician and nonphysician investors. (635)
9. Site and accreditation, multidisciplinary oversight, established patient safety-related standards of care, judicious patient and procedure selection, and a specialized workforce perpetuate the exceptionally low mortality rate of outpatient surgery. (635)

*Numbers in parentheses refer to pages, figures, boxes, or tables in Pardo MC, Miller RD, eds. *Basics of Anesthesia*. 7th ed. Philadelphia: Elsevier; 2018.

SELECTION: PATIENT, PRACTITIONER, PROCEDURE, PLACE

10. There is no list of acceptable patients or case types for outpatient venues, but rather the expertise and preparedness of each site dictates its ability to care for specific patients or procedures. A personalized patient plan that minimizes complexity and maximizes predictability should be developed incorporating existing guidelines from professional societies. If the site cannot provide the optimal level of care for a patient or the specific procedure, the procedure should be referred to a more appropriate care setting. (636)

11. Ambulatory anesthesiologists value standardized work as well as the patient's and surgeon's time. They are effective communicators and utilize cost-effective multimodal analgesia and minimally invasive short-acting anesthetics for rapid, safe recovery. They recognize that a specialized team can impact the duration and predictability of operative room time and recovery room stay. (636)

12. Responsibilities of an ASC medical director include maintenance of compliance with regulatory and legislative directives, adherence to regulations regarding keeping medical records, restrictions on facility size, maintenance of emergency equipment, sterilizing systems, personnel-to-patient ratios, and the availability of recovery beds. These duties are often fulfilled by an anesthesia provider. (636)

13. Unnecessary variation and a hierarchical culture typically contribute to unsafe, inefficient practice that results in a higher cost of health care delivery. Variation is limited through adherence to consistent, agreed-upon guidelines and standard care plans for the management of patients. (636)

14. The most frequently performed surgeries in the ambulatory surgical setting are lens and cataract surgery, orthopedic surgery, and laparoscopic cholecystectomy. (637)

15. The risk of unanticipated admission is increased after 60 minutes of surgery in patients with an American Society of Anesthesiologists (ASA) physical status of 3 or 4, advanced age, or obesity. (637)

16. Unanticipated admission and hospital transfer have been deemed quality measures by the AHRQ. Other ongoing quality improvement projects are conducted through the AHRQ as a part of the Ambulatory Surgery Center Quality Collaboration. (637)

17. Hospital-based acute care via the emergency department was found to be 30-fold higher than unanticipated admission in a study of 3.8 million patients treated at over 1200 ambulatory surgical centers. (637)

18. According to a recent study, office-based anesthesia is as safe as hospital- and ASC-based anesthesia; however, previous studies have suggested that office-based anesthesia has not always been as safe. (637)

19. Office accreditation, proper procedure and patient selection, provider credentialing, facility accreditation, patient safety checklists, and implementation of professional society guidelines have improved safety in office-based procedures. (637)

20. Inadequate patient monitoring appears responsible for the majority of cases of anesthesia-related injury in office-based anesthesia. (638)

21. Risk is increased by unqualified or insufficiently experienced surgical or anesthesia staff, a lack of proper equipment, insufficient training for resuscitation and other emergencies, and inadequate access to hospitals for continued treatment of life-threatening emergencies. (638)

THE PERIOPERATIVE JOURNEY OF AN AMBULATORY SURGICAL PATIENT

22. Essential social factors for successful ambulatory surgery are a driver or other arrangements for safe transport home, a caregiver for postsurgical care and assistance with activities of daily living, and a patient and family motivated for recovery at home. (638)

23. Of Medicare beneficiaries undergoing cataract surgery, 53% underwent preoperative evaluation, resulting in a $12.4 million increase in health care costs in the month before surgery compared to the 11 months before the preoperative month. (639)

24. According to a Cochrane review, routine testing before cataract surgery does not improve outcomes. (639)

25. Recent guidelines suggest risk stratification–driven testing to modify risk and stabilize specific existing medical conditions. In other words, will a result from ordering this test prompt an intervention that will reduce this patient's risk of perioperative injury? (639)

26. As part of the assessment of risk for major adverse cardiac events in patients undergoing noncardiac surgery, patient-specific and procedure-specific factors are assessed. The patient's functional capacity is determined, and a functional capacity of at least four metabolic equivalent (MET) values (e.g., ascending two flights of stairs) is adequate for most outpatient procedures. The ACC/AHA guidelines further recommend utilizing one of two risk-calculating methods to determine perioperative risk. The surgical risk calculator of the National Surgical Quality Improvement Program or the Revised Cardiac Risk Index can assist in risk stratifying patients. (639)

27. Cardiovascular patient clinical factors associated with an increased risk of perioperative complications include new-onset or unstable angina, malignant hypertension, myocardial infarction within 6 months, newly diagnosed cardiac dysrhythmia, decompensated heart failure, severe valvular disease, drug-eluting stent placement within 12 months, and bare metal stent placement within 4 weeks. (639)

28. Pulmonary patient clinical factors associated with an increased risk of perioperative complications include symptomatic bronchospasm, productive cough, increased work of breathing, severe obstructive sleep apnea, and decreased oxygen saturation. (640)

29. Renal, endocrine, and neurologic patient clinical factors associated with an increased risk of perioperative complications include symptomatic hyperglycemia or hypoglycemia, insufficient recent dialysis, recent cerebrovascular accident or unmanaged transient ischemic attack, and dementia or delirium. (640)

30. The STOP-BANG question screens for obstructive sleep apnea (OSA). (640–641)

31. Surgery type, opioid exposure, an inability to undergo local or regional anesthesia, and a lack of physician training or equipment to manage complications associated with undiagnosed or uncontrolled OSA and its comorbid conditions increase risk in a patient with OSA undergoing surgery. (640)

32. Patients with OSA are at increased risk for cerebrovascular events, myocardial infarction, bleeding, and perioperative respiratory events (e.g., difficult intubation). (641)

33. Yes. The Centers for Medicare and Medicaid Services has required that a preoperative assessment be performed prior to every anesthetic. Furthermore, physical status correlates with unanticipated admission and delayed discharge. A thorough assessment may mitigate this risk. (642)

34. Yes, brief motivational interviewing can increase postoperative smoking cessation when performed preoperatively by an anesthesiologist. (642)

35. Supraglottic edema, stridor, laryngospasm, desaturation, and coughing may occur during general anesthesia in the presence of active or recent upper respiratory infection. A supraglottic airway device may not fully reduce this risk. (643)

36. No, routine preoperative pregnancy testing is not mandatory. Based on two studies, the cost per positive result is between $1000 and $3000 per test, with an unknown benefit of not performing elective surgery on a parturient. Pretest probability of active pregnancy can be assessed before conducting the test in patients providing a reliable history. (643)

37. MAC is an anesthesia billing term describing sedation by an anesthesia provider. General anesthesia may occur during MAC because sedation is titrated with continuous monitoring to accommodate the needs of the patient and surgeon throughout a procedure. (645)

38. Paravertebral blockade as well as novel blocks of the chest wall (serratus anterior plane and pectoral nerve blocks) provide anesthesia and analgesia for breast surgery. (645)

39. Limited exposure (less than 90 minutes) of nitrous oxide exposure does not appear to increase the risk of postoperative nausea and vomiting (PONV). (645)

40. Robust opioid-sparing multimodal analgesia, adequate hydration, limited nitrous oxide exposure, evidence-based antiemetic therapy, not administering neostigmine with volatile anesthetics, and low-dose intraoperative propofol infusion have been suggested as techniques to reduce postoperative nausea and vomiting after general anesthesia. (646)

41. Phase I recovery lasts until anesthesia or surgically induced derangements in protective reflexes and motor function resolve. When resolved and pain, nausea, and vomiting are well controlled, patients may advance to phase II recovery. Phase II recovery persists until discharge criteria are met. During phase III recovery, which occurs at home, the patient returns to his or her preoperative physiologic state. (646)

42. Handoff forms or checklists can improve retention and transmission of relevant patient and perioperative information. (646)

43. Fast-tracking, or phase I bypass, refers to the transfer of a patient who has already met phase I discharge criteria directly from the operating room and is advanced immediately to the second phase of recovery. This may result in patient recovery in an ambulatory care unit with different nursing staffing from that in the postanesthesia care unit (PACU). (646)

44. A fast-tracking benefit is that patients are rapidly reunited with their friends and family. In some instances, fast-tracking has been shown to substantively decrease costs. (646)

45. Age less than 60 years, ASA physical status score less than 3, and nongeneral surgery are predictive of successful fast-tracking. (646)

46. Inaccurate patient selection for phase I bypass increases nursing workload and reduces potential cost savings as workload is shifted from the PACU to the phase II recovery area. (646)

47. The modified Aldrete criteria and White criteria are scoring systems for evaluating phase II readiness. Clinical patient characteristics assessed by these criteria include level of consciousness, physical activity, hemodynamic stability, respiration, oxygen saturation status, pain level, and nausea symptoms. (646)

48. Reduced PONV, decreased sedation, and reduced opioid requirements postoperatively result from not administering opioids before the postoperative period. (646)

49. Decreased pain, decreased opioid-related adverse effects, high patient satisfaction, and rapid throughput via fast-tracking are potential benefits of effective multimodal analgesia. (646)

50. Many nonopioids have been established as safe and effective in ambulatory surgery. They include preoperative pregabalin and gabapentin, COX-2 inhibitors, intraoperative β-blockers, ketorolac and other nonselective nonsteroidal anti-inflammatory drugs, subanesthetic-dose ketamine, magnesium, dexamethasone, dexmedetomidine, intravenous lidocaine infusion, and regional anesthesia. (648)

51. Four milligrams of dexamethasone is sufficient for PONV prophylaxis, although previously established regimens utilized 8 mg. (648)

52. After assessment, patients with persistent PONV following an initial 4-mg dose of ondansetron may be treated with low doses of alternative agents. In these cases promethazine or prochlorperazine may prove to be superior to repeat dosing of ondansetron. (648)

53. ASA practice guidelines delineate necessary and unnecessary criteria for discharge. The postanesthesia discharge scoring system (PADSS) is a validated scoring tool for assessing patient readiness for discharge and reduces the length of stay in the recovery room when compared to arbitrary recovery time requirements. (648)

54. In the event a patient does not meet discharge criteria, the patient should be continuously observed in a hospital facility or short-stay unit depending on the needs for monitoring and care of the patient. Outpatient procedural sites should have a well-defined plan for patient transfer in such unanticipated situations. (649)

55. Patients may suffer moderate to severe pain, cognitive impairment, nausea and vomiting, and impaired function in activities of daily living that may persist for several days after discharge from an outpatient surgical facility. (649)

56. Prolonged patient recovery or uncontrolled significant pain increases the burden on the caregiver. Caregiving by family and friends after outpatient surgery can result in emotional and physical disturbances in the lives of the family and friends providing such care. The stressors and challenges for caregivers after outpatient surgery are unique, but common themes have been described. (649)

57. Traditional antiemetics appear equally efficacious when compared to newer, longer-acting formulations. (649)

58. Predictors for postdischarge nausea and vomiting 3 to 7 days after ambulatory surgery include prolonged operating room time, history of PONV, use of ondansetron in the PACU, and pain during the 3 to 7 days after discharge. (649)

59. Although no guideline exists for contacting patients after outpatient regional anesthesia, tracking the patient experience, block success, or potential injury carries great benefit for patient care as well as continued process improvement. As postoperative iatrogenic nerve injury is not infrequent, the ability to assess mechanism of injury as well as dictate patient treatment are key to follow-up communication. Both define an expert consultant in regional anesthesia. (650)

60. Applying iterative design to a surgical facility's standardized work is only possible through outcomes tracking and reevaluation. A standardized follow-up phone interview assessing key factors in patient satisfaction and outcome should be conducted for quality reporting and benchmarking of the group's performance. This process may help control costs, reduce risk, and optimize the patient experience. Outcome measurement is a tenet of evidence-based medicine. (650)

38 ANESTHESIA FOR PROCEDURES IN NON-OPERATING ROOM LOCATIONS

Chanhung Z. Lee and Wilson Cui

1. What are some anesthesia-related concerns when performing non–operating room anesthesia (NORA)?

CHARACTERISTICS OF NORA LOCATIONS

2. What are some special challenges facing the anesthesiologist providing NORA?
3. What are some fundamental capabilities available in the operating room that must also be available for NORA?
4. What are some safety concerns facing the anesthesiologist during NORA?

SAFETY AND CONCERNS IN RADIOLOGY SUITES

5. How might the anesthesiologist limit his or her exposure to radiation during diagnostic and therapeutic radiologic procedures?
6. What is the federal guideline limit of annual occupational exposure to radiation in Sievert units? How does this compare to radiation exposure during a chest radiograph or a computed tomography (CT) scan of the head?
7. What are some signs and symptoms of anaphylactoid reactions that can occur after the administration of iodinated contrast agents? How can it be treated?
8. What prophylaxis may be administered to patients at risk of a serious adverse reaction to an intravenously administered contrast agent?
9. What is the potential serious adverse reaction that can occur in patients with severe renal impairment receiving gadolinium-based magnetic resonance imaging contrast agents?

MAGNETIC RESONANCE IMAGING

10. What is magnetic resonance imaging (MRI)?
11. What are some features of MRI that make it difficult for the patient to tolerate?
12. What are some MRI safety considerations?
13. How must anesthetic equipment and monitors in the MRI center be altered for MRI compatibility?
14. How should the patient be monitored when undergoing an anesthetic for MRI?
15. How must accidental extubation of the patient's trachea during MRI be managed?
16. Why is there an increased risk of hypothermia for patients in the MRI scanner?

ANESTHESIA FOR NONINVASIVE IMAGING PROCEDURES

17. What anesthetic techniques may be used for noninvasive imaging procedures?
18. How does the management of anesthesia for patients undergoing CT compare with the management of anesthesia for patients undergoing MRI?

INTERVENTIONAL RADIOLOGY

19. Is general anesthesia preferred over sedation for procedures in interventional radiology? What are the advantages and disadvantages of each technique?
20. Why might anticoagulation be necessary during interventional radiology procedures?

21. Why is blood pressure management crucial in interventional neuroradiology procedures?
22. What are some anesthetic concerns related to anesthesia for patients scheduled to undergo transjugular intrahepatic portosystemic shunt (TIPS) placement in interventional radiology?
23. What are some challenges related to anesthetizing patients with acute hemorrhage in interventional radiology?

ENDOSCOPY AND ENDOSCOPIC RETROGRADE CHOLANGIOPAN-CREATOGRAPHY

24. What is the advantage of performing endoscopy with minimal or moderate sedation delivered by an anesthesiologist?
25. What are some anesthetic considerations that may influence the choice of anesthesia technique for endoscopic procedures?
26. What complications may occur as a result of endoscopic procedures?
27. What are the anesthetic challenges in caring for a patient with acute upper gastrointestinal bleeding undergoing endoscopy?

CATHETER-BASED CARDIOLOGY PROCEDURES

28. Why might patients require anesthesia for interventional cardiology procedures? What adverse effects might the anesthetic have on cardiac function during these procedures?
29. What are some anesthetic considerations when caring for a patient during electrophysiology catheter-based ablation procedures?
30. What knowledge about the procedure should the anesthesiologist have when caring for patients undergoing placement of a cardiac implantable electronic device (CIED)?
31. Why does a patient undergoing elective electrical cardioversion require sedation and amnesia?
32. What is involved in the anesthetic management of a patient undergoing elective electrical cardioversion?
33. What are some advantages and challenges of general anesthesia for patients undergoing structural heart disease intervention in the radiology suite?
34. What are the specific challenges of caring for pediatric patients undergoing interventional cardiology procedures?
35. What are the implications of an intracardiac shunt on the anesthetic management of pediatric patients undergoing interventional cardiology procedures?
36. What are some potential complications the anesthesiologist may encounter in interventional cardiology procedures?
37. How might pericardial effusion or tamponade present during an interventional cardiology procedure? How should it be managed?

ELECTROCONVULSIVE THERAPY

38. Which patients are candidates for electroconvulsive therapy (ECT)?
39. How is ECT accomplished?
40. What are the absolute and relative contraindications to ECT?
41. How should patients with an implanted cardiac defibrillator or pacemaker be managed for an ECT?
42. Which premedication can be considered for ECT? Should any be given routinely?
43. What monitors should be used during the administration of anesthesia for ECT?
44. How can the airway of the patient undergoing ECT be managed? What equipment should be available to the anesthesiologist?
45. Which agents might be used for the induction of anesthesia in a patient undergoing ECT, and what are the advantages and disadvantages of each?
46. After unconsciousness is induced, what is the purpose of the administration of succinylcholine? Why should a tourniquet be applied on a distal limb?
47. What are the cardiovascular responses to ECT and their consequences?
48. What are some post-ECT manifestations in the patient?

ANSWERS*

1. Some anesthesia-related concerns when performing non–operating room anesthesia (NORA) include maintenance of patient immobility and physiologic stability, perioperative anticoagulation management, readiness for unexpected complications, provision of sedation and smooth and rapid emergence, and appropriate postprocedure monitoring and management during transport. (658)

CHARACTERISTICS OF NORA LOCATIONS

2. Some special challenges facing the anesthesiologist providing NORA include communication regarding the procedure and expectations, limited access to the patient's airway, poor availability of accessory help, and the potential difficulty in quickly obtaining emergency equipment. At the conclusion of anesthesia in remote locations there is typically a greater amount of distance the anesthesiologist must transport the patient before reaching the postanesthesia care unit. This results in a greater need for supplemental oxygen delivery and continuous monitoring. (659)

3. Anesthesia care provided in NORA must adhere to the same standards that apply to the operating room; the American Society of Anesthesiologists (ASA) has issued minimal guidelines for NORA care. Fundamental capabilities for monitoring, the delivery of supplemental oxygen, mechanical ventilation of the lungs, the availability of suction, the delivery and scavenging of inhaled anesthetics, and an adequate supply of anesthetic drugs and ancillary equipment must all be available for the delivery of anesthesia in remote locations. (660)

4. Some safety concerns the anesthesiologist faces when administering anesthesia in remote locations include the possibility of exposure to increased radiation, loud sound levels, heavy mechanical equipment, and the scavenging of waste anesthetic gases. Lead aprons, lead thyroid shields, portable lead-glass shields, earplugs, and elevator keys may be necessary. The locations of the nearest defibrillator, fire extinguisher, gas shutoff valves, and exits should all be noted. (660)

SAFETY AND CONCERNS IN RADIOLOGY SUITES

5. The anesthesiologist should attempt to limit his or her exposure to radiation by wearing a lead apron and thyroid shield, through the use of movable lead-glass screens, and by remaining as far away as possible from the radiation source, preferably at least 1 to 2 m. A recent study also highlighted the importance of eye protection for anesthesia providers working significant hours in the radiology suite. Finally, clear communication between the radiology and anesthesia teams is crucial for limiting radiation exposure. The radiation exposure can be monitored by wearing radiation exposure badges. (660)

6. Federal guidelines set a limit of 50 mSv (millisieverts) for the maximum annual occupational dose of radiation. By comparison, for patients receiving a chest radiograph the dose is 0.1 mSv, whereas for those receiving a computed tomography (CT) scan of the head the dose is 2 mSv. The average background radiation exposure in the United States is 3 mSv per year. (660)

7. Anaphylactoid reactions in response to the administration of iodinated contrast agents can range from mild to severe. Mild side effects may include nausea, a perception of warmth, headache, and pruritus. Moderate side effects may include faintness, emesis, urticaria, laryngeal edema, and bronchospasm. Severe reactions may include seizures, hypotensive shock, laryngeal edema, respiratory distress, and cardiac arrest. The newer nonionic contrast dyes of lower osmolarity tend to be associated with fewer incidences of allergic reactions. Treatment is relative to the reaction and may require the administration of oxygen, intravenous fluids, and epinephrine if necessary. (660)

---

*Numbers in parentheses refer to pages, figures, boxes, or tables in Pardo MC, Miller RD, eds. *Basics of Anesthesia.* 7th ed. Philadelphia: Elsevier; 2018.

8. Patients at risk for an adverse reaction to a contrast agent should be pretreated with steroid and antihistamine medicines on both the night before and the morning of the procedure to minimize the reaction. A typical regimen for a 70-kg adult is 40 mg prednisone, 20 mg famotidine, and 50 mg diphenhydramine. Adequate hydration is necessary in these patients to maintain their intravascular volume because the intravenous contrast medium also acts as an osmotic load for the patient, inducing diuresis. (661)

9. Nephrogenic systemic fibrosis (NSF) is a serious adverse reaction that can occur in patients with severe renal impairment receiving gadolinium-based MRI contrast agents. In NSF there is fibrosis of the skin, connective tissue, and sometimes internal organs. The severity of NSF can range from mild to severe and can also be fatal. (661)

MAGNETIC RESONANCE IMAGING

10. Magnetic resonance imaging (MRI) is a radiologic technology that provides digitalized tomographic images of the body by exposing the body to a very high-strength constant magnetic field and high-frequency alternating electric and magnetic fields. MRI does not produce any ionizing radiation. These studies are useful for the evaluation of neurologic and soft tissues because they can distinguish between fat, vessels, and tumor. (661)

11. MRI is difficult for the patient to tolerate because the patient must lie still for up to an hour or more on a long thin table. The table moves within a long thin tube that has walls close to the face of the patient, making some patients claustrophobic. In addition, the MRI scanner makes loud booming noises that may augment a patient's discomfort. (661)

12. MRI safety considerations include the potential for hearing loss from the loud booming noise during scans, the possibility of electrical burns, and the risk of missile injury with ferromagnetic objects. Contraindicated items containing metals that can be dangerously heated and cause injury are standard pulse oximeter probes, standard electrocardiogram electrodes, and temperature probes. A contraindication to MRI are patients who have any implanted metals that are attracted by a magnetic field or easily heated by alternating electromagnetic fields. Examples of metallic items include artificial cardiac pacemakers, some aneurysm or intravascular clips, some orthopedic hardware, wire-enforced epidural catheters, and pulmonary artery catheters with a temperature wire. Missile injury can occur because the MRI scanners are always surrounded by a large magnetic field gradient (up to 6 m away) that can pull metal objects into the magnet with alarming speed and force. (661)

13. Standard operating room monitors and anesthetic equipment must not be used in the MRI scanner. Plastic, nonmagnetic steel, and aluminum components replace metal ones within special anesthesia machines, ventilators, monitors, and intravenous infusion equipment specially made for MRI compatibility. Aluminum gas cylinders must be used instead of standard iron gas cylinders. Again, traditional pulse oximeters must not be used in the MRI scanner because they can cause very serious burns to the patient. (661)

14. The patient undergoing an anesthetic for MRI should have his or her blood pressure, oxygen saturation, and cardiac rhythm continually monitored with special MRI-compatible equipment. Capnograph monitors may also be used to detect end-tidal carbon dioxide, especially when monitoring from a distance. Extensions must be placed on all monitoring equipment because the patient moves into the MRI scanner during the study. Arterial lines may require long lengths of pressure tubing, and the pulse generated from the MRI may generate artificial spikes. Anesthesia providers can remain outside the magnet room during scans if they have access to vital sign displays and can view the patient through the window or by video camera. A primary anesthesia workstation must be located outside the magnet room, and the patient must be promptly transferred out of the scanner room if a life-threatening problem arises. (661)

15. Accidental extubation of the patient's trachea during MRI must be managed by immediate discontinuation of imaging, removing the patient from the scanner, and rapidly controlling the patient's airway. In the event that resuscitative equipment is necessary in an emergency, the patient must be moved far enough away from the MRI scanner to prevent metal components of the resuscitative equipment from becoming attracted to the magnet. (661)

16. The airflow through the MRI scanner increases the amount of heat loss from the patient, placing the patient at an increased risk of hypothermia. This risk is of particular concern for pediatric patients undergoing MRI. (661)

ANESTHESIA FOR NONINVASIVE IMAGING PROCEDURES

17. Anxiolysis, moderate sedation, and general anesthesia are all anesthetic techniques that may be used for noninvasive imaging procedures. For pediatric patients, deep sedation or general anesthesia may be required. In all cases, the ASA Standards of Basic Monitoring apply, capnography may be useful, and supplemental oxygen should be available. (662)

18. Anesthesia for CT scanning is similar to that for MRI. That is, access to the patient is limited and monitoring is remote. CT scanning differs from MRI in that the scans are typically shorter, the scanner is an open space making claustrophobia less likely, and the avoidance of ferromagnetic equipment is not necessary. CT scanners do emit ionizing radiation, however. (663)

INTERVENTIONAL RADIOLOGY

19. Anesthetic requirements of patients undergoing interventional radiology procedures vary. Evidence is limited on which technique is superior. General anesthesia ensures airway security, limits movement artifact, and guarantees patient comfort during prolonged cases. The ability to hyperventilate and produce mild hypocapnia may also be beneficial in patients with elevated intracranial pressures. Sedation with spontaneous respiration causes minimal perturbation to hemodynamics and allows faster recovery. The choice depends on the procedural need, the patient's comorbid conditions, and the anesthesiologist's clinical judgment. (663)

20. Interventional radiology procedures often involve the management of coagulation parameters depending on the anticoagulation status of the patient and the nature of the procedure. Procedures that involve catheters in the arterial tree require anticoagulation, often with heparin, to avoid thromboembolic complications. When the catheters are removed, the anticoagulation effect of heparin is usually reversed with protamine. Unexpected or excessive bleeding during the procedure may also occur and necessitate immediate heparin reversal. (664)

21. Blood pressure management and manipulation may be crucial in interventional neuroradiology procedures, making arterial line placement and communication with the interventional radiology team important. Deliberate hypertension may be necessary during occlusive cerebrovascular disease to promote collateral cerebral blood flow, in patients with a subarachnoid hemorrhage in whom vasospasm has developed, or in patients with compromised blood flow to spinal cord, kidneys, or other organs. Conversely, the prevention of arterial hypertension may be critical in patients with recently ruptured intracranial aneurysms or those who have undergone carotid artery angioplasty and stent placement who are susceptible to hyperperfusion injury. Predetermined arterial blood pressure ranges should be established prior to a procedure. (664)

22. Some anesthetic concerns related to anesthesia for patients scheduled to undergo transjugular intrahepatic portosystemic shunt (TIPS) placement in interventional radiology include the effects of liver failure on other organ systems, possible coagulopathy and thrombocytopenia requiring correction prior to the procedure, the possible need for general endotracheal anesthesia, and the potential for post-TIPS complications including altered mental status from encephalopathy, massive hemorrhage, and worsening liver failure from decreased portal vein blood flow. (665)

23. Challenges related to anesthetizing patients with acute hemorrhage in interventional radiology include the rapid and safe induction of anesthesia, the establishment of

adequate intravenous access with long tubing, and managing potential coagulopathy and thrombocytopenia due to acute factor and platelet losses with the administration of intravenous fluids and blood products. (665)

ENDOSCOPY AND ENDOSCOPIC RETROGRADE CHOLANGIOPANCREATOGRAPHY

24. Having an anesthesiologist dedicated to monitoring patients under minimal or moderate sedation enables the endoscopist to focus entirely on the invasive procedure. The use of propofol provides faster onset of adequate anesthesia and shorter recovery. However, severe respiratory depression can occur and limits its use to anesthesia providers. (666)

25. Anesthetic considerations that may influence the choice of anesthesia technique for endoscopic procedures include the patient's comorbid conditions (coagulopathy, thrombocytopenia, ongoing bleeding, cardiac instability, pulmonary disease), patient's airway examination or history of obstructive sleep apnea, limited access to the patient's airway during the procedure, the patient's position (prone, lateral), the importance of patient immobility during the procedure, and the duration of the procedure. (666)

26. Complications that may occur with endoscopy can be grouped by sedation and airway-related, procedure-related, and patient-related factors. Serious complications may include aspiration, laryngospasm, pharyngeal injury, esophageal or intestinal perforation, and bleeding. Clinical signs and symptoms associated with perforation can be nonspecific, such as neck, chest, or abdominal pain; tachycardia; tachypnea; hypotension; and abdominal distention. (666)

27. The challenges of caring for a patient with upper intestinal bleeding undergoing endoscopy include difficult endotracheal intubation, venous access, massive transfusion and volume resuscitation, correction of coagulopathy, and maintaining hemodynamic stability. The patient may have underlying medical issues such as cirrhosis and coagulopathy that require treatment. Anesthetic management of such critically ill patients is further complicated by the location being outside the operating room, where resources and help may not be nearby. (667)

CATHETER-BASED CARDIOLOGY PROCEDURES

28. Patients may undergo interventional cardiology procedures for diagnostic angiography, angioplasty with or without stent placement, electrophysiology study with possible ablation of dysrhythmia, implantation of pacemaker or defibrillators, and percutaneous intervention of valvular defects or other congenital structural heart diseases. The goal of the anesthesiologist is to ensure patient comfort and safety, to provide hemodynamic monitoring, and to assist in cardiopulmonary resuscitation during an emergency. In a cooperative patient, minimal sedation and analgesia are sufficient when local anesthetic is provided prior to percutaneous vascular access. However, general anesthesia is necessary if surgical exposure is anticipated or if the patient is uncooperative because of mental status. General anesthesia and positive-pressure ventilation can cause additional myocardial depression and cardiovascular instability in vulnerable patients. Coronary ischemia, sometimes induced by angioplasty, as well as dysrhythmia can lead to sudden instability. The use of vasoconstrictors or inotropic agents may be necessary during interventional cardiology procedures. (667)

29. When caring for a patient during electrophysiology catheter-based ablation procedures, the preprocedure evaluation should focus on their cardiopulmonary reserve, airway, comorbid conditions, and any relevant medications such as anticoagulants. It is useful to know the patient's symptoms when arrhythmias occur, because syncope or angina may suggest a decreased cardiac output and may warrant invasive arterial blood pressure monitoring. Local anesthetics and sedation are particularly useful during the initial cannulation and catheter insertion, and minimal sedation is usually necessary afterward. In fact, many electrophysiologists believe excessive sedation suppresses dysrhythmias and interferes with mapping. An exception is for atrial fibrillation procedures, in which general anesthesia with endotracheal intubation may be helpful so that respiratory movement is predictable, esophageal temperature may be monitored

(to avoid left atrial perforation), and phrenic nerve stimulation can be detected. (667)

30. When caring for a patient undergoing placement of a cardiac implantable electronic device (CIED), the anesthesiologist should know the type of CIED, its indication, the underlying cardiac rhythm, and whether the patient is pacemaker dependent. The management of the device should be discussed with the cardiologist or the electrophysiologist prior to the case. The anesthesiologist should have a functional knowledge of how to operate transcutaneous pacing and defibrillator devices. Finally, the anesthesiologist should be aware if a defibrillation threshold test will be performed during the procedure, in which the cardiologist intentionally induces fibrillation to test the device's ability to sense and terminate fibrillation. In this case, additional short-acting anesthetic may be indicated and possibly invasive arterial monitoring of the blood pressure. (668)

31. The electrical shock during cardioversion would be painful and can be traumatic to the patient if done without sedation and amnesia. Furthermore, elective electrical cardioversion may be preceded by transesophageal echocardiography (TEE) to examine the left atrium for thrombus, which may increase the length of the procedure. (668)

32. Before undergoing elective electrical cardioversion, the patient should have fasted according to the NPO guidelines. Standard monitors—pulse oximetry, electrocardiogram, blood pressure—are placed. Emergency medication and airway equipment for endotracheal intubation, suction, oxygen supply and methods of positive-pressure ventilation should be immediately available. Adequate preoxygenation should be achieved prior to the administration of sedative. The upper airway may be topically anesthetized with local anesthetics to suppress the gag reflex during probe insertion, but there is a potential drawback of lingering loss of airway reflex lasting longer than the procedure, making it difficult for the patient to handle secretions. With propofol the anesthesiologist can titrate the level of sedation to allow the passage of the TEE probe, maintain patient cooperation during the TEE examination, and ensure amnesia of the electric shock. During and immediately after sedation, the patient may require manual relief of airway obstruction. Monitoring of the patient is necessary until the recovery of mentation, airway reflexes, and unencumbered respiration. (668)

33. Advantages of general anesthesia for patients undergoing structural heart disease intervention include providing for an immobile patient, controlled ventilatory movement, ease of continuous TEE examination, and an already secured airway in the case of hemodynamic instability or emergent cardiac surgery. These cases are challenging given the significant cardiac defect and the remote location of the procedure. (669)

34. Most pediatric patients undergoing interventional cardiology procedures require general anesthesia. Specific challenges involve the understanding of complex congenital cardiac lesions, implications on the neonatal or transitional cardiopulmonary physiology, potential difficult airway, immature or altered drug metabolism and clearance, and the rapidity of cardiopulmonary instability during anesthesia. Because of their smaller size, there are additional challenges in obtaining vascular access and maintaining normothermia under anesthesia. (669)

35. The presence of a left-to-right shunt has minimal effect on the rate of induction of anesthesia in pediatric patients with either inhaled or intravenous agents. However, hyperoxia and hyperventilation with general anesthesia in these patients may lead to pulmonary vasodilation, increase of shunt fraction, pulmonary congestion, and decrease in systemic cardiac output. Conversely, the induction of anesthesia with inhaled agents in the presence of a right-to-left shunt is slowed owing to dilution by shunted blood, whereas the induction of anesthesia with intravenous agents is more rapid. Such patients are cyanotic, have right-sided heart dysfunction, and can be quite ill. In these patients deep sedation or general anesthesia can pose significant risk. Secondary polycythemia in cyanotic patients also

puts them at higher thrombotic risk. The rule of thumb is to have the cyanotic patient remain at preanesthetic hemodynamic and oxygenation baseline, which can be challenging. Hypoxia, hypercapnia, excessive positive airway pressure, metabolic acidosis, hypothermia, and painful stimulation can lead to increases in pulmonary vascular resistance and right-sided heart failure and are best avoided in pediatric patients undergoing interventional cardiology procedures. Judicious de-airing and intravenous fluid are essential to avoid paradoxical embolism regardless of the direction of shunt. (669)

36. Potential complications the anesthesiologist may encounter in interventional cardiology procedures include bleeding, hematoma, pneumothorax, vascular injury, arrhythmias, heart block, and cardiac perforation leading to pericardial effusion and tamponade. (669)

37. Pericardial effusions or tamponade during an interventional cardiology procedure may present as persistent hemodynamic instability unrelated to induced arrhythmias and refractory to medicines. The diagnosis is confirmed with echocardiography. After discussion with the cardiologist, blood products should be ordered, anticoagulation may be reversed, and volume resuscitation should be initiated. If the pericardial effusion is small and self-limiting, the plan may be to do nothing but wait and observe. Otherwise, a pericardial drain may be placed or rapid mobilization for surgical decompression of tamponade may be necessary. The vascular access placed by the cardiologist may be used for monitoring (arterial line) and fluid resuscitation (central venous line). (669)

ELECTROCONVULSIVE THERAPY

38. Patients who have severe clinical depression that is refractory to medicines, who have become acutely suicidal, who are acutely psychotic or schizophrenic, and with acute mania are all candidates for electroconvulsive therapy (ECT). The American Psychiatric Association also recommends ECT for maintenance therapy. (669)

39. ECT is accomplished by administering an electrical stimulus to the patient that is sufficient to induce a generalized seizure of greater than 15 seconds' duration but no longer than 2 minutes. The mechanism for the short-term benefit derived from ECT is unknown but is thought to be the result of changes in the neurobiology of neurotransmitter levels in the central nervous system and the suppression of the hypothalamic-pituitary-adrenal axis hyperactivity. (670)

40. There is no absolute contraindication to ECT. Relative contraindications include malignant hypertension, severe cardiomyopathy, hemodynamically significant dysrhythmia, recent cerebrovascular accident, and aortic or intracranial aneurysms. Patients with CIEDs and women with low-risk pregnancy can undergo ECT safely. (670)

41. Patients with an implanted cardiac defibrillator should have their defibrillator function deactivated prior to the procedure so that the device does not misinterpret the ECT stimulus as an arrhythmia. Patients who are pacemaker-dependent may also need to have their pacemaker set in an asynchronous mode in which the ECT stimulus doesn't lead to pacemaker inhibition and bradycardia. (670)

42. Preoperative medication is generally not recommended before an ECT procedure. Benzodiazepine anxiolytics are contraindicated because they may raise seizure threshold, shorten seizure duration, and delay awakening after the procedure. Prophylactic β-adrenergic antagonists such as esmolol or labetaolol are sometimes given if excessive sympathetic responses have been observed in previous ECT treatments. Preemptive analgesia with an opiate, acetaminophen, or nonsteroidal anti-inflammatory drugs and an antiemetic agent may be warranted if the patient had consistent complaints in past ECT treatments. (670)

43. Routine monitors must be used during an ECT procedure, including pulse oximetry, blood pressure monitoring, and a continuous electrocardiogram. In addition to these, a peripheral nerve stimulator may be useful to confirm neuromuscular blockade and the recovery of skeletal muscle from neuromuscular blockade. An electroencephalogram may also be used to confirm grand mal seizure activity during ECT. (670)

44. The airway of the patient undergoing ECT can be managed by hand with a mask, provided the patient is not at risk for the aspiration of gastric contents. Before the induction of anesthesia the patient must be well preoxygenated. The anesthesiologist must be prepared to mask ventilate by hand using supplemental oxygen before the onset of seizure activity and also in the postseizure period, given that apnea may follow seizure activity even after the termination of the effects of succinylcholine. A laryngeal mask airway may be useful to manage the airway of patients in whom bag-mask ventilation is predicted to be difficult or who have obstructive sleep apnea. The anesthesiologist must have all the equipment needed to intubate the trachea of the patient should it become necessary. Suction must also be available in the event that the regurgitation of gastric contents or excessive oral secretions should occur. (670–671)

45. Most induction agents for general anesthesia may be used to induce anesthesia in patients undergoing ECT. The most common agents are methohexital, propofol, etomidate, and ketamine. Intravenous methohexital is the agent of choice as it lowers seizure threshold and is rapidly cleared. Propofol increases seizure threshold and shortens seizure duration but also rapidly clears. Etomidate provides for hemodynamic stability and can decrease the seizure threshold but can also induce myoclonic activity, nausea and vomiting, and adrenal insufficiency after a single dose. Ketamine increases intracranial pressure and may cause post-ECT confusion and is the least likely choice. (671)

46. The administration of succinylcholine to induce paralysis reduces the risk of musculoskeletal injury during the generalized seizure. A tourniquet is applied to a distal limb to prevent succinylcholine blockade of the neuromuscular junction distally, thus allowing the monitoring of motor seizure in that isolated limb. (671)

47. Cardiovascular responses to ECT occur in two phases. The first (tonic) phase is characterized by profound parasympathetic discharge that can lead to bradycardia, atrioventricular block, atrial arrhythmias, premature atrial or ventricular contractions, and even asystole. Atropine or glycopyrrolate may be necessary treatment during this phase. The second (clonic) phase is characterized by sympathetic nervous system overstimulation. Therefore, after ECT bradycardia and hypotension may occur first, followed by tachycardia and hypertension, which may be severe and persistent. Myocardial ischemia and cardiac dysrhythmia can occur and are the most common causes of fatality after ECT. (671)

48. After ECT and the resultant grand mal seizure, the patient is likely to be postictal. Headache, confusion, agitation, cognitive impairment, and memory loss may be present after the procedure. (671)

Chapter

39 POSTANESTHESIA RECOVERY

Dorre Nicholau

ADMISSION TO THE POSTANESTHESIA CARE UNIT

1. How do the Standards for Postanesthesia Care adopted by the American Society of Anesthesiologists (ASA) differ from the ASA Practice Guidelines for Postanesthesia Care?
2. What are the five standards for postanesthesia care according to the Standards for Postanesthesia Care document adopted by the ASA?
3. What is the minimum time interval requirement for vital sign measurement and recording in the postanesthesia care unit (PACU)?

EARLY POSTOPERATIVE PHYSIOLOGIC DISORDERS

4. What are some postoperative physiologic disorders that may manifest in the PACU?

UPPER AIRWAY OBSTRUCTION

5. What is the most frequent cause and usual mechanism of upper airway obstruction in the PACU?
6. How does upper airway obstruction present clinically?
7. What is the initial intervention to treat upper airway obstruction?
8. Why might residual neuromuscular blockade not manifest until the patient is in the PACU?
9. What are two potential reasons for inadequate reversal of neuromuscular blockade?
10. How might residual neuromuscular blockade manifest in an awake patient?
11. How is residual neuromuscular blockade assessed in an awake patient?
12. What are some factors that can contribute to prolonged nondepolarizing neuromuscular blockade in the PACU?
13. What are some factors that can contribute to prolonged depolarizing neuromuscular blockade in the PACU?
14. What is laryngospasm, and when is it likely to occur?
15. How should laryngospasm be treated?
16. What operative factors may result in life-threatening airway edema in the immediate postoperative period?
17. What leak tests can be performed to evaluate airway patency in patients at risk for airway edema prior to extubation of the trachea?
18. What are some special considerations for patients with obstructive sleep apnea for postanesthesia care?
19. How should upper airway obstruction be managed in the PACU?
20. How can upper airway obstruction in the PACU due to the sedating effects of opioids or benzodiazepines be treated?

21. How can upper airway obstruction in the PACU due to the residual effects of neuromuscular blocking drugs be treated?
22. How can upper airway obstruction in the PACU due to hematoma after thyroid or carotid surgery be treated?
23. What are some methods by which upper airway patency can be monitored during patient transport from the operating room to the PACU?

HYPOXEMIA IN THE POSTANESTHESIA CARE UNIT

24. What are some potential causes of hypoxemia in the PACU? Which of these is most common?
25. What are some potential causes of postoperative hypoventilation?
26. In a patient with a normal A-a gradient, what would be the resultant Pa_{O_2} of a patient breathing room air if the patient's Pa_{CO_2} increases from 40 to 80 mm Hg?
27. What is the normal ventilatory response to elevated arterial carbon dioxide levels? How is this affected by residual anesthetic drugs?
28. In the PACU, how can arterial hypoxemia secondary to hypercapnia be reversed?
29. What is diffusion hypoxia?
30. Describe the hypoxic pulmonary vasoconstriction (HPV) response, and name some medications and conditions that may inhibit it.
31. What are some causes of a true shunt that may present as arterial hypoxemia in the PACU? What is the response to supplemental oxygen in these patients?
32. What is the most common cause of pulmonary shunting presenting as arterial hypoxemia in the PACU? How can it be treated?
33. What is the significance of an increased venous admixture in the PACU?
34. What coexisting lung diseases may result in a decreased diffusion capacity and subsequent arterial hypoxemia in the PACU?

PULMONARY EDEMA IN THE POSTANESTHESIA CARE UNIT

35. What are the typical causes of cardiogenic and noncardiogenic pulmonary edema in the PACU?
36. What is postobstructive pulmonary edema?
37. What are some possible causes of postobstructive pulmonary edema presenting in the PACU?
38. How might postobstructive pulmonary edema present in the PACU?
39. How is postobstructive pulmonary edema diagnosed and treated?
40. What is transfusion-related acute lung injury (TRALI)? When is it likely to present?
41. How is TRALI distinguished from transfusion-associated circulatory overload?

OXYGEN SUPPLEMENTATION

42. What is the $F_{I_{O_2}}$ that can be delivered through a simple nasal cannula? What are some other options for oxygen delivery in the PACU?
43. What is a high-flow nasal cannula? What is its advantage?
44. Is there a role for continuous positive airway pressure (CPAP) and noninvasive positive-pressure ventilation (NIPPV) in the PACU?

HEMODYNAMIC INSTABILITY

45. What are some factors associated with hypertension in the PACU?
46. What are some complications that can result from hypertension in the PACU?
47. What are some causes of hypotension in the PACU?
48. What are the most common causes of allergic reactions leading to hypotension in the perioperative setting?
49. How is myocardial ischemia detected in the PACU?
50. What are some factors that may contribute to cardiac arrhythmias in the PACU?
51. What are some possible causes of sinus tachycardia in the PACU?
52. How should new-onset atrial fibrillation be managed in the PACU?
53. What drugs may contribute to ventricular tachycardia in the PACU?
54. What are some possible causes of bradycardia in the PACU?

DELIRIUM

55. What is the incidence of postoperative delirium?
56. What are some risk factors and causes of postoperative delirium?
57. How should postoperative delirium be managed?

58. What is emergence agitation?

RENAL DYSFUNCTION

59. What is the differential diagnosis of postoperative renal dysfunction?
60. How is oliguria defined? What is the most common cause of oliguria in the PACU?
61. How should oliguria due to decreased intravascular volume be managed in the PACU?
62. What are the risk factors for postoperative urinary retention?
63. Which patients are at risk for acute renal dysfunction due to intra-abdominal hypertension?
64. Which patients are at risk for acute renal dysfunction due to rhabdomyolysis? How should it be managed?
65. Which patients are at risk for acute renal dysfunction due to contrast nephropathy? How should it be managed?

BODY TEMPERATURE AND SHIVERING

66. What is the incidence of postoperative shivering? How should it be treated?
67. What are some adverse effects of postoperative hypothermia?

POSTOPERATIVE NAUSEA AND VOMITING

68. What are some factors associated with an increased incidence of postoperative nausea and vomiting (PONV)?
69. What is the simplified risk score for identifying patients at risk for PONV?
70. How can PONV be prevented and/or treated?

DELAYED AWAKENING

71. What are some common causes of delayed awakening in the PACU? How should it be managed?

DISCHARGE CRITERIA

72. What are the principles used to determine PACU discharge criteria?

ANSWERS*

ADMISSION TO THE POSTANESTHESIA CARE UNIT

1. The Standards for Postanesthesia Care adopted by the American Society of Anesthesiologists (ASA) is a document that delineates the minimal requirements for monitoring and postanesthesia care in all locations. These are minimal standards that are to be exceeded when deemed appropriate by the judgment of the anesthesia caregiver. These differ from the ASA Practice Guidelines for Postanesthesia Care, which provide more specific recommendations for the clinical evaluation and therapeutic intervention for physiologic disorders that may present in the postanesthesia care unit (PACU). Unlike the ASA standards of care, these guidelines are recommendations, not requirements. (676)
2. There are five standards for postanesthesia care according to the Standards for Postanesthesia Care document adopted by the ASA. All patients who have received general anesthesia, regional anesthesia, or monitored anesthesia care shall receive postanesthesia management, which includes (1) appropriate staffing and equipment of the unit; (2) transportation to the PACU by the anesthesia caregiver with continual monitoring, evaluation, and treatment as necessary; (3) reevaluation of the patient in the unit, verbal report, and transfer of care from the anesthesia provider to the PACU nurse; (4) continual evaluation and monitoring of the patient in the unit with documented reports; and (5) discharge of the patient from the unit under the physician's responsibility. (676)
3. Vital signs must be measured and recorded as often as necessary but at a minimum every 15 minutes while in the PACU. (676)

---

*Numbers in parentheses refer to pages, figures, boxes, or tables in Pardo MC, Miller RD, eds. *Basics of Anesthesia.* 7th ed. Philadelphia: Elsevier; 2018.

EARLY POSTOPERATIVE PHYSIOLOGIC DISORDERS

4. A number of postoperative physiologic disorders may manifest in the PACU. Although airway problems and cardiovascular events account for the majority of recovery room serious events, more common events include nausea and vomiting, oliguria, hypoventilation, bleeding, hypothermia, delirium, pain, and delayed awakening. Hypertension or hypotension, cardiac dysrhythmia, upper airway obstruction, hypoventilation, and arterial hypoxemia require immediate attention and intervention. (676)

UPPER AIRWAY OBSTRUCTION

5. Upper airway obstruction in the PACU is most often due to the loss of pharyngeal tone resulting from the residual depressant effects of inhaled and intravenous anesthetics and the persistent effects of neuromuscular blocking drugs. In awake patients, the pharyngeal muscles contract synchronously with the diaphragm. This activity serves to pull the tongue forward and tent the airway open as the diaphragm creates the negative pressure for inspiration. In the PACU, this pharyngeal muscle activity may be lost, and the resultant compliant pharyngeal tissue collapses with negative inspiratory pressure causing obstruction. (676)

6. Upper airway obstruction presents clinically as collapse of the chest wall plus protrusion of the abdomen with inspiratory effort resulting in a rocking motion. When this occurs there is a characteristic paradoxic breathing pattern consisting of retraction of the sternal notch and exaggerated abdominal muscle activity. This rocking motion becomes more prominent with increasing airway obstruction. Airway obstruction can be associated with arterial hypoxemia and desaturation on pulse oximetry. (676)

7. The initial intervention to treat upper airway obstruction is the jaw thrust maneuver. (676)

8. Residual neuromuscular blockade might not manifest until the patient is in the PACU for several reasons. First, the diaphragm recovers from neuromuscular blockade before the pharyngeal muscles do. Second, while the endotracheal tube is in place the inability to maintain patency of the upper airway may be masked. Third, stimulation associated with awakening, extubation, patient transfer, and transport may all contribute to keeping the airway open during these times. Not until the patient is calmly resting in the PACU may upper airway obstruction become evident. (676)

9. Two potential reasons for inadequate reversal of neuromuscular blockade include inappropriate dosing of neostigmine and that qualitative measurement of the train-of-four (TOF) ratio may not accurately reflect recovery of neuromuscular function. (677)

10. Residual neuromuscular blockade in an awake patient may manifest as a struggle to breathe. In a patient whose mental status is not clear enough to communicate clearly the patient may appear agitated. (677)

11. In an awake patient, clinical assessment of residual neuromuscular blockade is preferred to the application of the painful measurements of the TOF ratio and tetanic stimulation. Clinical evaluation includes grip strength, tongue protrusion, the ability to lift the legs off the bed, and the ability to lift the head off the pillow for a full 5 seconds. Of these, the sustained head lift most directly reflects the ability of the patient to maintain and protect the airway. An extubated patient's ability to oppose and fix the incisor teeth against a tongue depressor is another clinically reliable indicator to pharyngeal tone. This maneuver correlates with an average TOF ratio of 0.85. (677)

12. Factors that may contribute to prolonged nondepolarizing neuromuscular blockade include drugs, diseases, and metabolic states. Drugs that prolong neuromuscular blockade include residual inhaled anesthetics, local anesthetics (lidocaine and other sodium channel blockers), cardiac antidysrhythmic drugs (procainamide), antibiotics (aminoglycosides most commonly), calcium channel blockers, furosemide, and corticosteroids. Metabolic states that may prolong

neuromuscular blockade include hypothermia, respiratory acidosis, renal or hepatic failure, hypermagnesemia, and hypocalcemia. Of these, hypothermia and respiratory acidosis are easily recognized and reversible. (677)

13. Factors that may contribute to prolonged depolarizing neuromuscular blockade include excessive doses of succinylcholine, reduced plasma cholinesterase activity, inhibited cholinesterase activity, and atypical plasma cholinesterase, which is a genetic variant. Plasma cholinesterase activity may be reduced due to decreased plasma levels, extremes of age, disease states (hepatic failure, malnutrition, uremia), pregnancy, plasmapheresis, glucocorticoids, and contraceptives. Inhibited cholinesterase activity may be reversible (neostigmine, edrophonium) or irreversible (echothiophate). (677)

14. Laryngospasm is bilateral vocal cord spasm that completely occludes the laryngeal opening. Laryngospasm usually occurs during emergence from anesthesia immediately after extubation in the operating room but can occur when patients are awakening after general anesthesia in the PACU. (677)

15. Laryngospasm can be treated initially with jaw thrust and continuous positive airway pressure (CPAP) (up to 40 cm H_2O). This typically is sufficient, but in cases in which laryngospasm persists a small dose of succinylcholine can be administered (0.1 to 1.0 mg/kg IV [intravenously] or 4.0 mg/kg IM [intramuscularly]) to relax the vocal cords. (678)

16. Operative factors that may result in life-threatening airway edema in the immediate postoperative period include prolonged procedure in the prone or Trendelenburg position; aggressive fluid resuscitation; surgical procedures on tongue, pharynx, and neck (most common examples are thyroidectomy, carotid endarterectomy, and cervical spine procedures); and hematoma at the surgical site (again, common examples include thyroidectomy and carotid endarterectomy). In the case of volume resuscitation and procedures requiring prone or Trendelenburg positioning, airway edema may be accompanied by facial or scleral edema. In cases such as neck dissection, carotid endarterectomy, and thyroidectomy, life-threatening airway edema may be the result of increased pressure from a hematoma that is not evident on external physical examination. (678)

17. Leak tests can be performed to evaluate airway patency in patients at risk for airway edema prior to extubation of the trachea. One leak test evaluates the patient's ability to breathe around an occluded endotracheal tube (ETT) with the cuff deflated. One can also measure the intrathoracic pressure required to produce an audible leak around the ETT with the cuff deflated. Another method is to measure the exhaled tidal volume before and after the ETT cuff is deflated during volume control ventilation. (678)

18. There are some special considerations for patients with obstructive sleep apnea in the PACU. These patients should not be tracheally extubated until they are fully awake. Because of their increased risk for airway obstruction, one should minimize the use of opioids and avoid benzodiazepines or any drugs that depress respiratory drive or promote sleepiness. To this end, the application of regional anesthesia and multimodal analgesia techniques should be used whenever possible. Patients should have CPAP available postoperatively. Patients' home CPAP or BiPAP (bilevel positive airway pressure) devices should be available for use upon admission to the unit. If they do not use CPAP at home or do not have their machines with them, a respiratory therapist may need to ensure the proper fit of a CPAP device as well as the positive airway pressure necessary to relieve the airway obstruction. The time in the PACU should be used to evaluate patients to determine the appropriate degree of monitoring required once discharged from the unit. As a general rule, patients should be monitored with continuous pulse oximetry on the surgical ward. However, because pulse oximetry will not detect carbon dioxide retention in a patient who is receiving supplemental oxygen, many patients with sleep apnea will require intensive care unit (ICU) level monitoring. (678)

19. The initial intervention to deal with upper airway obstruction is the jaw thrust maneuver. When this is not sufficient to relieve the obstruction, CPAP (5 to 15 cm H_2O) can be applied via face mask. If necessary, this can be followed by placement of nasal and oral airways and in extreme cases laryngeal mask airway or endotracheal tube placement. (678)

20. Upper airway obstruction in the PACU due to the sedating effects of opioids or benzodiazepines can be treated with persistent stimulation or small, titrated doses of naloxone or flumazenil, respectively. (678)

21. Upper airway obstruction in the PACU due to the residual effects of neuromuscular blocking drugs can be treated by pharmacologic reversal or by correcting contributing factors (e.g., hypothermia). (678)

22. Upper airway obstruction in the PACU due to hematoma after thyroid or carotid surgery can be treated through decompression of the airway by releasing the clips or sutures on the wound and evacuating the hematoma. This temporizing measure may be required because mask ventilation and endotracheal intubation through direct laryngoscopy can be difficult in these patients secondary to airway displacement. (678)

23. Some methods by which upper airway patency can be monitored during patient transport from the operating room to the PACU include watching for the appropriate rise and fall of the chest wall with inspiration, listening for breath sounds, or simply feeling for exhaled breath with the hand over the patient's nose and mouth. (679)

HYPOXEMIA IN THE POSTANESTHESIA CARE UNIT

24. There are multiple potential causes of hypoxemia in the PACU. These include right-to-left shunt, mismatching of ventilation to perfusion, congenital heart disease, congestive heart failure, pulmonary edema, alveolar hypoventilation, diffusion hypoxia, aspiration of gastric contents, pulmonary embolus, pneumothorax, posthyperventilation hypoxia, increased oxygen consumption (as from shivering), acute lung injury (e.g., sepsis or transfusion-related), advanced age, and obesity. Of these, atelectasis (shunt) and alveolar hypoventilation are the most common causes of postoperative hypoxemia in the PACU. (679)

25. Among the potential causes of postoperative hypoventilation are drug-induced central nervous system depression (volatile anesthetics, opioids), residual effects of neuromuscular blocking drugs, impaired ventilatory muscle mechanics, increased levels of carbon dioxide production, and coexisting pulmonary disease. Each of these causes of alveolar hypoventilation leads to a corresponding increase in arterial partial pressure of carbon dioxide ($Paco_2$). (679)

26. In a patient breathing room air at sea level, hypoventilation to a $Paco_2$ of 80 mm Hg will result in hypoxemia, even when the patient has normal lungs without a significant A-a gradient. This is demonstrated through the alveolar gas equation. Alveolar oxygen pressure (Pao_2) in this scenario is 50 mm Hg. Supplemental oxygen can mask alveolar hypoventilation by leading to normal saturation of oxygen detected by pulse oximetry. (679)

27. Minute ventilation increases in response to elevated $Paco_2$ in a linear manner. Normally minute ventilation increases by approximately 2 L/min for every 1 mm Hg increase in arterial Pco_2. In the PACU, this linear ventilator response to Pco_2 may be depressed by residual anesthetic drugs including inhaled anesthetics, opioids, and benzodiazepines. (680)

28. Reversal of arterial hypoxemia secondary to hypercapnia can be achieved by the addition of, or increase in, the concentration of supplemental oxygen or the normalization of Pco_2. Normalization of Pco_2 can be accomplished by stimulation of the patient to wakefulness; the pharmacologic reversal of the effects of narcotics, benzodiazepines, and muscle relaxants; or in some cases control of the airway and initiation of positive-pressure ventilation. (680)

29. Diffusion hypoxia refers to the rapid diffusion of nitrous oxide into the alveoli at the end of a nitrous oxide anesthetic. Nitrous oxide dilutes the alveolar gas, producing a transient decrease in alveolar oxygen pressure that can persist for

up to 5 to 10 minutes after discontinuation of nitrous oxide. In the absence of supplemental oxygen, arterial hypoxemia may ensue and contribute to arterial hypoxemia in the PACU. (680)

30. The hypoxic pulmonary vasoconstriction (HPV) response is the attempt of normal lungs to optimally match ventilation and perfusion by constricting vessels that perfuse poorly ventilated alveoli. This vasoconstrictive response shifts blood flow to well-ventilated regions of the lung. When the HPV response is inhibited arterial hypoxemia may result and may present in the PACU. Agents that produce pulmonary vasodilation and thus inhibit the HPV response include inhaled anesthetics, nitroprusside, and dobutamine. Physiologic conditions that inhibit the HPV response include pneumonia and sepsis. (680)

31. Some causes of a true shunt that may present as arterial hypoxemia in the PACU include atelectasis, pulmonary edema, gastric aspiration, pulmonary emboli, and pneumonia. Patients with arterial hypoxemia secondary to a true shunt will not respond to supplemental oxygen. (680)

32. The most common cause of pulmonary shunting presenting as arterial hypoxemia in the PACU is atelectasis. It can be treated through mobilization to the sitting position, incentive spirometry, and if necessary, positive airway pressure via a face mask. (680)

33. Increased venous admixture refers to the contribution of mixed venous blood to arterial hypoxemia. This effect is typically significant only in cases of low cardiac output when blood returns to the heart in a severely desaturated state. Normally, only 2% to 5% of the cardiac output is shunted through the lungs, but conditions that increase shunt fraction may significantly increase the effect of venous admixture on arterial oxygenation. (680)

34. Coexisting lung diseases such as emphysema, interstitial lung disease, pulmonary fibrosis, or primary pulmonary hypertension may result in a decreased diffusion capacity and subsequent arterial hypoxemia in the PACU. (680)

PULMONARY EDEMA IN THE POSTANESTHESIA CARE UNIT

35. Pulmonary edema in the immediate postoperative period is most often due to cardiogenic causes, increased intravascular fluid volume or cardiac dysfunction. Noncardiogenic causes of pulmonary edema in the PACU include the pulmonary aspiration of gastric contents, sepsis, postobstructive pulmonary edema, and transfusion-related acute lung injury (TRALI). (681)

36. Postobstructive pulmonary edema (also called negative-pressure pulmonary edema) is a transudative edema that results from one of two causes: from the exaggerated negative pressure generated by inspiration against an acutely obstructed airway (type I) or following the relief of a chronic partial airway obstruction (type II). The exaggerated negative intrathoracic pressure increases venous return, afterload, and pulmonary venous pressures, which contribute to transudation of fluid. Young, muscular, healthy males are most at risk owing to their increased muscle mass and ability to generate significant inspiratory force. (681)

37. The most common cause of postobstructive pulmonary edema presenting in the PACU is laryngospasm. Other possible causes include other causes of upper airway obstruction, including epiglottitis, bilateral vocal cord paralysis, goiter, and occlusion of the ETT. (681)

38. Postobstructive pulmonary edema presents clinically within 90 minutes after relief of the airway obstruction as arterial hypoxemia and respiratory distress. Other manifestations may include tachycardia, tachypnea, rales, rhonchi, and evidence of bilateral pulmonary edema. (681)

39. Objective data of postobstructive pulmonary edema include hypoxemia and associated bilateral diffuse infiltrates. The diagnosis depends on clinical suspicion once other causes of pulmonary edema are ruled out. Treatment is supportive with supplemental oxygen, may include diuresis, and if necessary, requires positive-pressure ventilation with CPAP or mechanical ventilation. (681)

40. TRALI refers to pulmonary edema associated with fever and systemic hypotension after the transfusion of plasma-containing blood products. Although fresh frozen plasma and whole blood are the obvious culprits, packed red blood cells and platelets also contain plasma and can trigger TRALI. Typically, the physiologic effects of TRALI are manifest within 1 to 2 hours after transfusion but can occur up to 6 hours after transfusion. A complete blood count obtained with the onset of symptoms would reveal an acute decrease in the white blood cell count, reflecting the sequestration of granulocytes within the lung and exudative fluid. The diagnosis is made by an increased alveolar-to-arterial oxygen difference and bilateral pulmonary infiltrates in a chest radiograph. If TRALI is suspected, the transfused blood container bag should be returned to the blood bank for evaluation. (681)

41. TRALI may be difficult to differentiate from transfusion-associated circulatory overload because both manifest as pulmonary edema after the transfusion of blood products. They can be distinguished by the fever and hypotension associated with TRALI, as well as by the characteristics of the resulting edema fluid, which is exudative in the case of TRALI and transudative in the case of transfusion-associated circulatory overload. In either case treatment is supportive, including supplemental oxygen and diuresis. (681)

OXYGEN SUPPLEMENTATION

42. As a general rule, each liter per minute of oxygen flow through a simple nasal cannula will increase the FiO_2 by 0.04. The delivery of oxygen by this method is limited by lack of humidification and temperature correction of the gas. The maximum rate of 6 L/min results in approximately 0.44 FiO_2. Other options for oxygen delivery in the PACU include a face mask, nonrebreather face mask, high-flow nebulizers, and high-flow nasal cannula. Other than the high-flow nasal cannula, each of these oxygen delivery methods is limited in the FiO_2 they can provide secondary to the entrainment of room air when the patient inhales. (681)

43. High-flow delivery systems, such as the high-flow nasal cannula, can deliver oxygen at a rate of 40 L/min. Patients tolerate such high flows because the inspired gas is humidified and warmed to 99.9% relative humidity and 37° C. These devices deliver oxygen directly to the nasopharynx throughout the respiratory cycle, and the high flow may enhance the FiO_2 by a CPAP effect. (681)

44. The decision to use noninvasive modes of ventilation in the PACU must be guided by careful consideration of both patient and surgical factors. Hemodynamic instability, refractory hypoxemia, and the inability to protect the airway due to altered mental status are standard contraindications to noninvasive positive-pressure ventilation (NIPPV). Additional contraindications to consider in this setting include an increased risk of aspiration due to the surgical procedure (e.g., esophagectomy), inability to properly apply the nasal or face mask delivery apparatus because of facial surgery (e.g., sinus surgery), or the need to avoid oropharyngeal and gastric distention by positive-pressure ventilation (e.g., esophageal and gastric operations). With the previous considerations in mind, home settings of CPAP are recommended routinely for patients with obstructive sleep apnea in the PACU. In the appropriate patient population, application of CPAP in the PACU has been shown to reduce the incidence of intubation, pneumonia, and sepsis in patients who undergo abdominal surgery. (682)

HEMODYNAMIC INSTABILITY

45. Patients with essential hypertension are at greatest risk for postoperative hypertension in the immediate postoperative period. Some additional factors to consider include pain, arterial hypoxemia, hypoventilation, hypercarbia, increased intracranial pressure, urinary retention, gastric distention, drug or alcohol withdrawal, emergence agitation, and shivering. Surgical procedures that predispose the patient to hypertension include craniotomy, carotid endarterectomy, cardiothoracic surgery, and head and neck procedures. (682)

46. Complications that can result from hypertension in the PACU include myocardial ischemia, cardia arrhythmia, congestive heart failure with pulmonary edema, stroke, encephalopathy, and postoperative bleeding at the surgical site. (682)

47. A combination of one or more of the following physiologic derangements may account for hypotension in the PACU: a decrease in preload (hypovolemia), intrinsic pump failure (cardiogenic), or a decrease in afterload (distributive). Decreased preload may be due to inadequate volume resuscitation in patients who undergo preoperative bowel preparation or whose surgical procedure results in ongoing translocation of fluid (most often major intra-abdominal procedures), unrecognized or ongoing blood loss, or loss of sympathetic tone as a result of neuraxial blockade (spinal or epidural). Intrinsic pump failure often results from exacerbation of preexisting cardiac conditions, such as cardiomyopathy, valvular disease, arrhythmias, or coronary artery disease. Cardiac tamponade, pulmonary embolus, and tension pneumothorax should be ruled out in at-risk patients, such as those who undergo intraoperative central-line placement, intrathoracic or mediastinal invasion, or total hip arthroplasty. Decreased afterload can be attributed to iatrogenic sympathectomy. This may be due to high neuraxial blockade (spinal or epidural) or blunting of sympathetic drive by narcotics and residual intravenous anesthetics (propofol or dexmedetomidine) in patients who rely on sympathetic tone to maintain blood pressure (examples include sepsis and patients with pericardial disease). Other causes include frank sepsis, burns, drug-induced (e.g., β-blockers, calcium channel blockers), spinal shock, and anaphylaxis. A high spinal anesthetic can lead to hypotension due to all three causes because it results in a sympathectomy that dilates venous and arterial vasculature to produce decreased preload and afterload. It also affects the cardioaccelerator fibers of T4, resulting in intrinsic cardiac failure secondary to bradycardia. (682–683)

48. The most common cause of allergic reaction leading to hypotension in the perioperative setting is neuromuscular blocking drugs, followed by latex and antibiotics. (683)

49. It is difficult to reliably detect myocardial ischemia in the PACU because patients are often unable to identify or communicate symptoms of cardiac ischemia in the immediate postoperative period. In one study, patients with postoperative myocardial infarction complained of chest pain only 35% of the time. Often PACU patients will attribute cardiac pain to incisional pain or vice versa. Furthermore, interpretation of the postoperative electrocardiogram (ECG) must be done with the patient's cardiac history and risk index in mind. In low-risk patients, ST-segment changes do not usually reflect myocardial ischemia. Relatively benign causes of ST-segment changes in low-risk patients include anxiety, esophageal reflux, hyperventilation, and hypokalemia. Conversely, in high-risk patients any ST-segment, T-wave, or rhythm changes compatible with myocardial ischemia prompts further evaluation (i.e., measurement of troponin) to rule out myocardial ischemia. Current American Heart Association/American College of Cardiology guidelines cite insufficient evidence regarding routine postoperative 12-lead ECG or troponin measurements in patients at high risk for perioperative myocardial ischemia who do not exhibit ongoing signs or symptoms of myocardial ischemia. These guidelines recommend against routine screening of an unselected patient population using troponin measurements. (683)

50. Factors that may contribute to cardiac arrhythmias in the PACU may include hypoxemia, hypoventilation and associated hypercarbia, pain, agitation, electrolyte abnormalities, myocardial ischemia, endogenous or exogenous catecholamines, hypertension, intravascular fluid overload, anemia, and substance withdrawal. (683)

51. Possible causes of sinus tachycardia in the PACU include pain, agitation, fever, hypercarbia, hypovolemia, anemia, and shivering. Less common and more

ominous causes include the onset of cardiogenic or septic shock, pulmonary embolism, thyroid storm, and malignant hyperthermia. (684)

52. New-onset atrial fibrillation that presents in the PACU should be treated. Control of the heart rate is a goal of treatment in these patients and can be achieved with β-adrenergic blockers or calcium channel–blocking drugs. Diltiazem is the calcium channel blocker of choice in this circumstance. If chemical conversion is indicated, an amiodarone loading dose can be initiated. Often rate control with a β-blocker such as metoprolol is enough to convert the heart rhythm from new-onset atrial fibrillation to sinus rhythm. If the patient is hemodynamically unstable, prompt electrical cardioversion is indicated. (684)

53. Premature ventricular contractions and ventricular bigeminy are common in the PACU. They are most often a result of increased sympathetic tone as may accompany pain or hypercarbia. Ventricular tachycardia is rare in the PACU and is indicative of underlying cardiac abnormality. In the case of torsades de pointes, the administration of drugs that prolong the QT interval, such as amiodarone, procainamide, droperidol, and serotonin uptake inhibitors to name only a few, may contribute to the cardiac abnormality. (684)

54. Bradycardia in the PACU is often iatrogenic. Drug-related causes include the administration of β-adrenergic blockers, calcium channel blockers, neostigmine reversal of neuromuscular blockade, narcotic administration, and treatment with dexmedetomidine. Procedure-related and patient-related causes include bowel distention, increased intracranial pressure or intraocular pressure, and high spinal anesthesia that blocks the cardioaccelerator fibers originating from T1 to T4. Underlying conduction abnormalities and myocardial ischemia are indications for emergent intervention. (684)

DELIRIUM

55. The incidence of postoperative delirium ranges between 4% and 75% of patients, depending upon patient characteristics and type of surgery. The incidence is highest in elderly patients and those undergoing certain procedures such as hip replacement, cardiac surgery, abdominal aortic aneurysm repair, and bilateral knee replacement. (685)

56. Postoperative delirium may be patient related, iatrogenic, or surgery related. The most significant predictors of postoperative delirium are advanced age (>70 years), preoperative cognitive impairment, decreased functional status, alcohol abuse, malnutrition, dehydration, and a previous history of dementia, depression or delirium. Intraoperative factors that are predictive of postoperative delirium include surgical blood loss and the number of intraoperative transfusions. Some precipitating factors include medication administration or withdrawal, pain, hypoxemia, electrolyte abnormalities, environmental change (e.g., ICU admission), sleep-wake cycle disturbances, bladder catheter placement, restraint use, and infection. Intraoperative hemodynamic derangements and the anesthetic technique do not seem to be predictors of postoperative delirium. (685)

57. Postoperative delirium should be managed initially through nonpharmacologic measures and environmental modifications, such as withdrawal of any inciting stimulus and frequent reorientation. Severely agitated patients may benefit from haloperidol (0.5 mg IV) as first-line therapy if there are no contraindications. Restraints and additional personnel may also be necessary in selected patients. (685)

58. Emergence agitation is a transient period of excitation characterized by inconsolable crying, agitation, and delirium that is associated with the emergence from general anesthesia. It is more common in children than adults, with a peak incidence in children between the ages of 2 and 4 years. More than 30% of children will experience delirium at some period during their PACU stay. It typically resolves quickly and is followed by an uneventful recovery. (686)

RENAL DYSFUNCTION

59. The differential diagnosis of postoperative renal dysfunction includes prerenal, renal, or postrenal causes. Prerenal causes include hypovolemia due to bleeding,

sepsis, third space fluid loss, and inadequate volume resuscitation. Other prerenal causes are hepatorenal syndrome, low cardiac output, renal vascular obstruction, or intra-abdominal hypertension. Intrarenal causes include acute tubular necrosis, radiographic contrast dyes, rhabdomyolysis, tumor lysis, and hemolysis. Postrenal causes include urinary retention, surgical injury or obstruction to the ureters, or mechanical obstruction to the urinary catheter. Frequently the cause is multifactorial, and a preexisting renal insufficiency may be exacerbated by an intraoperative insult. For example, preoperative infection, perioperative or intraoperative contrast radiologic studies, or hepatic dysfunction may put patients at risk for acute renal dysfunction. Intravascular volume depletion can exacerbate hepatorenal syndrome or acute tubular necrosis caused by sepsis. In the PACU, diagnostic efforts should focus on the identification and treatment of readily reversible causes of oliguria. (686)

60. Oliguria is defined as a urine output of less than 0.5 mL/kg/h. The most common cause of oliguria in the PACU is the depletion of intravascular volume. (686)

61. Oliguria due to decreased intravascular volume is usually responsive to a 500 to 1000 mL administration of intravenous crystalloid. Intravenous fluids should be continued as necessary to maintain renal perfusion, particularly if there is ongoing blood loss. A hematocrit should be measured under these circumstances. If oliguria persists despite an intravascular fluid challenge, or if an intravascular fluid challenge is contraindicated, evaluation by central venous monitoring or echocardiography may facilitate diagnosis. (686)

62. Postoperative urinary retention refers to the inability to void despite a bladder volume of more than 500 to 600 mL. Risk factors include age over 50, male gender, intraoperative volume resuscitation, duration of surgery, bladder volume on admission, and type of surgery, in particular anorectal procedures or joint replacement. Other contributors include perioperative medications such as anticholinergics, β-blockers, and narcotics. (686)

63. Persistently elevated intra-abdominal pressure impedes renal perfusion and leads to renal ischemia. Intra-abdominal hypertension is defined as a sustained intra-abdominal pressure higher than 12 mm Hg, and abdominal compartment syndrome is defined as a sustained intra-abdominal pressure of 20 mm Hg or higher that is associated with new organ dysfunction or failure. Patients who have had abdominal surgery, major trauma, or burns or who are critically ill are at risk. Intra-abdominal hypertension should be ruled out as a cause of oliguria by measuring the bladder pressure in any patient with a tense abdomen postoperatively. Prompt intervention is necessary in these patients to relieve intra-abdominal hypertension and restore renal perfusion. (687)

64. Rhabdomyolysis should be diagnosed and treated in oliguric patients who have suffered a major crush or thermal injury, including intraoperative thermoablation of tumors. Rhabdomyolysis should also be ruled out in morbidly obese patients who undergo prolonged surgical procedures; the risk is increased in patients of male gender and who have been positioned in lithotomy or lateral decubitus position. Patients may have severe pain in the areas of contact with the operating table. A creatine phosphokinase level can be measured in suspected patients. Volume loading and treatment with mannitol, urine alkalinization, and loop diuretics can be used to flush renal tubules and prevent ongoing renal tubular damage. (687)

65. Contrast nephropathy should be considered in patients who have undergone angiography with intravascular stent placement. These patients often have chronic renal insufficiency and are at increased risk to develop renal failure secondary to an intravenous contrast load. Perioperative aggressive hydration with normal saline and alkalinization with sodium bicarbonate have been shown to be effective renal protective measures. Sodium bicarbonate (154 mEq/L) infusions at a rate of 1 mL/kg/h should be continued for 6 hours after contrast agent exposure. Mucomyst can be given and is a relatively inexpensive and easily administered medication that may also provide renal protection. (687)

BODY TEMPERATURE AND SHIVERING

66. The incidence of postoperative shivering may be as high as 65% after general anesthesia and 33% with epidural anesthesia. Postoperative shivering is not always associated with a decrease in body temperature; shivering in normothermic patients is thought to result from uninhibited spinal reflexes manifested as clonic activity. Meperidine is the most effective treatment for postoperative shivering, but shivering can also be treated with other opioids and clonidine. (687)

67. Adverse effects of postoperative hypothermia include shivering, inhibition of platelet function, coagulation factor activity, and drug metabolism. These may result in exacerbation of postoperative bleeding, prolonged neuromuscular blockade, and delayed awakening. Forced air warmers can be used to actively warm patients with postoperative hypothermia. (687)

POSTOPERATIVE NAUSEA AND VOMITING

68. Patient-related factors associated with an increased incidence of postoperative nausea and vomiting (PONV) include female gender (postpuberty), nonsmoking status, age less than 50 years, and history of motion sickness or PONV. Anesthetic factors include use of volatile anesthetics or nitrous oxide, administration of large doses of neostigmine, and perioperative opioids. Significant surgical factors include type of procedure, such as eye muscle or middle ear surgery, gastric distention as in swallowed blood, and duration of surgery. (687)

69. There is a simplified risk score for identifying patients at risk for PONV. It is a four-point score that allots a single point for each of the following factors: (1) female gender, (2) history of motion sickness or PONV, (3) nonsmoking, and (4) use of postoperative opioids. A score of 0, 1, 2, 3, or 4 corresponds to an incidence of 10%, 21%, 39%, 61%, and 79%, respectively. (688)

70. Modifications of the anesthetic technique that may prevent PONV include avoidance of general anesthesia, preferential use of propofol infusions, avoidance of nitrous oxide and volatile anesthetics, minimization of opioid administration, and adequate hydration. Although prophylactic measures to prevent PONV are more effective than rescue drugs administered in the PACU, some patients have PONV despite prophylaxis. Several drugs are available for the treatment of PONV, including scopolamine, hydroxyzine, promethazine, droperidol, metaclopromide, ondansetron, dolasetron, and dexamethasone. Dexamethasone is most effective when given prophylactically at the start of surgery, and ondansetron is most effective when given 30 minutes before the end of anesthesia. (688)

DELAYED AWAKENING

71. Residual effects of anesthetic or sedating drugs are the most common cause of delayed awakening in the PACU. If narcotic or benzodiazepines are suspected, then careful titration of the reversal drugs naloxone and flumazenil can be used. For example, in adults 20- to 40-µg increments of naloxone are used to avoid abrupt reversal of analgesia and associated hypertension and tachycardia. The use of flumazenil should be done with caution to avoid precipitation of seizures. Both naloxone and flumazenil have short half-lives, so the patient should be carefully observed for resedation. Rarely physostigmine may be used to reverse the CNS effects of anticholinergic drugs. Hypothermia and hypoglycemia should also be considered as potential causes of delayed awakening postoperatively. In rare cases computed tomographic imaging may be indicated to rule out an intracerebral event. (689)

DISCHARGE CRITERIA

72. PACU discharge criteria are based on the principles that patients must be observed until they are no longer at risk for respiratory depression and their mental status has returned to baseline. No specific length of stay is required, and hemodynamic parameters are based on the patient's baseline measurements.

The Aldrete discharge scoring system is an objective measure assigning points, or a score, to a patient to determine readiness for discharge. Components of the Aldrete scoring system include activity, breathing, circulation, consciousness, and oxygen saturation. The patient must be able to breathe comfortably, clear secretions, and oxygenate adequately. (689)

40 PERIOPERATIVE PAIN MANAGEMENT

Meredith C.B. Adams and Robert W. Hurley

1. What are some potential adverse physiologic effects of acute postoperative pain?
2. What factors correlate with the severity of postoperative pain?
3. What are some potential benefits of the effective management of acute postoperative pain?
4. What is chronic postsurgical pain (CPSP)? How common is it?
5. What are the goals of an acute pain management service?

NEUROBIOLOGY OF PAIN

6. What is nociception?
7. What are nociceptors? How are they stimulated?
8. What is the neurologic pathway of afferent pain impulses?
9. Where along the neurologic pathway of afferent pain impulses can modulation of the painful stimulus occur?
10. How can the modulation of painful stimuli occur in the periphery? What pharmacologic agents may be particularly useful for the modulation of painful stimuli in the periphery?
11. How can the modulation of painful stimuli occur at the level of the spinal cord?
12. How can the modulation of painful stimuli occur above the level of the spinal cord?
13. Name some excitatory and inhibitory neurotransmitters believed to have a role in the modulation of painful stimuli.
14. What is the difference between preemptive analgesia and preventative analgesia? What is their clinical relevance?
15. What is opioid-induced hyperalgesia (OIH)?
16. What is multimodal perioperative analgesia?
17. What are the goals of multimodal perioperative analgesia?
18. Name some routes for the administration of analgesic drugs.

ANALGESIC DELIVERY SYSTEMS

19. Describe patient-controlled analgesia (PCA). What is the lockout interval?
20. What are some advantages of PCA?
21. What is a risk of PCA? How can this be monitored?

SYSTEMIC THERAPY

22. What is the limitation of the oral administration of opioids for the management of acute postoperative pain? When is this route of administration appropriate?
23. What is the role of oral analgesic medications as part of a perioperative multimodal approach to the treatment of pain?
24. What are some oral analgesic medications that can be administered as part of a perioperative multimodal approach to the treatment of pain?
25. What are some advantages and disadvantages of the intermittent intravenous administration of opioids to treat postoperative pain?

26. What are some intravenous nonopioid medications that can be administered to treat postoperative pain?
27. What role does ketamine have in the perioperative period? What are the side effects of low-dose ketamine therapy?
28. How do the efficacy and potency of acetaminophen compare between oral and intravenous administration?
29. What are some side effects of intravenous clonidine that limit its analgesic benefits in the treatment of postoperative pain?
30. What is the mechanism by which intravenous magnesium is thought to exert its analgesic effects?
31. What benefit does the intramuscular administration of analgesic agents have over oral administration? What are some problems with this method of administration?
32. What are the advantages and disadvantages of the subcutaneous, transdermal, and transmucosal administration of opioids?
33. What is buprenorphine? What is the concern regarding buprenorphine use in the patient scheduled to undergo surgery?
34. How should a patient taking oral buprenorphine be managed preoperatively, intraoperatively, and postoperatively?

NEURAXIAL ANALGESIA

35. What are some of the potential benefits of the neuraxial administration of opioids for postoperative analgesia?
36. What are the advantages and disadvantages of a single-dose administration of opioid in the intrathecal space for the management of acute postoperative pain?
37. What characteristic of an opioid administered into the intrathecal space determines its time of onset and its duration of action?
38. Why does the epidural administration of opioid require more drug than the intrathecal administration of the same opioid?
39. Why might a local anesthetic be added to the opioid for administration in the epidural space for the management of postoperative pain?
40. Why is it believed that fentanyl produces a more segmental band of anesthesia than morphine when administered in the epidural space?
41. How do the resulting plasma concentrations of fentanyl compare when the same dose of fentanyl is administered intravenously versus epidurally?
42. How do hydrophilic and lipophilic opioids administered by a continuous infusion in the epidural space exert their effect?
43. What are some of the potential adverse effects of neuraxial opioids for postoperative analgesia? What different potential adverse effects may be caused by neuraxial infusion of local anesthetics?
44. What is the early depression of ventilation that may be seen with the neuraxial administration of an opioid believed to be due to?
45. What is the delayed depression of ventilation that may be seen with the neuraxial administration of an opioid believed to be due to? Why might this effect be more pronounced with morphine than with fentanyl?
46. Which patients may be most at risk for delayed depression of ventilation from the administration of a neuraxial opioid?
47. How should a motor block in a patient with an epidural infusion for postoperative pain be managed?
48. What is the concern regarding the concurrent use of neuraxial analgesia and anticoagulants? What are some general concepts regarding this issue covered in the American Society of Regional Anesthesia guidelines?
49. What factors increase the risk of postoperative epidural abscess associated with epidural analgesia?

SURGICAL SITE (INCISION) INFILTRATION

50. What is the benefit of surgical site infiltration with liposomal bupivacaine?

INTRA-ARTICULAR ADMINISTRATION	51. What are the advantages and disadvantages of the intra-articular administration of analgesics?
INTRAPLEURAL REGIONAL ANESTHESIA	52. How is intrapleural regional analgesia achieved? What is an advantage and a disadvantage of this technique for the management of acute postoperative pain?
PARAVERTEBRAL BLOCKS	53. What are the benefits of the paravertebral blockade technique?
PERIPHERAL NERVE BLOCK	54. What is an advantage and a disadvantage of peripheral nerve blocks for the management of acute postoperative pain? 55. What are some adjuvant drugs that can be used for peripheral nerve blockade?
REGIONAL ANALGESIA	56. What are the advantages of perioperative continuous perineural catheters in upper extremity surgeries? 57. What are some advantages of perioperative continuous perineural catheters in lower extremity surgeries?
TRANSVERSUS ABDOMINIS PLANE BLOCK	58. What are the indications for a transversus abdominis plane block? What advantages does this peripheral block offer?

ANSWERS*

1. Potential adverse physiologic effects of acute postoperative pain include hypoventilation, atelectasis, ventilation-to-perfusion mismatching in the lungs, hypercapnia, pneumonia, systemic hypertension, tachycardia, cardiac dysrhythmias, myocardial ischemia, deep vein thrombosis, decreased immune function, ileus, nausea and vomiting, urinary retention, hyperglycemia, sodium and water retention, insomnia, fear, and anxiety. Poorly controlled postoperative pain may also be a factor in developing chronic postsurgical pain (CPSP). (692)

2. Factors that positively correlate with the severity of postoperative pain include preoperative opioid intake, increased body mass index, anxiety, depression, pain intensity level, characteristics of fibromyalgia, and the duration of surgery. Factors that are negatively correlated include the patient's age and the level of the surgeon's operative experience. A perioperative plan should be developed that encompasses these factors to lessen the severity of the patient's postoperative pain. (692)

3. Some potential benefits of the effective management of acute postoperative pain include improvement in patient comfort, a decrease in perioperative morbidity, enhanced postoperative rehabilitation, and a possible decrease in chronic postsurgical pain. It may also reduce cost by shortening the time spent in postanesthesia care units, intensive care units, and hospitals. (693)

4. CPSP is defined as pain after a surgery lasting longer than the normal recuperative healing time. Acute pain can transition to CPSP quickly in patients whose pain is poorly controlled postoperatively. It is thought to occur in 10% to 65% of postoperative patients, of whom 2% to 10% have severe CPSP. CPSP results in long-term behavioral and neurobiologic changes. (693)

5. The goals of an acute pain management service are to evaluate and treat postoperative pain to minimize the period of recuperation, decrease duration of hospital stay, improve patient satisfaction, and to inhibit the development of chronic (persistent) pain through early intervention. (694)

*Numbers in parentheses refer to pages, figures, boxes, or tables in Pardo MC, Miller RD, eds. *Basics of Anesthesia.* 7th ed. Philadelphia: Elsevier; 2018.

NEUROBIOLOGY OF PAIN

6. Nociception is used to describe the recognition and transmission of painful stimuli. Pain is described as an unpleasant sensory and emotional experience caused by actual or potential tissue damage. (694)

7. Nociceptors are the free nerve endings of afferent myelinated Aδ and unmyelinated C nerve fibers. Nociceptors are stimulated by thermal, mechanical, or chemical tissue damage. (694)

8. Nociceptors, on stimulation, send axonal projections to the dorsal horn of the spinal cord and synapse on second-order neurons there. The axonal projections of the second-order neurons cross to the contralateral half of the spinal cord and ascend the spinothalamic tract to the thalamus in the brain. In the thalamus, these second-order neurons synapse with third-order neurons that send axonal projections to the sensory cortex. Before reaching the thalamus, the second-order neurons divide and also send axonal branches to the reticular formation and periaqueductal gray matter. (694)

9. Modulation of the painful stimulus can occur at almost every level along the afferent neurologic pain pathway. It can occur at the site of stimulation of the nociceptors or at any synapse. In addition, modulation of nociception can even occur by the inhibition of the afferent sensory pathways by descending inhibitory pathways originating at the level of the brainstem. (694)

10. Modulation of painful stimuli can occur in the periphery by decreasing or eliminating the endogenous mediators of inflammation in the vicinity of the nociceptor. Examples of endogenous mediators of inflammation include prostaglandins, histamine, bradykinin, serotonin, acetylcholine, lactic acid, hydrogen ions, and potassium ions. These endogenous inflammatory mediators sensitize and excite nociceptors, leading to the conduction of the painful stimulus. Pharmacologic agents that are particularly useful for the modulation of painful stimuli in the periphery are aspirin and nonsteroidal anti-inflammatory drugs (NSAIDs). These agents modulate painful stimuli by decreasing the synthesis of prostaglandins. (694)

11. The modulation of painful stimuli can occur at the level of the spinal cord through the effects of excitatory or inhibitory neurotransmitters in the dorsal horn of the spinal cord. (694)

12. The modulation of painful stimuli can occur above the level of the spinal cord through the effects of a descending inhibitory pathway that originates in the brainstem. The descending inhibitory pathway synapses in the substantia gelatinosa region of the spinal cord. There are at least two types of descending inhibitory pathways, the opioid and α-adrenergic pathways. The opioid descending pathway releases endorphins and enkephalins, whereas the α-adrenergic descending pathway releases norepinephrine. Both these pathways work by hyperpolarizing the nerve fibers of the ascending pain pathway and potentially negate the action potential that would otherwise have resulted from the stimulation of the nerve by the painful stimulus. Neurotransmitters or second messenger effectors (e.g., substance P, protein kinase C-γ) may also play important roles in spinal cord sensitization and chronic pain. (695)

13. Examples of excitatory pain modulating neurotransmitters include glutamate, aspartate, vasoactive intestinal polypeptide, cholecystokinin, gastrin-releasing peptide, angiotensin, and substance P. Examples of inhibitory neurotransmitters that are believed to modulate painful stimuli include enkephalins, endorphins, and somatostatin. (695)

14. The precise definition of preemptive analgesia is one of the major controversies in perioperative pain medicine and contributes to the confusion regarding its clinical relevance. The concept is that the development of central or peripheral sensitization of pain transmission after a traumatic injury can result in amplification of the pain response in the postoperative period. Preemptive analgesia is defined as an analgesic intervention initiated before the noxious stimulus develops in order to block peripheral and central pain transmission at the time of

initial stimulation. Preventive analgesia is functionally defined as an attempt to block pain transmission prior to the injury (incision), during the noxious insult (surgery itself), and after the injury and throughout the recovery period. Unfortunately, few trials have examined the concept of preventive analgesia in a rigorous fashion. Confining the definition of preemptive analgesia to only the immediate preoperative or early intraoperative (incisional) period may not be clinically relevant or appropriate because the inflammatory response may last well into the postoperative period and continue to maintain peripheral sensitization. (695)

15. Opioid-induced hyperalgesia (OIH) is the exacerbation of pain following the administration of opioid analgesics. Short-term administration of opioids in the perioperative setting may lead to a paradoxical increase in the patient's pain severity and decrease in pain tolerance. This has been demonstrated in humans who received an intraoperative opioid infusion for operative analgesia as well as in human and animal experimental models. Although the clinical impact of OIH has not been fully elucidated, the possibility of its contributing to acute postoperative pain should be considered. OIH has also been implicated as a risk for the development of CPSP; the pronociceptive process involves the activation of the N-methyl-D-aspartate (NMDA) receptor. (695)

16. Multimodal perioperative analgesia is a broad definition that refers to managing postprocedural pain through multiple approaches. For example, postoperative pain can be managed through a combination of interventional analgesic techniques (epidural or peripheral nerve catheters) and systemic pharmacologic therapies (NSAIDs, α-adrenergic agonists, NMDA receptor antagonists, membrane stabilizers, and opioids). (696)

17. The goals of multimodal perioperative analgesia include sufficient diminution of the patient's pain to instill a sense of control over the pain, enable early mobilization, allow early enteral nutrition, and attenuate the perioperative stress response. The secondary goal of this approach is to maximize the benefit (analgesia) while minimizing the risk (side effects of the medication being used). This may lead to decreased perioperative morbidity, decreased length of hospital stay, and improved patient satisfaction. (696)

18. Routes for the administration of analgesic drugs include oral, transmucosal, transdermal, intramuscular, intrapleural, intravenous, subcutaneous, rectal, neuraxial, and by injection to block a peripheral nerve. (696)

ANALGESIC DELIVERY SYSTEMS

19. Patient-controlled analgesia (PCA) is a method of delivering medication that the patient controls. Medication delivery can be oral, intravenous, subcutaneous, neuraxial, or by peripheral nerve catheter. The most common is the intravenous route, in which the patient controls his or her own administration of the opioid by pressing a button connected to a pump. The pump is programmed to deliver a preset small intravenous dose of opioid when triggered by the patient. The lockout interval is the interval of time that must pass after the last self-administered dose before the patient can deliver another small dose of opioid to himself or herself. (696)

20. There are several advantages of PCA. There is high patient acceptance and for patients a sense of control when using a PCA. There is also improved titration of drug and subsequent patient comfort with less total drug administered, less sedation, improved sleep at night, and a more rapid return to physical activity after surgery. (696)

21. A risk of PCA is for respiratory depression. Many hospitals use continuous pulse oximetry monitoring for patients receiving PCA intravenous analgesia. It is important to recognize that respiratory depression is better monitored by continuous capnography and respiratory rate monitoring, but these are not readily available and not sufficiently sensitive and specific. Continuous pulse oximetry is better than no monitor, but it may not reveal respiratory depression, particularly in patients receiving supplemental oxygen. (696)

SYSTEMIC THERAPY

22. The limitation of the oral administration of opioids for the management of acute postoperative pain is the lack of ability to titrate it effectively to pain and the prolonged amount of time it takes to reach its peak effect. Patients are also limited by their perioperative NPO (nothing by mouth) status. The oral route of administration for opioids is appropriate when the pain the patient is experiencing has decreased and there is no longer a need for rapid adjustments in the level of analgesia. (697)

23. Oral analgesic medications, both opioid and nonopioid, are an integral component of a perioperative multimodal approach to the treatment of pain. The preoperative administration of analgesics may reduce postoperative pain and may help reduce the risk of CPSP. (697)

24. Oral analgesic medications that can be administered as part of a perioperative multimodal approach to the treatment of pain include membrane stabilizers (gabapentin and pregabalin), NSAIDs, and acetaminophen. Tricyclic antidepressants, serotonin-norepinephrine reuptake inhibitors, and vitamin C are also agents that may have some efficacy but have not received sufficient investigation. (697)

25. Advantages of the intermittent intravenous administration of opioids to treat postoperative pain include its short time delay for analgesia and less variability in plasma concentrations when titrated in small doses. Disadvantages include its short duration of action due to rapid redistribution and the requirement for continued nursing surveillance and monitoring. This administration route is useful for the treatment of acute and severe pain in the postanesthesia or intensive care unit. (699)

26. Some intravenous nonopioid medications that can be administered to treat postoperative pain include ketamine, acetaminophen, dexamethasone, clonidine, and magnesium. (699)

27. Ketamine can be effective in small doses for postoperative analgesia partly due to its NMDA antagonistic properties, which can attenuate central sensitization and opioid tolerance. Low-dose ketamine infusions have a low incidence of hallucinations or cognitive impairment. Ketamine is comparable to opioids with regard to its side effects of dizziness, itching, nausea, or vomiting. The use of ketamine in patients at high risk for the development of chronic postsurgical pain or who have opioid use disorders or significant opioid tolerance should be considered. (699)

28. No clinical trial has demonstrated a difference in efficacy or potency between oral and intravenous acetaminophen. There is a difference in bioavailability, however, and the time to onset of analgesia is shorter with the intravenous administration. (699)

29. Side effects of bradycardia and hypotension associated with intravenous clonidine limit its analgesic benefits in the treatment of postoperative pain. (699)

30. Intravenous magnesium likely exerts its analgesic effects through blockade of the NMDA receptor. (699)

31. The intramuscular injection of analgesic agents has a more rapid onset and more rapidly reaches its peak effect than the oral route of administration of analgesic agents. There are significant problems with the intramuscular administration of analgesics leading to its decline in use. Following intramuscular administration, the plasma concentration of the drug can vary among patients by three to five times, making dosing of the drug difficult. The use of this route has been replaced by intravenous PCA dosing, which provides a more standardized dosing interval. (699)

32. Opioids can be administered through subcutaneous, transdermal, and transmucosal routes. Subcutaneous delivery can be an effective method for patients without intravenous access or who need long-term access at home. Subcutaneous therapy is primarily used in palliative care patients. Transdermal fentanyl results in a variable range of serum concentrations and analgesic

response across patient populations and requires 24 to 48 hours to reach peak levels. These limitations can lead to adverse outcomes for patients in the perioperative period because of side effects such as respiratory depression. The primary indication for transmucosal opioid therapy is for the rapid onset of analgesia to treat breakthrough pain in an opioid-tolerant adult oncology patient. (699)

33. Buprenorphine is a long-acting partial agonist at the μ-opioid receptor, and when used with a full agonist, such as morphine or fentanyl, it acts as an antagonist. Therefore, the analgesia the patient experiences is less than what the patient would normally experience for a given dose of morphine or fentanyl. Buprenorphine is commonly used for detoxification or maintenance therapy for patients with opioid use disorders (addiction). It is now more frequently being prescribed for the treatment of pain in those without opioid use disorders as well. Its use poses additional challenges to the anesthesiologist in the operative setting because of its pharmacodynamics and pharmacokinetics. The pharmacokinetics of buprenorphine are somewhat unpredictable, making it hard to predict when its partial agonist properties will have worn off after the last dose of buprenorphine taken prior to surgery. This uncertainty leads to the risk of unexpected respiratory depression from the full opioid agonist as the buprenorphine unbinds from the opioid receptor. In addition, its antagonist properties can make opioid pain medicines ineffective, leading to poor postoperative pain control. (699)

34. There are numerous ways in which to handle the perioperative analgesic care of a buprenorphine patient. Ideally the patient should be weaned down or off buprenorphine at least 72 hours prior to surgery, recognizing the risk of withdrawal in high-dose patients. If there is no ability to wean the patient from buprenorphine preoperatively, the best approach is to maintain the buprenorphine therapy throughout the perioperative setting by converting the oral dose to intravenous and continuing to administer it intraoperatively and postoperatively while the patient is NPO. Any additional analgesic needs made necessary by the surgical operation can be addressed with an additional full agonist opioid, as well as through a multimodal approach. In this manner, the complex pharmacokinetic properties of buprenorphine can be avoided. (699)

NEURAXIAL ANALGESIA

35. Potential benefits of the neuraxial administration of opioids for postoperative analgesia include superior pain control, improved postoperative pulmonary function, decreases in cardiovascular complications, decreases in infectious complications, and decreases in total hospital costs. (699)

36. Typically, the intrathecal administration of opioid is administered as a single dose in conjunction with a local anesthetic block for a surgical procedure. An advantage of this method of opioid delivery is its placement in small concentrations near its site of action. Disadvantages of a single-dose intrathecal administration of opioid for the management of acute postoperative pain include the lack of ability to titrate and the need for other analgesic options after the initial intrathecal opioid effect subsides. (700)

37. The lipid solubility of intrathecal opioids is the primary determinant of its time of onset and duration of action. The onset time is shorter with more lipid-soluble drugs, and the duration of action is shorter. Conversely, less lipid-soluble drugs have a longer onset time and a prolonged duration of action. For example, intrathecal hydrophilic morphine produces a peak analgesic effect in 20 to 60 minutes and postoperative analgesia for up to 36 hours. Fentanyl, which is more lipid soluble, can be injected concurrently to shorten the onset time of analgesia. (700)

38. The epidural administration of opioid requires more medication to be administered than if it were administered intrathecally because the drug must diffuse across the dura to reach the spinal cord and exert its effect. In addition, fat, connective tissue, and the epidural veins all take up opioid that is deposited in the epidural space. In contrast, the intrathecal administration of opioid places the opioid

directly at its site of action. The dose of epidurally administered opioid is approximately 10 times the dose of intrathecally administered opioid to produce an equipotent effect. (700)

39. Local anesthetic added to the opioid solution for administration in the epidural space results in a synergistic analgesic effect. This is believed to occur because of the blockade of painful stimuli at two different sites at the spinal cord. The opioid administered acts by binding to opioid receptors. The local anesthetic administered acts at the nerve roots and in the dorsal root ganglia by blocking the transmission of afferent impulses. The synergistic effect of these two classes of drugs allows for a decreased dose of each to be administered to the patient. This has the added benefit of a decreased risk of the potential side effects of both drugs. (700)

40. Fentanyl administered in the epidural space is believed to produce a more segmental band of anesthesia than morphine because of its increased lipid solubility. The increased lipid solubility of fentanyl causes it to bind to opioid receptors in the spinal cord adjacent to the area in which it enters the intrathecal space. Morphine, being more hydrophilic, binds less readily and instead diffuses in the intrathecal space. This results in a wider distribution of anesthesia with morphine than with fentanyl when administered in the epidural space. (700)

41. The plasma concentration of fentanyl when administered intravenously is similar to the plasma concentration of fentanyl when the same dose is administered epidurally. This is thought to occur from the systemic absorption of epidural fentanyl by the vasculature in the epidural space. This implies that at least part of the analgesic effect of fentanyl administered epidurally is through its systemic effects. (700)

42. The analgesic site of action of the epidural administration of a continuous infusion of opioids can be primarily spinal or systemic, depending on their lipid solubility. There are mechanistic differences between continuous epidural infusions of lipophilic (e.g., fentanyl, sufentanil) and hydrophilic (e.g., morphine, hydromorphone) opioids. For continuous epidural infusions of lipophilic opioids the analgesic site of action is not clear, although several randomized clinical trials suggest that it is systemic. Hydrophilic opioid epidural infusions have a primarily neuraxial mechanism of action. (700)

43. Potential adverse effects of the neuraxial administration of opioids for postoperative analgesia include pruritus, urinary retention, nausea and vomiting, sedation, and early and delayed depression of ventilation. Local anesthetic infusions are more likely to cause hypotension and motor block than opioid infusions. (700)

44. The early depression of ventilation that is seen with the neuraxial administration of opioids usually occurs in the first 2 hours after the administration of the opioid. Early respiratory depression is believed to occur as a result of vascular uptake and redistribution of the opioid. (701)

45. The delayed depression of ventilation that is seen with the neuraxial administration of opioids usually occurs 6 to 24 hours after the administration of the opioid. It is believed to be due to the cephalic spread of the opioid in the cerebrospinal fluid to the medullary centers of the brain. The medullary centers are in the area of the fourth cerebral ventricle. This effect may be more pronounced with the less lipid-soluble opioids, such as morphine, than with the more lipid-soluble drugs, such as fentanyl. The more lipid soluble the opioid is, the more readily it will attach to opioid receptors on the spinal cord. This makes less medication available for diffusion to the brain. The opposite occurs with the less lipid-soluble drug, leaving more drug available for diffusion to the medullary centers. (701)

46. Patient characteristics contribute to the risk of depression of ventilation from the administration of neuraxial opioid. Factors that increase the risk for the depression of ventilation include larger dose, geriatric age group, concomitant administration of systemic opioids or sedatives, the possibility of prolonged or extensive surgery, the presence of comorbid conditions, and thoracic surgery. (701)

47. A patient with a motor block associated with an epidural catheter should be promptly evaluated and have the epidural infusion discontinued. The motor block should resolve within 2 hours of discontinuing the infusion. Causes of a persistent or increasing motor block in patients with an epidural infusion that should be considered and excluded include hematoma, abscess, and migration of the epidural catheter. (701)

48. The concern regarding the concurrent use of neuraxial analgesia and anticoagulants is for the formation of a spinal or epidural hematoma. The incidence of spinal or epidural hematoma related to neuraxial analgesia is rare, but it can be catastrophic and requires immediate surgical attention. General concepts for the management of neuraxial analgesia with anticoagulation include (1) the timing of neuraxial needle or catheter insertion or removal should reflect the pharmacokinetic properties of the specific anticoagulant, (2) frequent neurologic monitoring is essential, (3) concurrent administration of multiple anticoagulants may increase the risk of bleeding, and (4) the analgesic regimen should be tailored to facilitate neurologic monitoring, which may be continued in some cases for 24 hours after epidural catheter removal. (701)

49. Factors that increase the risk of postoperative epidural abscess associated with epidural analgesia include a longer duration of anesthesia and the presence of coexisting immunocompromising or complicating diseases (e.g., malignancy, trauma). The overall incidence of postoperative epidural abscess associated with epidural analgesia is extremely rare, however. (701)

SURGICAL SITE (INCISION) INFILTRATION

50. Liposomal bupivacaine has been approved for surgical site infiltration by the FDA (Food and Drug Administration). It is an extended-release formulation that is designed to provide analgesia for over 96 hours after injection. (701)

INTRA-ARTICULAR ADMINISTRATION

51. Intra-articular injection of opioids may provide analgesia for up to 24 hours postoperatively and prevent the development of chronic postsurgical pain. However, superiority of this delivery method over systemic administration has not been demonstrated and has been associated with joint damage. Continuous intra-articular administration of bupivacaine has been associated with chondrolysis in the glenohumeral joint. (702)

INTRAPLEURAL REGIONAL ANESTHESIA

52. Intrapleural regional analgesia is most frequently used for the management of acute postoperative pain after a thoracotomy. It is achieved by the injection of a local anesthetic solution through a catheter placed in the intrapleural space. The catheter is often placed intraoperatively by the thoracic surgeon one interspace lower than that of the surgical incision. The local anesthetic diffuses to the intercostal nerves and produces a multilevel, unilateral intercostal nerve block. Unfortunately, this technique provides little analgesia for patients unless it is actually placed in the paravertebral space from the intrathoracic approach. An advantage of this technique for postoperative pain management is the potential for pain relief without hemodynamic changes associated with epidural analgesia. A disadvantage of this technique is that the local anesthetic may be lost through the pleural drainage tubes that are placed after a thoracotomy. Complications associated with this technique include pneumothorax and high plasma concentrations of local anesthetic. The majority of local anesthetic infused into the intrapleural space flows to the dependent aspect of the patient, which is most often the lung bases where analgesia is not needed. The efficacy of this technique for postoperative pain management is therefore highly variable and has mostly been abandoned. This technique is less frequently used than epidural catheters or paravertebral blocks. (702)

PARAVERTEBRAL BLOCKS

53. Paravertebral blockade has been directly correlated with improved outcomes for patients undergoing breast surgery. This technique has also been found to

decrease the development of chronic postsurgical pain, as well as the acute pain associated with the procedure. Paravertebral blocks are now also being used for thoracic, cardiac, and pediatric procedures. (702)

PERIPHERAL NERVE BLOCK

54. An advantage of peripheral nerve blocks for the management of acute postoperative pain is their ability to provide good management of intraoperative and postoperative pain while not affecting the patient systemically. Thus the patient is not at risk for any of the negative effects of systemic opioids. A disadvantage of single-administration peripheral nerve blocks for postoperative pain is their relatively short duration of action. (702)

55. Adjuvant drugs that can be used for peripheral nerve blockade include epinephrine, clonidine, opioids, and more recently dexmedetomidine. Epinephrine significantly increases the duration of blockade with minimal side effects. Clonidine is beneficial in extending the duration of preoperative blockade by about 2 hours but has less utility with perineural catheters. The mechanism is most likely peripheral α_2-adrenergic receptor mediated, and dose dependent. Clonidine is a better preemptive analgesic when added to a local anesthetic block than when used as a single drug. Side effects, including hypotension, bradycardia, and sedation, are less likely to occur with lower doses. (702)

REGIONAL ANALGESIA

56. Continuous perineural catheters for upper extremity procedures have been associated with increased pain relief with minimal opioid supplementation. Patients also have increased satisfaction and sleep quality. An example is continuous interscalene blockade for shoulder surgery. (702)

57. Continuous perineural catheters for lower extremity surgery (e.g., hip, knee, ankle, foot) are associated with an earlier discharge from the postanesthesia care unit. Lumbar plexus catheters can be used as part of a multimodal regimen with better pain scores at rest and during physical therapy. The advantage over epidural anesthesia is that there is unilateral blockade rather than unnecessary bilateral blockade. (702)

TRANSVERSUS ABDOMINIS PLANE BLOCK

58. The transversus abdominis plane block has been used for many abdominal procedures, including abdominal hysterectomy, cesarean section, and laparoscopic cholecystectomy. Theoretical advantages of this technique over other modalities include avoidance of both neuraxial involvement and lower extremity blockade, decreased urinary retention, and decreased systemic side effects. Ultrasound guidance has made this a more reliably achieved peripheral blockade. (703)

41 CRITICAL CARE MEDICINE

John H. Turnbull and Wendy Smith

The authors would like to thank the authors of the previous version of this chapter for their contribution.

RESPIRATORY FAILURE

1. How can respiratory failure be categorized?
2. What are some common causes of hypoxemic respiratory failure?
3. What are some common causes of hypercapnic respiratory failure?
4. List the typical goals for mechanical ventilation in the ICU.
5. What are some common modes of mechanical ventilation?
6. Compare and contrast assist control (AC) with synchronized intermittent mandatory ventilation (SIMV).
7. What is pressure support ventilation, and when can it be used?
8. Describe the key ventilator settings in volume control ventilation mode.
9. Describe the key ventilator settings in pressure control ventilation mode.
10. Describe the key ventilator settings in synchronized intermittent mandatory ventilation mode.
11. How does the set inspiratory flow rate influence the inspiratory and expiratory times?
12. How does a ventilator switch between inspiration and expiration in volume control, pressure control, and pressure support modes?
13. What is positive end-expiratory pressure (PEEP)?
14. How does PEEP improve oxygenation?
15. What are some possible adverse effects of PEEP?
16. What is the function of the trigger on the ventilator?
17. What occurs when the ventilator flow trigger is set too low?

NONINVASIVE POSITIVE-PRESSURE VENTILATION

18. What is noninvasive positive-pressure ventilation (NIPPV)?
19. What are some indications for NIPPV?
20. What are three contraindications to NIPPV?
21. What are the physiologic benefits of high-flow nasal cannula?
22. What are indications for high-flow nasal cannula?
23. What are some patient characteristics that indicate readiness for a trial of weaning from mechanical ventilation?
24. What A-a gradient measurement indicates readiness for a trial of weaning from mechanical ventilation?
25. What is the rapid shallow breathing index? What value is associated with successful weaning from mechanical ventilation?
26. What maximum inspiratory force (MIF) measure is associated with successful weaning from mechanical ventilation?
27. What is the endotracheal tube cuff leak test?
28. What is protocol-driven weaning from mechanical ventilation? What is its advantage?

29. How are spontaneous breathing trials used as a strategy for weaning patients from mechanical ventilation?
30. Which patients may include the use of NIPPV for weaning from mechanical ventilation?

ACUTE RESPIRATORY DISTRESS SYNDROME

31. What are the hallmarks of acute respiratory distress syndrome (ARDS)?
32. What are the Berlin criteria for the definition of ARDS? How does this differ from the previous definition of ARDS?
33. List three direct causes and three indirect causes of acute lung injury.
34. What are the basic principles for the treatment and management of mechanical ventilation of patients with ARDS?
35. In addition to lung protective ventilation, what other therapies should be considered for patients with severe ARDS?

TRACHEOSTOMIES

36. What is the optimal timing for tracheostomy placement for intubated patients in the intensive care unit (ICU)?
37. When a tracheostomy is dislodged within the first 7 days of placement, what is the most appropriate method to secure the airway? How does this differ in a more mature tracheostomy?

SHOCK

38. What defines shock?
39. List three major categories of shock. How can they be differentiated using central venous pressure (CVP) and cardiac output (CO) measurements?
40. What are some common causes of hypovolemic shock?
41. What are the common clinical findings in hypovolemic shock?
42. What is the treatment for hypovolemic shock?
43. What are the causes of cardiogenic shock?
44. What are the common clinical findings in cardiogenic shock?
45. What is the treatment for cardiogenic shock?
46. Which antiarrhythmic agent is preferred to treat tachyarrhythmia in a patient with cardiogenic shock?
47. What are some common causes in vasodilatory shock?
48. What are the common clinical findings of vasodilatory shock?
49. What is the treatment for vasodilatory shock?

HEMODYNAMIC MONITORING

50. Is arterial waveform analysis, CVP measurement, or pulmonary artery occlusion pressure (PAOP) measurement the most accurate measurement to predict fluid responsiveness in a hypotensive patient?
51. Describe three indications for the use of bedside ultrasonography in the intensive care unit (ICU).
52. How can fluid responsiveness be assessed using echocardiography?

SEPSIS

53. What is the current fundamental approach to the management of patients with sepsis?
54. Describe key components of the updated Surviving Sepsis Campaign bundle.

ACUTE RENAL FAILURE

55. What are the RIFLE criteria that are used to describe the spectrum of acute kidney injury (AKI)?
56. Describe prerenal, intrarenal, and postrenal causes of AKI.
57. What are the treatment options for AKI?
58. Is continuous renal replacement therapy or intermittent hemodialysis the most appropriate renal replacement therapy for a critically ill patient?

PAIN AND SEDATION

59. What are some indications for, and benefits of, treating pain and agitation in the ICU?
60. What are the options for analgesia in the ICU? Which opioid is most commonly used and why?

61. What are the specific considerations for the use of methadone in the ICU?
62. What are some adjunctive medicines that can be used along with opioids as a multimodal approach to treating pain and agitation in critically ill patients?
63. What role do benzodiazepines play in the sedation of critically ill patients? What are their limitations?
64. What are the advantages and disadvantages of the use of propofol as a sedative in the ICU?
65. What is propofol infusion syndrome, and what are some of the common clinical findings?
66. What are the advantages of dexmedetomidine as a sedative in the ICU?
67. What are the advantages of ketamine as a sedative in the ICU?
68. What is the potential benefit of sedation interruption in the ICU?

DELIRIUM

69. How is delirium defined? What are the two types of delirium encountered in the ICU?
70. How is mortality risk impacted by the presence of delirium in the critically ill?
71. What are some common causes of delirium in a patient in the ICU?
72. What is the common method of delirium assessment in the ICU?
73. What is the treatment for delirium in a patient in the ICU?
74. What is post-ICU syndrome?

NUTRITIONAL SUPPORT AND GLUCOSE MANAGEMENT

75. What are some important clinical benefits of providing optimal nutrition to patients in the ICU?
76. What are some considerations regarding enteral nutrition in patients who are scheduled to undergo surgery?
77. What is the most appropriate glycemic management for critically ill patients?

PROPHYLAXIS

78. What are some risk factors for venous thromboembolism in critically ill patients? What are some pharmacologic and nonpharmacologic methods of prophylaxis?
79. What medicines may be used for prophylaxis against gastrointestinal stress ulcers and bleeding?

HOSPITAL-ACQUIRED INFECTIONS

80. What are some common hospital-acquired infections, and how can their risk be minimized?

ANSWERS*

RESPIRATORY FAILURE

1. Respiratory failure can be categorized based on the underlying physiologic disease. Respiratory failure can result in hypoxemia or hypercapnia, and it can be an acute or a chronic process. The distinctions may blur in patients with multiple ongoing processes. (707)
2. Hypoxemic respiratory failure generally occurs because of ventilation/perfusion ($\dot{V}/\dot{Q}$) mismatch leading to a large A-a gradient. Causes may include trauma, acute respiratory distress syndrome (ARDS), sepsis, pneumonia, pulmonary embolism, cardiogenic pulmonary edema, and obstructive lung disease. Additional causes include intrapulmonary shunt, hypoventilation, and increased O_2 extraction. (707)
3. Hypercapnic respiratory failure may be due to increased dead space ventilation, as can occur with chronic obstructive pulmonary disease (COPD) or asthma. Another cause includes hypoventilation, as can occur with neuromuscular weakness or drug intoxication. Finally, hypercapnia can result from a severe infiltrative pulmonary process, such as ARDS. (707)

---

*Numbers in parentheses refer to pages, figures, boxes, or tables in Pardo MC, Miller RD, eds. *Basics of Anesthesia*. 7th ed. Philadelphia: Elsevier; 2018.

4. Patients receive mechanical ventilatory support to (1) reduce the work of breathing, (2) improve oxygen delivery, and (3) facilitate carbon dioxide elimination. Finally, strategies are undertaken to reduce the risk of ventilator-associated lung injury. (708)

5. Common modes of mechanical ventilation include assist control (AC), synchronized intermittent mandatory ventilation (SIMV), and pressure support ventilation (PSV). (708)

6. With assist control ventilation all breaths delivered to the patient are fully supported and consistent, whether initiated by the ventilator or by the patient. With SIMV, the ventilator is set to deliver a minimum number of fully supported breaths, and attempts to synchronize the mandatory breaths with the patient's spontaneous breaths. Patient initiated breaths that fall between the preset mandatory breaths are not fully supported, but they can be augmented with pressure support. (708)

7. With PSV the driving pressure (ΔP) is set to augment the patient's tidal volume. PSV can only be used with spontaneously ventilating patients because the patient initiates all breaths. Neither a preset tidal volume nor a respiratory rate is programmed. (708)

8. In volume control ventilation mode, the key ventilator settings are a set tidal volume and respiratory rate. This ensures a predictable, minimum minute ventilation. Positive end-expiratory pressure (PEEP) and fraction of inspired oxygen (F_{IO_2}) are also set. (708)

9. In pressure control ventilation mode the driving pressure (ΔP) must be set. Also, the inspiratory time or the inspiratory/expiratory (I:E) ratio time is set. It is important to note in this setting that tidal volumes are influenced by lung compliance and could vary should lung compliance change quickly. Vigilance is necessary to make sure minute ventilation is maintained. (708)

10. In SIMV mode, the ventilator is programmed to deliver a set tidal volume and respiratory rate. The ventilator attempts to synchronize mandatory breaths to the patient's own spontaneous breaths. Often, SIMV is combined with pressure support to support the breaths that exceed the mandatory minimum. Therefore, a ΔP is also set in this circumstance. (708)

11. The set inspiratory flow rate regulates the amount of time that the ventilator spends cycling in inspiration and expiration. By increasing inspiratory flow, the set tidal volume is delivered in a shorter time, which allows more time for exhalation. The inspiratory flow rate is usually set by the respiratory therapist and is typically 60 L/min. (709)

12. For volume control ventilation, inspiration ends when the tidal volume has been achieved and then expiration begins. In pressure control modes, inspiration ends when the set inspiratory time ends. In pressure support mode, inspiration ends when the inspiratory flow rate decreases to a predefined level. At this point, expiration begins. (709)

13. PEEP is positive airway pressure that is applied throughout the respiratory cycle and maintained during expiration. The typical PEEP range is between 5 and 20 cm H_2O pressure. (709)

14. PEEP increases mean airway pressure and therefore minimizes atelectasis. PEEP increases the functional residual capacity of the lungs and, in patients with a lung injury, results in improved pulmonary compliance. The recruitment of alveoli, or the inflation of previously collapsed alveoli, by PEEP can lead to improved oxygenation in a mechanically ventilated patient. (709)

15. Excessively high levels of PEEP can overdistend and damage alveoli. Excessive PEEP may also cause hemodynamic instability by reducing preload to both the right and the left ventricles, resulting in hypotension. Finally, if there is inadequate time allowed for the exhalation of the delivered tidal volume, there can be a buildup of end-expiratory pressure. This is often referred to as auto-PEEP and can lead to hemodynamic collapse. (709)

16. The trigger is how the ventilator detects the patient's inspiratory effort to deliver a positive-pressure breath. The trigger can be based on flow (typically a change of flow of 2 L/min) or pressure (change of pressure of 2 cm H_2O). The ventilator trigger is usually managed by respiratory therapists. (709)

17. If the ventilator flow trigger is set too low, the ventilator may trigger despite the lack of a patient-initiated breath. This can occur with bronchopleural fistulas or in a hyperdynamic state when cardiac movements transmitted through the precordium trigger the ventilator. In such cases increasing the flow trigger may decrease the occurrence of inappropriately initiated breaths. (709)

NONINVASIVE POSITIVE-PRESSURE VENTILATION

18. Noninvasive positive-pressure ventilation (NIPPV) is the application of positive pressure to provide support of oxygenation and ventilation without an endotracheal tube. Ventilation is provided via a face mask, nasal pillows, or a helmet. Two modes of NIPPV are CPAP (continuous positive airway pressure) and BiPAP (bilevel positive airway pressure). (710)

19. NIPPV is indicated in a patient who has a potentially rapidly reversible pulmonary process that requires ventilatory support. In patients with acute exacerbations of COPD, there is strong evidence that appropriate use of NIPPV is an effective treatment that can reduce the need for subsequent endotracheal intubation and reduce mortality rate. NIPPV has been used successfully to treat other forms of acute respiratory failure such as pneumonia, congestive heart failure, and postsurgical respiratory failure. NIPPV may be just as effective as conventional ventilation with respect to oxygenation and removal of carbon dioxide in these patients, and it is associated with fewer serious complications and a shorter ICU stay. (710)

20. There are specific contraindications to the use of NIPPV. The patient must be alert and compliant. Because NIPPV requires a tight-fitting mask for effective ventilation, many patients find it uncomfortable, and those who are claustrophobic poorly tolerate the mask. Facial lesions or trauma that prevents proper fit of nasal or facial masks is a contraindication. Other contraindications include shock or severe cardiovascular instability, respiratory arrest or upper airway obstruction, inability to protect the airway from aspiration, severe upper gastrointestinal bleeding, excessive airway secretions, vomiting, neuromuscular weakness, and recent gastroesophageal surgery. (710)

21. High-flow nasal cannula provides heated, humidified supplemental oxygen at flow rates that are greater than can be provided by traditional nasal cannula, thereby increasing the effective F_{IO_2} achieved. Higher flow rates also provide a low level of PEEP and flushes expired carbon dioxide from the upper airways. This decreases anatomic dead space and reduces the work of breathing. (710)

22. High-flow nasal cannula has shown benefit in patients with acute hypoxemic, nonhypercarbic respiratory failure compared to standard oxygen therapy and NIPPV. High-flow nasal cannula is more comfortable for patients, so it is beneficial for those who cannot tolerate NIPPV. (710)

23. To consider weaning from mechanical ventilation, a patient must have recovered from the process that originally required mechanical ventilatory support, have an intact mental status, be hemodynamically stable, have an intact gag and cough reflex, be able to manage airway secretions, be able to protect the airway against the aspiration of gastric contents, and lack excessive airway edema. (710)

24. The A-a gradient is measured to determine readiness for a trial of weaning from mechanical ventilation to ensure that the level of oxygen required can be delivered by face mask or nasal cannula. The patient should be maintaining adequate oxygen saturation with a Pa_{O_2}/F_{IO_2} of more than 150 mm Hg with PEEP less than 8 cm H_2O. (710)

25. The rapid shallow breathing index (RSBI) is the ratio of respiratory rate (breaths/min) to tidal volume in liters and is the most commonly used weaning predictor. The patient with an RSBI of less than 105 breaths/min/L is associated with weaning success. The RSBI is actually a better predictor of those who are likely to fail weaning than those who will succeed. A negative RSBI of more than 105 breaths/min/L identifies those who are likely to fail weaning from mechanical ventilation. (710)

26. The patient's respiratory strength is usually considered sufficient for weaning if the patient is able to generate a negative inspiratory force of at least −20 cm H_2O. The maximum inspiratory force (MIF) is not routinely measured as it is a challenge to obtain a correct measurement, and therefore it has poor predictive value. (710)

27. The endotracheal tube (ETT) cuff leak test is used to assess the degree of airway edema prior to extubation of the trachea. The ETT cuff is deflated and positive pressure gradually delivered until an audible leak of air escaping around the ETT is heard. A leak pressure of less than 10 cm H_2O suggests the absence of airway edema, whereas a leak pressure greater than 20 cm H_2O may indicate significant airway edema. (711)

28. Protocol-driven weaning from mechanical ventilation has been shown to reduce the length of time that patients remain on mechanical ventilatory support when compared to traditional physician weaning methods. Protocol-driven weaning is managed by bedside providers (nurses and respiratory therapists) without the need for continuous physician input. In this method, patients are weaned to a spontaneous breathing trial with low levels of pressure support, CPAP, or T-piece via a standard protocol. When a patient meets extubation criteria, a physician is notified, and if the physician agrees, the patient's trachea is extubated. (711)

29. Spontaneous breathing trials can be used as a weaning strategy in mechanically ventilated patients who are deemed ready. The trial of spontaneous breathing can be for 30 minutes up to 2 hours, while assessing the patient's respiratory, hemodynamic, and mental statuses. While spontaneously breathing, the patient may be placed on pressure support mode or T-piece. No single mode has been shown to be more beneficial. Some patients may require trials in excess of 2 hours, such as those with chronic respiratory failure or prolonged intubation of the trachea. (711)

30. Weaning from mechanical ventilation may include the use of NIPPV in select patients, such as those with easily managed airway anatomy, minimal secretions, intact mental status, and patients who would be compliant with the face mask. (711)

ACUTE RESPIRATORY DISTRESS SYNDROME

31. ARDS is usually caused by a specific event that results in direct or indirect lung injury. ARDS presents as diffuse, inflammatory lung injury with noncardiogenic pulmonary edema, $\dot{V}/\dot{Q}$ mismatch, hypoxemia, and poor pulmonary compliance. ARDS may resolve in some patients or may progress to chronic alveolitis leading to pulmonary fibrosis, increased physiologic dead space, chronic hypoxemia, and ventilator dependence. (711)

32. The Berlin criteria for the definition of ARDS include (1) new or worsening respiratory symptoms (2) with bilateral opacities as evidenced on chest imaging (3) that are not due to cardiac failure or volume overload (4) with Pao_2/Fio_2 of less than 300 mm Hg. Rather than differentiate acute lung injury from ARDS, the Berlin criteria divide ARDS into mild, moderate, and severe categories based on Pao_2/Fio_2. Pulmonary artery occlusion pressure measure is no longer required to meet criteria. When no inciting factor for lung injury is identified, a cardiogenic cause of pulmonary edema must be excluded with objective data (e.g., echocardiography). (712)

33. Direct causes of acute lung injury include pneumonia, the aspiration of stomach contents, pulmonary contusion, reperfusion pulmonary edema, amniotic fluid embolus, and inhalational injury. Indirect causes of acute lung injury include sepsis, severe trauma, cardiopulmonary bypass, drug overdose, acute pancreatitis, near drowning, and transfusion-related acute lung injury (TRALI). (712)

34. The treatment of ARDS generally remains supportive, with a focus on preventing further lung injury. The use of low tidal volume ventilation in patients with ARDS (6 mL/kg) versus the traditional standard tidal volumes (12 mL/kg) has been shown to decrease mortality rate. Lower tidal volumes function to "protect" the lung by preventing overdistention of remaining normal lung regions. Patients who are ventilated with lower tidal volumes and lower airway pressures tend to have lower arterial oxygen tension and higher arterial carbon dioxide tension. This is termed *permissive* hypoxemia and hypercapnia, in recognition of the fact that to normalize arterial blood gas significantly, more harmful mechanical ventilation may be required. (712)

35. For patients with severe ARDS, the administration of neuromuscular blocking drugs, such as cisatracurium, has been shown to improve survival. Prone positioning and extracorporeal life support may also be indicated, although the latter intervention has yet to objectively demonstrate improved outcomes in this population. (712)

TRACHEOSTOMIES

36. Tracheostomies are generally deferred until 10 to 14 days after endotracheal intubation to allow opportunity for weaning and extubation. Tracheostomies performed early (≤4 days) have not demonstrated improved outcomes, and physicians have been shown to be poor predictors of patients who will require long-term mechanical ventilation. Prior to placement of a tracheostomy the patient must be stable without high PEEP or oxygen requirements, because tracheostomy placement can lead to the loss of mean airway pressure and decruitment of alveoli. (712)

37. When accidental dislodgment of a tracheostomy tube occurs within the first 7 days after placement, orotracheal intubation is the safest way to secure the airway when feasible. A new tracheostomy tube should not be blindly inserted into the tracheostomy site as this may result in the false tract into subcutaneous tissue. If orotracheal intubation is not feasible, a pediatric laryngoscope blade may be inserted into the stoma and a new ETT inserted when tracheal rings are directly visualized. With more mature tracheostomies, a well-established tract allows for the blind passage of a tube. (713)

SHOCK

38. Shock is a clinical condition in which there is inadequate tissue perfusion and oxygenation to end organs such as the brain, heart, liver, kidneys, and abdominal viscera. Early in its course, shock may be reversible, but ongoing shock results in anaerobic metabolism, multiorgan system failure, and ultimately death. (713)

39. The major categories of shock include hypovolemic, cardiogenic, and vasodilatory (septic, anaphylactic, or neurogenic). In hypovolemic shock, both central venous pressure (CVP) and cardiac output (CO) are reduced owing to decreased venous return. Cardiogenic shock is typified by an increase in CVP, but CO is decreased as a result of poor pump function. In vasodilatory shock, CVP is usually decreased because of profound vasodilation and pooling of blood in the splanchnic beds, and CO is typically increased in early vasodilatory shock. However, CO may be normal or even depressed later in more advanced vasodilatory shock. (713)

40. The most common cause of hypovolemic shock is major blood loss, as can occur in trauma, during surgery, or with massive gastrointestinal hemorrhage. (713)

41. Hypovolemic shock is caused by inadequate circulating blood volume, and therefore decreased preload and CO. Fluid shifts from the interstitial space in the intravascular space. With continued decreased CO, there is a baroreceptor-mediated reflex tachycardia and an increase in systemic vascular resistance. Gluconeogenesis is induced, as is sodium reabsorption from the kidneys. In addition to being hypotensive, the patient may appear cool, clammy, and pale with increased plasma glucose levels and decreased urine output. (713)

42. The treatment for hypovolemic shock requires adequate intravenous access and aggressive isotonic fluid therapy to restore intravascular volume. Ideally, intravenous access is with short, large-bore intravenous peripheral catheters of 16 gauge or greater. Central venous catheters should be used in patients for whom large-bore peripheral access cannot be obtained. Fluid resuscitation can be guided by vital signs as well as laboratory measurements. Vasopressors and blood products may also be administered as necessary. When hypovolemic shock is due to acute blood loss, empiric blood product administration may be prudent. In the event of massive transfusion (defined as the need for 10 units packed red blood cells in 24 hours or 4 units in 1 hour), fresh frozen plasma and platelets should be administered in a 1:1:1 ratio to packed red blood cells. (713)

43. Cardiogenic shock occurs when the heart is not able to pump an adequate CO. The most common cause of cardiogenic shock is myocardial infarction. Other causes include severe cardiomyopathy, myocarditis, arrhythmia, endocarditis, valvular rupture, or a tear or rupture of a portion of the heart. (714)

44. Initially in cardiogenic shock, compensatory tachycardia helps to maintain CO, but this leads to increased myocardial oxygen consumption and decreased oxygen supply and cannot be sustained. If the right ventricle is the initial site of failure, the increased right-sided preload will be noted as increased CVP, detected clinically as distended neck veins, peripheral edema, or hepatic congestion. If the left ventricle fails, the increased preload can be detected as increased pulmonary capillary wedge pressure, which causes cardiogenic pulmonary edema and rales on physical examination. In either scenario, CO is low, and systemic blood pressure is therefore reduced. On physical examination, a patient in cardiogenic shock appears cool and pale secondary to the high systemic vascular resistance and shunting of blood away from the skin and skeletal muscle beds. (714)

45. The goal for treatment of cardiogenic shock is to improve CO, improve cardiac filling pressures, decrease afterload, and reduce myocardial oxygen demand. Resuscitation should be guided by the use of central venous monitors, invasive arterial blood pressure measurements, and echocardiography. Dobutamine is often given to provide inotropic support, as it improves forward flow and perfusion of the vital organs. Dobutamine, which often decreases systemic vascular resistance, can be given alone when hypotension is absent, or in combination with a vasopressor when the patient is also hypotensive. Norepinephrine is often chosen as the vasopressor of choice as it has better outcomes and fewer arrhythmias associated with use than dopamine. In patients in cardiogenic shock accompanied by hypertension, vasodilators such as nitroprusside and nitroglycerin may help with forward flow by decreasing afterload and preload. Treatment with diuretics must be done with caution. If the patient is in cardiogenic shock due to an acute myocardial infarction, early revascularization with angiography (if it can be accomplished within 90 minutes) or fibrinolytic therapy (if not contraindicated) can reduce mortality risk. In patients with severe heart failure refractory to treatment (left ventricular ejection fraction <25% and hemodynamic compromise), mechanical support with an intra-aortic balloon counterpulsation (IABP), extracorporeal life support (ECLS), or ventricular assist device (VAD) may be indicated. (714)

46. In a patient with stable hemodynamics, amiodarone is the preferred agent for treatment of a tachyarrhythmia complicating cardiogenic shock. Amiodarone has less negative inotropic affects than β-blocking or calcium channel blocking agents. However, if the patient's vital signs are unstable, immediate electrical cardioversion should be performed. (714)

47. The most common cause of vasodilatory shock is sepsis. Other causes of vasodilatory shock include anaphylaxis and neurogenic shock that occurs following a high spinal cord injury. Vasodilatory shock is also the final common pathway for late-shock stages of cardiogenic and hypovolemic shock. (714)

48. In vasodilatory shock there is dilation of the arterial vascular system leading to decreased systemic vascular resistance and hypotension. Capillary leakage may also result in fluid movement from the intravascular to extracellular space, resulting in hypovolemia. Initially, increases in heart rate and stroke volume increase CO and may compensate for the decrease in systemic vascular resistance, with the patient appearing warm and vasodilated. With worsening hemodynamics, tissue hypoperfusion, anaerobic metabolism, and lactic acidosis result. The patient will become increasingly cool and clammy, and eventually multiorgan ischemia and organ failure can occur. (717)

49. The treatment for vasodilatory shock involves adequate fluid volume resuscitation in conjunction with possible vasopressor therapy. Norepinephrine is the preferred vasopressor for septic shock, and in extreme cases epinephrine or vasopressin can be added. Vasopressin is not recommended as the initial single agent. For anaphylactic shock epinephrine is the vasopressor of choice. Epinephrine helps to also alleviate bronchospasm that may accompany severe anaphylaxis while also increasing SVR, stroke volume, and heart rate. Secondary treatments for anaphylaxis (such as histamine blockers) should not delay the administration of epinephrine, as they do not prevent airway edema or hypotensive shock. In neurogenic shock, treatment is directed to prevent secondary injury to the spinal cord through maintaining adequate spinal cord perfusion pressures. Initially this may be through intravascular fluid volume resuscitation, but it may require vasopressors with both α-adrenergic and β-adrenergic activity. (715)

HEMODYNAMIC MONITORING

50. Arterial waveform analysis, specifically pulse pressure variation (PPV), is a more accurate predictor of intravascular fluid responsiveness in critically ill patients than CVP or pulmonary artery occlusion pressure (PAOP) measurements. As a result of this, central venous catheters and pulmonary artery catheters are being placed less frequently for the monitoring of intravascular volume. (715)

51. Bedside ultrasonography is frequently used in the ICU for the placement of invasive catheters, including peripheral intravenous lines, arterial lines, and central venous catheters. Use of real-time ultrasound for the placement of internal jugular central venous catheters is associated with fewer failed attempts, fewer complications, and shorter procedure times. Ultrasound use may improve success rates for placing arterial and subclavian catheters as well. Echocardiography in the ICU provides valuable clinical information during the assessment of a patient's hemodynamics. Cardiac ventricular function, valvular and pericardial evaluation, and fluid volume status may be assessed to inform clinical decision making. Pulmonary ultrasound may help identify pneumonia, pleural effusions, pulmonary edema, and pneumothorax. (715)

52. Fluid responsiveness can be assessed using echocardiography in patients being mechanically ventilated. Inferior vena cava size alone can be an indicator of volume status. However, IVC diameter variation greater than 15% with positive-pressure ventilation is an indicator of fluid responsiveness (i.e., CO improvement after a fluid challenge). Patients must be ventilated with a tidal volume of at least 8 mL/kg and in sinus rhythm. (715)

SEPSIS

53. The fundamental approach to the management of patients with sepsis is early recognition, rapid cardiopulmonary resuscitation, immediate antibiotic administration, and identification and treatment of the infectious source. Excess fluid administration has not been shown to be beneficial when it is not needed physiologically and may be detrimental in the established phase of sepsis in patients with acute lung injury. (716)

54. The updated Surviving Sepsis Campaign bundle describes actions that must be taken within 3 hours and then within 6 hours of patient presentation with sepsis. Within 3 hours of presentation, patients should have a measured lactate level and blood cultures obtained prior to the administration of antibiotics. Following blood cultures, antibiotics must be administered, and the patient should receive

a 30-mL/kg crystalloid bolus for either hypotension or a lactate level 4 mmol/L or greater. Within 6 hours of presentation, vasopressors should be initiated for continued hypotension unresponsive to fluid administration with a MAP goal of 65 mm Hg or more. Volume status and tissue perfusion should be assessed if hypotension persists or for an initial lactate level 4 mmol/L or greater. A lactate level should also be repeated if the initial value was elevated. (716)

ACUTE RENAL FAILURE

55. The RIFLE criteria describe the spectrum of acute kidney injury (AKI). The first three stages are characterized by changes in glomerular filtration rate (GFR), creatinine (Cr), and urine output (UO).
    a. *R*isk: Cr increased × 1.5 or GFR decreased greater than 25%, UO less than 0.5 mL/kg/h × 6 h
    b. *I*njury: Cr increased × 2 or GFR decreased greater than 50%, UO less than 0.5 mL/kg/h × 12 h
    c. *F*ailure: Cr increased × 3 or Cr more than 4 mg/dL or GFR decreased greater than 75%, UO less than 0.3 mL/kg/h × 24 h, or anuria × 12 h
    The last two stages represent overall outcomes.
    d. *L*oss: loss of renal function longer than 4 weeks
    e. *E*SRD: end-stage renal disease (717)

56. The evaluation of AKI should focus on differentiating between prerenal, intrarenal, and postrenal causes. Prerenal causes include hypovolemia or low effective circulation volume, as with decompensated heart failure or liver disease. Intrarenal causes include glomerulonephritis, nephrotoxins (nonsteroidal anti-inflammatory drugs, aminoglycosides, myoglobin), vasculitis, acute interstitial nephritis, and tubular disease. Postrenal causes can result from obstructive nephropathy. Evaluation should include a careful physical examination, assessing volume status, measuring serum and urine electrolytes, urinalysis, and examining the urine sediment. (717)

57. Treatment for AKI is mainly supportive. The goal is to maintain euvolemia, eliminate/avoid nephrotoxic drugs, adjust all medications based on current creatinine clearance, and close monitoring and correction of electrolyte abnormalities. In cases of significant uremia, DDAVP may be given to improve platelet function. Dialysis may be required in patients with more advanced failure. Of note, pharmacologic agents administered to improve renal function such as low-dose dopamine and diuretics have not shown any benefit. (717)

58. Renal replacement therapy is an often necessary, lifesaving procedure in the ICU. Although patients receiving continuous renal replacement therapy (CRRT) are more hemodynamically stable than similar patients receiving intermittent hemodialysis, trials have failed to show a mortality risk benefit in patients receiving CRRT. The appropriate dose of dialysis, regardless of the method, appears to be a more significant factor in outcome, as patients who are underdosed for dialysis fare worse. (717)

PAIN AND SEDATION

59. Pain and agitation in the ICU can be unrecognized because many patients are not able to report it. Treatment of pain and agitation can provide analgesia, anxiolysis, and amnesia. Appropriately addressing pain and sedation may also help protect the patient from removing intravenous lines, catheters, drains, or tubes as well as prevent the impaired wound healing, increased levels of catecholamines, and development of posttraumatic stress disorder (PTSD) that are associated with undertreated pain and agitation. In certain circumstances sedation may be administered to prevent seizures, decrease intracranial pressure, treat alcohol withdrawal, and assist with ventilator dyssynchrony. (717)

60. The most widely used analgesics in the ICU are opioids. They may be administered via an infusion or as an intermittent bolus. The most commonly used opioid in the ICU is fentanyl, given its relatively short duration of action and lack of active metabolites. (718)

61. Although fentanyl is the most commonly used opioid in the ICU, methadone may prove useful in patients who have been receiving fentanyl infusions for long periods of time as well as in patients with difficult to control pain or a chronic pain history. Because of its long half-life the dose must be titrated slowly. Daily electrocardiograms are recommended, as methadone has been associated with prolonged QT interval and torsades de pointes. (718)

62. Adjunctive pain medications may help limit the exposure to opioids and their associated side effects when treating pain and agitation in critically ill patients. Options include acetaminophen, ketamine, antiepileptics, α_2-adrenergic agonists, tramadol, antidepressants, and topical lidocaine. Regional techniques may also be useful in specific circumstances. (718)

63. Benzodiazepines provide anxiolysis and anterograde amnesia while producing less ventilatory and cardiac depression compared to propofol. They are first-line therapy for patients with alcohol withdrawal and in patients presenting with seizures. However, they may contribute to ICU delirium, particularly in elderly patients, and increased mechanical ventilation days compared to other sedative medications. (718)

64. Propofol has many advantageous properties for use as a sedative in the ICU. It has rapid onset and short duration of action, making it useful for neurologic evaluations. It can also treat seizures and decrease intracranial pressure. Despite its ease of use, propofol has many significant side effects, which may limit its use in the ICU. Propofol causes hypotension by decreasing myocardial contractility and reducing systemic vascular resistance. Propofol is also a profound respiratory depressant. It should only be used for continuous sedation in intubated patients. Propofol may be used for procedural sedation in nonintubated patients as long as an anesthesia provider is continuously present to monitor the airway and other vital signs. Propofol is formulated in a lecithin base and therefore has a high fat content. Patients who are receiving long-term infusions of this drug must be periodically checked for hypertriglyceridemia. There have been many case reports of patients developing severe pancreatitis after prolonged propofol administration. The fat content of propofol should be accounted for in patients on total parenteral nutrition. (718)

65. Propofol infusion syndrome (PRIS) is a rare syndrome associated with the prolonged use of propofol. PRIS is caused by mitochondrial dysfunction. It is most common in children but can be seen in the adult population. The syndrome presents as metabolic acidosis, hyperkalemia, rhabdomyolysis, and fatty liver infiltration. Refractory bradycardia and a right bundle branch block indicate cardiac involvement. The development of PRIS is associated with an infusion rate of greater than 5 mg/kg/h for more than 48 hours in a critically ill patient in the setting of vasopressor or glucocorticoid adminsitration. When PRIS is suspected, the propofol infusion must be discontinued immediately, and supportive care is provided. Renal replacement therapy may be necessary. PRIS has a reported mortality rate as high as 80%. (718)

66. Dexmedetomidine is an α_2-receptor agonist whose use in critically ill patients may reduce the duration of mechanical ventilation and ICU length of stay when compared to more traditional sedatives. Unlike with propofol, patients may be extubated while sedated with dexmedetomidine to smooth the extubation process as dexmedetomidine does not blunt respiratory reflexes. Additionally, compared to other sedatives it promotes a more physiologic sleep state as evidenced by electroencephalogram. (719)

67. In critically ill patients ketamine is a useful pain adjunct that is associated with less respiratory depression than opioids. It may be used as a continuous infusion to limit the development of opioid tolerance and act as an adjunctive pain medication. Ketamine is also useful in small bolus doses to alleviate the pain of short-lived, frequent procedures, such as burn dressing changes. (719)

68. Sedation interruption describes daily sedation discontinuation and wake-up followed by retitration of sedatives. Sedation interruption in combination with protocol-driven ventilator weaning leads to shorter durations of mechanical ventilation, reduced mortality rate, and shorter ICU length of stay when compared to weaning without protocols. (719)

DELIRIUM

69. Delirium is defined as acute waxing and waning mental status with reduced ability to focus or sustain attention that is not accounted for by a preexisting dementia. ICU patients may present with hyperactive or hypoactive delirium. Patients with hyperactive symptoms appear agitated, restless, and emotionally labile, whereas patients with hypoactive symptoms may appear calm or with a flat affect or apathy but still suffer from cognitive deficits. (719)

70. Delirium is not a benign condition. Numerous studies have shown an increased risk of mortality among ICU patients who develop delirium. These risks vary from a greater than threefold increase in 6-month mortality rate to a 10% increase in the risk of death for every day spent in a state of delirium in the ICU. Delirium is associated with an increased number of days mechanically ventilated, increased length of stay in both ICU and hospital, and increased cost of care. In addition, delirium is associated with an increased risk of developing dementia in later life. It is unclear whether delirium may actually cause dementia, or if patients who are at greatest risk of dementia or have an early subclinical form of dementia are more likely to have episodes of delirium in the ICU. (719)

71. The causes and conditions associated with delirium in the ICU setting are numerous. They include preexisting cognitive impairment, advanced age, increasing severity of illness, multiorgan dysfunction, sepsis, immobilization, sleep deprivation, pain, mechanical ventilation, and the use of psychoactive drugs, particularly benzodiazepines. (719)

72. To actively treat delirium, it must be diagnosed first. The most widely used method of monitoring for delirium is the CAM-ICU assessment for delirium. CAM stands for confusion assessment method, and this tool should be used daily to assess for delirium in all ICU patients except those who are deeply sedated or comatose. The overall CAM-ICU is considered positive if a patient has mental status changes (acute onset or waxing and waning) and inattention plus one or both of the following: disorganized thinking or altered level of consciousness. (719)

73. Identifying and correcting underlying causes of ICU-related delirium is the first-line treatment of this syndrome. Attempts should be made to actively orient the patient to the surroundings. Physical and occupational therapy with early mobilization programs can help improve and prevent symptoms. If delirium still occurs, haloperidol or atypical antipsychotics may be helpful in improving orderly thought processes, although their efficacy has not been objectively studied. (719)

74. Post-ICU syndrome (PICS) describes a range of new or worsening disorders that may affect patients surviving critical illness and ICU stay. PICS can be one or more of physical dysfunction (weakness), cognitive dysfunction (poor concentration and memory, slower mental processing speed), or mental health problems (anxiety, depression, PTSD). (719)

NUTRITIONAL SUPPORT AND GLUCOSE MANAGEMENT

75. Providing optimal nutrition to patients in the ICU is important for wound healing, to maintain skeletal muscle mass and strength, and for the prevention of infection. Optimal nutrition may facilitate weaning from mechanical ventilation and rehabilitation. (720)

76. Considerations regarding enteral nutrition in patients who are scheduled to undergo surgery include their gastric residual volume, risk of vomiting and aspiration of gastric contents, and duration of NPO (nothing by mouth) status prior to the start of surgery. Because of the concern of vomiting and aspiration, gastric residual volumes of patients on enteral nutrition were measured and

feedings held for high volumes. Larger gastric residual volumes (500 mL or more) are now acceptable. Traditionally, patients were to have enteric feedings held for 8 hours prior to surgery, but there is now a shift to decreasing that amount of time in order to increase enteral nutrition. At some institutions there may be decreased NPO times, with the added step of aspiration of the gastric tube to empty the stomach prior to transfer to the operating room. Another approach is to continue enteral feedings until the time of transport to the operating room for patients whose feedings are postpyloric, such as jejunal feedings. Finally, if the surgery requires tracheostomy or airway manipulation, standard NPO guidelines may still be necessary. (720)

77. The optimal glucose range for critically ill patients is not known. Initially, it was thought that intensive insulin therapy to achieve a blood glucose level between 80 and 100 mg/dL would improve survival in ICU patients. More recent evidence suggests that such tight glycemic control may be associated with severe hypoglycemia and increased mortality risk in critically ill patients. A more moderate approach to glycemic control, targeting a range of 140 to 180 mg/dL, may be more appropriate to avoid the risks of severe hypoglycemia (less than 40 mg/dL) and hyperglycemia (greater than 200 mg/dL). (720)

PROPHYLAXIS

78. Independent risk factors for venous thromboembolism specific to critically ill patients include mechanical ventilation, central venous catheterization, vasopressor administration, and platelet transfusion. Pharmacologic prophylaxis significantly reduces this risk. Unfractionated heparin or low-molecular-weight heparin can be used, but in high-risk patients such as trauma and orthopedic patients low-molecular-weight heparin is recommended. Although not as effective, nonpharmacologic methods (compression stockings, intermittent pneumatic compression devices) can be used in patients at risk for bleeding complications. (720)

79. H_2 blockers or proton-pump inhibitors can be used for prophylaxis against gastrointestinal stress ulcers and bleeding in critically ill patients. The enteral route is preferred to reduce cost. (721)

HOSPITAL-ACQUIRED INFECTIONS

80. The most common hospital-acquired infections in ICU patients are urinary tract infections (31%), pneumonia (27%), and primary bloodstream infections (19%). Urinary tract infections can be minimized by adhering to sterile techniques for placement and limiting the duration of the indwelling catheter by assessing the need daily. Ventilator-associated pneumonia can be minimized by elevating the head of the bed 30 degrees, and use of endotracheal tubes with subglottic suctioning apparatus. Catheter-related bloodstream infections can be minimized by ultrasound guidance for catheter placement, adhering to sterile techniques with placement, and use of antimicrobial-impregnated central lines. (721)

42 ANESTHESIA FOR TRAUMA

Marc Steurer, Tony Chang, and Benn Lancman

INTRODUCTION

1. Trauma is the leading cause of death in what age group?
2. What is the most common cause of hypotension in trauma?
3. In early hemorrhage, what physiologic mechanisms exist in order to compensate for hypovolemia?
4. What are the differences between compensated and progressive shock?
5. What is acute traumatic coagulopathy?

INITIAL MANAGEMENT

6. What information regarding the patient's injury and status are usually provided to the emergency department staff prior to the arrival of the patient?
7. What is the purpose of a prearrival briefing in a major trauma?
8. What is ATLS? How is this approach used in trauma?
9. What are the components of the primary survey in the ATLS approach to the trauma patient?
10. What are some trauma patient injuries or indications that endotracheal intubation may be required?
11. What factors can undermine the effectiveness of preoxygenation in the trauma patient?
12. Why is a rapid sequence induction of anesthesia considered the standard of care for trauma patients undergoing endotracheal intubation?
13. Why should the doses of anesthesia induction drugs be reduced in unstable trauma patients?
14. How should trauma patients with suspected cervical spine injury be managed during endotracheal intubation?
15. What are three potential advantages of the use of video laryngoscopy in the trauma patient?
16. After securing the trauma patient's airway with endotracheal intubation, what needs to be addressed as part of postintubation care?
17. Which patient group and injury mechanisms need special considerations for their airway management?
18. What are some clinical signs that a trauma patient may have potential airway burns?
19. What are the components of the Glasgow Coma Scale (GCS)? In an example in which a male patient has been injured in a motorcycle accident, calculate his GCS score if he is moaning but not making any sense and he opens his eyes when the nurse attempts to insert an intravenous (IV) line while pulling his arm away.
20. What is a hybrid operating room? What advantage does this setting have over a traditional operating room?
21. What are some behaviors that demonstrate a good leader? What are some behaviors demonstrated by a good follower?

22. What is graded assertiveness? Describe how the PACE (probe, alert, challenge, and emergency action) technique of graded assertiveness might be used to communicate concerns about an inappropriately hypotensive patient with a head injury.

INTRAOPERATIVE MANAGEMENET

23. What are the three phases of major trauma resuscitation?
24. How should phase one (life-threatening uncontrolled hemorrhage) of major trauma resuscitation be managed?
25. What is damage control resuscitation, and what are the principles?
26. What is the purpose of a massive transfusion protocol? What types and quantity of products should be provided?
27. What is permissive hypotension? Why is it beneficial in major trauma?
28. Why should crystalloid and synthetic colloid administration be limited in the actively bleeding patient?
29. What is the role of cryoprecipitate and tranexamic acid during phase one of major trauma resuscitation (life-threatening uncontrolled hemorrhage)?
30. What is a concern regarding the use of vasopressors during phase one major trauma resuscitation?
31. How should phase two (ongoing, not life-threatening hemorrhage under partial surgical control) of major trauma resuscitation be managed?
32. What are some methods to assess the coagulation status of the trauma patient intraoperatively?
33. What is the difference between surgical and nonsurgical bleeding? How does the treatment differ?
34. What are some limitations of standard laboratory coagulation testing compared with point-of-care testing (POCT)?
35. What is the clinical utility of viscoelastic coagulation testing in major trauma resuscitation?
36. What are the three parts of the graphical output readout in the thromboelastograph (TEG) and rotational thromboelastometry (ROTEM) testing for coagulation? What intervention is indicated by each of the three parts?
37. What techniques or tools are available to prevent hypothermia during major trauma resuscitation in the operating room (OR)?
38. How should phase three (hemorrhage controlled) of major trauma resuscitation be managed?

SPECIAL GROUPS

39. What are some common causes of secondary injury in traumatic brain injury (TBI) patients?
40. What are some indications for endotracheal intubation of TBI patients?
41. What considerations should be taken during endotracheal intubation of TBI patients?
42. What are some considerations when choosing the induction agents for endotracheal intubation of TBI patients?
43. Which volatile agent is preferred during intraoperative management of TBI patients?
44. What are some principles for the intraoperative management of TBI patients?
45. What is Cushing reflex? What clinical implication can this have intraoperatively?
46. What are some considerations when caring for patients with acute spinal cord injury?
47. What are the components of "spinal shock," and how should it be managed?
48. How is the burn surface area estimated? What is the clinical significance of this?
49. What are some special considerations in the acute management of chemical burns, electrical burns, and thermal burns?
50. What are some considerations in the management of patients with acute burn injury?

51. What are some special considerations in the acute management of the pediatric trauma patient?
52. What are some special considerations in the acute management of the elderly trauma patient?
53. What are some special considerations in the acute management of the pregnant trauma patient?
54. What are some normal physiologic changes in pregnancy that can impact the presentation and management of the pregnant trauma patient?
55. What is the role of fetal monitoring in the pregnant trauma patient?

ANSWERS*

INTRODUCTION

1. Trauma is the leading cause of death among those younger than 45 years old. An estimated 5 million people worldwide die each year from injuries. (724)
2. Hemorrhagic shock is the most common cause of hypotension in trauma, though other causes must also be considered during the evaluation. These causes include relative hypovolemia from obstructed venous return as in the cases of tension pneumothorax or cardiac tamponade, cardiogenic shock, and neurogenic shock. (725)
3. Compensatory reflexes via the sympathetics, carotid sinus and aortic arch baroreceptors, and other low-pressure receptors may mask early hemorrhage and result in normotension. These reflexes lead to increased total peripheral resistance via vasoconstriction of the arterioles, increased venous return via venoconstriction, and increased heart rate. (725)
4. Intact physiologic compensatory mechanisms may be able to sustain adequate perfusion to vital organs in compensated shock. It is estimated that this may compensate for a blood loss of up to 15%. Progressive shock occurs as these mechanisms fail to provide adequate end-organ perfusion. If progressive shock is not corrected, the hemorrhage eventually leads to generalized tissue and cellular necrosis, metabolic acidosis, cardiac dysfunction, and ultimately death. (725)
5. Acute traumatic coagulopathy is characterized by factor deficiency, hyperfibrinolysis, and platelet dysfunction. It is the result of tissue hypoperfusion, which leads to a complex interaction among inflammatory factors, cellular dysfunction, and intrinsic anticoagulants. Acute traumatic coagulopathy can be exacerbated by iatrogenic factors of resuscitation including hemodilution, hypocalcemia, hypothermia, and acidosis. These processes lead to a positive feedback loop that can result in death if not corrected. (725)

INITIAL MANAGEMENT

6. Information provided to the emergency department staff prior to the arrival of the patient typically includes patient identifiers, mechanism of injury, injuries, vital signs, other signs, Glasgow Coma Scale (GCS) score, treatments, and responses to treatments. The awaiting health care team can then anticipate and prepare clinical needs accordingly. (726)
7. The purpose of a prearrival briefing in a major trauma is to maximize team efficiency and performance. By introducing each other communication barriers are broken down. Specific preparation and roles can be discussed and skill mix identified. (726)
8. ATLS is Advanced Trauma Life Support, an approach to the trauma patient developed by the American College of Surgeons. It provides a shared and consistent approach to a major trauma patient. It is based on a Primary Survey

---

*Numbers in parentheses refer to pages, figures, boxes, or tables in Pardo MC, Miller RD, eds. *Basics of Anesthesia*. 7th ed. Philadelphia: Elsevier; 2018.

(to identify immediately life-threatening injuries), a Secondary Survey (to identify serious but not immediately life-threatening injuries), and a Tertiary Survey (to assess for any additional injuries). (726)

9. The components of the primary survey in the ATLS approach to the trauma patient are organized into the ABCDE mnemonic: Airway and cervical spine control, Breathing and oxygenation, Circulation and hemorrhage control, Disability, and Exposure. Disability refers to a neurologic assessment to identify potentially catastrophic injuries that require prompt management. Exposure refers to inspecting the patient on all sides for other injuries, while simultaneously avoiding hypothermia. (726)

10. Some trauma patient injuries or indications that endotracheal intubation may be required include maxillofacial trauma, major hemodynamic instability, low oxygen saturation, burns, head injury, altered mental status (intoxication, behavioral, safety concerns), and need to transport (radiology, operating room [OR], intensive care unit [ICU], other). (727)

11. Preoxygenation can be difficult in the trauma patient as a result of a multitude of factors. These include direct pulmonary injury (hemothorax or pneumothorax, aspiration, pulmonary contusion, rib fractures), patient compliance (agitation associated with traumatic brain injury [TBI] or intoxication), and preexisting illness (pulmonary disease, and reduced functional residual capacity [FRC] from lying flat or increased intra-abdominal pressure). (727)

12. All trauma patients are assumed to have a "full stomach," so a rapid sequence induction of anesthesia is the standard of care when these patients undergo endotracheal intubation. (727)

13. The hemodynamic effects of induction agents are exaggerated in the trauma patient for two reasons: acute intravascular volume loss from bleeding, and sympathetic overstimulation caused by pain, distress, and hypovolemia that can mask the true volume status. Also, blood is relatively shunted toward the essential organs during a shock state, and thus the relative volume of distribution of induction drugs is reduced. For all these reasons, reducing the doses of anesthesia induction drugs helps minimize their potential exaggerated hemodynamic effect in trauma patients. (727)

14. Trauma patients with suspected cervical spine injury should have a hard collar placed to stabilize their spine. During laryngoscopy the front of the collar should be loosened and an additional clinician should manually stabilize the head and neck in alignment to minimize cervical spine movement. (728)

15. Video laryngoscopy provides several advantages over traditional direct laryngoscopy in the trauma patient. It offers enhanced group situational awareness and the potential for reduced force required for adequate visualization of the glottis and is part of many difficult intubation strategies, thus improving visualization on the first attempt. In a teaching context it also allows improved supervision and guidance to novice laryngoscopists. (728)

16. Following endotracheal intubation of the trauma patient, postintubation care consists of placing the patient on a ventilator and adjusting ventilator settings, implementing an ongoing sedation plan to avoid potential hypertension associated with awareness, assessing the need for additional venous or arterial access, and determining the disposition of the patient to definitive care (i.e., to the OR, radiology department, or the ICU). (728)

17. Patients with airway burns, oral trauma, or direct airway trauma need extra caution and thought for their airway management. Patients with airway burns need an expedited assessment and management of their airway because they can develop airway compromise because of edema. Oral and airway trauma can result blood in the upper airway or tracheal disruption. Video laryngoscopes and fiberoptic scopes are not as effective when blood obscures the field of view, creating more difficult endotracheal intubating conditions. These patients should be managed by experienced clinicians, and a surgical team should be available to provide a surgical airway if necessary. (728)

18. Some clinical signs that a trauma patient may have potential airway burns include facial burns, soot in the mouth or nose, carbonaceous sputum, explosion injuries to the upper body, and stridor. (728)

19. The components of the GCS are the patient's responses with the eyes (1-4), verbal response (1-5), and motor response (1-6). The maximum score is 15, and the minimum score is 3. In this example the patient's GCS score is 8, calculated as eyes = 2 (to pain), verbal = 2 (incomprehensible sounds), and motor = 4 (withdraws to pain). (729)

20. A hybrid operating room is one that is set up to function as a complete angiography suite as well as a fully functional traditional operating room. The advantage is that in a hybrid operating room a single location can provide the entirety of emergency interventional services that any major trauma may require. They are also usually located within the broader operating suite, providing a more familiar environment with assistance closer at hand. (730)

21. A good leader synthesizes information and helps focus the energies of a team to produce a desired outcome. The leader listens to the team, provides clear direction and expectations for patient care, shares uncertainty, delegates appropriately, and stands back and maintains the "big picture" (doesn't micromanage). A good follower is alert and communicative about the perspective on patient issues. The followers assist the leader to have the best, most current information to guide decision making. They use closed-loop communication; offer suggestions; alert the leader to changes in the clinical picture; provide feedback of any personal limitations, skills, or experience; and use techniques such as graded assertiveness when appropriate. (730)

22. Graded assertiveness is a communication strategy that allows team members to express their concerns about decisions to the team leader in a stepwise, structured way that maintains constructive group performance. An example is the PACE technique of graded assertiveness that uses four communication statements in the following order: probe, alert, challenge, and emergency action. For example, concern about an inappropriately hypotensive patient with a head injury might be initially communicated as a *probe*, such as "Don't we try to keep the blood pressure a little higher in head injury?" If this is ineffective or insufficient, then an *alert* should be used. An *alert* could be presented as, "Have you noticed the blood pressure has drifted down? Would you like me to treat it?" If this is still not addressing the concern, then a *challenge* followed by an *emergency action* statement may be appropriate. An example of a *challenge* statement is "Is there a reason you don't want to treat the hypotension?" and an example of *emergency action* is "I am going to treat the blood pressure. The blood pressure is too low." (730)

INTRAOPERATIVE MANAGEMENT

23. There are three phases of major trauma resuscitation. Phase one is characterized by life-threatening uncontrolled hemorrhage, and the clinical goal is to maintain end-organ perfusion and oxygenation and stop the bleeding. Phase two is ongoing hemorrhage under partial surgical control that is not immediately life threatening, and the clinical goal is tailored resuscitation. Phase three is hemorrhage under control, and the clinical goal is to restore physiology. (731)

24. During phase one (life-threatening uncontrolled hemorrhage) of major trauma resuscitation the patient is extremely volume depleted, requiring rapid, large volume resuscitation to maintain cardiac output. The goal of the medical team is to stop the bleeding as soon as possible. During this time the airway should be controlled, 100% F_{IO_2} administered, large-bore intravenous (IV) access obtained, damage control resuscitation and massive transfusion protocol instituted, emergency uncrossmatched blood administration considered, minimal use of crystalloids and colloids, rapid infusing systems used, and the administration of calcium chloride at a dose of 1 gram for every 3 blood products. (731)

25. Damage control resuscitation is a resuscitation strategy during life-threatening uncontrolled hemorrhage to provide circulatory support to prevent end-organ damage. The principles of damage control resuscitation are permissive hypotension, rapidly achieving hemostasis, early use of hemostatic and blood products, and minimal crystalloid and colloid use. These factors combine to minimize total blood loss while maximizing the use of endogenous compensatory mechanisms to bleeding. (731)

26. The purpose of a massive transfusion protocol is to facilitate communication, optimize blood bank response time, and minimize errors. Protocols for massive transfusions should initially focus on a ratio of 1:1:1 of packed red blood cells, fresh frozen plasma, and platelets. This restores oxygen-carrying capacity and the patient's ability to form blood clots. (732)

27. Permissive hypotension is temporarily targeting a lower than normal blood pressure (systolic blood pressure 80 to 90 mm Hg) in an actively hemorrhaging patient until hemostasis is achieved or until the patient's condition further deteriorates. This makes use of the body's physiologic compensatory mechanisms to hemorrhage (vasoconstriction in nonvital regions and redirection of the blood flow to vital organs) and supports hemostasis. Permissive hypotension can be used in all trauma patients with severe hemorrhage, but with adjustment of the tolerable systolic blood pressure in the elderly or those with preexisting cardiac disease or hypertension. (732)

28. Crystalloid administration has two main negative impacts in the actively bleeding trauma patient: hemodilution and increasing the rate of bleeding. Hemodilution is a concern as the administration of crystalloids dilutes out all the important functional components of the blood, reducing its ability to transport oxygen and support hemostasis. Crystalloids also increase the bleeding rate as volume resuscitation in the absence of hemorrhage control will result in a short-lived improvement in the hemodynamics followed by an increased rate of bleeding (due to higher blood pressure), followed by a worsening of acidosis, coagulopathy, and volume status. Large volumes of crystalloid will also worsen reperfusion injury and augment inflammatory responses. Synthetic colloid administration in the acutely bleeding patient increases coagulopathy by impairing both fibrinogen polymerization and platelet function. (732)

29. During phase one of major trauma resuscitation packed red blood cells, fresh frozen plasma, and platelets can be given in a 1:1:1 ratio. With ongoing life-threatening uncontrolled hemorrhage and large volume transfusions, the addition of cryoprecipitate to provide fibrinogen and tranexamic acid (an antifibrinolytic) to prevent coagulopathy may be helpful for clotting and hemostasis. (733)

30. The use of vasopressors during phase one major trauma resuscitation to support hemodynamics is controversial, as there is concern that in the severely volume-depleted patient the use of vasopressors may further constrict vessels supplying blood to vital organs. (733)

31. Phase two of major trauma resuscitation is characterized by ongoing hemorrhage that is not immediately life threatening and only under partial surgical control. During this phase the rate of transfusion slows down, and there is time to tailor the patient's resuscitation by point-of-care testing (POCT), and laboratory analysis of arterial blood gases (ABGs), hemoglobin, and electrolytes. Crystalloids and colloids may be used, cell salvage can be started, extra monitoring can be considered (arterial line, transesophageal echocardiography [TEE]), ventilatory adjustments can be made, and steps can be taken to avoid hypothermia, and it is possible to start titrating the dose of anesthetic. (734)

32. To assess the coagulation status of the trauma patient intraoperatively the clinician must know the patient's medical history, use standard laboratory coagulation tests and POCT, and correlate these findings with the clinical presentation. (734)

33. Surgical bleeding occurs as a result of tissue or vessel injury that is beyond the capabilities of the endogenous hemostatic system to stop. The treatment for surgical bleeding is for the surgeon to gain access to, and control of, the bleeding through mechanical hemostasis. Nonsurgical bleeding often presents as a diffuse ooze in a widespread pattern from exposed tissues that are bleeding from minimal trauma. For nonsurgical bleeding, correction of the appropriate coagulation abnormalities will help improve the bleeding. (735)

34. Standard laboratory coagulation tests consist of the prothrombin time, international normalized ratio, activated partial thromboplastin time, platelet count, and fibrinogen concentration. As measures of perioperative coagulopathy in the acutely bleeding patient, these have significant limitations such as a lack of sensitivity, specificity, validation, and timeliness. For this reason viscoelastic POCT of coagulation, such as the thromboelastograph (TEG) and rotational thromboelastometry (ROTEM), have become the mainstay for assessing the magnitude and nature of coagulation abnormalities and help guide procoagulant therapies. POCT provides rapid information in close proximity to the patient, thus facilitating serial measurements and tailoring treatments. (735)

35. Viscoelastic testing (TEG/ROTEM) has a role in phase two of major trauma resuscitation when there is some hemostatic control but ongoing significant transfusion requirements. The TEG/ROTEM can be used to assess the magnitude and nature of coagulopathy, and can help tailor the resuscitation of a patient's individual coagulopathy at that point in time. (735)

36. The three parts of a TEG/ROTEM graphical readout are the preclot formation phase, the clot formation phase, and the clot stability phase. In the preclot formation phase, which lasts less than 5 minutes, the plasma coagulation cascade is triggered and platelets are activated. Deficiencies in this phase indicate a need for prothrombin complex concentrate and fresh frozen plasma. In the clot formation phase the clot is formed and reaches maximum clot firmness, thus testing for platelet mass and fibrinogen availability. Deficiencies in this phase can be corrected with the transfusion of cryoprecipitate, fibrinogen concentrate, and platelet concentrates. In the clot stability phase fibrinolysis is detected and quantified. Deficiencies in this phase can be corrected with an antifibrinolytic. (735)

37. Hypothermia during major trauma resuscitation can be prevented through the use of warmed IV fluids and blood, forced air warming blankets (Bair Hugger), heat/moisture exchange filters for the airway, and raising the operating room temperature. Temperature monitoring helps the clinician to assess the success of these maneuvers. (736)

38. During phase three of major trauma resuscitation the patient's hemorrhage is controlled and physiology is restored. Hemodynamics and intravascular fluid volume are normalized, there is stepwise deepening of anesthesia, the massive transfusion protocol is deactivated, the metabolic status can be improved (lactate, base deficit), and there is communication with team members and the ICU. (736)

SPECIAL GROUPS

39. The most common causes of secondary injury in TBI patients include intracranial hypertension, arterial hypotension, hypoxia, hyperthermia, coagulopathy, hyperglycemia, hypoglycemia, and acidosis. The focus of TBI management is to limit secondary injury by avoiding and treating these potential causes. (737)

40. A secured airway should be established in TBI patients if they do not have the ability to maintain a patent airway owing to loss of reflexes or cannot adequately oxygenate or ventilate. Other indications for endotracheal intubation in these patients include signs of intracranial hypertension, uncontrollable seizure activity, or progressively worsening mental status. These factors often correlate with a deteriorating GCS score, usually 8 or less, or other concurrent injury. (737)

41. Inadequate fasting, hypoxia, uncertain intravascular fluid volume status, and presumed cervical spine injury in blunt trauma should be taken into consideration prior to endotracheal intubation of TBI patients, as with all other trauma patients. In addition, TBI patients may have increased intracranial pressure (ICP), pending herniation, or concurrent airway injuries or may be uncooperative or combative. Special attention must also be paid to cervical spine immobilization during airway manipulation, because TBI patients are at higher risk of having concurrent cervical spine injuries. (738)

42. The effect of induction agents on the TBI patient's hemodynamics and cerebral perfusion pressure must be cautiously considered. Propofol and etomidate both reduce cerebral blood flow and are frequently chosen for the induction of anesthesia. Nondepolarizing neuromuscular blocking drugs have no effect on cerebral hemodynamics, whereas succinylcholine may increase ICP. The effect of succinylcholine on ICP has not been shown to be clinically significant, however, and may be attenuated with a defasciculating dose of a nondepolarizing drug. (738)

43. Volatile agents decrease cerebral oxygen metabolism but increase cerebral blood flow because of direct vasodilating effects. This is known as "uncoupling" and occurs in a dose-dependent manner. This effect of increased cerebral blood flow of volatile anesthetics does not occur until after 0.5 minimum alveolar concentration (MAC), and over 1 MAC for sevoflurane. For this reason, sevoflurane causes the least vasodilation and is therefore preferred if volatile agents are used. (738–739)

44. The goal of management of TBI patients intraoperatively is to reduce ICP and maintain a cerebral perfusion pressure of 50 to 70 mm Hg. This involves arterial line monitoring to ensure a sufficient systolic blood pressure and to promptly treat systemic hypotension, administering mannitol and antiseizure medicines, maintaining euvolemia, facilitating venous drainage through reverse Trendelenburg positioning, and the avoidance of high peak inspiratory pressures and positive end-expiratory pressure. Generally hyperventilation is not recommended within the first 24 hours of injury unless treating impending herniation. Another factor pertinent for management is the availability of blood products to treat bleeding, which can be profound from disrupted venous sinuses, and to treat coagulopathy. (739)

45. Cushing reflex is the intense sympathetic nervous system response to a high ICP in an attempt to maintain cerebral perfusion. Cushing reflex is characterized by systemic hypertension and may mask intravascular fluid volume depletion. Profound intraoperative hypotension may occur after decompression and normalization of the ICP due to a sudden decrease in systemic sympathetic activity. Prior to decompression, the patient's intravascular fluid volume should be repleted, anesthetic agents should be decreased, and vasopressors and inotropes should be available for administration. Blood should also be available in case of abrupt bleeding. (739)

46. Spinal cord precautions must be undertaken immediately in patients with acute spinal cord injury, including cervical collar placement and strict roll precautions when moving. Adequacy of ventilation and oxygenation should be evaluated. Patients with cervical or thoracic spinal cord injuries, especially those with complete injuries, may have diaphragmatic, intercostal, and abdominal weakness. This leads to decreased vital capacity and the inability to cough and clear secretions. Signs include rapid, shallow breathing, increased work of breathing, and paradoxical abdominal movement. Succinylcholine can safely be used for neuromuscular blockade for endotracheal intubation within the first 24 hours of injury in acute spinal cord injury patients. (740)

47. Spinal shock describes the acute cardiovascular effects of high thoracic or cervical injury (usually T4 and above) due to disruption of the sympathetic cardioaccelerator fibers and sympathetic blockade. This results in significant bradyarrhythmias, atrioventricular block, systemic vasodilation and hypotension,

and motor and sensory findings below the level of the lesion. Spinal shock treatment is supportive with isotonic fluid, vasopressors and inotropes as necessary, with care not to overresuscitate the patient with IV fluids. The mean arterial blood pressure should be maintained at 85 to 90 mm Hg to maintain adequate spinal cord perfusion, unless contraindicated by concurrent injuries. The American Association of Neurological Surgeons no longer recommends the administration of large-dose steroids, which has been associated with negative effects, including death. (740)

48. Burn surface area is estimated by the "rule of nines," in which the front and back of the torso are each 18%, the front and back of each leg is 9%, each whole arm is 9%, and the whole head is 9%. Only partial-thickness (epidermis and part of the dermis) and full-thickness (entire epidermis and dermis) burns are included in the burn surface area. Superficial burns involving only the dermis (e.g., sunburn) are not included in the burn surface area estimate. Burn surface area estimation is important as it guides future management and the potential need for transfer to a tertiary center. (740)

49. The initial treatment of burn patients is to halt the burning process. In the acute management of chemical burns irrigation should be continued until the measured skin pH or fluid pH is neutral, with care not to allow irrigation fluid to run across unaffected skin. Mineral oil should be used instead of water in elemental metal burns to avoid worsening the burn. In the acute management of electrical burns entry and exit points must be identified to determine the course of the burn. Underlying muscle damage can lead to rhabdomyolysis and compartment syndrome, and increased fluid requirements may be necessary. In the acute management of thermal burns there should be continued prolonged irrigation with cold fluid and evaluation for the potential for inhalational injury. (740)

50. Considerations in the management of patients with acute burn injury include intravascular fluid volume resuscitation, the potential for airway edema and total airway obstruction, providing adequate analgesia, the risk of inhalation injury and carbon monoxide poisoning, potential for infection, potential for compartment syndrome due to reduced compliance of circumferentially burned tissues, and the potential need for transfer to a tertiary care center. Intravascular fluid volume resuscitation is commonly with a balanced salt solution, such as lactated Ringer or Plasma-Lyte, and can be guided by multiple available formulas. There is increasing recognition of the risk of precipitating acute respiratory distress syndrome (ARDS) 3 to 5 days after burn injury with excessive volume administration. Supplemental high-concentration oxygen is essential for the treatment of inhalational injuries if carbon monoxide poisoning is suspected, because standard pulse oximetry monitors can read an erroneously normal value despite tissue hypoxemia in patients with carbon monoxide poisoning. The administration of high-concentration oxygen significantly decreases the half-life of carbon monoxide in the blood and should be used as an initial measure until carbon monoxide poisoning has been excluded through laboratory analysis. (740)

51. Special considerations in the acute management of the pediatric trauma patient include late physiologic decompensation because pediatric patients can mask significant hemodynamic compromise as a result of their physiology, potentially difficult IV access and the need for potential interosseous access, achieving patient compliance with testing, and dosing drugs and blood transfusions based on weight. In pediatric patients any blood loss can be significant. There should also be the awareness of the potential of nonaccidental injury. Some indications of nonaccidental injury include injuries inconsistent with developmental milestones, multiple injuries (especially if over a period of time), frequent presentations, and an inconsistent history of the incident. (742)

52. Special considerations in the acute management of the elderly trauma patient include preexisting illness and reduced physiologic reserve, medications the patient may have taken or missed, the potential for the masking of blood loss by

the lack of tachycardia as a result of β-adrenergic blockade, the increased risk of trauma from minimal impact including fractures and subdural hematoma, an awareness of the potential for elder abuse, and the consideration of end-of-life care and the patient's wishes concerning interventions that would be acceptable to the patient. (743)

53. Special considerations in the acute management of the pregnant trauma patient include the fact that normal signs of blood loss may occur late, that fetal distress may be the first sign of maternal compromise, left uterine displacement reduces aortocaval compression, a reduced functional residual capacity can lead to rapid oxygen destaturation, improper seatbelt use can affect the injury pattern, and the awareness that intimate partner violence increases during pregnancy. Other considerations include the changes in maternal physiology, the higher likelihood of having difficulty intubating the trachea of a pregnant patient, the need for anti-D immunoglobulin in Rh-negative mothers with major trauma (ideally within 72 hours of the trauma), reducing radiation exposure (without delaying diagnosis), the potential need for fetal heart rate monitoring, and the potential need for delivery of the fetus to control massive uterine bleeding or to optimize maternal or fetal survival. In addition, the nature of the maternal and fetal injury changes as the fetus develops during the pregnancy. Starting in the second trimester the uterus moves to an extrapelvic position, and there is a progressive increased risk of direct injury to the fetus until term, while the maternal organs become more shielded. In the third trimester there is an increased risk of injury to the bladder and an increased likelihood of precipitating early labor. (744)

54. There are some normal physiologic changes in pregnancy that can impact the presentation and management of the pregnant trauma patient. These include an increased circulating volume that can mask significant blood loss, having a compensated respiratory alkalosis with a normal P_{CO_2} of about 30 mm Hg, and having increased clotting factors leading to a hypercoagulable state. At term a fibrinogen level of 300 mg/dL would be abnormally low. (744)

55. Fetal monitoring in the pregnant trauma patient can be used for determining fetal viability, as an early sign of maternal deterioration, and to assist in assessing for obstetric injuries. Continuous fetal monitoring should be considered after 24 weeks of gestation. (745)

43 HUMAN-INDUCED AND NATURAL DISASTERS

Catherine Kuza and Joseph H. McIsaac, III

DISASTER TYPES AND NOMENCLATURE

1. What is a disaster?
2. What constitutes a mass casualty event (MCE)?
3. What are the types of disasters that may result in an MCE?

EPIDEMIOLOGY

4. What has been the trend in the numbers of disastrous events over the past century? What are explanations for this trend?
5. Does mortality rate reflect the severity of a disaster? Why or why not?

DISASTER PREPARATION AND RESPONSE

6. What are the goals of disaster management?
7. What are the four phases of a disaster? What are examples of the actions performed in each of these phases?
8. What are some of the items in a personal and family emergency preparedness plan?
9. What are some examples of U.S. government agencies involved in disaster response? What are their responsibilities?
10. What group of medical professionals comprises the U.S. government agency Medical Specialty Enhancement Teams (MSETs)? What is the role of MSETs?
11. Which U.S. government emergency medical response team requires response personnel to complete one weekend of training each month?
12. What is a Hospital Incident Command System (HICS)? What is its purpose? What is a job action sheet?
13. What is the purpose of a hospital emergency management plan?
14. What are the main principles of a hospital emergency management plan?
15. Who should participate on the hospital disaster/emergency management committee?
16. What is the purpose of a postdisaster debriefing?
17. What are some examples of disaster training and education courses that providers can take to improve their disaster management skills and knowledge?

MASS CASUALTY EVENTS

18. What are some mechanisms of injury that can result in an MCE?
19. What is the role of anesthesiologists in MCEs?
20. What are the goals of patient triage in MCEs?
21. How are patients classified and managed during triage for MCEs?
22. What are some roles for the anesthesiologist in the prehospital setting during an MCE?
23. What are some considerations for airway management in an MCE?
24. What are some roles for the anesthesiologist in the hospital setting during an MCE?

25. What is the benefit of balanced resuscitation? What is the role of tranexamic acid in treating bleeding patients? When should it be given and why?

NUCLEAR EXPOSURE

26. What are some possible sources of exposure to ionizing radiation?
27. What are some examples of injuries resulting from radiation exposure?
28. What is the first step in the management of patients with radiation exposure?
29. Where does decontamination of mass casualty patients occur?
30. What are the typical findings in acute radiation syndrome? What can be done to minimize the risk?

CHEMICAL AND BIOLOGICAL TERRORISM

31. How is decontamination achieved for chemical and biological agents?
32. Why are education and training about personal protective equipment important for anesthesiologists?
33. What are the four levels of personal protective equipment? In most cases of toxin poisoning, what level of personal protective equipment is adequate for the health care provider?
34. What are the three categories of bioterrorism agents and diseases? Name an example of an agent or disease in each category.
35. What are some epidemiologic features of disease or infection that may suggest exposure or infection with biological weapons?
36. What is the mechanism of transmission of anthrax? Describe the signs, symptoms, and treatment of anthrax exposure.
37. What is the mechanism of transmission of smallpox? Describe the signs, symptoms, and treatment of smallpox exposure.
38. What is the mechanism of transmission of plague? Describe the signs, symptoms, and treatment of plague exposure.
39. What is the mechanism of transmission of tularemia? Describe the signs, symptoms, and treatment of tularemia exposure.
40. What is the mechanism of transmission of botulism? Describe the signs, symptoms, and treatment of botulin exposure.
41. What is the mechanism of transmission of ricin? Describe the signs, symptoms, and treatment of ricin exposure.
42. What is the mechanism of transmission of viral hemorrhagic fevers? Describe the signs, symptoms, and treatment of viral hemorrhagic fever exposure.
43. What is a toxic industrial chemical (TIC)?
44. What is a nerve agent? What are some signs and symptoms of nerve agent exposure?
45. What is the treatment for exposure to a nerve agent?
46. What is the mechanism by which a pulmonary agent causes death when used as a chemical weapon? Describe the signs, symptoms, and treatment of exposure to phosgene gas.
47. What is the mechanism by which the blood toxin hydrogen cyanide causes death when used as a chemical weapon? Describe the signs, symptoms, and treatment of exposure to weaponized hydrogen cyanide.
48. What is the mechanism by which vesicants cause harm when used as a chemical weapon? Describe the signs, symptoms, and treatment of exposure to weaponized vesicants.

INFECTIOUS DISEASE DISASTERS AND PANDEMICS

49. What is a pandemic? What are examples of infectious diseases that have resulted in pandemics?
50. What is the role of the anesthesiologist in infectious disease disasters?
51. What is the role of the Centers for Disease Control and Prevention (CDC) in infectious disease disasters?

CYBER ATTACKS AND HIGH-ALTITUDE ELECTROMAGNETIC PULSE EVENTS

52. What are the consequences of cyber attacks?
53. What is a high-altitude electromagnetic pulse (HEMP) event? What are its potential consequences?

54. What are some measures that can be implemented to provide protection against HEMP events?

55. What is the purpose of postdisaster syndrome surveillance?
56. What are some of the diseases that have emerged after natural disasters, such as the typhoon in the Philippines and the earthquake in Haiti in 2010?

RECOVERY

57. What are elements of the recovery phase? When should planning for the recovery phase begin?
58. What is the major limiting factor of how quickly a region can recover from a disaster? What is the duration of the recovery phase?

ANSWERS*

DISASTER TYPES AND NOMENCLATURE

1. A disaster is an event that overwhelms the usual capacity of the facility or geographic area, often requiring outside resources in management. It can be human induced (terrorism, war) or caused by natural phenomena (weather, earthquakes); a single event in time or extended over months to years (i.e., droughts); or localized or widespread over a large area. Available resources may not be sufficient to supply needs; examples of such resources include medical supplies, pharmaceuticals, food and water, shelter, and skilled responders. (748)

2. A mass casualty event (MCE) occurs when the number of victims surpasses the treatment ability and resources provided by a medical center. Even at Level I trauma centers with an activated disaster plan, it is difficult to provide care to more than seven casualties per hour. (749)

3. The disasters that may result in MCEs can be natural (hurricanes, floods, earthquakes, rain, ice, snow, bacterial/viral pandemics), unintentional (public transportation accident, nuclear or industrial accident), intentional (bombing, nuclear/biological/chemical attack), and human induced (oil spills, fires, terror attacks, chemical/nuclear plant explosion). (749)

EPIDEMIOLOGY

4. There has been an increasing number of disastrous events over the past century. The growing global population, improved methods to report events, advances in technology, increased number of transportation vehicles available and in use, biochemical and nuclear weapon development, and the evolution of new viruses all contribute to this rising number of disasters and mass casualties. Natural and human-induced disasters occurring in less developed countries may result in higher death tolls owing to lack of emergency preparedness plans and resources. (749)

5. It is important to recognize that mortality rate does not reflect the severity of the disaster. Communities can be affected by interrupting employment, education, transportation, food resources, and security. The vast damage created by disasters may also affect health care workers by preventing them from safely reporting to work. Power failures or floods can damage hospital equipment and cause secondary health hazards. (749)

DISASTER PREPARATION AND RESPONSE

6. The goals of disaster management are to reduce or prevent the potential losses from hazards, provide prompt and appropriate assistance to victims, and achieve rapid and effective recovery. (749)

7. The four phases of a disaster are mitigation, preparedness, response, and recovery. The actions performed in the mitigation phase include predisaster

---

*Numbers in parentheses refer to pages, figures, boxes, or tables in Pardo MC, Miller RD, eds. *Basics of Anesthesia.* 7th ed. Philadelphia: Elsevier; 2018.

planning, prevention, and minimizing the effects of the disaster. Preparedness requires establishing preparedness plans, performing emergency drills, and having warning systems in place. The response phase includes emergency relief, search and rescue efforts, and employing interventions aimed at minimizing the hazards created by a disaster. The recovery phase is returning a community to normal and entails reconstruction, establishing health care resources, providing temporary housing, and rebuilding the economy. (753)

8. Some items in a personal and family emergency preparedness plan include having at least a 3-day of supply of medications, food and water, pet care, and batteries. Families should have first aid and disaster kits, battery-powered radios, cash, and an alternative to power and lighting. In the event of an evacuation, families should devise preplanned evacuation routes and alternatives, have fuel for the car, establish family meeting places, and have supplies ready in a waterproof container (e.g., clothing, cash, food, and important documents). Families should perform drills for unanticipated emergencies. (753)

9. Some examples of U.S. government agencies involved in disaster response include the Federal Bureau of Investigation (FBI), the Federal Emergency Management Agency (FEMA), Department of Health and Human Services (HHS), Department of Defense (DOD), Centers for Disease Control and Prevention (CDC), and various medical response teams. These agencies generally provide domestic terrorism and crisis management, coordinate emergency responses and relief to affected areas, assist with the management of chemical terrorism, and coordinate and provide support for public health and medical treatment. (753)

10. The Medical Specialty Enhancement Team (MSET) is a U.S. government emergency response team comprising 30 surgeons, 30 anesthesiologists, and pediatricians that respond to domestic and international crises through deployment to either a disaster site or specific facility. This team is federally employed during deployments that last a minimum of 2 weeks. (753)

11. The Disaster Medical Assistance Team (DMAT) is a U.S. government emergency response team that requires its personnel to complete one weekend of training each month. This response team is trained to rapidly mobilize and sets up staff with physicians, nurses, and support personnel, emergency facilities, and pharmaceutical dispensaries near the disaster site. (753)

12. The Hospital Incident Command System (HICS) is an adaptable system that can be used at any hospital during emergencies, for planned events, or in managing threats. It highlights the importance of the mission areas of prevention, protection, mitigation, response, and recovery. It facilitates smooth transitions of care between hospitals and outside responding providers, assigns responsibilities to personnel and designated teams, plans and coordinates support requirements, emphasizes efficient communication, and obtains necessary equipment or supplies from outside sources. A job action sheet is a personalized document created by the HICS that defines a list of the tasks needed to be performed for the various responders' roles. There are different job action sheets created for each role in emergency/disaster response. (754)

13. The purpose of a hospital emergency management plan is to provide prompt medical care, justly allocate resources, and minimize deaths from disasters or MCEs in which a large number of victims require treatment. (755)

14. The main principles of a hospital emergency management plan are to be comprehensive, simple, flexible with organizational charts applicable to various disasters, and adaptable; have a predictable chain of management; clearly define authority, roles, and responsibilities; and be a part of the regional health plan in disasters. (755)

15. The hospital disaster/emergency committee should be multidisciplinary, composed of members who have different jobs and roles in the hospital. This may include, but is not limited to, personnel from hospital administration, chiefs of clinical divisions (e.g., surgery, orthopedics, anesthesiology, emergency medicine, pathology, blood bank, radiology, nutrition, nursing), clinical support

services (e.g., radiology, laboratory, blood bank, and social services), and hospital operations (e.g., engineering, material management, security, environmental services). (755)

16. After deactivation of the hospital disaster/emergency management plan there should be a postdisaster debriefing. This is done to evaluate the hospital's performance, identify areas of strength and weakness, and modify the plan accordingly to improve future performance. (755)

17. Examples of disaster training and education courses that providers can take to improve their disaster management skills and knowledge include educational materials designed by the World Association for Disaster and Emergency Management (WADEM) and the International Society for Disaster Medicine (ISDM). Additionally, there are courses such as Advanced Trauma Life Support (ATLS), Basic and Advanced Disaster Life Support, Emergency and Trauma Care Training courses through the World Health Organization, Primary Trauma Care courses, and the Disaster Management and Emergency Preparedness (DMEP) course offered through the American College of Surgeons Committee on Trauma (ACS COT), which are available to anesthesia providers. The teaching methods employed include self-study materials, problem-based learning, case discussions, disaster drills, simulation exercises, and mock field exercises using real resources, vehicles, staff, and equipment. (756)

MASS CASUALTY EVENTS

18. Mechanisms of injury that can result in an MCE include blunt and penetrating trauma, burns, and chemical and radiation injuries. (756)

19. Anesthesiologists are valuable members of disaster/MCE response teams due to their broad knowledge base ranging from physiology to pharmacology, familiarity with surgical injuries and procedures, ability to manage critically ill patients, and technical skills. Their training teaches them to be adaptable and provide care for patients in different hospital settings. During an MCE the role of anesthesiologists can be expanded to the prehospital setting to help with triage and to stabilize, resuscitate, and provide life support to patients. They can also provide care in the emergency department, operating room (OR), and postoperative/intensive care unit (ICU) environment. Furthermore, anesthesiologists can facilitate communication between surgeons, OR staff, and hospital personnel. Anesthesiologist responsibilities during an MCE may be designated in hospital emergency management plans. Anesthesiologists should therefore be familiar with protective equipment, decontamination processes, and antidotes to specific toxic exposures. (756)

20. The goals of patient triage in MCEs are to quickly prioritize injuries based on severity of injury and likelihood to survive so that limited resources can be distributed to those who are likely to survive and benefit. Resource allocation is thus distributed to achieve the greatest population benefit. This concept of population-based resource allocation can be difficult for providers who are used to utilizing every possible resource for each patient under their care. (757)

21. Two examples of triage systems for an MCE are SALT (sort, assess, lifesaving interventions, treatment/transport) and START (simple triage and rapid treatment for mass casualties). Patients are classified into one of four possible groups: those requiring immediate care, delayed care, first aid (minimal), and expectant management. Expectant management is employed when patients are unlikely to survive their injuries. These patients are isolated in a quiet area focusing on comfort and end-of-life care. (757)

22. Anesthesiologists can have great utility in the prehospital setting during an MCE. Airway management, intravenous line placement, resuscitation, and medication management are some examples. During damage control surgery performed at the disaster site, as in combat situations, the anesthesiologist may provide "field block anesthesia" or "on-site" anesthesia. Damage control surgery is rapid control of bleeding followed by abdominal packing. It is done to address and treat life-threatening injuries and stabilize the greatest number of patients in the

shortest amount of time possible. Anesthesiologists can also help stabilize and provide anesthesia and analgesia to patients who are trapped under rubble, as they did during the London subway bombings. (757)

23. Endotracheal intubation is the gold standard for airway management during MCEs. Usually, a rapid-sequence intubation is recommended; manual in-line neck stabilization should be provided when applicable, and cricoid pressure is considered optional (it is no longer a Level I recommendation). Anesthesiologists should take care to wear personal protective equipment as appropriate, which may inhibit dexterity and make endotracheal intubation more challenging. Supraglottic airway devices are acceptable alternatives when endotracheal intubation is not practical or available. Biological or chemical agents should be taken into considerations as well. For example, with nerve agent poisoning, neuromuscular blockers should be used with caution. (757)

24. Anesthesiologists can provide care during MCEs to patients in the emergency room, OR, and postoperatively in the ICU and postanesthesia care units. Patients may require airway and mechanical ventilation management, vascular access placement, decontamination, cardiopulmonary resuscitation, and treatment for chemical or biological toxicity. The OR is typically utilized for the treatment of life-threatening injuries and stabilization during MCEs. Damage control operations are performed only, and less urgent surgeries are deferred, so other patients who require surgery are able to be treated in a timely manner. Anesthesiologists in this situation should perform balanced resuscitation as during trauma surgeries with massive hemorrhage. (758)

25. Balanced resuscitation is employed as a bridge to definitive interventional bleeding control and minimizes the amount of fluids and blood products administered to maintain and tolerate a lower-than-normal blood pressure (systolic pressures of 80 to 100 mm Hg). The goal is to maintain organ perfusion while minimizing the risk of bleeding. Large fluid loads can worsen acidosis, activate the inflammation cascade, and cause hypothermia and coagulopathy. In hemorrhagic shock, blood products are favored over colloids and crystalloids and should be given in a packed red blood cell to fresh frozen plasma to platelet ratio of 1:1:1, as it improves survival. Vasopressors can impair tissue perfusion, and their use should be minimized. Tranexamic acid, an antifibrinolytic, may be given in bleeding trauma patients within 3 hours of injury to reduce the risk of death from bleeding; administration after 3 hours is harmful and increases mortality rate. (759)

NUCLEAR EXPOSURE

26. Exposure to ionizing radiation is likely to occur from terrorist attacks, nuclear power plant accidents, and nuclear weapon attacks. Radiation exposure may result from external sources (beta particles, gamma rays), contaminated debris, or inhaled gases and particulates. (759)

27. Examples of injuries resulting from radiation exposure include radiation burns, bone marrow suppression, destruction of the gastrointestinal tract mucosa, and bleeding with translocation of bacteria resulting in septic shock. (759)

28. Life-threatening injury treatment should precede the treatment of radiologic injuries in patients who have had radiation exposure. The first step in the management of radiation exposure is decontamination by removing all clothing and rinsing the skin with warm soapy water. Any wounds should be irrigated. Once stabilized and externally decontaminated, internal decontamination may need to be performed through gastric lavage, emetics, laxatives, and diuretics to prevent continued injury from retained nuclear material. During decontamination providers should wear personal protective gear and dosimeters to gauge their exposure to radiation. (759)

29. Decontamination of mass casualty patients is typically performed at the scene before transportation. Hospitals set up a secure area outside the main hospital area to complete decontamination and triage of patients. Out-of-hospital

decontamination reduces ongoing exposure injuries and minimizes the risk of secondary exposure to health care providers and other patients. (759)

30. Acute radiation syndrome is characterized by thrombocytopenia, granulocytopenia, nausea, vomiting, and diarrhea. Risk is minimized by limiting the duration of exposure through external and internal decontamination. Medications can be given to facilitate renal excretion and chelation. Potassium iodide can also be given within the first 24 hours to prevent radiation-induced thyroid abnormalities after nuclear power plant disasters. (760)

CHEMICAL AND BIOLOGICAL TERRORISM

31. Decontamination for chemical and biological agents is performed by emergency personnel wearing proper protective attire. It should take place in a designated decontamination area with its own water outlet using triage algorithms. All hazardous clothing and materials should be removed and stored in specific bags. Decontamination involves washing the skin using a soft brush or sponge and mild soap and warm water. Hot water is contraindicated because it can increase the absorption of chemicals, and cold water is avoided as it may cause hypothermia. The final step is flushing the whole body with running water for at least 1 minute. (760)

32. Because anesthesiologists may have a key role in the management of trauma and MCE victims, education and training about personal protective equipment is important to help limit their personal exposure. Anesthesiologists should know the location of decontamination areas in their hospital, be familiar with basic decontamination techniques, and be aware of what proper protective equipment is indicated in a given situation. (761)

33. There are four levels of personal protective equipment. Level A includes a positive-pressure self-contained breathing apparatus (SCBA), fully encapsulating chemical-resistant suit, double layer of chemical-resistant gloves, chemical-resistant boots, and an airtight seal between suit and gloves and boots. Level B includes a positive-pressure SCBA, chemical-resistant long-sleeved suit and boots, and a double layer of chemical-resistant gloves. Level C includes a full face air purification device (respirator) and a chemical-resistant suit, outer gloves, and boots. Level D equipment does not provide specific respiratory or skin protection but may include gloves, gowns, or safety glasses or face shield. In most cases of toxin poisoning, level C personal protective equipment is adequate for the health care provider at a fixed facility (first receiver). Level A protection is required when the greatest potential for exposure to hazards exists such as at a field site (first responders). (761)

34. Bioterrorism agents are as classified into three categories by the CDC. Category A agents are the highest priority. They are easily distributed or transmitted to victims, have a high mortality rate, and create public panic if released. Examples of category A diseases are anthrax, smallpox, plague, and hemorrhagic fevers (i.e., Ebola virus). Category B agents have moderate dissemination and morbidity rates and low mortality rates. Examples of category B agents are Q fever, *Vibrio cholerae*, ricin, and various enteric pathogens such as *Escherichia coli*, *Salmonella*, and *Shigella*. Category C agents are emerging pathogens that are not yet mass engineered. Examples of category C agents include various equine encephalitic viruses. (761)

35. Any clustering of unusual illness should be treated as bioterrorism until proved otherwise. Indications suggesting exposure or infection with biological weapons include an unusually high incidence or mortality rate from a disease cluster, a single pathogen in a cluster of patients with a suspicious clinical illness, the occurrence of a disease outside its natural geographic boundary, and the clustering of diseases that affect animals as well as humans. (761)

36. There are three mechanisms of transmission of anthrax: cutaneous, inhalational, and gastrointestinal. When weaponized anthrax inhalation causes flu-like symptoms followed by chest pain, cyanosis, hemoptysis, and profound

respiratory distress leading to respiratory failure. Shock and meningitis may also be present. A chest radiograph may reveal a widened mediastinum due to mediastinal adenopathy. Death can occur within 2 days once severe dyspnea develops, so prompt treatment is imperative. Treatment includes antibiotic therapy (ciprofloxacin or doxycycline), endotracheal intubation and mechanical ventilation, and hemodynamic support. These patients should initially be isolated, although there is little to no risk of secondary spread in patients affected by inhalational anthrax, and cases should be reported to the appropriate health care officials. Exposed individuals should receive prophylactic treatment with a fluoroquinolone alone for 60 days or a vaccination plus a fluoroquinolone for 30 days. (761)

37. Smallpox is highly infectious, with transmission occurring through aerosolized droplets that have been in direct contact with pustules. Smallpox initially causes fatigue, headache, and high fevers, with cutaneous lesions appearing over the next 3 to 4 days as the fever resolves. Smallpox lesions present at the same time and stage. Patients should be immediately isolated, and exposed contacts should be vaccinated within 3 to 7 days after exposure to be effective. (762)

38. Bubonic plague is spread primarily by flea bite, and after 2 to 6 days the patients develops sudden fevers, chills, headache, weakness, and painful lymph node enlargement. If untreated, bubonic plague can lead to gangrene and septic shock. When the infection seeds into the lungs it can cause pneumonic plague, manifesting as pneumonia and rapidly developing respiratory failure. Aerosolized plague (*Yersinia pestis*) is viable for approximately 60 minutes. If an individual develops pneumonic plague, management includes strict isolation and exposure precautions because pneumonic plague is highly contagious. Early antibiotic treatment is also critical, as the mortality rate of untreated individuals is over 50%. Streptomycin is preferred, but gentamicin, tetracycline, and chloramphenicol are also effective therapies for plague. (762)

39. Tularemia is caused by a gram-negative coccobacillus carried by several animal hosts. It can be transmitted through direct contact with an infected animal, ingestion of infected food, infected tick or deerfly bite, or aerosolization of the bacteria. Infected individuals present with acute respiratory symptoms, fevers, pleuritic pain, hilar lymphadenopathy, and pneumonia 3 to 5 days following exposure. Patients do not need to be isolated and can be treated with streptomycin. Prophylaxis with streptomycin, doxycycline, or ciprofloxacin can be given to exposed individuals. (763)

40. *Clostridium botulinum* toxin is a category A agent that causes diplopia, dysphagia, dysarthria, and dyspnea, progressing to skeletal muscle weakness between 12 and 36 hours after ingestion or inhalation of the toxin. Botulism results from the inhibition of acetylcholine release. The muscarinic effects of botulinum lead to decreased salivation, ileus, urinary retention, and decreased salivation. The toxin is not contagious; therefore, health care providers do not need to follow any additional special precautions. Treatment is with trivalent antitoxin and possible toxin removal through cathartics, enema, and gastric lavage. Endotracheal intubation and mechanical ventilation may also be required. (763)

41. Ricin causes the profound inhibition of protein synthesis and presents as fever, diarrhea, weakness, seizures, respiratory failure, cardiovascular collapse, and multiple organ failure within 36 to 72 hours after inhalation. There is no specific antidote for humans, so treatment is supportive ICU care. (763)

42. There are several viral hemorrhagic fevers that can be transmitted through contact with infected bodily fluids or by inhalation. Infected patients will present with fever, myalgia, generalized mucous membrane hemorrhage, edema, and death after an incubation period ranging from 2 to 18 days. Initial treatment is supportive; early isolation and reporting are imperative as mortality rates can be high. Vaccines are being researched and developed for the most life-threatening agents, such as Ebola. (763)

43. A toxic industrial chemical (TIC) or hazardous material (HAZMAT) is defined as a substance with potentially harmful effects due to the nature of its biochemical properties that is used for industrial purposes; when improperly stored or accidentally released it may cause damage to the environment, community, or animals and can cause significant injuries or death in humans. The toxicity of TICs is significantly lower than traditional chemical warfare agents, but the release of large quantities of TICs can result in significant damage and destruction. TICs may be released in natural disasters, terrorist attacks (toxic war or infiltrating chemical plants), and accidentally during transportation or industrial site accidents. There are about 70 known chemical warfare agents and 70,000 TICs produced, stored, and transported through countries. TICs can be broadly classified into corrosives (acids, alkalis, and reactive metals), asphyxiants that displace oxygen (carbon dioxide, argon, nitrogen, etc.), airway irritants (ammonia, phosgene), and metabolic poisons (cyanide, carbon monoxide, etc.). (763)

44. Nerve agents were developed for military purposes after World War II, were originally used as pesticides, and have a structure similar to organophosphates. Sarin is a potent nerve agent that has been used recently in chemical terrorist attacks. It is also referred to by the two-letter NATO military code "GB." Nerve agents are typically lipophilic clear liquids that vaporize at room temperature and are absorbed through the skin, mucous membranes, lungs, or gastrointestinal tract. They can also penetrate clothing and leather. Nerve agents act by inhibiting acetylcholinesterase, increasing acetylcholine in the nerve terminal, and producing cholinergic effects. Patients present with increased salivation and airway secretions, rhinorrhea, bronchoconstriction, miosis, sweating, nausea, diarrhea, altered mental status, bradycardia, muscle cramping and weakness, fasciculations, hyperthermia, and respiratory failure. (764)

45. Exposure to a nerve agent should be treated with atropine 2 to 6 mg intravenously or intramuscularly every 5 to 10 minutes until secretions decrease and ventilation improves. Diazepam can be used to prevent seizures. 2-Pralidoxime is a longer acting anticholinergic drug that unbinds the nerve agents from acetylcholinesterase and reactivates the enzyme. Pyridostigmine is a medication that reversibly binds to acetylcholinesterase. Administration of pyridostigmine 30 minutes before exposure therefore provides protection by occupying the binding sites that the nerve agents target. It then dissociates from the acetylcholinesterase enzyme after the exposure risk has passed. Most patients exposed to nerve agents will require endotracheal intubation and supportive ICU care. Other care is dictated by the type of nerve agent. For example, patients exposed to the G-series agents should undergo decontamination, although it is not recommended for the V-series. The V-series permeates leather and clothing, so care providers should wear the appropriate personal protective equipment made of rubber or synthetic materials resistant to this nerve agent. (764)

46. A weaponized chemical pulmonary agent (e.g., phosgene, chlorine) used for terrorism when released in sufficient quantities can cause death by displacing oxygen, resulting in asphyxia. After exposure to phosgene gas, there may be a symptom-free period of 1 to 24 hours, but during this time lung injury is occurring and acute lung injury, pulmonary edema, and adult respiratory distress syndrome (ARDS) eventually follow. There is no antidote, and the treatment is supportive with endotracheal intubation and lung-protective mechanical ventilation similar to ARDS treatment protocols. (764)

47. Aerosolized hydrogen cyanide disrupts the electron transport chain in the mitochondria by binding to cytochrome c oxidase, thus preventing electron transfer to oxygen and hindering adenosine triphosphate (ATP) production; this results in cellular hypoxemia and metabolic acidosis, leading to death. Patients present with dyspnea and restlessness and may develop seizures, coma, and cardiac arrest. Death can occur within minutes if victims are exposed to

high concentrations. The treatment is supportive with endotracheal intubation, mechanical ventilation, and cardiovascular support with vasopressors and inotropes. As with nitroprusside toxicity, the antidote is thiosulfate and hydroxocobalamin administered intravenously to promote the conversion of cyanide to the less toxic thiocyanate. (765)

48. Vesicants, known as "blister agents," are chemicals that produce burns and blisters on contact or can cause pulmonary damage and multisystem organ failure on inhalation. Examples of vesicants include sulfur mustard (the most common vesicant), nitrogen mustard, lewisite, and phosgene oxime. The onset of symptoms varies from immediate to delay by 2 to 24 hours depending on the type of vesicant. Symptoms range from mild symptoms including erythema, tearing, hoarseness, and cough to severe poisoning causing respiratory failure, blindness, erythematous and bullous skin lesions, leukopenia, central nervous system effects, and permanent respiratory damage. Initial treatment is through decontamination with health care providers in appropriate personal protective gear, then guided by the severity of symptoms. Dimercaprol is the antidote for lewisite poisoning, whereas combination treatment with thiosulfate, vitamin E, and dexamethasone may improve outcomes in patients exposed to sulfur mustard. (765)

INFECTIOUS DISEASE DISASTERS AND PANDEMICS

49. Infectious agents, such as viruses, can mutate, infect humans, and result in high death tolls after human-to-human transmission. A pandemic is rampant disease prevalent over the whole country or world. Examples of infectious diseases that have resulted in pandemics include influenza A, severe acute respiratory syndrome (SARS), and West Nile virus. (765)

50. Anesthesiologists must be prepared to recognize potential infectious disease outbreaks, wear protective gear, employ appropriate contact and isolation precautions, and notify public health organizations while managing patients with contagious infectious diseases. Although oseltamivir, zanamivir, and peramivir can be used in the treatment of influenza A, there are few other antiretroviral treatments. Supportive ICU care, endotracheal intubation, and mechanical ventilation may be required when treating these patients. (765)

51. The CDC, infectious disease experts, and epidemiologists help develop vaccines, create treatments, and provide educational materials and resources for hospitals, communities, and health care providers. Information provided by the CDC is on disease transmission and prevention strategies to prepare for and mitigate infectious disease disasters. The CDC website also provides a list of infectious organisms, modes of transmission, and the types of precautions that need to be employed when patients are infected. (765)

CYBER ATTACKS AND HIGH-ALTITUDE ELECTROMAGNETIC PULSE EVENTS

52. Cyber attacks can compromise computer infrastructures of governmental and local agencies, as well as those used to coordinate responses and communicate during disasters. Disruption of these computer systems can interfere with operational decision making and allocation of resources. Communication among fire, law enforcement, hospitals, and public heath agencies can also be disrupted. They can compromise our economic and national security, impede response teams' efforts during disaster management, cause chaos, and even result in death. (765)

53. High-altitude electromagnetic pulse (HEMP) events result from nuclear weapon detonation above the earth's surface. They produce gamma-radiation that interacts with the atmosphere, creating an electromagnetic energy field that disrupts the earth's magnetic field but is harmless to people. Over a period of days to weeks a HEMP event can affect entire continents and cause power surges; disrupt equipment connected to power grids, telecommunication infrastructures, and communication systems; damage voltage and currents in electronic devices; disable computers, infrastructure, and power grids; melt circuitry; or cause equipment to fail. The effects may be severe enough to cause

a blackout lasting months to years. These events can also destroy transformers and generators in critical electrical grid infrastructures that may take years to replace. These attacks can affect hospital equipment and computer systems. (765)

54. Measures that can be implemented to protect against a HEMP event include shielding and filtering of a few key devices such as monitors and pulse oximetry, unplugging and turning off unused electronic equipment, rotating backup equipment to keep batteries charged, and having backup power systems, batteries, and solar-powered equipment. Storing small items such as pulse oximetry in bubble wrap surrounded by aluminum foil may also protect them from most HEMP events. (766)

POSTDISASTER SYNDROME SURVEILLANCE

55. Disease patterns emerge after severe natural disaster because of destruction of homes, disruption of health care systems, and limited available resources. By using surveillance tools to monitor postdisaster disease trends, data can be obtained that demonstrate the degree to which the health care system was disrupted as a result of the disaster, identify various health needs, and recognize diseases associated with a specific region or disaster type. The data obtained from postdisaster syndrome surveillance can help identify necessary public health interventions, determine resource allocation, guide decision making, and identify interventions that can prevent the postdisaster diseases observed. (766)

56. After the natural disasters that occurred in the Philippines, several disease syndromes emerged. Communicable disease was the most predominant syndrome. Other syndromes include diarrheal disease (leptospirosis), acute respiratory infections, hypertension, fever, and skin disease. Similarly, after the 2010 earthquake in Haiti, respiratory infections, injuries, suspected malaria, and fever of unknown origin were the most commonly reported conditions. (766)

RECOVERY

57. The recovery phase includes providing support services (medical and psychological) to victims, cleaning and reconstruction of damaged structures, and rebuilding the economy. It is important to begin planning the recovery phase during the response phase. (767)

58. The financial resources needed to rebuild a community are the major limiting factor of how quickly a region can recover from a disaster. The recovery period duration depends on the type of disaster and the country's resources and can take anywhere from days to years. Complete recovery from more devastating disasters and disasters that occur in underdeveloped countries with limited resources, financial support, and lack of insurance plans can take years. (767)

CLASSIFICATION OF CHRONIC PAIN	1. What is the cause of nociceptive pain? Provide some examples of clinical conditions with nociceptive pain. 2. What is the cause of neuropathic pain? Provide some examples of clinical conditions with neuropathic pain.
MULTIDISCIPLINARY PAIN MANAGEMENT	3. Why is multidisciplinary teamwork beneficial for managing chronic pain? What are the components of such a multidisciplinary team? 4. What is the role of the chronic pain physician in multidisciplinary pain management? 5. What is the role of the psychologist in multidisciplinary pain management? 6. What is the role of the physical therapist in multidisciplinary pain management?
COMMON PAIN SYNDROMES	7. What is meant by the term *low back pain* (LBP)? What is the overall prognosis at 6 weeks and at 12 weeks for patients presenting with acute LBP? 8. With regard to the capacity to return to work, what is the prognosis for patients with LBP lasting 6 months compared to 2 years? 9. What are common risk factors for developing chronic LBP? 10. What is the basic pathophysiology of radiculopathy? 11. What are the histologic changes associated with internal disk disruption (IDD)? Describe how IDD can progress to a herniated nucleus pulposus and how this may cause pain. 12. List the "red flag" findings on history and physical examination in a patient with acute LBP that warrant immediate evaluation with diagnostic imaging. 13. What are the physical examination findings associated with radiculopathy? 14. What is radicular pain? 15. What medicines are used in the initial management of chronic radicular pain? What is the rationale for use of these medications? 16. What are some potential causes of acute lumbosacral pain? 17. How should patients with acute lumbosacral pain be managed? 18. Which anatomic structures are most commonly the cause of chronic lumbosacral pain? 19. How should patients with chronic lumbosacral pain be managed? 20. What is believed to the cause of neuropathic pain? 21. What are some characteristics of neuropathic pain? 22. What are the physical examination findings consistent with diabetic peripheral neuropathy (DPN)? 23. Describe the effects of poor glycemic control on the development and progression of DPN.

24. What is sympathetically mediated pain? What are some examples of sympathetically mediated pain?
25. What is postherpetic neuralgia (PHN)?
26. How does the lifecycle of the varicella-zoster virus explain the dermatomal distribution of PHN symptoms?
27. What is the role of antiviral therapy in the management of herpes zoster, and what effect does this therapy have on the subsequent development of PHN?
28. What is complex regional pain syndrome (CRPS)?
29. What are some signs and symptoms of CRPS? What distinguishes type 1 from type 2 CRPS?
30. How should patients with CRPS be managed? What is the primary goal in the management of these patients?
31. What is myofascial pain syndrome? How should it be managed?
32. What is fibromyalgia? How should it be managed?
33. What are some of the mechanisms by which cancer can cause pain?
34. Describe the World Health Organization (WHO)'s pain treatment ladder.
35. Provide an example of an analgesic medication used at each step of the WHO's pain treatment ladder.

PHARMACOLOGIC MANAGEMENT OF CHRONIC PAIN

36. What are some clinical uses for acetaminophen and nonsteroidal anti-inflammatory drugs (NSAIDs) for the management of chronic pain?
37. What are some clinical uses of antidepressants for the management of chronic pain? What are some side effects that may limit their use?
38. What are some clinical uses of anticonvulsants for the management of chronic pain? What are some side effects that may limit their use?
39. What are some arguments for and against the use of long-term opioid therapy for chronic noncancer pain?
40. What are some of the strategies that the pain physician can employ to prevent opioid misuse and abuse?
41. What are some of the criteria that are used to identify patients who will likely benefit from tapering off of long-term opioids?
42. What is the role for psychological interventions, such as cognitive behavioral therapy, in tapering off of long-term opioids?

INTERVENTIONAL PAIN THERAPIES

43. What is meant by the term *interventional pain therapy*? Name some of the commonly performed interventional procedures and the type of pain they are intended to treat.
44. What is the proposed mechanism of action of epidural steroid injections?
45. What is the efficacy of epidural steroid injections?
46. Describe the process of radiofrequency ablation (RFA) of a facet joint sensory nerve. What is the expected duration of analgesia following a lumbar RFA?
47. Which two ganglia fuse to form the stellate ganglion? Describe the location of the stellate ganglia relative to the cervical vertebral bodies, longus colli muscle, subclavian artery, the first rib, and the recurrent laryngeal nerve.
48. What are some indications for a stellate ganglion block?
49. What are the clinical signs of a successful stellate ganglion block?
50. What are some minor and major complications of a stellate ganglion block?
51. From which spinal levels do the greater, lesser, and least splanchnic nerves arise?
52. Which abdominal organs will not receive analgesia from a celiac plexus block?
53. What are some indications for a celiac plexus block?
54. What is the efficacy, and what are some expected side effects of a celiac plexus block?
55. What are some complications of a celiac plexus block? Contrast the clinical manifestations of inadvertent intravascular injection of ethanol and phenol following a celiac plexus block.
56. From which spinal nerves do the lumbar sympathetic nerves arise?
57. What are some indications for a lumbar sympathetic block?

58. What are some complications of a lumbar sympathetic block?
59. What are some indications for spinal cord stimulator therapy?
60. What are some indications for intrathecal drug delivery therapy in managing chronic pain syndromes?

ANSWERS*

CLASSIFICATION OF CHRONIC PAIN

1. Nociceptive pain is pain following injury or damage to tissue and occurs during the course of ongoing tissue injury or before healing is complete. Nociceptive pain is pain that is sensed by peripheral nociceptors and transmitted by ascending fibers first to the spinal cord, then to the thalamus, and ultimately to the cerebral cortex. Examples of nociceptive pain include osteoarthritis, a broken bone, a cut, or postsurgical pain. (770)

2. Neuropathic pain is pain that appears following injury or dysfunction to the nervous system and persists despite what appears to be complete healing of the initial tissue injury. Neuropathic pain may be caused by a lesion of either the central nervous system (CNS), such as poststroke pain or spinal cord injury pain, or a lesion of the peripheral nervous system. The three most common types of neuropathic pain include postherpetic neuralgia (PHN), diabetic peripheral neuropathy (DPN), and complex regional pain syndrome (CRPS). These are all examples of peripheral neuropathic pain. (770)

MULTIDISCIPLINARY PAIN MANAGEMENT

3. Chronic pain is a complex disorder, and patients usually have biological disease that coexists with cognitive, affective, behavioral, and social factors. The effective management of such a disease process requires the expertise of health care providers from a range of medical specialties. The teams practicing at comprehensive pain management centers consist of a pain physician, who is often an anesthesiologist, a psychologist, and a physical therapist working together. Although a crucial component of the patient's care, the primary care physician is usually not a direct member of the chronic pain management team. (771)

4. The chronic pain physician in multidisciplinary pain management is tasked with coordinating the evaluation, diagnosis, and treatment of patients through appropriate interventions, such as procedures and medications. The chronic pain physician should maintain good communication with the patient's primary care physician regarding the plan of care and overall progress. (771)

5. The psychologist in multidisciplinary pain management incorporates patient education, cognitive behavioral therapy, and relaxation training. (771)

6. The physical therapist in multidisciplinary pain management plans various exercise regiments to optimize the patient's overall function. (771)

COMMON PAIN SYNDROMES

7. Low back pain (LBP) refers to pain in the region of the spine from the T12 vertebrae to the sacrococcygeal joint. LBP is among the most common forms of pain seen in both primary care clinics and outpatient pain clinics. Most patients who present with acute LBP recover with no treatment or conservative measures alone. The majority of patients recover by 6 weeks (60% to 70%), and nearly all subjects have recovered by 12 weeks (90%). Although somewhat arbitrary, LBP persisting for more than 12 weeks is usually classified as "chronic LBP" rather than "acute LBP." Once LBP is chronic (persisted for more than 12 weeks after initial onset), the recovery is slow and variable, with decreasing potential for recovery as the course prolongs. (772)

---

*Numbers in parentheses refer to pages, figures, boxes, or tables in Pardo MC, Miller RD, eds. *Basics of Anesthesia.* 7th ed. Philadelphia: Elsevier; 2018.

8. In general, the longer that a patient has not been working as the result of LBP, the lower the chances of achieving a meaningful recovery (as measured by the capacity to return to the same job) in spite of appropriate therapy. Although published estimates vary and are highly dependent on a number of factors, patients who are out of work for 6 months have a less than 50% chance of returning to work. Patients out of work for 2 years or more have a probability that approaches zero of ever returning to work. (771)

9. A number of risk factors have been identified from epidemiologic studies to be associated with the development of chronic LBP. They include age, gender, socioeconomic status, education level, presence of certain psychological or personality disorders, obesity, tobacco use, perceived general health status, repetitive physical activity (e.g., bending, lifting, twisting), jobs that require heavy lifting or use of heavy equipment, job dissatisfaction, depression, spinal anatomic variations and deformities, and imaging abnormalities. (771-772)

10. Radiculopathy is an objective neurologic deficit, such as weakness, numbness, or loss of deep tendon reflexes, that results from a cascade of pathologic events resulting in the blockade of transmission at the level of the spinal nerve. The loss of neural conduction may result from physical compression by an adjacent intervertebral disk fragment, osteophyte, or rarely, a neoplasm. Other causes include inflammatory, vascular, or neurodegenerative changes affecting one or more spinal nerves. (772)

11. Internal disk disruption (IDD) occurs when dehydration causes the hydrolytic pressure exerted by the nucleus pulposus to gradually overcome the counteracting tensile strength of the annulus fibrosis. This results in a degradation of the annulus fibrosus, starting with the innermost layers. Histologically, this degradation is described as annular fissures. The chronic stress applied to disks results in the ingrowth and sensitization of nociceptive pain fibers into the annulus fibrosus, which can then lead to the development of vague and poorly localized pain in the low back. With repeated chronic stress, an annular fissure can extend beyond the peripheral-most extent of the annulus, and inflammatory disk material can come into close proximity to spinal nerves, causing nerve irritation and pain (termed *herniated nucleus pulposus*, or, more commonly, a ruptured disk). Structural changes may also be observed, such as spinal nerve compression by a herniated disk or bone hypertrophy and sclerosis from adjacent vertebral bodies. It should be noted that nonpainful disk herniations are frequently observed and can spontaneously regress with time. (772)

12. The high prevalence of the development and rapid resolution of LBP, and the infrequency of a serious underlying disease of the spine, such as a malignancy, infection, or unstable fractures, obviate the need to obtain diagnostic imaging in most new cases. However, several "red flag" findings noted during a routine history and physical examination should prompt immediate diagnostic imaging. These signs include age less than 20 or greater than 50, history of trauma including minor falls in the elderly population, history of a serious systemic illness such as cancer, intravenous drug use, immunosuppression, organ transplantation, and long-term corticosteroid use. Pain that occurs at rest, keeps patients awake through the night, and does not respond to analgesics should raise a suspicion for nonbenign pain. Cauda equina compression, including the classic triad of saddle anesthesia, subjective bilateral lower extremity pain with objective weakness/gait disturbances, and decreased anal sphincter tone, usually with overflow urinary and bowel incontinence, is also concerning. Loss of Achilles reflexes may be observed and may be due to compression of the S1 nerve root. (772)

13. Radiculopathy is an objective physical examination finding of dysfunction including weakness, numbness, or loss of deep tendon reflexes originating from decreased neural transmission of a specific spinal nerve. (772)

14. Radicular pain refers to pain occurring in a dermatomal distribution and arising from the ectopic discharge of painful impulses in ascending pain fibers. The pain usually occurs in band-like patterns, which typically follow the distribution of a single dermatome. Radicular pain does not always occur with radiculopathy. (772)

15. Chronic radicular pain is a persistent, neuropathic pain that follows the distribution of one or more spinal nerves. There is a lack of consensus on how to treat chronic radicular pain. First-line medications for the management of chronic radicular pain include medicines used in the treatment of nerve injuries, such as gabapentin, pregabalin, tricyclic antidepressants (TCAs), and serotonin-norepinephrine reuptake inhibitors (SNRIs). Neuropathic pain medications often require several weeks of dosing prior to observing effects. (772)

16. Potential causes of acute lumbosacral pain include traumatic sprain of the lumbar spine or joint muscles and ligaments, or early IDD. (773)

17. Patients with acute lumbosacral pain without radicular symptoms and no obvious abnormal physical findings are unlikely to benefit from radiologic studies. These patients are best managed symptomatically. (773)

18. The lumbar intervertebral disks, lumbar facet joints, and sacroiliac joints are the anatomic structures most commonly associated with chronic lumbosacral pain. In chronic LBP the incidence of IDD is estimated to be 29% to 49%. The lumbar facet and sacroiliac joints each account for about 15% of chronic LBP. (773)

19. Patients with lumbar facet joint sacroiliac joint pain can be diagnosed with diagnostic local anesthetic blocks, although the placebo effect can complicate results. If relief is achieved with the block, radiofrequency treatment can provide pain reduction for 3 to 6 months. Degenerating intervertebral disks can be treated with spinal cord stimulators or with implanted epidural electrodes when medical and surgical therapies have failed. (774)

20. Neuropathic pain is thought to arise when the sensitization of peripheral and central nervous systems (that provide protection during the healing process) persists after injured tissues have healed. (774)

21. Characteristics of neuropathic pain include spontaneous pain that occurs without stimulus, hyperalgesia, and allodynia. Hyperalgesia is an exaggerated response of pain to a stimulus that is normally only very mildly uncomfortable (e.g., severe pain caused by a pinprick). Allodynia is an abnormal response of pain to a stimulus that is usually not painful, such as brushing or light touch. (774)

22. DPN most often presents as lower extremity sensory disturbances including numbness, paresthesias, dysesthesias, and allodynia. The symptoms will gradually affect more proximal areas of the lower extremities and eventually involve the distal upper extremities. A loss of sensation and proprioception may predispose patients to the development of poorly healing foot ulcers and diabetic arthropathies (Charcot joints), which may present as a unilateral pain. (774)

23. The incidence, severity, and rate of progression of the symptoms of DPN are closely related to a patient's ability to maintain a normal blood sugar level. (774)

24. Sympathetically maintained pain is a subset of neuropathic pain in which sympathetic stimulation augments chronic pain and loss of function. Blockade of the sympathetic nervous system transmission may reduce chronic pain development. Examples of sympathetically mediated pain include PHN, chronic regional pain syndrome, and stump neuroma in amputees. (774)

25. Acute herpes zoster secondary infections (shingles) in aging immune systems or immunosuppressed patients manifests as a painful vesicular rash that is typically limited to a dermatomal distribution over the thorax or face. PHN is pain that persists after the onset of a vesicular rash and continues after the resolution of cutaneous symptoms. The pain associated with PHN is characterized as episodic lancinating pain with severe allodynia in the affected dermatome. (774)

26. The dermatomal distribution of the rash seen in herpes zoster and the subsequent development of PHN pain in the same distribution may be attributed to the varicella-zoster virus (VZV) life cycle. Following initial infection and the

development of a diffuse rash, commonly called *chickenpox*, the virus goes dormant in the sensory dorsal root ganglia. With aging or other causes of senescence of the immune system, reactivation is believed to cause damage to small unmyelinated C fibers within an affected dermatome. Central and peripheral neural sensitization may also occur. (774)

27. Antiviral therapy, including acyclovir, famciclovir, and valacyclovir, has been demonstrated to decrease the amount of time for the acute herpes zoster vesicular rash to heal, in addition to decreasing the severity and duration of acute pain. The early initiation of antiviral therapy for the treatment of zoster is associated with a decreased progression to PHN. However, about 20% of patients still progress to develop PHN, which is difficult to treat. (774)

28. CRPS is persistent neuropathic pain that develops within 4 to 6 weeks following a trauma to an extremity. The pain is disproportionate to any inciting event and may involve sensory, vasomotor, edema or sudomotor, and motor or trophic abnormalities. (774)

29. Some signs and symptoms of CRPS include neuropathic pain, asymmetric temperature or skin color changes, edema or sweating changes, decreased range of motion, weakness, tremor, dystonia, or trophic changes in the hair, nails, or skin. Type 1 CRPS is differentiated from type 2 CRPS depending on the identification of an inciting nerve injury. CRPS type 1, formerly known as reflex sympathetic dystrophy, may develop following minor injury or without obvious nerve damage. CRPS type 2, formerly known as causalgia, develops following identified nerve injury. Examples of CRPS type 2 injuries may range from major trauma to relatively minor events, such as venipuncture. (774-775)

30. The primary goal in the management of CRPS patients is to facilitate functional restoration through physical and occupational therapy. The complete elimination of pain is often not possible. However, reductions in pain are possible, such that the patient can regain basic function of the affected area and have improved well-being. Medications have not been shown to have any efficacy except to manage the neuropathic pain. Sympathetic blocks, such as stellate ganglion block and lumbar sympathetic block, have demonstrated analgesia lasting for 3 to 5 days—well beyond the expected pharmacologic half-life of local anesthetics but not long term. The brief reprieve in symptoms may allow the patient to more fully participate in physical therapy or a functional restoration program. Spinal cord stimulation for the treatment of CRPS has been shown to provide long-term benefits of reduced pain, facilitation of physical and occupational therapy, and restoration of function. Optimal management of these patients is best achieved with a multidisciplinary team of providers. (775)

31. Myofascial pain syndrome is acute, recurrent, or chronic regional musculoskeletal pain characterized by exquisite tenderness and hyperirritability in muscles or fascia. Trigger point injections and physical therapy are often used to manage the symptoms. (775)

32. Fibromyalgia is defined by widespread, chronic (more than 3 months) musculoskeletal pain accompanied by symptoms such as fatigue, waking unrefreshed, and cognitive dysfunction. It affects up to 2% of the U.S. population, women more than men. Fibromyalgia can occur in patients with rheumatic diseases, such as rheumatoid arthritis, systemic lupus erythematosus, and ankylosing spondylitis. Management emphasizes promotion of physical activity through nonpharmacologic means. Medications that can be used to treat fibromyalgia include a TCA, SNRIs, and tramadol. (775)

33. Patients with cancer commonly experience chronic pain, especially if untreated or unresponsive to treatment. The nature of the pain may be somatic, neuropathic, visceral, ischemic, or mixed. Pain may arise directly from the tumor through spread into visceral, osseous, or neural structures. Pain may also be the result of treatment of the cancer such as chemotherapy-induced painful neuropathies, radiation-induced plexopathies or neuropathies, or postoperative surgical pain. (776)

34. The World Health Organization (WHO)'s pain ladder is a simple algorithm devised by the WHO in 1986 for the treatment of cancer pain. The ladder is simple to use, provides adequate analgesia in 70% to 90% of patients, and provides a rational basis for the use of strong opioids in cancer patients with ongoing pain. The three-step ladder starts with the use of a nonopioid with or without an adjuvant (an agent aimed at treatment of neuropathic pain symptoms) and progresses to include a weak opioid in step 2 and a strong opioid in step 3. Treatment progresses up the ladder until adequate pain relief is achieved. (776)

35. Examples of medications on the "first step" of the WHO pain ladder include nonsteroidal anti-inflammatory drugs (NSAIDs), acetaminophen, and adjuvant analgesics including gabapentin, TCAs, lidocaine, calcitonin, bisphosphonates, and SNRIs. Examples of medications on the "second step" of the WHO pain ladder include codeine, hydrocodone, and tramadol. Examples of medications on the "third step" of the WHO pain ladder include oxycodone, hydromorphone, transdermal fentanyl, and methadone. (776)

PHARMACOLOGIC MANAGEMENT OF CHRONIC PAIN

36. Clinical uses for acetaminophen and NSAIDs include the treatment of mild to moderate pain including headache and acute muscle strain and sprain. NSAIDs may be helpful for the long-term management of pain and stiffness associated with osteoarthritis and chronic LBP. These analgesics are also used as the initial drug to treat mild or moderate cancer pain or as an adjunct with other medicines. (776)

37. Antidepressants used for the first-line management of neuropathic pain include TCAs and SNRIs. TCA doses are less than those used for depression. Side effects of TCAs that may limit their use in the management of chronic pain are due to their anticholinergic and antihistaminic side effects. Some of the commonly reported side effects include sedation, orthostatic hypotension, dry mouth, constipation, blurred vision, cutaneous flushing, urinary retention, and confusion or delirium. TCAs can also worsen preexisting heart block. (776)

38. Anticonvulsants are effective for the first-line treatment of neuropathic pain. Although generally well tolerated, some common side effects include dizziness, somnolence, and peripheral edema. (776)

39. The use of opioids in acute pain conditions allows for greater functionality during recovery and rapid resolution of acute pain states. However, the long-term use of opioids for the management of chronic noncancer pain presents a dilemma for the pain physician. Opponents of such therapy point to a lack of scientific evidence supporting their long-term use and high risks for physiologic side effects such as tolerance, constipation, sedation, opioid-induced hyperalgesia, and psychological side effects such as cognitive dysfunction, misuse, abuse, and addiction. There is also an increased risk of overdose-related morbidity and mortality associated with long-term opioid therapy. Organizations have released guidelines recommending against the long-term use of opioids for noncancer pain, including the 2016 Centers for Disease Control and Prevention Guidelines and the 2014 American Academy of Neurology Position Paper. Advocates of chronic opioid use point to a prolonged history of patient-reported benefit with chronic opioids and a lack of any clear alternatives. (777)

40. Opioid abuse and misuse are among the most feared complications of chronic opioid therapy. Tools (e.g., the Screener and Opioid Assessment for Patients with Pain) can be used by trained professionals to assess risk among candidates for opioid therapy. In addition, frequent and periodic urine or saliva toxicology screening, opioid therapy agreements, motivational counseling, and use of state or regional opioid prescription monitoring programs may also aid in risk reduction with long-term opioid use. (777)

41. The tapering of opioids may be initiated for a number of reasons such as therapeutic failure despite reasonable dose escalation, intolerance of side effects, persistent lack of adherence to a patient treatment agreement,

nonphysiologic side effects such as social or professional deterioration, or the resolution of the pain. Prior to discontinuation, physicians must consider the possibility that failure of opioid therapy is the result of underdosing, progression of the underlying condition, or another ongoing condition complicating the pain disorder, such as physiologic comorbid conditions. Opioid rotation rather than tapering may be considered in those with persistent or worsening pain. (778)

42. The use of cognitive behavioral therapy (CBT) in patients undergoing opioid taper has been demonstrated to provide patient support and to more thoroughly address potential underlying issues. Some of the more common reasons for CBT include treatment of anxiety regarding tapering off opioids after long-term use, the development of coping strategies for both anxiety and pain, and the treatment of any underlying conditions, such as depression. (778)

INTERVENTIONAL PAIN THERAPIES

43. "Interventional pain therapy" refers to a series of interventional procedures in which a nerve or other structure presumed to be responsible for the generation or conduction of painful signals is identified and targeted with local anesthetic, steroid, or controlled energy such as that achieved with radiofrequency treatment. Some of the more common interventional therapies performed on the spine include epidural steroid injections to treat radicular pain, sacroiliac joint injections to treat sacroiliitis, and facet joint injections and medial branch blocks to treat pain originating from the facet joints. A number of peripheral nerve and sympathetic blocks are frequently employed to treat chronic pain. Examples of interventions utilizing directed energy rather than pharmacologic therapy include medial branch radiofrequency ablation (RFA) to treat facet joint pain or the use of spinal cord stimulation to treat failed back surgery syndrome or CRPS. (778)

44. Epidural steroid injections are among the most frequently performed interventional pain procedures and are used to treat lumbar and sacral radicular pain. The exact mechanism of action is poorly defined but may be related to the anti-inflammatory properties of steroids on localized irritated or injured spine nerves, such as from a herniated disk. The rationale for epidural, rather than systemic, use of steroids is to target a particular pain generator while avoiding systemic side effects of steroids. (779)

45. Epidural steroids are most effective if administered between 3 and 6 weeks of the onset of radicular pain and have been demonstrated to reduce the severity and duration of leg pain. Beyond 3 months from treatment there is no long-term reduction in pain or improvement of function. Epidural steroid injections are not helpful for lumbosacral pain without radicular symptoms. (779)

46. The facet joints are true synovial joints with the potential to develop arthritis, and pain from these joints affects up to 15% of patients with chronic LBP. A diagnostic block of the sensory nerve at the same spinal level with local anesthetic is used to identify the facet joint generating pain. If the test block produces pain relief, RFA of the sensory nerve at the identified levels is applied. Radiofrequency energy can result in the disruption of neural transmission, and hence pain, for approximately 6 to 12 months. (779)

47. The stellate ganglion is formed by the fusion of the inferior cervical and first thoracic sympathetic ganglia. The ganglion is located anterior to the longus colli muscle, anterior to the neck of the first rib and transverse process of the seventh cervical vertebrae. It is posterior and superior to the first branch of the subclavian artery and posterior to the dome of the lung, carotid artery, and jugular vein. The most common approach to the stellate ganglion is at the level of C6, using the anterior paratracheal approach. (780)

48. The stellate ganglion conducts all sympathetic fibers from the head, neck, and upper extremities. Some indications for a stellate ganglion block include to manage the sympathetically mediated pain of CRPS of the upper extremity, neuropathic pain syndromes, shingles, early PHN, postradiation neuritis,

Raynaud disease, frostbite, vasospasm, occlusive and embolic vascular disease, and hyperhidrosis. (782)

49. Signs of a successful stellate ganglion block include the traditional triad of miosis, ptosis, and anhydrosis. Additional findings may include enophthalmos, nasal congestion, venodilation in the hand and forearm, and an increase in temperature of the blocked limb by at least 1° C. These are expected outcomes of the block and are not considered adverse effects. (782)

50. Minor complications of a stellate ganglion block include blockade of the recurrent laryngeal nerve through the diffusion of local anesthetic, phrenic nerve block leading to unilateral diaphragmatic paresis, and somatic block of the upper extremity, which can be a small localized area or complete brachial plexus block. Major complications associated with a stellate ganglion block include a neuraxial block and seizures. A neuraxial block can lead to a high spinal or epidural block with loss of consciousness and apnea. Because a high epidural block may not maximally manifest for 15 to 20 minutes following the injection of local anesthetic, patients should be monitored for at least 30 minutes following the procedure. Intravascular injection of local anesthetic into the adjacent vertebral or carotid artery can result in immediate generalized seizures. Seizures are usually brief and don't require treatment. (782)

51. Nociceptive information from the abdominal viscera is transmitted via the sympathetic fibers anterior to the fifth through twelfth thoracic vertebral bodies. These nerves travel to the celiac ganglia as the greater splanchnic nerve originating from T5 to T9, the lesser splanchnic nerve originating from T10 to T11, and the least splanchnic nerve originating from T12. The celiac ganglia are located anterior to the aorta and surround the superior mesenteric and celiac arteries at the level of T12-L1. (783)

52. The pelvic viscera, descending colon, sigmoid colon, and rectum are innervated by the hypogastric plexus rather than the celiac plexus (the viscera distal to the splenic flexure of the colon). All other abdominal organs are innervated through the celiac plexus. (783)

53. A celiac plexus or splanchnic nerve block can be used to control pain from the pancreas, liver, gallbladder, omentum, mesentery, and alimentary tract from the stomach to the transverse colon. Neurolysis of celiac plexus or splanchnic nerves can provide dramatic improvement to patients with pancreatic cancer or other intra-abdominal malignancies. (783)

54. Neurolytic celiac plexus block can provide long-lasting benefit for 70% to 90% of patients with pancreatic cancer or other intra-abdominal malignancies. Two physiologic side effects of a neurolytic celiac plexus block include diarrhea accompanied by abdominal cramping and orthostatic hypotension through the effects of unopposed parasympathetic nervous system activity. (783)

55. Complications of a celiac plexus block include hematuria, intravascular injection, and pneumothorax. Ethanol and phenol are commonly injected into the area of the celiac plexus in the setting of painful malignancies in order to produce long-lasting pain relief and improved quality of life through the chemical destruction of nerves. Large systemic doses of phenol will cause a constellation of symptoms similar to local anesthetic systemic toxicity, including CNS excitation, generalized seizures, and cardiovascular collapse. Ethanol is utilized in a highly concentrated form, and the intravascular injection of ethanol will produce intoxication above the legal limit but below the danger level for severe alcohol toxicity. The consequences of this intoxication may be magnified by the use of sedation during a celiac plexus block procedure. A rare but devastating complication of celiac plexus neurolysis with either phenol or ethanol is paraplegia. (784)

56. The cell bodies from T11 to L2, with variable contributions from T10 and L3, travel to the lumbar sympathetic ganglia that lie over the anterolateral surface of the L2 through L4 vertebrae. (784-785)

57. The most common indications for a lumbar sympathetic block is CRPS type 1 and 2 of the lower extremity. Other indications include peripheral vascular insufficiency due to small vessel occlusion, which can improve microvascular circulation and reduce accompanying ischemic pain. Variable success has been seen in patients with neuropathic pain, shingles, and early PHN. (785)

58. Some complications of a lumbar sympathetic block include intravascular injection, hematuria (as a result of direct needle placement in the kidney), and nerve root, epidural, or intrathecal injection (minimized with radiographic guidance). Following a neurolytic lumbar sympathetic block, as many as 10% of patients can have postsympathectomy pain arising from the L1 and L2 nerve root distribution over the anterior thigh. (786)

59. Spinal cord stimulator therapy has become widely utilized for the treatment of conditions including CRPS, failed back surgery syndrome with a neuropathic component, and unilateral radiculopathy. The indications for spinal cord stimulation therapy continue to expand while existing indications become more refined with the development of new technology. (786)

60. Intrathecal drug delivery therapy is typically reserved for patients with or without cancer with severe pain that doesn't respond to conservative management, or who have had escalation of oral analgesics for many years. Intrathecal drug delivery therapy has shown improvement in analgesia and a reduction of opioid-related side effects, such as somnolence and fatigue, in patients with cancer-related pain. (786)

45 CARDIOPULMONARY RESUSCITATION

Krishna Parekh and David Shimabukuro

INTRODUCTION

1. Who developed the guidelines for cardiopulmonary resuscitation (CPR) and emergency cardiovascular care (ECC)?

BASIC LIFE SUPPORT

2. What are the four major components of Basic Life Support (BLS)?
3. According to the American Heart Association (AHA) algorithm, what is the sequence of steps a health care provider should take after recognizing an unresponsive patient in the health care setting?
4. What are some differences between laypersons and health care providers in the sequence of events for recognition and management of an unresponsive patient?
5. What is proper rescuer positioning and hand placement for maximal effectiveness of cardiac compressions in the adult patient?
6. By how much is the sternum of an adult patient depressed during each cardiac compression?
7. What is the recommended rate of chest compressions for adult CPR? What is the ratio of cardiac compressions to ventilation during one-rescuer or two-rescuer CPR?
8. What is the head tilt–chin lift maneuver? How can it be modified in a patient with a possible neck injury?
9. What are the current recommendations regarding ventilation during CPR?
10. What have out-of-hospital studies shown comparing CPR involving compression-ventilation versus CPR with compression only?
11. How are health care providers expected to manage ventilation during CPR in the health care setting?
12. Where on the chest is the appropriate placement of defibrillator pads?
13. How many joules (J) of electricity should be delivered during an attempt at external defibrillation?
14. What is the definitive treatment for ventricular fibrillation (VF) and ventricular tachycardia (VT)?
15. What is the most important determinant of return of spontaneous circulation in a patient with VF/VT when performing external defibrillation?
16. What are the recommendations regarding the routine use of extracorporeal CPR (venoarterial extracorporeal membrane oxygenation) for patients in cardiac arrest?

ADULT ADVANCED CARDIOVASCULAR LIFE SUPPORT

17. What are some physiologic variables that can be used to monitor CPR?
18. What are the recommendations for the technique and timing of airway management in patients in cardiac arrest?

19. What are some methods by which to confirm advanced airway placement in patients in cardiac arrest?
20. What are the advantages of a cuffed endotracheal tube for ventilation of the lungs in a patient receiving CPR?
21. What are some possible causes of VF/VT?
22. What is the appropriate treatment for VF/VT?
23. What is torsades de pointes? What are some causes of torsades de pointes?
24. What is the treatment for torsades de pointes?
25. What is pulseless electrical activity (PEA)? What are some causes of PEA?
26. What is the appropriate treatment for PEA and asystole?
27. What is the goal of initial drug therapy during CPR? What are the mainstays of treatment for the patient in cardiac arrest?
28. What actions of epinephrine are thought to be responsible for its beneficial effects during cardiac arrest?
29. What is the dose of amiodarone administered during cardiac arrest?
30. What is the advantage of the delivery of drugs by a centrally placed intravenous catheter during CPR?
31. How long should the rescuers wait for drug administered via a peripheral vein to reach the central circulation?
32. What are two alternatives for drug delivery when vascular access is not available?

PEDIATRIC ADVANCED CARDIOVASCULAR LIFE SUPPORT

33. How does the algorithm for CPR compare between children and adults?
34. How should cardiac compressions be performed in infants?
35. How should cardiac compressions be performed in children?
36. Which artery should be used to palpate the pulse in infants up to 1 year of age?
37. Which artery should be used to palpate the pulse in children older than 1 year of age?
38. How many joules should be delivered for external defibrillation in pediatric patients?
39. Can standard adult automated external defibrillators (AEDs) and external defibrillators be used in pediatric patients?
40. What is the role of extracorporeal membrane oxygenation in pediatric cardiac arrest patients?

POSTRESUSCITATION CARE

41. How should a cardiac arrest patient be managed after the return of spontaneous circulation?
42. What is the goal for hemodynamic management in postresuscitation care?
43. What is the goal for oxygenation and ventilation management in postresuscitation care?
44. What is the goal for temperature management in postresuscitation care?
45. What is the goal for serum glucose management in postresuscitation care?

SPECIAL PERIOPERATIVE CONSIDERATIONS

46. What has the American Society of Anesthesiologists (ASA) published regarding the common causes of perioperative cardiac arrest in each of the following categories: medication, respiratory, and cardiovascular?
47. What has the ASA published regarding the initial steps of resuscitation for intraoperative cardiac arrest?
48. What are some drugs used in the operating room that can precipitate an anaphylactic reaction?
49. What is the treatment for intraoperative anaphylaxis?
50. What is the treatment for an intraoperative gas embolism?
51. What is the treatment for local anesthetic toxicity?
52. How should cardiovascular collapse in a patient who has received neuraxial anesthesia be managed?

ANSWERS*

INTRODUCTION

1. The American Heart Association (AHA), in conjunction with the International Liaison Committee on Resuscitation, published updated guidelines in 2015 for cardiopulmonary resuscitation (CPR) and emergency cardiovascular care (ECC) based on evidence from the medical and basic science literature. This multinational committee will continuously evaluate new evidence and publish revised guidelines at ECCguidelines.heart.org, rather than give periodic updates as they had in the past. (788)

BASIC LIFE SUPPORT

2. The four major components of Basic Life Support (BLS) are the recognition of an unresponsive patient and cardiac arrest, activation of an emergency medical system, early administration of CPR, and early defibrillation if indicated. (788–789)

3. According to the AHA algorithm, after recognizing an unresponsive patient in the health care setting a health care provider should ensure safety, check for response, activate the resuscitation team, check for adequate breathing and pulse, retrieve an automated external defibrillator (AED) and emergency equipment, begin CPR and defibrillate when available, and provide two-person CPR as help arrives. (789)

4. The AHA guidelines allow for a larger role for dispatcher-guided CPR for laypersons. In contrast, health care providers have more flexibility for when to activate the resuscitation, either before or after assessment of breathing and pulse. Health care providers should check for a pulse while simultaneously evaluating for adequate ventilation. The pulse is assessed at either the carotid or femoral artery. The elapsed time for the pulse check should not exceed 10 seconds, in order to minimize the time to start chest compressions. (790)

5. For cardiac compressions in the adult patient, the heels of the rescuer's hands should be placed on the lower half of the patient's sternum, between the nipples. This provides for maximum compression to the underlying cardiac ventricles and optimizes blood flow produced by the compressions. If the rescuer's hands are placed incorrectly during cardiac compressions, not only is blood flow not optimized, but the patient may suffer from internal injury as well. During cardiac compressions, the rescuer's upper body should be directly over the patient's chest. The shoulders are positioned directly over the hands, and the elbows are kept straight. This position enables the rescuer to use the weight of his or her upper body for compression and may prevent fatigue. (790)

6. The sternum of an adult patient should be depressed at least 5 cm, but no more than 6 cm, during cardiac compression. Excessive compression depth has been associated with an increased rate of thoracic injury. (790)

7. The recommended rate for chest compressions for adult CPR is 100 to 120 compressions per minute. The rescuer needs to push hard and push fast but allow for full chest recoil. Rates higher than 120 have been associated with inadequate compression depth. The ratio of cardiac compressions to ventilation during CPR is 30 compressions to 2 breaths, regardless of the number of rescuers. (790)

8. Upper airway obstruction in an unconscious patient can be due to the tongue falling against the posterior pharynx. The head tilt–chin lift maneuver involves extension of the head and displacement of the mandible to an anterior position, thereby moving the tongue forward away from the posterior pharynx. For many individuals, this is adequate to provide a patent airway. For patients with suspected neck trauma, the rescuer needs to modify the head tilt–chin lift maneuver to avoid exacerbating a potential spinal cord injury. The head tilt

---

*Numbers in parentheses refer to pages, figures, boxes, or tables in Pardo MC, Miller RD, eds. *Basics of Anesthesia.* 7th ed. Philadelphia: Elsevier; 2018.

should be excluded from the maneuver and only the chin lift performed in these patients. (790)

9. Since 2010, chest compressions are the priority over ventilation in an effort to increase the likelihood of a return of spontaneous circulation. Airway maneuvers can still be attempted, but they should be done quickly to minimize any interruptions in chest compressions. (790)

10. Several large out-of-hospital studies have shown that CPR involving compression-ventilation has similar outcomes to CPR with compression only. (790)

11. Health care providers are expected to provide assisted ventilation during CPR in the health care setting. Excessive positive-pressure ventilation should be avoided to allow for adequate preload and cardiac output. When possible, an advanced airway should be established in patients during in-hospital cardiac arrest. Tidal volumes of 400 to 600 mL should be given over 1 second at a rate of 10 breaths per minute. (790)

12. The defibrillator pads should be applied to the chest with firm pressure ensuring good skin contact in a position that will maximize the flow of electrical current through the myocardium. The standard placement is with one pad below the right clavicle and to the right of the upper sternum and the second pad at the level of the apex of the heart in the midaxillary line. (790)

13. The amount of joules (J) delivered for external defibrillation depends on whether the defibrillator is monophasic (360 J) or biphasic (120 to 200 J). Biphasic defibrillators are thought to be more successful at terminating ventricular fibrillation (VF) and ventricular tachycardia (VT) and require less energy and may therefore cause less myocardial damage. (790)

14. The definitive treatment for VF/VT is external defibrillation. (791)

15. The most important determinant of the success of external defibrillation in VF/VT is the duration of the time lapse between cardiopulmonary arrest and external defibrillation. For this reason, the current recommendation is to apply external defibrillation as soon as possible in these patients. Delayed defibrillation results in slower rates of return of spontaneous circulation and survival to hospital discharge, with worse outcomes associated with each minute of delay. (791)

16. Although there may be some benefit of extracorporeal CPR (venoarterial extracorporeal membrane oxygenation) in selected patients with witnessed and reversible causes of cardiac arrest, there is not enough evidence to recommend its routine use in patients in cardiac arrest. (791)

ADULT ADVANCED CARDIOVASCULAR LIFE SUPPORT

17. Continuous monitoring of end-tidal carbon dioxide ($ETco_2$) with waveform capnography can be beneficial during resuscitation as confirmation of advanced airway placement and also as a guide for the adequacy of chest compressions. Alternative physiologic measures include arterial pressure monitoring, central venous oxygen saturation, and bedside cardiac ultrasound by an experienced sonographer with minimal interruptions in CPR. (791)

18. The 2015 AHA guidelines recommend either a bag-mask ventilation device or advanced airway (endotracheal tube or supraglottic airway) for providing oxygenation and ventilation during CPR. The choice of technique for ventilation and airway management depends on the skill of the provider and the patient's clinical course. There are no formal recommendations for the timing or type of airway management. For placement of an advanced airway chest compressions should not be interrupted for longer than 10 seconds and should be resumed immediately following securing the airway. (791)

19. Methods by which to confirm advanced airway placement in patients in cardiac arrest include continuous waveform capnography (recommended), auscultation of bilateral breath sounds, visualization of bilateral chest rise, an esophageal detection device, nonwaveform capnogram, and ultrasound. (792)

20. Advantages of a cuffed endotracheal tube for ventilation of the lungs in a patient receiving CPR include the reliable administration of supplemental oxygen, compressions and ventilations are no longer necessarily synchronous and compressions can be performed without interruption, assurance of proper ventilation and ET_{CO_2} monitoring, and protection against the aspiration of gastric contents. (792)

21. Possible causes of VF/VT include hypovolemia, hypoxia, hydrogen ion excess (acidosis), hypokalemia/hyperkalemia, hypothermia, tension pneumothorax, cardiac tamponade, toxins, thrombosis (pulmonary and coronary). (792)

22. Patients in VF/VT should receive immediate defibrillation of 120 to 200 J with a biphasic defibrillator. Good quality CPR should also be instituted and maintained throughout the resuscitation. Epinephrine 1 mg intravenously may be administered every 3 to 5 minutes if VF or VT persists after one to two sets of CPR-defibrillation cycles. Amiodarone, an antiarrhythmic, can be considered for persistent VF/VT as well. (793)

23. Torsades de pointes is an atypical form of VT with a characteristic twisting of the QRS complex around the baseline such that it appears as a sine wave. Causes of torsades de pointes include drugs that prolong the QT interval, such as quinidine, procainamide, disopyramide, phenothiazines, and tricyclic antidepressants; other causes include bradycardia, hypokalemia, hypomagnesemia, and acute myocardial ischemia or infarction. (793)

24. The treatment for torsades de pointes may include overdrive pacing of the cardiac atria or ventricles and treatment with magnesium sulfate for stable patients. A patient whose condition is unstable should undergo defibrillation. (793)

25. Pulseless electrical activity (PEA) is a term used to describe the presence of a cardiac rhythm on the electrocardiogram (ECG) with little or no cardiac output. In patients with PEA there is an absence of peripheral pulses or systemic blood pressure. Cardiac rhythms that may be present include organized electrical activity, idioventricular rhythms, and ventricular escape rhythms. Causes of PEA are identical to those of VF and VT. (793)

26. PEA and asystole are managed similarly. Both are treated with effective CPR with minimal interruptions, identifying and treating reversible causes, the administration of epinephrine, and establishment of an advanced airway. Defibrillation provides no benefit for patients in PEA or asystole. The cardiac rhythm should be checked after every 5 cycles or 2 minutes of CPR, and if a pulse is present the rescuer should identify the rhythm and treat accordingly. (795)

27. The goal of initial drug therapy during CPR is the increasing of coronary and cerebral perfusion pressures. The mainstay for treatment of the patient in cardiopulmonary arrest is the administration of oxygen and epinephrine. (796)

28. Epinephrine is a combined direct α- and β-adrenergic receptor agonist. Epinephrine has been shown to be beneficial in establishing the return of spontaneous circulation in multiple animal studies. Epinephrine also increases coronary perfusion pressure by increasing diastolic blood pressure. However, increases in heart rate and afterload increase myocardial oxygen consumption. (796)

29. Amiodarone, a class III antiarrhythmic, can be used in the treatment of VF/VT at an initial dose of 300 mg intravenously. If VF/VT persists, an additional bolus of 150 mg can be administered. (796)

30. The advantage of the administration of drugs by a centrally placed intravenous catheter during CPR is the rapid delivery of drugs to the heart. CPR should not be interrupted for placement of central venous access unless peripheral access and intraosseous access cannot be obtained. (796)

31. When a peripheral intravenous site is used for the administration of drugs during cardiopulmonary arrest, drug administration should always be followed by at least 20 mL of normal saline, and a period of 1 to 2 minutes should be allowed for drugs to reach the central circulation. (796)

32. Two alternatives for drug delivery when vascular access is not available include an endotracheal tube or the placement of an intraosseous line. Drugs that can be absorbed across the alveolar epithelium include epinephrine, lidocaine, atropine, and naloxone. The endotracheal tube dose is 2 to 10 times the recommended intravenous dose, and the drug should be diluted into 5 to 10 mL of sterile water before instillation down the endotracheal tube. The intraosseous line should be treated as any other peripheral or central intravenous line. (796)

PEDIATRIC ADVANCED CARDIOVASCULAR LIFE SUPPORT

33. The algorithm for CPR in pediatric patients is basically the same as that for adults, which is chest compressions are initiated before airway in breathing. One distinct difference is that, because most pediatric cardiac arrests are due to arterial hypoxemia, compressions and ventilation are recommended over compression-only resuscitation. The pattern should be 30 compressions to 2 breaths for single-rescuer and 15 compressions to 2 breaths for two-rescuer CPR. (796)

34. Hand placement during cardiac compressions in infants is with the rescuer's one hand to support the back while compressions are performed with two fingers of the other hand. Cardiac compression in the infant should be performed at a rate of 100 to 120 compressions per minute. The sternum of the infant patient during cardiac compressions should be depressed by at least one third of the anteroposterior diameter of the chest, or 4 cm. (797)

35. Cardiac compressions in children can be accomplished with the heel of one hand directly over the lower half of the sternum, between the nipples and above the xiphoid process. The recommended rate for cardiac compressions in children is the same as that for infants and adults, 100 to 120 compressions per minute. Depression of the sternum should also be one third to one half the anteroposterior diameter of the chest, or 5 cm. In infants up to 1 year of age, the brachial artery in the mid-upper arm or the femoral artery are best for pulse palpation. (797)

36. In infants up to 1 year of age, either the brachial artery in the mid-upper arm or the femoral artery is best for pulse palpation.

37. In children older than 1 year of age, the carotid artery and the femoral artery are the preferred arteries for pulse palpation. (797)

38. The number of joules delivered for external defibrillation in pediatric patients is directly related to the body weight. The recommended initial setting is 2 to 4 J/kg. If the initial attempt at defibrillation is unsuccessful, the subsequent attempt should be made with at least 4 J/kg but no more than 10 J/kg. (798)

39. Standard biphasic AEDs can be used in children older than 1 year outside the hospital setting. For inpatient external defibrillation, the AHA guidelines recommend the use of a pediatric dose attenuator system, if available. If this is not available, a standard external defibrillator can be used in pediatric patients. (798)

40. Extracorporeal membrane oxygenation can be considered in all pediatric cardiac arrest patients who have failed standard resuscitative therapies. (798)

POSTRESUSCITATION CARE

41. The management of the cardiac arrest patient after the return of spontaneous circulation should include transfer to the ICU for close monitoring and optimization of hemodynamics, oxygenation, and ventilation. In addition, correction of electrolyte and glucose derangements, neurologic evaluation, and temperature management should be instituted. A cardiac evaluation with ECG, echocardiogram, and serial cardiac enzymes should be obtained. Patients should be transferred for percutaneous coronary intervention or angiography as indicated. Prognosis is usually best delayed until at least 72 hours following return of spontaneous circulation and targeted temperature management. (798)

42. There is no specific goal for hemodynamic management in the postresuscitation phase. Hypotension should be treated as necessary with vasoactive drugs and fluids, with the target of arterial blood pressure as indicated by the clinical scenario. (798)

43. In the postresuscitation phase the goal for oxygen saturation is more than 94%. The goal for ventilation is normocapnia, with a target Pa_{CO_2} between 35 and 45

mm Hg. Hyperventilation is not recommended and may be harmful because of its effects on cerebral blood flow. (798)

44. Hyperthermia is known to worsen brain injury. The 2015 guidelines recommend that all comatose patients following cardiac arrest and return of spontaneous circulation be treated with targeted temperature management with a goal temperature between 32° C and 36° C. Patient factors should be taken into account when choosing the temperature, as therapeutic hypothermia can cause impaired coagulation and increased risk of infection at lower temperature levels. (799)

45. In the postresuscitation phase, both hypoglycemia and hyperglycemia should be avoided. Although tight serum glucose control has not been shown to improve neurologic outcome, hyperglycemia after resuscitation from cardiac arrest is associated with poor neurologic outcome. (799)

SPECIAL PERIOPERATIVE CONSIDERATIONS

46. The American Society of Anesthesiologists (ASA) has published the common causes of perioperative cardiac arrest. Medication-related causes include anesthetic overdose, high neuraxial blockade, local anesthetic toxicity, and drug administration errors. Respiratory-related causes include hypoxemia, auto-positive end-expiratory pressure, and acute bronchospasm. Cardiovascular-related causes include vasovagal shock, hypovolemic/hemorrhagic shock, distributive shock, obstructive shock, right ventricular failure, left ventricular failure, arrhythmia, and acute coronary syndrome. (800)

47. The ASA has published the following sequence of initial steps of resuscitation for intraoperative cardiac arrest: call for help, initiate chest compressions, discontinue anesthetic, discontinue surgery, retrieve emergency equipment, increase the fraction of inspired oxygen to 100%, manually ventilate the lungs, open all intravenous lines, and use capnography to assess CPR. (800)

48. Drugs used in the operating room that can precipitate an anaphylactic reaction include latex, β-lactam antibiotics, succinylcholine, all muscle relaxants, and intravenous contrast material. (800)

49. The main treatment for anaphylaxis is epinephrine. The causative drug should be discontinued or removed if possible. Epinephrine and vasopressin can be used to support the arterial blood pressure. Intravenous fluids may be necessary, and steroids and antihistamines are often administered. In the event of complete cardiovascular collapse, CPR and Advanced Cardiovascular Life Support (ACLS) should be started, and larger doses of epinephrine may be required. (800)

50. The treatment of an intraoperative gas embolism is to stop insufflation, occlude open veins, and flood the surgical field with saline. The patient should also be placed in a Trendelenburg position with the left side down. In the case of complete cardiovascular collapse, CPR and ACLS should be started. (800)

51. Local anesthetic toxicity is characterized by neurologic symptoms prior to cardiac manifestations, and if noted the local anesthetic should be immediately discontinued if possible. Cardiac manifestations can range from premature ventricular contractions to asystole. In the event of cardiovascular toxicity, intralipid should be administered. Prolonged resuscitation can result in good neurologic recovery in these patients. (800)

52. Cardiac arrest from neuraxial anesthesia should be managed with standard CPR and ACLS. (801)

46 OPERATING ROOM MANAGEMENT

Amr E. Abouleish

ANESTHESIOLOGY STAFFING	1. What are the major determinants of the number of anesthesia clinicians needed to staff clinical needs?
	2. Why is benchmarking or comparing productivity using per full-time equivalent (FTE) physician measurements not always meaningful?

OPERATING ROOM EFFICIENCY	3. Why is having an operating room (OR) with 100% efficiency not the most cost-effective goal?
	4. Which surgeon should be given more surgical block time: the surgeon with 60% utilization of current block time or the surgeon with 130% utilization of current block time?
	5. Will focusing on turnover time increase OR throughput?

ANSWERS*

ANESTHESIOLOGY STAFFING

1. For anyone who has to make daily assignments of anesthesia clinicians (physician anesthesiologists, resident anesthesiologists, nurse anesthetists, and anesthesiologist assistants), the answer is obvious and easy. The major determinants are the number of clinical sites that need to be staffed (especially at the beginning of the day) and the concurrency or staffing ratio of medical direction or supervision. Additional factors that impact the number of clinicians include any late-arriving clinicians (such as for late shifts or call) who are not available at the start of day to cover sites, number of postcall clinicians, and "support" clinicians (e.g., nurse anesthetist to help with breaks, resident for blocks or postanesthesia care unit coverage). To the dismay of administrators and accountants, what is not a determinant is the amount of work (cases, billed units, charges, etc.) scheduled at the site. (804)

2. As noted previously, the need to have a clinician is not based on the actual work that is to be done but rather on what sites need to be covered. Despite this, administrators and consultants want to measure clinical productivity just like other specialties. The most common measurements rely on "per physician" or "per FTE" (full-time equivalent). For anesthesiologists, nonanesthesia factors affect productivity "per FTE" measurements including the type of case, surgical duration, and utilization of the site covered. But the most confounding factor

---

*Numbers in parentheses refer to pages, figures, boxes, or tables in Pardo MC, Miller RD, eds. *Basics of Anesthesia*. 7th ed. Philadelphia: Elsevier; 2018.

is that staffing ratios vary within a group and from hospital to hospital. When an anesthesiologist medically directs care of more than one room, his or her "per FTE" numbers will be higher than those of the anesthesiologist who personally performs care (i.e., one room at a time). When trying to benchmark productivity, if concurrency is not accounted for, then comparisons may be meaningless. On the other hand, if productivity is measured by clinical site covered, then comparison of group productivity can be done (Abouleish AE, Prough DS, Barker SJ, et al. Organizational factors affect comparisons of the clinical productivity of academic anesthesiology departments. *Anesth Analg.* 2003;96:802-812). (804)

OPERATING ROOM EFFICIENCY

3. Intuitively, one would think that having a 100% efficient operating room (OR) would be the ideal setting. The simplest way to understand why this is not ideal is to look at utilization of OR time as a surrogate for efficiency. First, if OR time is 100% utilized on average, then this does not mean that every day the OR time is 100% utilized exactly. The reality is that some days the OR time will be less than 100% and other days it will be higher. From an economic perspective, keeping staff past their scheduled time (when OR utilization is greater than 100%) is very costly in both direct costs (overtime) and indirect costs (employee dissatisfaction and resulting attrition). On the other hand, if the OR finishes consistently before the staff shift ends, then one could argue that employees are being "underutilized" or paid to "sit around." But this view is missing the major point, which is that the underutilized time is less costly than overutilized time. So, in the long run, it is more efficient and cost effective to have underutilized time than overutilized time. (806)

4. It depends! As noted in the chapter, simply basing block allocation on utilization can result in wrong incentives. The best method to determine block allocation is the hospital contribution margin by OR day per surgeon. In the question, the two surgeons may actually be doing the exact same types of cases and numbers of cases, but one is faster than the other. So it makes no sense to punish the fast surgeon who completes the work quickly and provides an opportunity for the OR to do an add-on case and reward the slow surgeon who is keeping staff over their shift. (806)

5. Invariably at some point (and often multiple times) every OR suite will undergo a "turnover" initiative. Intuitively, reducing the time the patient is out of the OR would result in more cases. The reality is that reducing turnover time alone cannot allow for additional cases to be done. It can reduce overutilized time. In order to improve OR throughput, one needs to look at the whole process from the time the patient is scheduled for surgery until the time the patient has left the perioperative area. Multidisciplinary quality improvement projects will improve OR throughput, but often they can be labor intensive, expensive, and unsustainable. An excellent example of this process is reported from the Mayo Clinic (Cima RR, Brown MJ, Hebl JR, et al; Surgical Process Improvement Team, Mayo Clinic, Rochester. Use of lean and six sigma methodology to improve operating room efficiency in a high-volume tertiary-care academic medical center. *J Am Coll Surg.* 2011;213:83-94). (807)

47 AWARENESS UNDER ANESTHESIA

Daniel J. Cole

INCIDENCE

1. What is the difference between explicit and implicit memory?
2. Can the incidence of intraoperative awareness be reliably determined in the recovery room or through patient self-reporting?
3. What are the components of the "structured interview" used to evaluate the occurrence of intraoperative awareness?
4. When studied prospectively, and when using a structured interview, what is the approximate incidence of intraoperative awareness?

ETIOLOGY AND RISK FACTORS FOR INTRAOPERATIVE AWARENESS

5. What are the three major causes of intraoperative awareness?
6. What are some risk factors for intraoperative awareness?
7. What procedures are associated with an increased risk of intraoperative awareness?

PSYCHOLOGICAL SEQUELAE

8. What are some of the most common recalled awareness experiences of patients who have had intraoperative awareness?
9. If a patient has an episode of intraoperative awareness, what is the approximate risk of late psychological sequelae?
10. What are the potential psychological sequelae of intraoperative awareness?
11. What percentage of patients who self-identified to the Anesthesia Awareness Registry created in 2007 mistakenly believed they had experienced intraoperative awareness under general anesthesia, when in fact they had received regional anesthesia or sedation?
12. What percentage of patients who complained of intraoperative awareness under regional anesthesia or sedation experienced psychological sequelae?

PREVENTION OF AWARENESS

13. What are some conventional monitors used to assess anesthetic depth?
14. What are some limitations of brain function monitors for assessing anesthetic depth and the risk for intraoperative awareness?
15. What measures can be taken to help prevent intraoperative awareness?
16. What are the elements that The Joint Commission recommends to prevent and manage intraoperative awareness?
17. What do the data on brain function monitors suggest regarding the efficacy of these monitors to prevent intraoperative awareness?

THE ASA'S PRACTICE ADVISORY ON INTRAOPERATIVE AWARENESS AND BRAIN FUNCTION MONITORS

18. According to the Practice Advisory from the American Society of Anesthesiologists (ASA) on Intraoperative Awareness and Brain Function Monitoring, what should the preoperative evaluation include to minimize the risk of intraoperative awareness?
19. According to the Practice Advisory from the ASA on Intraoperative Awareness and Brain Function Monitoring, what should the preinduction phase include to minimize the risk of intraoperative awareness?

20. According to the Practice Advisory from the ASA on Intraoperative Awareness and Brain Function Monitoring, what should intraoperative monitoring include to minimize the risk of intraoperative awareness?

21. According to the Practice Advisory from the ASA on Intraoperative Awareness and Brain Function Monitoring, what should intraoperative and postoperative management include to minimize the risk of intraoperative awareness and associated sequelae?

MEDICOLEGAL SEQUELAE OF AWARENESS

22. Why is there a large disparity between the incidence of intraoperative awareness and associated malpractice claims?

23. What factors influence a patient's decision to initiate a malpractice claim?

24. What is the percentage of malpractice claims for intraoperative awareness in the Anesthesia Closed Claims Project database?

25. What demographics are associated with a malpractice claim for awareness in the Anesthesia Closed Claims Project database?

26. What are the causes of intraoperative awareness in the Anesthesia Closed Claims Project database?

ANSWERS*

INCIDENCE

1. Explicit memory, or conscious memory, refers to the recollection of previous experiences and is equivalent to remembering (intraoperative awareness). Implicit memory, or unconscious memory, is the ability of a patient to respond to commands, yet lack conscious recall of intraoperative events. (812)

2. The incidence of intraoperative awareness is best estimated by formally interviewing patients postoperatively, well after discharge from the postanesthesia recovery room. Patients will not reliably, or voluntarily, report awareness if they were not disturbed by it, or if embarrassed to do so. A structured interview is recommended to evaluate the incidence of awareness. (812)

3. The structured interview used to evaluate the occurrence of intraoperative awareness consists of the following components:
   - What was the last thing you remember before you went to sleep?
   - What is the first thing you remember after your operation?
   - Can you remember anything in between?
   - Can you remember if you had any dreams during your procedure?
   - What was the worst thing about your procedure? (813)

4. Prospective studies using a structured interview postoperatively estimate the incidence of intraoperative awareness to be 1 to 2 occurrences per 1000 patients undergoing a general anesthetic. (813)

ETIOLOGY AND RISK FACTORS FOR INTRAOPERATIVE AWARENESS

5. The three major causes of intraoperative awareness include light anesthesia, increased patient requirements for anesthesia, and anesthetic delivery problems. (813)

6. Risk factors for intraoperative awareness include hemodynamic intolerance of anesthetic drugs; patients who are hypovolemic; patients with limited cardiovascular reserve; ASA (American Society of Anesthesiologists) Physical Status 3 to 5; emergency surgery; administration of small doses of volatile anesthetics; a nitrous oxide or intravenous-based anesthetic; chronic use of alcohol, opioids, amphetamines, or cocaine; genetic resistance to anesthetics; and anesthesia delivery equipment problems. Children have a higher incidence of awareness. (813)

---

*Numbers in parentheses refer to pages, figures, boxes, or tables in Pardo MC, Miller RD, eds. *Basics of Anesthesia*. 7th ed. Philadelphia: Elsevier; 2018.

7. Cesarean delivery and open heart procedures are associated with an increased risk of intraoperative awareness. (813)

PSYCHOLOGICAL SEQUELAE

8. Some of the most common recalled awareness experiences of patients who have had intraoperative awareness include auditory sounds, feelings of paralysis, seeing lights, and feelings of helplessness, fear, or anxiety. Pain is less common but is more likely to occur in patients who have experienced paralysis with the inability to move. (814)

9. Approximately one third of patients who have an episode of intraoperative awareness have late psychological sequelae. Patients who experience muscle paralysis have an increased chance of long-term psychological sequelae. (814)

10. Potential psychological sequelae of intraoperative awareness include flashbacks, anxiety/nervousness, loneliness, nightmares, and fear/panic attacks that vary from bothersome to distressing. Some patients develop severe, persistent symptoms (posttraumatic stress disorder) that profoundly interfere with interpersonal relationships and daily activities. (814)

11. One third of patients who self-identified to the Anesthesia Awareness Registry created in 2007 mistakenly believed they had experienced intraoperative awareness under general anesthesia, when in fact they had received regional anesthesia or sedation. (814)

12. Approximately 40% percent of patients who complained of intraoperative awareness under regional anesthesia or sedation experienced psychological sequelae, similar to those experiencing intraoperative awareness under general anesthesia. (814)

PREVENTION OF AWARENESS

13. Conventional monitors of anesthetic depth include patient movement, tachycardia, hypertension, tearing, perspiration, and clinical instinct. One could also include anesthetic gas analyzers, which assess the dose of volatile anesthetic delivered to the patient. (814)

14. Limitations of brain function monitors include the following: (1) There is not a unitary mechanism of general anesthesia, and thus various anesthetics are likely to produce unique electrical activity at a given anesthetic depth. Consequently, a unique algorithm to each specific anesthetic regimen would likely be required for optimal correlation between electrical signals in the brain and anesthetic depth. (2) General anesthesia occurs on a continuum without a quantitative dimension, and there is considerable interpatient pharmacodynamic variability to a specific anesthetic. Attempting to translate a conscious or unconscious state into a quantitative number can at best be limited to the art of probability with an expectation of false positive and false negative data. (3) There is less than an optimal likelihood of cortical electric activity having reliable sensitivity and specificity to a biochemical event that occurs at a distant subcortical structure. (815)

15. Suggestions for the prevention of intraoperative awareness include premedication with an amnesic drug such as a benzodiazepine, giving adequate doses of drugs to induce anesthesia, avoiding muscle paralysis unless necessary, administering a volatile anesthetic at a dose of 0.7 minimum alveolar concentration (MAC) or more with monitoring of end-tidal levels to ensure delivery of adequate levels of a volatile anesthetic, and consideration of a brain function monitor on a case-by-case basis. (815)

16. The Joint Commission's recommendations to prevent and manage intraoperative awareness include development and implementation of an anesthesia awareness policy, staff education, informed consent for high-risk patients, timely maintenance of anesthesia equipment, postoperative follow-up of all patients who have undergone general anesthesia, and postoperative counseling for patients with awareness. (815)

17. The results of five randomized, controlled trials that evaluated the effect of brain function monitoring on the incidence of intraoperative awareness are

mostly derived from studies in patients at high risk for awareness. These studies show that bispectral index score (BIS)-guided anesthesia (BIS levels 40 to 60) reduced the incidence of awareness compared to routine care. However, the incidence of awareness in trials comparing BIS-guided anesthesia to end-tidal anesthetic gas–guided (0.7-1.3% MAC) anesthesia was not different. During total intravenous anesthesia (TIVA), BIS-guided anesthesia reduced the incidence of awareness compared to routine care, suggesting that BIS-guided anesthesia may be especially useful during TIVA. (816)

THE ASA'S PRACTICE ADVISORY ON INTRAOPERATIVE AWARENESS AND BRAIN FUNCTION MONITORS

18. According to the ASA Practice Advisory on Intraoperative Awareness and Brain Function Monitoring, the preoperative evaluation for preventing intraoperative awareness should include the identification of potential risk factors for intraoperative awareness, an interview of the patient and review of past medical records, and obtaining informed consent for those patients at high risk for intraoperative awareness. (816)

19. According to the ASA's Practice Advisory on Intraoperative Awareness and Brain Function Monitoring, the preinduction phase of anesthesia should include the use of a checklist for machine/equipment function, verification of function of intravenous access and infusion equipment, and consideration of a preoperative benzodiazepine for the patient. (816)

20. According to the ASA's Practice Advisory on Intraoperative Awareness and Brain Function Monitoring, intraoperative monitoring should include multiple modalities to monitor the depth of anesthesia. Clinical and conventional monitoring should be utilized. Brain function monitoring can be used on a case-by-case basis. If a volatile anesthetic is the primary anesthetic, the use of end-tidal anesthetic concentration of more than 0.7 age-adjusted MAC should be used in high-risk patients. During TIVA a BIS level of 40 to 60 may help reduce awareness compared to routine care. (816)

21. According to the ASA's Practice Advisory on Intraoperative Awareness and Brain Function Monitoring, intraoperative and postoperative management should include consideration of a benzodiazepine if the patient unexpectedly becomes conscious, a postoperative visit, consideration of a structured interview to determine the patient's anesthetic experience, an occurrence report for continuous quality improvement, and offering the patient psychological counseling if intraoperative awareness is reported. (817)

MEDICOLEGAL SEQUELAE OF AWARENESS

22. The large disparity between the incidence of intraoperative awareness and actual malpractice claims is multifactorial and includes the nature and severity of the injuries associated with awareness, as well as the medicolegal and injury compensation system. (817)

23. Factors influencing a patient's decision to initiate a malpractice claim are poor communication between the patient and physician, unmet expectations, and financial pressure on the patient. One study reported that 50% of potential plaintiffs had a poor relationship with their physician. (818)

24. Claims for intraoperative awareness represent a small fraction (2.6%) of all malpractice claims in the Anesthesia Closed Claims Project database. (818)

25. Demographics associated with a malpractice claim for intraoperative awareness in the Anesthesia Closed Claims Project database include female gender, ASA status 1 or 2, younger than 60 years of age, and elective surgery. (818)

26. The two main causes of intraoperative awareness in the Anesthesia Closed Claims Project database were light anesthesia and anesthetic delivery problems (medication errors, vaporizer malfunction, and intravenous catheter infiltration). (818)

48 QUALITY AND PATIENT SAFETY IN ANESTHESIA CARE

Avery Tung

DEFINITIONS: QUALITY VERSUS SAFETY	1. Define quality in reference to health care systems.
	2. Define safety in reference to health care systems.
	3. Provide an example of a perioperative health care process that improves only quality.
	4. Provide an example of a perioperative health care process that improves only safety.
	5. Provide an example of a perioperative health care process that improves both quality and safety.
SPECIFIC APPROACHES TO ANESTHESIA SAFETY	6. Describe how anesthesiologists can learn from experience to improve patient safety.
	7. Describe how anesthesiologists can use the adoption of specialty-wide standards to improve patient safety.
	8. Describe how anesthesiologists can use patient safety–focused programs to improve patient safety.
FROM SAFETY TO QUALITY: MAKING ANESTHESIA BOTH SAFER AND BETTER	9. Define and give an example of quality measures focusing on process in anesthesiology.
	10. Define and give an example of quality measures focusing on structure in anesthesiology.
	11. Define and give an example of quality measures focusing on outcome in anesthesiology.
TOOLS FOR IMPROVING LOCAL OUTCOMES	12. What are the common elements of the structured quality improvement programs PDSA (plan, do, study, act) and DMAIC (define, measure, analyze, improve, control)?
	13. Define a never event.
	14. Define a sentinel event.
	15. What is a root cause analysis?
	16. What is FMEA (failure mode effects analysis)?

ANSWERS*

DEFINITIONS: QUALITY VERSUS SAFETY	1. Quality describes the degree to which health care systems increase the likelihood for positive health outcomes. In contrast to safety (see item 2), quality incorporates an "optimization" element and targets specific health outcomes. Such outcomes may include traditional morbidity/mortality rates but also include "softer" outcomes such as efficiency, cost, and patient satisfaction. Unlike safety, quality may but usually does not, focus on adverse events. (821)

---

*Numbers in parentheses refer to pages, figures, boxes, or tables in Pardo MC, Miller RD, eds. *Basics of Anesthesia*. 7th ed. Philadelphia: Elsevier; 2018.

2. Safety in health care systems refers to a lack of harm and an absence of adverse events. Almost by definition, a process is safe if patient injury is avoided. It is easy to see that a process can always be made incrementally safer. Insulin administration, for example, which requires a two-provider check on dose prior to administration, could be made incrementally safer by requiring a three-, four-, or even five-provider check. (821)

3. An example of a perioperative health care process that improves quality is improved postoperative pain management techniques that result in shorter hospital stays. Another example is the provision of an email address for patients to contact their anesthesiologists after the care is completed. Such a process may improve patient satisfaction but by itself is unlikely to improve safety. These measures improve quality but may not affect safety. (822)

4. Examples of a perioperative health care process that improves only safety include increased availability of fiberoptic capability and pin indexing for cylinders. Such practices improve safety (by reducing adverse events) but may not improve quality. (822)

5. An excellent example of a perioperative health care process that improves both quality and safety is ultrasound-guided central line insertion. By reducing the incidence of carotid puncture, ultrasound reduces adverse events and thus improves safety. By reducing the time to successful insertion and the number of misses, ultrasound improves efficiency, thus improving quality. (822)

SPECIFIC APPROACHES TO ANESTHESIA SAFETY

6. Anesthesiologists can learn from experience to improve patient safety. Although inefficient, this pathway consists of collating the collective experience of administered anesthetics and identifying patterns relating anesthesia practices to adverse events. Examples include the relationship between muscle relaxant use and greater perioperative morbidity, hypertension and tachycardia with desflurane use, specific shapes for oxygen flowmeter knobs, and the lack of sensitivity of auscultation in detecting esophageal intubation (or visual inspection for $Spo_2 < 90\%$). (822)

7. In part as a response to cumulative experiences of millions of anesthetics, anesthesiology was the first medical specialty to produce specialty-wide standards to improve safety. These standards were driven in part by mounting malpractice settlements and had the explicit goal of reducing adverse anesthesia-related events. Although not grounded in formal studies of benefit, the original standards (for monitoring) met common sense rules, were associated with better outcomes when adopted, and have stood the test of time. Among these standards are the presence of an anesthesiologist in the operating room at all times; continuous monitoring of ventilation, circulation, and electrocardiogram; continuous monitoring for circuit disconnect and oxygen concentration; and minimum durations between blood pressure measurements. Since their adoption, these standards have been widely accepted and joined by two other society standards: preoperative evaluation and postoperative care. The overall efficacy of the three anesthesiology standards on perioperative outcomes remains unclear. But existing data from large databases and closed claims analyses suggest a clear reduction in adverse anesthesia-related events. (822)

8. Anesthesiology was one of the earliest specialties to sponsor formal programs targeted at patient safety. Among these are the Anesthesia Patient Safety Foundation and the Anesthesia Closed Claims project. The former supports newsletters, instructional videos, and grants for patient safety research. The latter examines "closed" (settled) malpractice claims to identify potentially unsafe practices. Examples of such practices include the severe consequences of esophageal intubation, presenting signs of cardiac arrest after spinal anesthesia, the risk of fire during monitored anesthesia care for upper airway surgery, and risk factors for adverse outcome after obstetric hemorrhage. (823)

FROM SAFETY TO QUALITY: MAKING ANESTHESIA BOTH SAFER AND BETTER

9. Process quality measures refer to specifications regarding how clinical care should be delivered. Usually derived from published literature, examples of process measures in anesthesiology include perioperative use of β-blockers for patients at risk for heart disease, use of ultrasound for central line insertion, and antibiotics within 1 hour of incision. Note that, as with structural quality measures, process measures are relatively easy to measure, but success or failure at a process measure does not require that the outcome of care improve. (824)

10. Structural quality measures refer to the presence or absence of specific organizational features considered relevant to the delivery of quality medical care. Examples of structural measures in anesthesiology include the presence (or absence) of round-the-clock in-house intensive care coverage, an electronic medical record, and rapid response teams. Note that structural quality measures are easy to measure, but their link to outcome improvements may be difficult to discern. (825)

11. Outcome quality measures refer to changes in the result or outcome of medical care. Such outcomes may include both intermediate and long-term results and can encompass medical, efficiency, and satisfaction domains. Examples of outcome measures in anesthesiology can include perioperative renal failure or myocardial infarction rates, length of stay, readmissions, and pain at 3 months. Note that outcome measures may be very difficult to measure and can have a wide range of definitions and target ideals, even for a single organ system. For example, renal failure rates on days 3, 7, 21, and 30 may vary widely in their ease of measurement, relevant therapeutic requirements, and "ideal" value. Unlike structural and process measures of quality, which do not require adjustment for patient-specific comorbid conditions and issues, outcome measures are inherently linked with patient comorbid conditions. Outcome measures thus require risk adjustment to be used for comparisons between caregivers or health care systems. Variability between risk adjustment systems may then result in skewed estimates of quality. (825)

TOOLS FOR IMPROVING LOCAL OUTCOMES

12. PDSA (plan, do, study, act) is perhaps the most common structural framework for quality improvement. The words describe the four steps in any quality improvement process. "Plan" refers to identifying a goal (be it structure, process, or outcome) and developing a plan to improve that goal. "Do" involves implementing that plan. "Study" involves measuring the results of the plan, and "act" collates the learning elements identified during the three previous phases and using them to influence the next cycle. DMAIC (define, measure, analyze, improve, control) recapitulates the PDSA process with slightly more detail. "Define" refers to defining the problem, "measure" refers to establishing a current baseline, "analyze" refers to targeting the cause or defining the specific intervention, "improve" refers to actual implementation, and "control" refers to monitoring, ongoing tweaking, and improvement. Both structured quality improvement programs involve the following common elements: evaluate, implement, and measure. (825)

13. The term *never event* was first used in 2001 by the National Quality Forum to describe a medical error considered so preventable that its very occurrence is a marker of poor quality. Never events may be defined by national or regional regulatory agencies and usually are promulgated as part of a regulatory framework. Never events are almost always associated with a required regulatory response by the health care system responsible for the event. Examples include wrong side surgery, inpatient suicide, postoperative retained foreign objects, and hemolytic transfusion reaction. Never events may differ from one regulatory authority to another. Currently, most U.S. hospitals participate in the program run by The Joint Commission, an accrediting agency for U.S. hospitals. (826)

14. A "sentinel event" is an adverse event type designated for special attention by The Joint Commission. Such events include retained foreign objects and hemolytic transfusion reaction. These events, when they occur in a hospital accredited by The Joint Commission, mandate a special response including a root cause analysis (RCA) (see next), development of an action plan, and report back to The Joint Commission. In keeping with an empiric, experience-based approach to quality, The Joint Commission produces a Sentinel Event Alert newsletter that compiles rare events to provide physicians with experience-based cues for avoidance. An example of such a cue is the observation that nearly one half of cases of retained foreign object occur without the official equipment count being incorrect. (826)

15. An RCA is an approach to improving safety not unlike a case study in business school. The RCA process is mandated by The Joint Commission for certain adverse events but can be employed for any process the health care system deems relevant. RCAs are typically multidisciplinary and are convened after an adverse event to identify fixable system causes. The overriding goal is to modify the system so that the chances of a second event are lower. An example of an RCA (and the topic of the first ever Joint Commission Sentinel Event Alert) is a potassium overdose as a result of an intravenous injection of concentrated KCl. An important root cause in such an event would be the availability of concentrated KCl on the floor. A drawback to RCA is that it is retrospective in nature. (826)

16. FMEA stands for failure modes effects analysis. An FMEA is a prospective analysis of a specific process to identify potential weak spots that may predispose to an adverse event. An example would be a process to improve insulin ordering and administration. An FMEA might identify variability in ordering, differences in vial shape and size, unavailability of syringes, and an absence of standardized sliding scales as potential issues. Properly done, an FMEA is extremely time consuming as it must consider all possible adverse events that may result from a process. In contrast, an RCA need focus only on the event that did occur. (827)

Chapter

49 PALLIATIVE CARE

Sarah Gebauer

24. What is an advance directive?
25. What are the criteria used to determine whether a person has capacity to make medical decisions?
26. If a patient does not have capacity to make medical decisions, what should be done to obtain consent for anesthesia?
27. What does a surrogate decision maker do?
28. What are the three intraoperative treatment scenarios for patients with perioperative limitations on treatment (such as a DNR [do not resuscitate] order) described by the American Society of Anesthesiologists (ASA)?
29. When should the patient's preexisting DNR order be reinstated if changes are made in the perioperative period?
30. Why are all DNR orders not suspended during the perioperative period?

ANSWERS*

INTRODUCTION

1. *Palliative care* is defined as "an approach that improves the quality of life of patients and their families facing the problems associated with life-threatening illness, through the prevention and relief of suffering by means of early identification and impeccable assessment and treatment of pain and other problems, physical, psychosocial, and spiritual." (829)
2. *Palliative medicine* refers to the medical expertise provided within a palliative care team. (829)

PALLIATIVE CARE

3. Patients are considered hospice candidates if two physicians determine that they have a life expectancy of 6 months or less. (829)
4. Palliative care is a more inclusive term that is appropriate at any age and any stage in a serious illness and can be provided together with curative treatment. Services may be provided in the clinic, inpatient, or home settings. In contrast, hospice in the United States refers to an insurance benefit that provides patients with 6 months or less with a variety of medical and ancillary services with a focus on comfort rather than cure. Most hospice care is provided at home, with a small portion provided on an inpatient basis. (829)
5. Shared decision making in palliative care means talking to patients and families, eliciting their values and goals, and making medical recommendations and decisions based on those values and goals. (830)
6. Personnel provided by hospice include a nurse, aide, social worker, spiritual counselor, volunteers, and access to a physician. (830)
7. Goods and services provided by hospice include nursing support available around the clock, access to short-term inpatient or continuous care, bereavement support for family members for 1 year after the patient's death, medical equipment, and medical supplies. (830–831)

WHAT DO PALLIATIVE CARE TEAMS DO?

8. Physicians, nurses, social workers, and chaplains commonly make up palliative care teams. Physicians provide symptom management and facilitate communication about goals of care. Nurses help manage symptoms, communication issues, and assess the psychosocial and spiritual needs of the patient and family. Social workers address the psychosocial needs of families and may help with discharge planning needs. Chaplains assist patients and families in identifying and addressing spiritual distress and help facilitate religious rituals. (832)

---

*Numbers in parentheses refer to pages, figures, boxes, or tables in Pardo MC, Miller RD, eds. *Basics of Anesthesia*. 7th ed. Philadelphia: Elsevier; 2018.

9. Consultations for palliative care generally address goals of care and symptom management. During goals of care consultations, palliative care specialists share information, get a sense of what a patient's goals and values are, and make medical recommendations based on those goals and values. During symptom management consultations, palliative care specialists query the patient about common palliative care symptoms, evaluate possible medical and psychosocial causes for those symptoms, and treat the symptoms based on their cause. (832)

10. Benefits associated with palliative care in the intensive care unit (ICU) include decreased time in the ICU, decreased hospital length of stay, no increase in mortality, decreased family member posttraumatic stress disorder (PTSD) and anxiety, decreased disagreements between families and providers, and decreased disagreements among providers. (832–833)

11. The surgical covenant is a belief in which the surgeon has an exaggerated sense of accountability for a patient's outcome. The American College of Surgeons encourages integration of palliative care in a range of surgical patients, not just those at the end of life. (833)

12. Opioids and benzodiazepines are often administered during the withdrawal of ventilator support to treat respiratory distress and anxiety during the process. Examples include fentanyl and midazolam. (833)

13. Prior to withdrawing the ventilator, physicians should ensure that the patient is not paralyzed, prepare opioids and benzodiazepines to be readily available at bedside, discontinue any unnecessary lines or tubes, contact the hospital chaplain for help accommodating spiritual and religious rituals, and ensure family support. (833)

14. It is helpful to ask patients about their spirituality for at least two reasons. Many patients say that religion is important in helping them adjust to, and cope with, the diagnosis of serious illness. Also, there may be religious rituals, such as the way a patient's body should be handled after death, that are important for the health care team to know. (833)

PALLIATIVE CARE AND PAIN

15. The ethical principle of double effect of opioid use in palliative care states that a physician can treat symptoms that may hasten death as a secondary effect, as long as the doctor's intention is to have a good outcome. This is often applied in relation to giving opioids at the end of life, in which the good outcome is pain relief and the bad outcome is death. (834)

16. Nonopioid approaches to the treatment of bony pain include intrathecal catheters, hormonal therapy, bone-modifying agents, and radiotherapy. The choice of which treatment may be helpful for bony pain may depend on the cause of the pain. (834–835)

CHALLENGES IN THE PALLIATIVE CARE PATIENT

17. Palliative care or hospice consultation criteria may depend on hospital or community norms. A palliative care consultation may benefit seriously ill patients without clear treatment preferences or decision makers, patients with refractory symptoms, or patients whose care causes conflict among staff members. Inpatients with life-threatening disease or with an illness with a high probability of leading to death are also candidates. Outpatients who have complex symptoms, difficult to manage symptoms (e.g., pain or nausea), psychosocial issues, or advance care planning needs may also benefit from a palliative care consultation. Hospice consultation should be sought for patients with a life expectancy of 6 months or less who are interested in focusing on symptom-related treatments rather than treatments with intent to cure. (836)

18. The four main disease trajectories of dying include sudden death, terminal illness, organ failure, and frailty. In sudden death a patient is healthy and functional, and then a catastrophic event, like being in a car accident, occurs. Terminal illness, in which a functional patient undergoes a decline over a period of weeks to months, occurs in most cancers. Organ failure, in which patients

have repeated decreases in functionality owing to illness and then improve but never quite back to their previous baseline, occurs in illnesses like chronic obstructive pulmonary disease (COPD). Frailty, in which a patient with a long-term, chronic illness slowly loses function over a period of years, occurs in dementia. (837)

19. The SPIKES protocol was originally developed as a mnemonic to help physicians deliver bad news, but its steps can be used in a variety of situations. The first step, setting, is a reminder to choose a quiet, private space with sufficient chairs for all those attending the meeting. During the second step, perception, the physician asks about and assesses the patient's and family's understanding of the patient's condition. The third step, invitation, reminds the physician to ask how much detail the patient wants. The fourth step, knowledge, is when the physician uses plain language to communicate medical information. The fifth step, empathy, emphasizes the importance of acknowledging emotions. During the sixth step, sequelae, all participants agree on next steps. (839)

20. The way a family meeting is begun sets the tone for the crucial information that follows. A premeeting with other members of the medical team is usually helpful to make sure everyone is on the same page. Physicians should remember to introduce family and team members, give an explanation for why the meeting is being held, and display empathy when appropriate. (838)

21. Recordings of physicians show that they tend to focus on technical detail, avoid emotional topics, and dominate conversations. (838)

22. A time-limited trial is an agreement between clinicians and a patient/family to use certain medical therapies over a defined period to see if the patient improves or deteriorates according to agreed-on clinical outcomes. Time-limited trials are useful when it is unclear whether a patient's condition will improve with additional time, therapies, or both. (839)

23. Mandibular movement with breathing, peripheral cyanosis, and Cheyne-Stokes breathing are specific for patient death within 3 days but occur in less than 60% of patients. Unfortunately, predicting when death will occur is difficult and poorly studied. (839)

PERIOPERATIVE MANAGEMENT OF THE PALLIATIVE CARE PATIENT

24. An advance directive is a legal document that describes a person's wishes for medical intervention and care, such as attempted resuscitation, life support, or artificial hydration or nutrition. Many advance directives include the naming of a surrogate decision maker as part of the form. Living wills, Five Wishes, and state-specific advance directives are examples. (840)

25. The criteria used to decide whether a person has the capacity to make medical decisions are "the ability to communicate a choice, to understand the relevant information, to appreciate the medical consequences of the situation, and to reason about treatment choices." (840)

26. If a patient does not have the capacity to make medical decisions and the procedure is not an emergency, anesthesiologists should determine who the patient's surrogate decision maker is according to the patient's advance directive or state law. That person should then be contacted to obtain informed consent. (841)

27. A surrogate decision maker makes medical decisions on the patient's behalf, with substituted judgment. Substituted judgment means the surrogate tries to decide what the patient would prefer based on the patient's goals and values, not what the surrogate would want in the same situation. (841)

28. The American Society of Anesthesiologists (ASA) has published guidelines for the care of patients with DNR orders and limitations on treatment. The guidelines describe three scenarios for the care of these patients. One is *full attempt at resuscitation*, which means that the preexisting order is completely reversed and any procedures may be used. The second is *limited attempt at resuscitation defined with regard to specific procedures*, in which a patient may request that interventions such as chest compressions, for example, not be used. The third is *limited attempt at resuscitation defined with regard to the patient's goals and*

values, in which the patient may give the physician authority to use clinical judgment to decide which resuscitation procedures are appropriate. (841)

29. As per ASA guidelines, the patient's preexisting DNR order, or other limitations on treatment like an advance directive, should be reinstated upon leaving the postanesthesia care unit (PACU) or when the patient has recovered from the side effects of anesthesia. This should be discussed with the patient and clearly documented. (841)

30. Not all DNR orders are suspended in the perioperative period. The ASA and the American College of Surgeons consider the automatic suspension of DNR orders to not address a patient's right to self-determination. Those two groups, in addition to the Association of Perioperative Registered Nurses, recommend discussing the risks and benefits of changes in the patient's DNR order prior to surgery. (841)

50 SLEEP MEDICINE AND ANESTHESIA

Mandeep Singh, Rami A. Kamel, and Frances Chung

HUMAN SLEEP
1. How is the sleep-wake cycle controlled?
2. What are the electroencephalogram (EEG) features of wakefulness?
3. What are the EEG features of the different stages of normal sleep?

GENERAL ANESTHESIA
4. What are the EEG features of different stages of general anesthesia?

SLEEP AND ANESTHESIA: HOW DIFFERENT ARE THEY?
5. What are the main differences between sleep and anesthesia?

FUNCTIONAL NEUROANATOMY OF SLEEP AND AROUSAL PATHWAYS
6. What are the key neural pathways engaged in sleep and arousal?

SLEEP-DISORDERED BREATHING OR SLEEP-RELATED BREATHING DISORDERS
7. What are the characteristics of sleep-disordered breathing? What are the common types of sleep-disordered breathing?
8. What characterizes obstructive sleep apnea (OSA)?
9. What characterizes central sleep apnea (CSA)?

PATHOPHYSIOLOGY OF UPPER AIRWAY COLLAPSE IN OBSTRUCTIVE SLEEP APNEA
10. What is the pathophysiology of upper airway collapse in OSA?

CLINICAL DIAGNOSTIC CRITERIA
11. What test is the gold standard for the definitive diagnosis of OSA?
12. Based on the American Academy of Sleep Medicine, how are apneas and hypopneas defined?
13. How is obstructive hypopnea distinguished from central hypopnea?

14. What is the apnea-hypopnea index (AHI)?
15. What defines severe, moderate, and mild OSA?
16. What are the clinical diagnostic criteria for OSA?
17. What is measured during laboratory polysomnography?
18. What are the various home sleep testing devices currently available?

POLYSOMNOGRAPHY AND PORTABLE DEVICES

PREVALENCE OF OSA IN THE GENERAL AND SURGICAL POPULATION

19. What is the prevalence of OSA in the general population?
20. What approximate number of people in the general and surgical populations with moderate-to-severe OSA are undiagnosed?

OSA AND COMORBID CONDITIONS

21. What comorbid conditions are commonly found in patients with OSA?

SURGERY AND OSA SEVERITY

22. What factors predict postoperative increased AHI from baseline, and on what postoperative day does the AHI peak?
23. According to the American Society of Anesthesiologists (ASA) Closed Claims Project database, on what postoperative day is opioid-induced respiratory depression most likely to occur? What are some contributory factors?
24. What are some factors associated with fatality following life-threatening critical respiratory events with opioids in the postoperative period?

OSA AND POSTOPERATIVE COMPLICATIONS

25. What is the risk of postoperative complications in patients with diagnosed and undiagnosed OSA?

PREOPERATIVE ASSESSMENT

26. What are some of the principles of preoperative assessment of OSA?
27. What are some types of positive airway pressure (PAP) devices used for treating patients with OSA?
28. What is the benefit of perioperative PAP therapy in patients with diagnosed or undiagnosed OSA?
29. What are some tools that can be used for preoperative screening of patients for OSA?
30. What is the STOP-BANG questionnaire? What score indicates a high risk of OSA on the STOP-BANG questionnaire?
31. What are some important perioperative strategies used to mitigate the risk of OSA?
32. What is the best management strategy for a patient who scored a 7 when screened with the STOP-BANG questionnaire and is scheduled for an emergency laparotomy for a ruptured abdominal aortic aneurysm?
33. What is the best management strategy for a patient with OSA with significant daytime sleepiness, who has been noncompliant to continuous positive airway pressure (CPAP) therapy for the past 10 years, and who has gained 20 kg in the past 2 years? The patient also has severe chronic obstructive pulmonary disease (COPD) requiring home oxygen at 2 L/min and moderate pulmonary hypertension. He is scheduled to undergo a coronary artery bypass grafting for progressively worsening dyspnea.
34. What is the best management strategy for a patient with severe OSA with good CPAP compliance, no daytime sleepiness, and well-controlled hypertension who is scheduled for open reduction and internal fixation of fractures of both bones of the forearm under axillary brachial plexus block?

POSTOPERATIVE DISPOSITION OF OSA PATIENTS

35. What are some factors that contribute to the disposition of the OSA patient?
36. For how long should a patient with diagnosed or suspected OSA be monitored in the postanesthesia care unit (PACU) postoperatively?
37. What is the definition of recurrent respiratory events in the PACU?
38. What is pain-sedation mismatch?
39. How should patients with suspected OSA (i.e., scored as high risk on screening questionnaires) who develop recurrent respiratory events in the PACU be managed?
40. What is the proper management of a patient with a moderate risk of OSA (STOP-BANG score 4) who underwent knee arthroscopy under general anesthesia? Postoperatively, he is awake and breathing well with a respiratory rate of 16 breaths per minute. His vital signs are stable, and the oxygen saturation is at 98% on room air. His pain score is 3/10 at rest and 4/10 on movement without the need for intravenous analgesics.
41. What is the proper management of the following patient: a morbidly obese patient (BMI [body mass index] of 45 kg/m^2) who underwent laparoscopic cholecystectomy under general anesthesia and is diagnosed with OSA but noncompliant with CPAP therapy. The intraoperative course was uneventful. Postoperatively, she remained in the PACU for 2 hours. Her pain score is 8/10 at rest and 9/10 on movement despite treatment with hydromorphone 10 mg administered intravenously while in the PACU. She is drowsy and is noted to have repeated obstructive events that are associated with arousals terminating the events. Her respiratory rate is 7 breaths per minute.
42. What is the proper management of a patient who underwent total knee replacement under spinal anesthesia with an adductor canal block and local infiltration analgesia? The patient was diagnosed with severe OSA and is noncompliant with her CPAP therapy. Postoperatively, she is awake and is breathing well with a respiratory rate of 14 breaths per minute. Her oxygen saturation is at 96%, pain is well controlled, and she has only required hydromorphone 0.2 mg intravenously over the past 2 hours.

ANSWERS*

HUMAN SLEEP

1. Sleep is believed to be under the control of two processes: the circadian drive (process C) and a homeostatic drive (process S). The circadian drive regulates the appropriate timing of sleep and wakefulness across the 24-hour day, such that people get sleepy during their accustomed sleep times during a 24-hour cycle. The homoeostatic drive regulates sleep need and intensity according to the time spent awake or asleep; hence, sleep deprivation leads to increasing sleepiness. These two sleep drives are additive, and temporal organization must be preserved to obtain a subjective experience of being refreshed and rested. (845)
2. The American Academy of Sleep Medicine (AASM) has classified wakefulness and sleep into various stages based on characteristic electroencephalogram (EEG) patterns. *Wakefulness* is characterized by *beta activity* with eyes open (low amplitude, 12 to 40 Hz) and *alpha activity* with eyes closed (low amplitude, 8-13 Hz). (846)
3. The EEG features of sleep can be divided into non–rapid eye movement (NREM) sleep and rapid eye movement (REM) sleep. *NREM sleep* has three characteristic patterns on the EEG: *stage N1 sleep* is characterized by attenuation of alpha activity during wakefulness, to low amplitude, mixed frequency signal and vertex sharp waves; *stage N2 sleep* is characterized by the presence of *K-complexes* (well-delineated, negative, sharp waves followed by a positive deflection, lasting

*Numbers in parentheses refer to pages, figures, boxes, or tables in Pardo MC, Miller RD, eds. *Basics of Anesthesia.* 7th ed. Philadelphia: Elsevier; 2018.

0.5 second) and *sleep spindles* (high-frequency bursts with tapering ends, distinct from the background rhythm and last ≥0.5 second); *stage N3 sleep* is characterized by *delta waves* (higher amplitude lower frequency rhythms) accompanied by waxing and waning muscle tone, decreased body temperature, and decreased heart rate. *REM sleep* is characterized by rapid eye movements, dreaming, irregular breathing and heart rate, and skeletal muscle hypotonia. In REM sleep, the EEG shows active high-frequency, low-amplitude rhythms. (846)

GENERAL ANESTHESIA

4. General anesthesia could be described as a reversible drug-induced coma. The EEG patterns of general anesthesia–induced consciousness are described in three periods—induction, maintenance, and emergence. *Induction* by small doses of hypnotic agents acting on the γ-aminobutyric acid type A (GABA$_A$) receptors induces a state of sedation in which the patient is calm and easily arousable, with the eyes generally closed. This is followed by a brief period of paradoxic excitation, characterized by an increase in *beta activity* on the EEG. During *maintenance* four distinct phases have been described. *Phase I*, a light state of general anesthesia, is characterized by a decrease in EEG beta activity and an increase in EEG *alpha activity* and *delta activity*. During *phase II*, the intermediate state, beta activity decreases and *alpha and delta activity* increases, with so-called anteriorization—that is, an increase in alpha and delta activity in the anterior EEG leads relative to the posterior leads. *Phase III* is a deeper state, in which the EEG is characterized by flat periods interspersed with periods of alpha and beta activity (burst suppression). As this state of general anesthesia deepens, the time between the periods of alpha activity lengthens, and the amplitudes of the alpha and beta activity decrease. During *phase IV*, the most profound state of general anesthesia, the EEG is isoelectric (completely flat), indicated in conditions such as induced coma, neuro-protection during neurosurgery, or status epilepticus. *Emergence* from general anesthesia sees the EEG patterns proceed in approximately reverse order from phases II or III of the maintenance period to an active EEG that is consistent with a fully awake state. (846–847)

SLEEP AND ANESTHESIA: HOW DIFFERENT ARE THEY?

5. Sleep is a natural state of decreased arousal, controlled by circadian and homeostatic drives. Sleep states are amenable to disruptive influences such as psychological and environmental factors. In the presence of significant sensory stimulation, the sleep state gets disrupted, and the subject arouses. Sleep is characteristically a nonhomogeneous state with distinct stages, periodic arousals, and variable body postures, occurring in a cyclic pattern. Sleep state reversal occurs spontaneously after putative restorative functions are completed. Anesthesia, on the other hand, is a drug-induced state that is independent of intrinsic rhythms and immune to environmental and psychological factors. Anesthesia is a more or less homogeneous state, the depth and duration of which is directly dependent on drug pharmacokinetics and pharmacodynamics. A basic tenet of anesthesia is suppression of arousals, rendering the subject insensate to bodily injury during surgery. Anesthesia state reversal requires voluntary stoppage of drug administration as well as effective drug elimination. (847)

FUNCTIONAL NEUROANATOMY OF SLEEP AND AROUSAL PATHWAY

6. Sleep state modulation is regulated by two groups of neural centers: the wakefulness-promoting centers (locus coeruleus [LC], dorsal raphe, and tuberomammillary nucleus) and the sleep-promoting center (hypothalamic ventrolateral preoptic nucleus [VLPO]). During wakefulness, the LC is active and exerts an inhibitory influence on the hypothalamic VLPO. At sleep onset, the LC activity decreases, disinhibiting the VLPO, which now exerts an inhibitory influence on key brainstem and thalamic centers, blocking the ascent of arousal-promoting pathways to the cortex through them. The mutual inhibition between VLPO and LC acts to produce switch-like, *bistable states* of wakefulness and sleep at a certain threshold. (847)

SLEEP-DISORDERED BREATHING OR SLEEP-RELATED BREATHING DISORDERS

7. Sleep-disordered breathing (SDB) is characterized by abnormalities of respiration patterns during sleep. The abnormal patterns of breathing are broadly grouped into obstructive sleep apnea (OSA) disorders, central sleep apnea (CSA) disorders, sleep-related hypoventilation disorders, and sleep-related hypoxemia disorder. (848)

8. OSA disorders are characterized by complete or incomplete upper airway closure during sleep in the presence of respiratory effort during some portion of the event. This results in varying severity of hypoxemia and hypercapnia. There are repeated episodes of complete or partial closure of the pharynx, associated hypoventilation, and termination by EEG arousal. (848)

9. CSA disorders are characterized by reduction (hypopnea) or cessation (apnea) of airflow due to absent or reduced respiratory effort. Central apnea or hypopnea may occur in a cyclic, intermittent, or irregular (ataxic) fashion. (848)

PATHOPHYSIOLOGY OF UPPER AIRWAY COLLAPSE IN OBSTRUCTIVE SLEEP APNEA

10. Upper airway (UA) collapsibility and patency are dependent on a continuous balance between collapsing and expanding forces influenced by sleep-wake arousal. During sleep, UA collapse in OSA patients is due to multiple factors such as loss of UA dilating muscle tone, impaired response to mechanoreceptors sensing intrapharyngeal pressures, ventilator overshoot (high loop gain of the respiratory control system), and an increased arousal threshold. Moreover, patients with OSA have a UA that is predisposed to collapse, as seen by the presence of smaller UA cross-sectional areas and higher critical closure pressures than patients without OSA. During NREM sleep and anesthesia, reduction of wakeful cortical influences, reflex gain, and ventilatory drive predisposes to UA collapse and hypoventilation. (848)

CLINICAL DIAGNOSTIC CRITERIA

11. Classically, the gold standard for the definitive diagnosis of OSA requires an overnight polysomnography (PSG) or sleep study. (848)

12. Based on the American Academy of Sleep Medicine, apneas and hypopneas are defined as a reduction in the rate of airflow from intranasal pressure of at least 90%, or between 50% and 90%, respectively, for at least 10 seconds accompanied by either a 3% to 4% decrease in oxygen saturation or EEG arousal. (848)

13. Obstructive hypopnea is present if thoracoabdominal motion is out of phase or if airflow limitation is observed on the nasal pressure signal. Central apnea is present if thoracoabdominal motion is in phase and there is no airflow limitation on the nasal pressure signal. Mixed apneas begin as central for at least 10 seconds and end as obstructive, with a minimum of three obstructive efforts. (849)

14. The apnea-hypopnea index (AHI) is the average number of abnormal breathing events per hour of sleep. (849)

15. OSA severity is determined by the AHI as follows: mild, 5 to 15 events per hour; moderate, 15 to 30 events per hour; and severe, more than 30 events per hour. (849)

16. The clinical diagnosis of OSA requires either an AHI of 15 or more or an AHI greater than or equal to 5, with symptoms such as excessive daytime sleepiness, unintentional sleep during wakefulness, unrefreshing sleep, loud snoring reported by a partner, or observed obstruction during sleep. (849)

POLYSOMNOGRAPHY AND PORTABLE DEVICES

17. All laboratory PSG tests are performed using central, occipital, and frontal EEG; right and left electro-oculogram; electrocardiogram; and chin and bilateral anterior tibialis muscle electromyogram. Thoracoabdominal motion is usually monitored by respiratory inductance plethysmography, and airflow is monitored using either a nasal pressure transducer or nasal thermistor. Arterial oxygen saturation is monitored by pulse oximetry. Body position and snoring are recorded manually. (849)

18. Home sleep testing may be a viable alternative to standard PSG for the diagnosis of OSA in certain subsets of patients. The Portable Monitoring Task Force of the AASM has classified level 2 (full unattended PSG with 7 or more recording channels), level 3 (devices limited to 4 to 7 recording channels), and level 4 (monitors with 1 to 2 recording channels including nocturnal oximetry) devices. In particular, the level 2 portable PSG device has a diagnostic accuracy similar to that of standard PSG, whereas nocturnal oximetry is both sensitive and specific for detecting OSA in high-risk surgical patients. Portable devices may be considered when there is high pretest likelihood for moderate-to-severe OSA without other substantial comorbid conditions, and proper standards for conducting the test and interpretation of results are met. (850)

PREVALENCE OF OSA IN THE GENERAL AND SURGICAL POPULATION

19. The prevalence of moderate-to-severe OSA is 13% among men and 6% among women in the general population. The estimates are higher with increasing age and body mass index (BMI). (850)

20. Approximately 80% of people in the general population with moderate-to-severe OSA are undiagnosed. The prevalence of undiagnosed moderate-to-severe OSA among surgical patients is difficult to assess but appears to be higher than in the general population. Over 60% of patients with moderate-to-severe OSA were not diagnosed by the anesthesia provider preoperatively. (850)

OSA AND COMORBID CONDITIONS

21. OSA is associated with long-term cardiovascular morbidity including myocardial ischemia, heart failure, hypertension, arrhythmias, cerebrovascular disease, metabolic syndrome, insulin resistance, gastroesophageal reflux, and obesity. It is important to be mindful of craniofacial deformities (e.g., macroglossia, retrognathia, midfacial hypoplasia), endocrine disorders (e.g., hypothyroidism, Cushing disease), demographic group (male, age over 50 years), and lifestyle factors (e.g., smoking, alcohol consumption) that are closely associated with OSA. Perioperative physicians should be aware of these possible comorbid conditions because further optimization and risk stratification may be indicated at the time of surgery. (850)

SURGERY AND OSA SEVERITY

22. Preoperative AHI, age, and opioid dosage were significant predictors of increased postoperative AHI. Although AHI significantly increases from baseline on the first night after surgery, peak increase occurs on the third postoperative night. These findings are clinically significant for surgical patients, as they are not monitored as closely during the second and third postoperative nights. It is well known that postoperative complications like myocardial infarction, congestive heart failure, and pulmonary embolus are more likely to occur during the second and third postoperative days, which is coincident with the increased AHI and decreased oxygen saturation. (850)

23. According to the American Society of Anesthesiologists (ASA) Closed Claims Project database, postoperative opioid-induced respiratory depression is most likely to occur within the first 24 hours of surgery. Contributory factors include multiple prescribers, concurrent administration of nonopioid sedating medications, and inadequate nursing assessments or response. As many as 97% of these events were considered preventable. (851)

24. Factors such as OSA, deep levels of sedation, nighttime events, and postoperative acute renal failure have been shown to be associated with fatality following life-threatening critical respiratory events with opioids. (851)

OSA AND POSTOPERATIVE COMPLICATIONS

25. A meta-analysis of 13 studies demonstrated that patients with OSA versus non-OSA were associated with a twofold increased risk of postoperative events, such as acute respiratory failure, desaturation, and intensive care transfer. Large population-based studies using a national database have shown that patients with a diagnosis of OSA have increased risk of perioperative complications, such as emergent intubation, noninvasive or mechanical ventilation, aspiration

pneumonia, pulmonary embolism, and atrial fibrillation. Patients with undiagnosed OSA were found to have a threefold higher risk of postoperative cardiovascular complications, primarily cardiac arrest and shock, compared to diagnosed OSA patients. (851)

PREOPERATIVE ASSESSMENT

26. A thorough history and physical examination are essential for assessing OSA preoperatively. Focused questions regarding nature and severity of OSA symptoms should be asked. Previous consultations with sleep physician and sleep reports should be reviewed. Patients may present with signs and symptoms of significant comorbid conditions including morbid obesity, metabolic syndrome, uncontrolled or resistant hypertension, arrhythmias, cerebrovascular disease, and heart failure. Preoperative assessment should also rule out the presence of significant nocturnal hypoxemia, hypercarbia, polycythemia, and cor pulmonale. Obesity hypoventilation syndrome (OHS) and pulmonary hypertension should be ruled out in OSA patients. A serum bicarbonate level of 28 mmol/L or more is a useful screening tool for chronic hypercapnia and potentially for OHS. A preoperative transthoracic echocardiogram may be considered in patients suspected to have severe pulmonary hypertension and if intraoperative acute elevations in pulmonary arterial pressures (high-risk or long-duration surgery) are anticipated. (851)

27. OSA patients may be using positive airway pressure (PAP) devices for treatment, such as continuous positive airway pressure (CPAP), bilevel positive airway pressure (BiPAP), and auto-titrating positive airway pressure (APAP) machines. APAP devices provide upper airway stability while asleep based on airflow measurements, fluctuations in pressure, or airway resistance based on internal algorithms and has the potential to account for night-to-night variability of OSA severity. (852)

28. The use of perioperative CPAP significantly reduces the postoperative AHI from baseline preoperative AHI and offers modest reduction of hospital length of stay. Currently guidelines recommend that surgical patients with moderate-to-severe OSA who are compliant with PAP therapy should bring the device to the hospital and continue its use. Patients who are noncompliant with use of PAP therapy should be counseled at minimum to resume therapy preoperatively. Patients with diagnosed OSA and recent exacerbation of symptoms and those who were lost to follow-up care may benefit from a preoperative reassessment from a sleep medicine physician. Patients with significant comorbid conditions, a high serum bicarbonate level (indicating chronic hypercapnia), and preoperative hypoxemia in the absence of respiratory disease are candidates for preoperative evaluation and initiation of PAP therapy. (852)

29. An overnight PSG is the gold standard diagnostic test for OSA, but routine screening with PSG can be costly and resource intensive. As a result, simple, economical, and sensitive screening tests using clinical criteria to identify and risk-stratify potential OSA patients have been developed. The ASA "Practice Guidelines for the Perioperative Management of Patients with Obstructive Sleep Apnea" recommends a comprehensive preoperative evaluation including a review of the medical records, patient/family interview and screening, and physical examination. Other tools that have been validated for screening surgical patients are the STOP-BANG questionnaire, the Berlin Questionnaire, and the Perioperative Sleep Apnea Prediction (P-SAP) score. (854)

30. The STOP-BANG questionnaire is a concise and easy-to-use screening tool for OSA consisting of eight questions with the acronym STOP-BANG (www.stopbang.ca). This screening tool includes four "yes/no" questions with a mnemonic (S-snoring, T-tiredness, O-observed you stop breathing, P-blood pressure), and it combines demographic data of *B*MI (>35 kg/m^2), *a*ge (>50 years), *n*eck circumference (>40 cm), and *g*ender (male). Patients are deemed to be at low risk for OSA with scores of 0 to 2, intermediate risk with 3 to 4, and high risk with scores of 5 to 8. In patients whose STOP-BANG scores are the

mid-range (3 or 4), further criteria are required for classification. For example, a STOP score of 2 or more plus BMI criteria (BMI >35 kg/m² or male or neck circumference >43 cm in males, and >41 cm in females) or a STOP-BANG score of 3 or more plus serum HCO_3 of 28 mmol/L or more would classify that patient as having a high risk for moderate-to-severe OSA. (854)

31. To mitigate the risk of OSA, preoperative sedative premedication should be avoided. Intraoperatively, the anesthesiologist should be prepared for difficult mask ventilation, laryngoscopy, and endotracheal intubation. Adequate preoxygenation, head elevated body position, and measures to decrease the risk of aspiration of gastric acid should be considered. Short-acting agents such as propofol, remifentanil, and desflurane are preferred over long-acting agents. Multimodal analgesia with nonopioid analgesics should be used to decrease the opioid requirement. Extubation should take place when the patient is fully conscious, able to obey commands, has no residual neuromuscular blockade, and is able to maintain a patent airway. After extubation of the trachea, patients should be recovered in a semiupright or lateral position. Local or regional anesthesia techniques may be of benefit as they avoid manipulation of the airway and reduce the postoperative requirement for sedating analgesic medication. Patients previously on PAP therapy at home may continue using their PAP devices during procedures under mild to moderate sedation. (855)

32. The patient scored a 7 when screened with STOP-BANG questionnaire and is therefore at high risk of having undiagnosed the moderate-to-severe OSA. However, the surgery is emergent so the sound management is to proceed with surgery but with risk mitigation strategies during the entire perioperative period. After hospital discharge, this patient should be considered for referral to a sleep physician for assessment. (855)

33. The best management strategy for a patient with OSA who is noncompliant to CPAP therapy for the past 10 years, has significant weight gain, has oxygen-dependent chronic obstructive pulmonary disease (COPD), and has moderate pulmonary hypertension who is scheduled to undergo coronary artery bypass grafting for progressively worsening dyspnea is to refer the patient for preoperative assessment by a sleep physician. In this scenario, the patient is already diagnosed with moderate-to-severe OSA as evidenced by his daytime sleepiness. He has significant comorbid conditions (COPD, pulmonary hypertension, heart failure) and is scheduled for major elective surgery. This patient may benefit from institution of optimal PAP therapy to reduce this risk of perioperative adverse events. (855)

34. The best management strategy for a patient diagnosed with severe OSA who is compliant with CPAP and antihypertensive therapy is to proceed with elective surgery. This patient additionally benefits from regional rather than general anesthesia. (855)

POSTOPERATIVE DISPOSITION OF OSA PATIENTS

35. Factors that contribute to the disposition of the OSA patient include the nature of surgery, OSA severity, and the requirement of postoperative parenteral opioids. The attending anesthesiologist is responsible for the final decision of patient disposition. (856)

36. Patients with diagnosed or suspected OSA should be monitored in the postanesthesia care unit (PACU) for an extended period of time. It is reasonable to observe these patients in the PACU for an additional 60 minutes in a quiet environment after criteria for discharge have been met. (856)

37. Recurrent respiratory events in the PACU are defined as (1) episodes of apnea for 10 seconds or more, (2) bradypnea fewer than 8 breaths per minute, (3) pain-sedation mismatch, and (4) repeated oxygen desaturation to less than 90%. (856)

38. Pain-sedation mismatch is the simultaneous occurrence of high pain scores and high sedation levels. The patient is found to be drowsy and when aroused complains of severe uncontrolled pain. In this scenario, it is important to be cautious with prescribing more sedating medications. For these patients opioid-

sparing techniques should be instituted, and arrangement should be made for postoperative monitoring after transfer from the PACU. (856)

39. Patients with suspected OSA (i.e., scored as high risk on screening questionnaires) who develop recurrent respiratory events in the PACU are at increased risk of postoperative respiratory complications. These patients should be monitored after transfer from the PACU with continuous pulse oximetry, and PAP therapy may be instituted for recurrent obstructive events associated with significant hypoxemia. Patients with preoperative PAP therapy should continue PAP therapy postoperatively. (856)

40. This patient with a moderate risk of OSA has no evidence of recurrent PACU respiratory events (normal respiratory rate and room air oxygen saturation) after an extended stay in the PACU. His pain is also well controlled without the need for significant doses of intravenous opioid analgesia. Because knee arthroscopy is a minor procedure, this patient may be discharged home safely. (856)

41. This clinical scenario describes an already diagnosed OSA patient who is noncompliant with her CPAP treatment. She has a significant comorbid condition (morbidly obese), and postoperatively, she shows pain-sedation mismatch as evidenced by her high pain scores despite high-dose intravenous opioid analgesia and excessive sedation. She also exhibits recurrent PACU respiratory events (upper airway obstructive events associated with arousals for termination and a respiratory rate of 7 breaths per minute). All these factors call for PAP therapy as well as a postoperative monitored bed in the interest of comprehensive and diligent perioperative care. (856)

42. This patient diagnosed with severe OSA, noncompliant with her CPAP therapy, who underwent major surgery needs a postoperative monitored bed. Because she shows no pain-sedation mismatch and no other PACU respiratory events, she does not need immediate treatment with PAP therapy in the PACU. However, she may require additional analgesics after transfer to the floor when the regional anesthetic starts to wear off. In this setting, it is in the best interest of the patient to be monitored postoperatively. (856)

51 NEW MODELS OF ANESTHESIA CARE: PERIOPERATIVE MEDICINE, THE PERIOPERATIVE SURGICAL HOME, AND POPULATION HEALTH

Neal H. Cohen and Lorraine M. Sdrales

1. What is meant by a health care system? How is this evolving?
2. What is an accountable care organization?
3. What is the difference between a fee-for-service payment system and a value-based payment system?
4. What are bundled payments for health care?
5. What are some new potential roles for anesthesiologists in an evolving health care system?
6. How has anesthesiology practice expanded to perioperative medicine in recent years?
7. What is a potential downside to having the preoperative evaluation of a patient done by an anesthesia care provider (anesthesiologist or advanced practice nurse) in the clinic and subsequently having a different anesthesia provider administer anesthesia on the day of surgery?
8. What is enhanced recovery after surgery (ERAS)?
9. What is the concept of the perioperative surgical home?
10. What is the concept of population health?
11. What are some potential roles of an anesthesiologist in population health?
12. What are some implications of the evolving changes in health care delivery for anesthesia training programs?

ANSWERS*

1. A health care system refers to an organized business model that may include multiple hospital sites and other facility-based services, including ambulatory surgery centers and physician practices. It is the organization of

---

*Numbers in parentheses refer to pages, figures, boxes, or tables in Pardo MC, Miller RD, eds. *Basics of Anesthesia*. 7th ed. Philadelphia: Elsevier; 2018.

people, institutions, and resources to provide health services for their target population. Health care systems are evolving from traditional hospital-based organizations to include a variety of health care facilities and, in some cases, physician practices. The extension of the hospital-based system to one that includes a number of different delivery models and levels of care has been stimulated by the changes in health care financing and the need to better coordinate care across the continuum of services provided to patients. In addition, as changes in clinical care as well as health care payment models have been implemented, many services historically delivered in the inpatient setting are now being provided in ambulatory settings. The goal for consolidation in the health care industry is to provide care in the most cost-effective settings, minimize use of high-cost facilities, and potentially reduce risks associated with inpatient care (e.g., infection control). These integrated health systems are theoretically designed to provide coordinated health care to a target population, including outpatient care for prevention and wellness, high-intensity inpatient services, and posthospitalization care (rehabilitation, skilled nursing care, and home health services). The implications of these changes on anesthesia practices are significant. In many cases local practices are being consolidated; some are being purchased by large anesthesia or multispecialty physician organizations that are better able to provide diverse clinical services, contract and negotiate more successfully on behalf of the providers, and develop and manage clinical practice guidelines to optimize (and standardize) clinical management. (860)

2. An accountable care organization (ACO) is an organization that includes both hospitals and providers collaboratively sharing the responsibility for delivering comprehensive care to a population of patients. Most important, not only do the providers have responsibility for overall care of this group of patients, but the ACO also assumes full financial risk for delivering the care. Members of the ACO, which may include multiple hospitals, medical groups, and extended care facilities, manage and coordinate care for their defined group of patients to ideally provide high-quality comprehensive care at a reduced cost. Because the ACO assumes both clinical and financial risk, the organization should be motivated to deliver the care in the most patient-centric, efficient way. The financial model for an ACO includes payment for all clinical services to be provided to the patients in the organization with incentives tied to quality and cost. If a patient receives care from a provider or at a facility not a member of the ACO, the ACO retains financial responsibility to compensate the outside providers for the services rendered to the patient. Under an ACO model, each individual provider or, in the case of an anesthesia practice, the practice receives payment in proportion to the numbers of services provided, quality metrics, costs of care, and other measures. Under this model of care, the anesthesia practice must work closely with other providers and negotiate for the practice's fair share of the compensation for clinical care. The payment may or may not be directly related to relative value units generally used to compensate for physician services. A successful ACO requires close communication, cooperation, and coordination among physicians, ancillary providers, hospitals, extended care facilities, and home health agencies. (861–862)

3. A fee-for-service payment system is the traditional payment model in which providers are reimbursed for the specific clinical services they provide. For anesthesia services, payment from both government and private payers is based on the American Society of Anesthesiologists relative value system (ASA RVG) that includes base unit value and time. In a value-based payment system, providers are compensated based on the "value" and "quality" of the health care service provided. In a value-based system, each practice is required to identify specific measures of value and quality that support payment. (862)

4. A bundled payment for health care is a predefined, fixed, single payment to a health care system (hospital, providers, etc.) or to individual physician practices on the basis

of expected costs for an individual episode of care. In bundled payments there is a financial incentive for coordination of care within the health system, and the burden of unnecessary services is shared by all within the health care system. Under this model each provider will be reimbursed based on the "value" of contribution to the patient's care. The distribution of payment requires each practice to define metrics of cost, quality, and outcome related to the individual service in order to negotiate for an appropriate portion of the bundled payment. (863)

5. The changes in health care delivery and payment have created significant opportunities for anesthesiologists to extend their role beyond the traditional operating room environment and to participate in care across the entire spectrum of delivery. Some of the new roles for anesthesiologists in an evolving health care system include perioperative patient management in addition to the preoperative evaluation, expanded roles in critical care and pain medicine, participation in the perioperative surgical home (PSH) or enhanced recovery after anesthesia (ERAS) programs, expansion of roles to include the continuum of care (population health) and a number of administrative roles in perioperative care, medical direction, information management, and quality improvement initiatives. (863)

6. Anesthesiologists have assumed a broader role in health care delivery in many practices over the past decade. Building on the experiences of anesthesiologists in pain medicine and critical care medicine, the knowledge, clinical skills and broad-based perioperative (and periprocedural) perspective, many anesthesiologists have taken on responsibilities for optimizing the clinical condition of patients with comorbid conditions such as chronic obstructive pulmonary disease, diabetes mellitus, and sleep apnea in the preoperative period and taking greater responsibility for participating in care postoperatively. The expansion of preoperative evaluation clinics that has occurred as fewer patients are admitted until the day of surgery has had significant impact on defining some of these new models of care, as have other changes in the role of surgeons and hospitalists in perioperative management. In addition to redefining the role of anesthesiologist in preoperative optimization and traditional perioperative care, many anesthesiologists and anesthesia practices have identified new roles in clinical service lines, ERAS programs, and the PSH, building on a similar concept of the medical home for primary care patients. Under each of these models, the anesthesiologist works collaboratively with the surgeon, hospitalists, and other providers to coordinate care, taking into account issues related to the surgical procedure and anesthetic management and improving transitions of care beyond the immediate postoperative period. (863)

7. The changing roles of anesthesiologists and other providers in the perioperative period has been the need to differentiate roles and responsibilities across the continuum of care. The traditional model of an individual anesthesiologist managing the entire perioperative course from preoperative evaluation through the procedure and postoperative course is no longer viable for a number of reasons. In most current models of care the preoperative assessment (and management) is performed by an anesthesia provider in a preoperative evaluation setting or by phone. The provider performing the assessment is not the one who will provide anesthesia care for the procedure. This model, which has advantages, also creates fragmentation of care and limits the opportunity for the anesthesiologist to develop a meaningful relationship with the patient. The coordination of care across the perioperative period can be challenging under this new model. To be effective the providers involved in the perioperative care of the patient must ensure good communication and, when transitions of care take place, that the information generated at each stage of the evaluation is transmitted and that the transitions are seamless for both patient and all providers. (863–864)

8. ERAS is an evidence-based practice applied to a specific surgical procedure to better coordinate care throughout the perioperative period. The model is designed to improve both quality of care and outcomes for a patient. ERAS is a multidisciplinary approach for which a provider, most commonly the

anesthesiologist, coordinates the care across the continuum. Most ERAS models of care have ensured use of evidence-based practices during and after surgery, including implementation of clinical pathways to optimize goal-directed fluid management, pain management techniques, postoperative rehabilitation, and other aspects of care. These approaches have been very effective in reducing costs of care, hospital length of stay, and postoperative complications. (864)

9. The PSH is a model of perioperative management of patients incorporating all aspects of the perioperative course of a patient undergoing a surgical procedure. The anesthesia team provides preoperative optimization of underlying medical conditions, defines and implements evidence-based perioperative clinical management strategies, coordinates transitions of care (e.g., home, rehabilitation, skilled nursing facility), and facilitates communication among all providers to ensure that all clinical issues are defined and addressed in a timely and evidence-based manner. In addition, under the PSH model, the anesthesiologists and surgeons can more effectively evaluate and refine performance measures and provide documentation of quality, safety, and costs based on predefined metrics. Most of the clinical programs that have demonstrated successful implementation of the PSH model of care are focused on an individual procedure, surgical practice, or service line, providing the opportunity for the surgeon, anesthesiologists, and other providers to collaborate effectively with consistent goals and metrics to guide management. (864)

10. The concept of population health has gained increasing emphasis, in large part as hospitals and health systems assume greater roles in ensuring the health of a population of patients. The concept of population health is based on the theory that health care delivery can be most effectively improved if providers assume a broader perspective in addressing the needs of a population of patients across the continuum of care. The goal of population health is to improve quality of care and outcomes by focusing on the wellness of a population, efforts on prevention, management of chronic and acute disease, coordination of care, and managing costs. It is an outcome-based, proactive approach to the management of a population of patients rather than a reaction to an individual's health needs. The roles for anesthesiologists in population health are extensive, building on some of the concepts defined in the PSH and ERAS and extending the skills of anesthesiologists in other aspects of care based on the improvements in care that have been implemented in the operating room environment. (865)

11. Potential roles of an anesthesiologist in population health are an extension of some of the roles assumed as part of the PSH. These roles include clinical management of the patient from preoperative medical optimization to actively coordinating postoperative clinical management and transition of care beyond the hospital setting. Anesthesiologists can also be involved in administrative roles, health policy development, implementation of multimodal approaches to acute and chronic pain, defining appropriate management strategies and sites for long-term care (e.g., mechanical ventilatory support), and palliative care. Finally, anesthesiologists can participate in developing strategies for optimizing care and resource use for patients based on objective quality metrics and documented outcomes. (865)

12. The changes in health care delivery and expansion of the role for anesthesia providers in the evolving health care environment require that each resident completing an anesthesia training program understand the various models of care and develop broad-based clinical skills and a perspective that extends beyond the operating room. To accomplish these goals, anesthesia residents should be provided with both didactics incorporating concepts of the PSH, ERAS, and population health. They should participate in quality improvement projects and root cause analyses, as required by the Accreditation Council for Graduate Medical Education (ACGME). In addition, the residents needs to have an understanding of the concepts underlying the transition to value-based incentive compensation models and bundled payments and their implications for the scope of practice of anesthesia. Because the electronic health record will be the source

of most of the data to document quality, efficiency, and patient safety, residents should have an understanding of how data are collected, the accuracy and limitations of the data, and the overall benefits and limitations of the electronic health record. To successfully address some of the challenges confronting practices in expanding the roles and scope, residents should learn how to utilize clinical data to optimize resource use and clinical management. Finally, and as important, the residency programs must ensure access to the broad range of practices and clinical expectations of anesthesiologists and be given some training and experience in some of the new clinical and administrative roles that anesthesiologists can assume. (866)

INDEX

Note: Page numbers followed by "b", "f", and "t" indicate boxes, figures, and tables, respectively.